# Monographs on Pathology of Laboratory Animals

Sponsored by the
International Life Sciences Institute

The following volumes have appeared so far

Endocrine System
1983. 346 figures. XV, 366 pages. ISBN 3-540-11677-X

Respiratory System
1985. 279 figures. XV, 240 pages. ISBN 3-540-13521-9

Digestive System
1985. 352 figures. XVIII, 386 pages. ISBN 3-540-15815-4

Urinary System
1986. 362 figures. XVIII, 405 pages. ISBN 3-540-16591-6

Genital System
1987. 340 figures. XVII, 304 pages. ISBN 3-540-17604-7

Nervous System
1988. 242 figures. XVI, 233 pages. ISBN 3-540-19416-9

Integument and Mammary Glands
1989. 468 figures. XI, 347 pages. ISBN 3-540-51025-7

Hemopoietic System
1990. 351 figures. XVIII, 336 pages. ISBN 3-540-52212-3

Cardiovascular and Musculoskeletal Systems
1991. 390 figures. XVII, 312 pages. ISBN 3-540-53876-3

Eye and Ear
1991. 141 figures. XIII, 170 pages. ISBN 3-540-54044-X

Nonhuman Primates I
1993. 235 figures. XIII, 221 pages. ISBN 3-540-56465-9
0-944398-15-4

Nonhuman Primates II
1993. 264 figures. XVI, 248 pages. ISBN 3-540-56527-2
0-944398-16-2

2nd editions to follow

Endocrine System
1996. 521 figures. XVIII, 521 pages. ISBN 3-540-59477-9
0-944398-64-2

T.C. Jones D.L. Dungworth
U. Mohr (Eds.)

# Respiratory System

## Second Edition

Completely Revised and Updated
with 382 Figures and 32 Tables

Springer

Thomas Carlyle Jones, D.V.M., D.Sc.
Professor of Comparative Pathology
Emeritus, Harvard Medical School
ILSI Research Foundation
1126 Sixteenth Street, N.W., Washington, DC 20036, USA

Donald L. Dungworth, B.V.Sc., Ph.D., M.R.C.V.S.
Professor of Veterinary Pathology, Emeritus
University of California, Davis
6260 Cape George Road
Port Townsend, WA 98368, USA

Ulrich Mohr, M.D.
Professor of Experimental Pathology
Medizinische Hochschule Hannover
Institut für Experimentelle Pathologie
Konstanty-Gutschow-Strasse 8
30625 Hannover, Germany

Distribution rights for North America, Canada, and Mexico by
International Life Sciences Institute (ILSI)
1126 Sixteenth Street NW, Washington, DC 20036, USA

2nd Edition
ISBN-13: 978-3-642-64667-6 e-ISBN-13: 978-3-642-61042-4
DOI: 10.1007/978-3-642-61042-4

1st Edition

Library of Congress Cataloging-in-Publication Data. Respiratory system / T.C. Jones, D.L. Dung-worth, U. Mohr (eds.).—2nd ed. p. cm.—(Monographs on pathology of laboratory animals) Includes bibliographical references and index. 1. Laboratory animals—Diseases. 2. Respiratory organs Diseases. 3. Rodents—Diseases. 4. Rodents as laboratory animals. 5. Pathology, Comparative. I. Jones, Thomas Carlyle. II. Dungworth, D.L. (Donald L.) III. Mohr. U. (Ulrich) IV. Series. [DNLM: 1. Respiratory System—pathology. 2. Animals, Laboratory. 3. Rodent Diseases. WF 140 R43463 1996] SF996.5.R47 1996 599.32'3—dc20 DNLM/DLC for Library of Congress 95-45938 CIP



Typesetting: Best-set Typesetter Ltd., Hong Kong

SPIN: 10128630 25/3134/SPS – 5 4 3 2 1 0 – Printed on acid-free paper

# Foreword to the Second Edition

The International Life Sciences Institute (ILSI) is a nonprofit, worldwide foundation established in 1978 to advance the understanding of scientific issues relating to nutrition, food safety, toxicology, risk assessment, and the environment. By bringing together scientists from academia, government, industry, and the public sector, ILSI seeks a balanced approach to solving problems of common concern for the well-being of the general public. This volume is the second of the Second Edition of *Monographs on Pathology of Laboratory Animals*. The series is designed to facilitate communication among those involved in the safety testing of foods, drugs, and chemicals. The complete set covers cardiovascular/musculoskeletal, digestive, endocrine, genital, hemopoietic, nervous, respiratory and urinary systems, eye and ear, integument and mammary glands, and nonhuman primates. The series is intended for use by pathologists, toxicologists, and others concerned with evaluating toxicity and carcinogenicity studies. ILSI is committed to supporting programs to harmonize toxicologic testing, to advance a more uniform interpretation of bioassay results worldwide, to promote a common understanding of lesion classifications, and to encourage wide discussion of these topics among scientists. Scientific understanding and cooperation will be improved worldwide through the series and this international project.

ILSI accomplishes its work through its branches and institutes. ILSI's branches currently include Argentina, Australasia, Brazil, Europe, Japan, Korea, Mexico, North America, Southeast Asia, and Thailand, and a focal point in China. The ILSI Health and Environmental Sciences Institute focuses on global environmental issues. ILSI Research Foundation includes the ILSI Allergy and Immunology Institute, ILSI Human Nutrition Institute, ILSI Pathology and Toxicology Institute, and ILSI Risk Science Institute.

Alex Malaspina
President
International Life Sciences Institute

# Preface to the Second Edition

Approximately ten years have elapsed since the second volume of the International Life Sciences Institute (ILSI) Monographs on Pathology of Laboratory Animals, Respiratory System, was first completed. New information of interest to pathologists has developed at a rather remarkable pace during these years. Exceptional progress has been made in the routine identification of enzymes and cell products in respiratory cells. A better understanding has developed on the functions of cells of the respiratory tract and of the mechanisms involved in cell metabolism, particularly those involving toxins and carcinogens. Clear concepts have developed concerning the significance of pathologic lesions, particularly in the upper respiratory tract and their relation to human health and risk assessment. Standardized nomenclature has developed significantly during the 10-year period since the first edition and is being utilized on an international basis. This has resulted in significant improvement in communication of pathologic data to regulatory agencies and in scientific publications worldwide. This monograph series and others sponsored by ILSI have had significant effects on these improved communications and the international acceptance of standardized nomenclature. In this second edition, new formats have been used where more appropriate for the subjects to be covered. The format used in the first edition, however, retains its usefulness as it is still necessary to recognize the morphologic features of pathologic lesions in order to identify them precisely, an essential first step toward achieving insights into pathogenetic mechanisms and making them relevant for decisions eventually applicable to public health.

The functional roles of different cells of the upper respiratory tract are now much better appreciated and their varying responses to inhaled toxicants are now more clearly evident. New approaches to the study of the cells and tissues of the nasal apparatus, as reiterated in this volume, will surely add to our knowledge of the pathologic aspects of this system.

We are very grateful to the dedicated scientists from lands all around the world who have contributed to this volume. The authors are named in the table of contents, the list of contributors, and the heading of each individual manuscript. The members of the editorial board, listed on the frontispiece, are particularly to be thanked for their efforts in identifying authors and for the scientific review of individual manuscripts. The editors are especially grateful to Dr. Alex Malaspina for his steadfast support and to the members of the ILSI staff and others who have helped in so many ways. We particularly wish to mention Ms. Sherri Lopez, former Associate Editor and Manager of the ILSI Pathology and Toxicology Institute; Ms. Sharon Weiss, the Associate Director of the ILSI Pathology and Toxicology Institute; as well as Ms. Frances DeLuca, Executive Assistant, ILSI Pathology and Toxicology Institute and ILSI Research Foundation.

We are grateful to Prof. Dietrich Goetze, Ms. Barbara Montenbruck, and others on the staff of Springer-Verlag for the quality of the finished book.

November 1995

T.C. Jones
D.L. Dungworth
U. Mohr

# Contents

# Contributors

Ian Y.R. Adamson, Ph.D.
Professor of Pathology, The University of Manitoba, Winnipeg, Manitoba, Canada

Jürgen Althoff, M.D.
Professor of Experimental Pathology, Senior Sanofi-Winthrop Fellow (Toxicology), Sanofi-Winthrop Inc., Collegeville, Pennsylvania, USA

Gerhard Bargsten, Dr.rer.nat.
Institute of Anatomy, Hannover Medical School, Hannover, Germany

Josep A. Bombi, M.D.
Associate Professor, Department of Anatomic Pathology, Hospital Clinic, University of Barcelona, Medical School, Barcelona, Spain

Gary A Boorman, D.V.M., M.S., Ph.D.
Chief, Pathology Branch, National Institute of Environmental Health Sciences, Research Triangle Park, North Carolina, USA

Drummond H. Bowden, M.D.
Professor Emeritus, The University of Manitoba, Winnipeg, Manitoba, Canada

David G. Brownstein, D.V.M.
Professor of Comparative Medicine, Yale University School of Medicine, New Haven, Connecticut, USA

Antonio Cardesa, M.D.
Professor and Chairman, Department of Anatomic Pathology, Hospital Clinic, University of Barcelona, Medical School, Barcelona, Spain

Gerald E. Dagle, D.V.M., Ph.D.
Adjunct Associate Professor, Washington State University, Tri-Cities, United States Transuranium Registry, Richland, Washington, USA

Jerry K. Davis, D.V.M., Ph.D.
Director, Division of Comparative Medicine, Professor, Pathobiology, University of Florida, Gainesville, Florida, USA

Donald L. Dungworth, B.V.Sc., Ph.D., M.R.C.V.S.
Professor Emeritus, University of California, Davis, Davis, California, USA

Makito Emura, Prof.Dr.rer.nat.
Head, Tissue Culture Unit, Institute of Experimental Pathology, Hannover Medical College, Hannover, Germany

Heinrich Ernst, D.V.M.
Fraunhofer Institute of Toxicology and Aerosol Research, Hannover, Germany

J.K. Frenkel, M.D., Ph.D.
Professor Emeritus, University of Kansas, Adjunct Professor, University of New Mexico, Santa Fe, New Mexico, USA

Fletcher F. Hahn, D.V.M., Ph.D.
Head, Pathology Group, Inhalation Toxicology Research Institute, Lovelace Biomedical and Environmental Research Institute, Albuquerque, New Mexico, USA

Rick Hailey, D.V.M.
Head, Morphologic Pathology, National Institute of Environmental Health Sciences, Research Triangle Park, North Carolina, USA

Jack R. Harkema, D.V.M., Ph.D.
Michigan State University, East Lansing, Michigan, USA

Martin Heinrichs, D.V.M.
Department of Experimental Pathology and Toxicology, Boehringer Ingelheim KG, Ingelheim am Rhein, Germany

Ronald A. Herbert, D.V.M., Ph.D.
National Institute of Environmental Health Sciences, Research Triangle Park, North Carolina, USA

Ryuichi Higashiguchi, M.D.
Assistant, Department of Oncological Pathology, Cancer Center, Nara Medical University, Nara, Japan

Alexander Kast, D.V.M., Priv.-Doz
Priv.-Doz. of Toxicologic Pathology, Gießen University, Germany

Birgit Kittel, Dr.med.vet.
BASF AG, Department of Toxicology, Ludwigshafen, Germany

Yoichi Konishi, M.D.
Professor, Department of Oncological Pathology, Cancer Center, Nara Medical University, Nara, Japan

J. Russell Lindsey, D.V.M., M.S.
Professor and Chairman, Department of Comparative Medicine, University of Alabama at Birmingham, Veterinary Medical Officer, Veteran's Administration Medical Center, Birmingham, Alabama, USA

Annabel G. Liebelt, Ph.D.
Registry of Experimental Cancers, National Cancer Institute, National Institutes of Health, Bethesda, Maryland, USA

Rodney A, Miller, D.V.M., Ph.D.
Technical Group Leader, Pathology, Battelle, Pacific Northwest Laboratory, Richland, Washington, USA

Ulrich Mohr, M.D.
Director, Institute of Experimental Pathology, Hannover Medical School, Hannover, Germany

Kevin T. Morgan, D.V.Sc., Ph.D.
Chemical Industry Institute of Toxicology, Research Triangle Park, North Carolina, USA

Thomas Nolte, D.V.M.
Institute of Toxicology, ASTA Medica AG, Halle/Westfalen, Germany

Charles G. Plopper, Ph.D.
Professor, School of Veterinary Medicine, University of California, Davis, Davis, California, USA

H.-B. Richter-Reichhelm, D.V.M.
Priv.Doz. for Experimental Pathology, Bundesinstitut für gesundheitlichen Verbraucherschutz und Veterinärmedizin, Berlin, Germany

Sabine Rehm, Dr.med.vet.
SmithKline Beecham Pharmaceuticals, King of Prussia, Pennsylvania, USA

Roger A. Renne, D.V.M.
Manager, Toxicology Department, Battelle, Pacific Northwest Laboratory, Richland, Washington, USA

Susanne Rittinghausen, D.V.M.
Fraunhofer Institute of Toxicology and Aerosol Research, Hannover, Germany

Trenton R. Schoeb, D.V.M., Ph.D.
Professor, University of Florida, Gainesville, Florida, USA

A. Schulte, D.V.M.
Bundesinstitut für gesundheitlichen Verbraucherschutz und Veterinärmedizin, Berlin, Germany

Alfred P. Wehner, D.M.D., Sc.D., cand.med., D.A.T.S.
President, Biomedical and Environmental Consultants, Inc., Richland, Washington, USA

Prof. W. Weller
Silikose-Forschungsinstitut der Bergbau-Berufsgenossenschaft, Bochum, Germany

# The Upper Respiratory System

# HISTOLOGY, ULTRASTRUCTURE, EMBRYOLOGY, FUNCTION

## Normal Morphology of the Nasal Passages in Laboratory Rodents

Jack R. Harkema and Kevin T. Morgan

### Introduction

The nasal passages are the portal of entry of the respiratory tract. Because laboratory rodents are obligate nose breathers and highly dependent on the sense of smell, normal structure and function of the upper airways are critical to the health and well-being of these animals. The rodent nose is a structurally complex organ with multiple functions. Besides housing the essential components of the olfactory system, the nasal passages filter, humidify, and warm the inspired air preparing it for the delicate gas exchange tissues in the lung. The nasal cavity has been described as an efficient "scrubbing tower" that removes most, but not all, inhaled chemicals potentially harmful to the lower respiratory airways and pulmonary parenchyma (Brain 1970).

Because the nose is a common site for particle deposition (Anderson and Proctor 1982; Brain and Valberg 1979; Hounam and Morgan 1977; Lippman 1970; Swift 1981) and the site for absorption of many gases and vapors (Aharonson et al. 1974; Brain and Valberg 1979; Morgan and Frank 1977; Stott and McKenna 1984), this organ is a common site of injury induced by inhaled irritants. Laboratory rodents have been shown to be susceptible to injury from a wide range of xenobiotics such as: formaldehyde, chlorine, ozone, and cigarette smoke (Buckley et al. 1984; Harkema et al. 1989; Monticello et al. 1990; Walker 1983). These toxicant-induced lesions generally exhibit characteristic, site-specific distribution patterns (Morgan and Monticello 1990).

Therefore toxicant-induced nasal lesions can be assessed only with a good understanding of the normal morphology of the rodent nose. Although the gross anatomy of the nasal airways in several animal species has been known for a long time, only recently have studies been conducted to characterize systematically the cells lining this important airway in laboratory animals. Current knowledge of nasal cell and tissue morphology is primarily the result of animal studies that were designed to examine quantitatively the response of the entire nasal epithelium to various toxicants. In this chapter we provide a brief outline of the normal morphology of the nasal passages in laboratory rodents (e.g., rats and mice). In addition, we discuss how to prepare nasal tissue for microscopic examination. Since the surface epithelia lining the nasal airways are often the principal sites of injury from exposure to inhaled chemical toxicants, special emphasis is placed on the normal morphology and distribution of these tissues. Nasal anatomy of rats and mice is also compared to those of other laboratory animal species (e.g., monkeys, dogs) and humans. After this discussion of normal nasal structure, the following three chapters in this monograph focus on the histopathology of the nasal passages in laboratory rodents.

### Preparation of Nasal Tissues for Microscopic Examination

Detailed descriptions of how to process the noses of laboratory animals for morphological assessment of toxicant-induced injury have been published (Mery et al. 1994; Uraih and Maronpot 1990; Morgan et al. 1991; Harkema et al. 1987; Young 1981). Because of the complex and variable structure of the nasal passages and the encasement of the nose within a bony shell, special attention to fixation, decalcification, and careful sampling is required for obtaining uniform, high-quality sections from each laboratory rodent evaluated. The first systematic approach for sectioning the nasal passages of laboratory rodents in toxicological studies was described by Young (1981). Figure 1 illustrates the set of four transverse sections of the nose as proposed by Young representing proximal, middle and distal locations. Other investigators have proposed more numerous section levels (Morgan 1991). In all the proposed methods specific dental or palatine landmarks are used to identify the sites for sectioning. Because nasal lesions are usually site specific, section-level selection is critical in assessing the extent, severity, and relevance of the alterations.

Immediately after the death of the animal the head is removed from the carcass and the nasal cavity is gently flushed retrograde through the nasopharyngeal orifice with the appropriate fixative. The eyes, skin, musculature, and brain are removed, and the head is immersed in a large volume of the fixative. For routine light microscopic evaluation 10% neutral buffered formalin is commonly used to fix the nasal tissues for at least 24 h. If electron microscopy is to be used for ultrastructural analysis, the nasal tissues are routinely fixed with 2% glutaraldehyde in cacodylate buffer (pH 7.4; Harkema, unpublished) or Fowler's fixative (Fowler et al. 1983; Uraih and Maronpot 1990).

After fixation the head is decalcified. In our laboratories 13% formic acid for 4–5 days with frequent changes of the solution (Harkema et al. 1989) or 5% formic acid with ion-exchange resin for 2–3 days (Uraih and Maronpot 1990) is generally adequate to decalcify the nasal cavity of a 10- to 14-week rat (Harkema et al. 1989). The decalcification time, however, depends on the age and

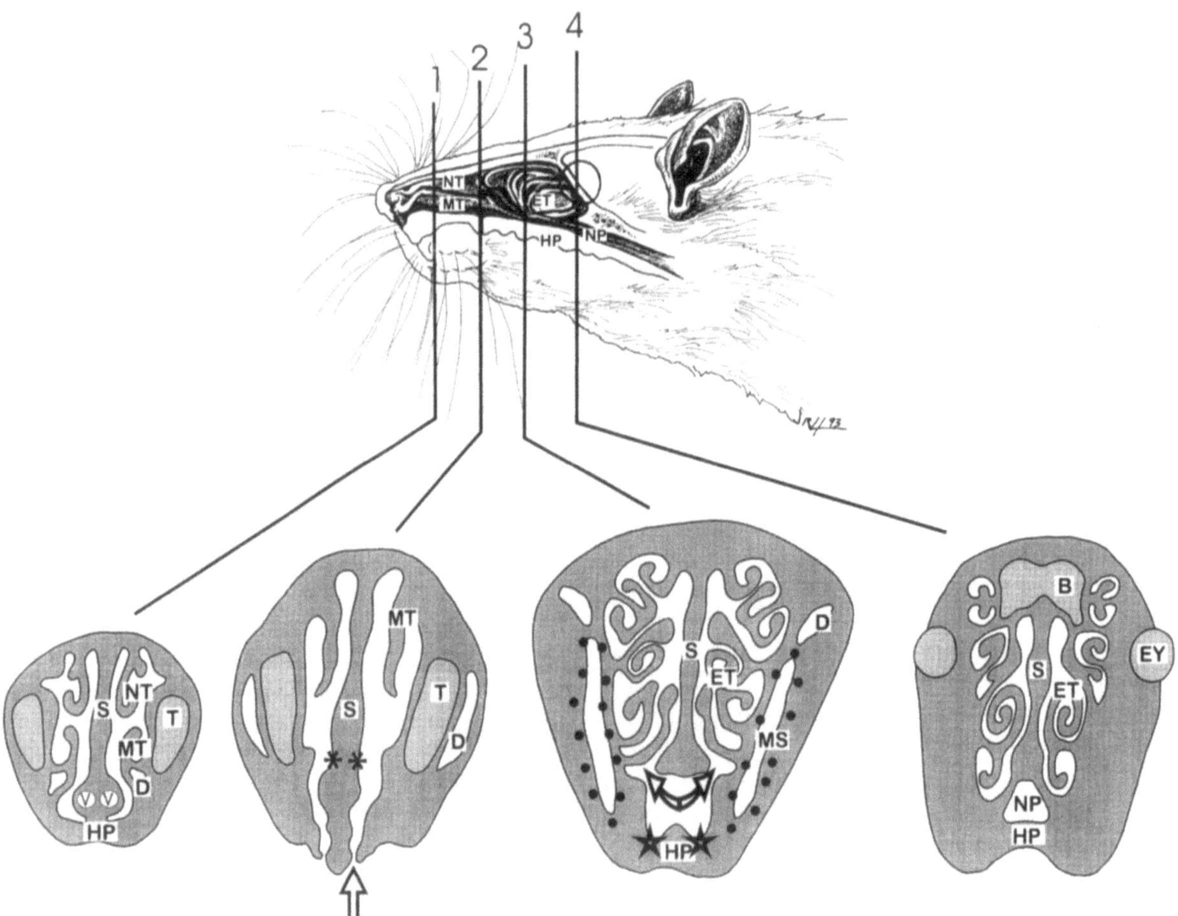


**Fig. 1.** Diagram of the exposed mucosal surface of the nasal lateral wall and turbinates of the rat. *Vertical lines*, levels of the proximal surfaces of the transverse tissue blocks (1–4) proposed by Young (1981) for microscopic examination. *S*, Septum; *NT*, nasoturbinate; *MT*, maxilloturbinate; *ET*, ethmoid turbinates; *T*, root of incisor tooth; *D*, nasolacrimal duct; *V*, vomeronasal organ; *HP*, hard palate; *EY*, eye; *B*, brain; *MS*, maxillary sinus; *NP*, nasopharynx; *asterisks*, location of Masera's organ; *straight open arrow*, nasopalatine duct at the level of the incisive papilla; *curved open arrows*, location of septal window; *stars*, location of nasal associated lymphoid tissue

size of the laboratory rodent and the fixative. If nasal tissues have been fixed for electron microscopy, the head should be decalcified with 10% ethylene diaminetetraacetate (EDTA) in 0.1 *M* cacodylate buffer (pH 7.4) at 4°C for 4–5 weeks. Decalcification with EDTA preserves the ultrastructural detail of cells in the nasal mucosa and bone. A detailed tissue processing and selection method for ultrastructural evaluation of the rodent nose has been described by Monteiro-Riviere and Popp (1984).

As mentioned above, a consistent tissue sampling scheme is crucial for adequate histopathological evaluation of rodent nasal passages. The number of section levels selected may vary with the study, but it is important that the regions selected for examination are the same for each animal, and that they adequately represent the entire nasal airway. Section level selection is a critical issue in nasal toxicology, and availability of suitable sections is essential for adequate assessment of the distribution, severity, and importance of the nasal lesion (Mery et al. 1994). The four transverse sections of the rodent nose proposed by Young (1981) are taken at specific anatomic locations that can be identified by dental or palatine landmarks: (a) immediately posterior to the upper incisor teeth, (b) at the level of the incisive papilla, (c) at the level of the second palatal ridge, and (d) at the level of the first molar teeth (Fig. 1). The tissue blocks sampled from each location are routinely embedded in paraffin or glycol methacrylate. Sections 4–6 μm thick are cut from the paraffin-embedded blocks and stained with hematoxylin and eosin. Sections of 1–2 μm thickness are cut from the anterior surfaces of the glycol methacrylate-embedded tissues and stained with toluidine blue.

## Gross Anatomy of the Nose

Major structural differences exist in the gross anatomy of the nasal passages among animal species. These differences have been emphasized in previous reviews of comparative nasal anatomy (Negus 1958; Proctor and Chang 1983) and demonstrated in studies using silicone rubber casts of the nasal airways (Schreider and Raabe 1981). With these casts the total volume of the nasal cavity of a 250-g, Sprague-Dawley rat has been estimated to be 0.4 $cm^3$. In comparison, an adult rhesus monkey has a nasal cavity volume of 8 $cm^3$. Using morphometric data, Gross et al. (1982) estimated the volume of the nasal cavity in a 288-g F344 rat to be 0.3 $cm^3$ and that in a 33-g B6C3Fl mouse to be 0.03 $cm^3$. Using magnetic resonance imaging of a human subject (adult male), the human nasal cavity in vivo has been estimated to be 16 $cm^3$ (Guilmette et al. 1989).

In addition to the obvious differences in nasal cavity size and volume, species vary in luminal surface area of the nasal cavity, due to the size and complexity of turbinate structures projecting from the lateral walls. The total surface area of a 16-week-old B6C3Fl mouse is estimated, using morphometric techniques, to be 289 $mm^2$ ± 13.1 $mm^2$, compared to 1343.5 $mm^2$ ± 55 $mm^2$ in a 16-week-old F344 rat (Gross et al. 1982). The surface area of the nasal airways of an adult baboon has been estimated to be 15680 $mm^2$ using measurements of a nasopharyngeal silicone cast (Patra et al. 1986). Differences in the architecture of the nasal lateral wall of rats, macaque monkeys, dogs, and humans are illustrated in Fig. 2. Turbinate structures are more complex in rats and dogs, compared to the two primate species.

In rodents the two nasal passages are structurally symmetric and separated by a septum. Nasoturbinate, maxilloturbinate, and ethmoid turbinates project into the lumen from the lateral wall of each airway (Fig. 1). Each turbinate has a central bony core overlaid by a richly vascularized and innervated mucosa composed of a inner lamina propria and an outer surface epithelium. A septal window provides a direct connection between the left and right nasal passages and an airway into the nasopharyngeal meatus (Fig. 1). This posterior opening in the septum is a point of convergence for both luminal air and surface mucous streams. Inspired air flows through four main intranasal routes (dorsal, ventral, medial, and lateral meatuses. In the rat the bulk of the inspired airflow is through the lateral, middle medial, and dorsal medial meatuses (Morgan et al. 1991; Kimbell et al. 1993). Each lateral meatus has a characteristic curved profile and a curved lateral recess reflecting its close anatomical association with the root of the incisor tooth.

The nasal and buccal cavities are connected by bilaterally symmetric nasopalatine ducts that pass through the incisive canals of the hard palate (Fig. 1). In the adult F344 rat these ducts are approximately 0.5 mm in diameter and have valvelike flaps on the buccal side which prevent passage of food material from the oral cavity into the nasal

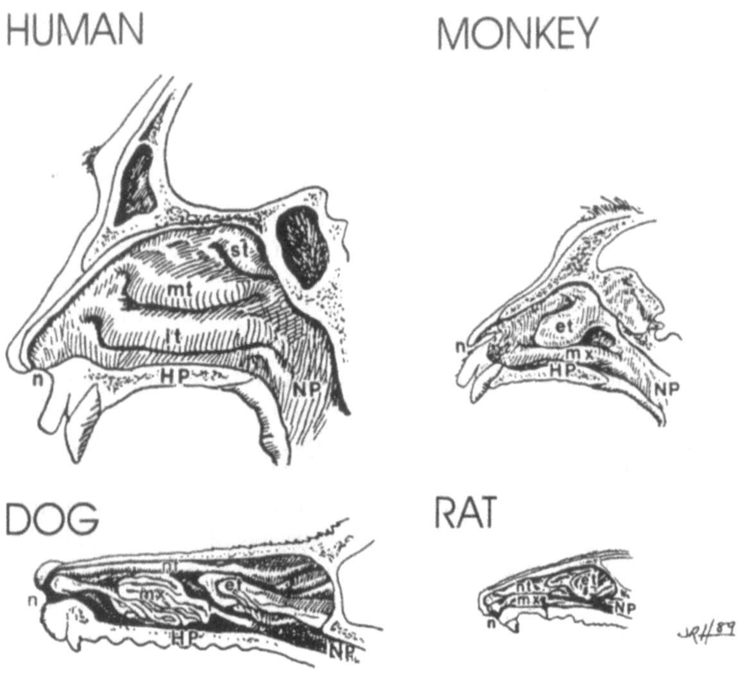


**Fig. 2.** Diagrammatic representation of the exposed mucosal surface of the nasal lateral wall of the human, monkey, dog, and rat. *HP*, Hard palate; *n*, naris; *NP*, nasopharynx; *ET*, ethmoid turbinates; *nt*, nasoturbinate; *mx*, maxilloturbinate; *mt*, middle turbinate; *it*, inferior turbinate; *st*, superior turbinate

passages. The role(s) of the nasopalatine ducts is unknown, but they may provide a passageway for air or nasal secretions. These patent oronasal ducts are not present in humans or nonhuman primates (Negus 1958).

## Nasal Surface Epithelium

Besides differences in the gross architecture of the nose among animal species, species-specific differences arise in the amount and distribution of surface epithelial populations lining the nasal passages. There are, however, four distinct nasal epithelial types in all animal species. These are stratified squamous epithelium, which is primarily restricted to the nasal vestibule; ciliated, pseudostratified, respiratory epithelium in the main nasal chamber and nasopharynx; nonciliated or poorly ciliated transitional epithelium lying between squamous epithelium and respiratory in the proximal aspect of the main chamber; and olfactory epithelium located in the dorsal and distal aspects of the nasal cavity. Figure 3 illustrates the distribution of these distinct epithelial cell populations in the lateral nasal wall and septum of the F344 rat. Detailed maps of the distribution of the epithelia lining the nasal passages of the F334

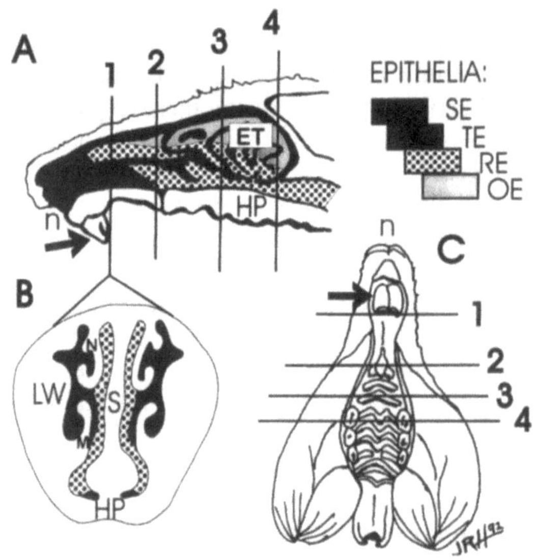


**Fig. 3. A** Distribution of the four principal epithelial types (*SE*, squamous epithelium; *TE*, transitional epithelium; *RE*, respiratory epithelium; *OE*, olfactory epithelium) lining the nasal lateral wall and turbinates in the rat. *n*, Naris; *HP*, hard palate; *ET*, ethmoid turbinates. **B** Anterior face of the tissue block from level 1 of the proximal nose illustrating the intranasal airways that are lined by SE, TE, and RE. *M*, Maxilloturbinate; *N*, nasoturbinate; *S*, septum; *LW*, lateral wall (nasal). **C** Ventral view of the head of a rat with the lower jaw removed and exposing the hard palate. The horizontal lines identify the levels of the four transverse tissue sections of Young (1981) that are also illustrated in **A**. *Closed, straight arrows*, incisor tooth. Alcian blue (pH 2.5), H&E

rat and the B6C3Fl mouse have recently been provided by Mery et al. (1994). In addition to these four conspicuous nasal epithelia, there is a fifth, less conspicuous epithelial type in laboratory rodents. Lymphoepithelium overlying nasal-associated lymphoid tissues (NALT) is located in the ventral aspects of the distal lateral wall at the entrance to the nasopharyngeal duct and near the septal window (Fig. 1).

### Squamous Epithelium

The nares and nasal vestibule in rats and mice are completely lined by a lightly keratinized, stratified squamous epithelium (Fig. 4). It is composed of basal cells along the basal lamina and several layers of squamous cells which become progressively flatter toward the luminal surface. Only 3.5% of the entire nasal cavity of the F344 rat is lined by squamous epithelium, while 21% of the nasal cavity of the B6C3Fl mouse is lined by this epithelium (Gross et al. 1982). Squamous epithelium of the nasal vestibule extends from the floor of the ventral meatus to the nasopalatine ducts and merges with the squamous epithelium of the buccal mucosa.

Of the four main epithelial populations lining the nasal cavity, squamous epithelium has the greatest number of cells in the S phase of the cell cycle (Johnson et al. 1990). In the F344 rat squamous epithelium contains no histochemically detectable mucosubstances (Harkema et al. 1989). This region of the nasal mucosa probably functions as does the epidermis in the skin, to protect the underlying tissues from potentially harmful atmospheric agents.

### Transitional Epithelium

Distal to the stratified squamous epithelium and proximal to the ciliated respiratory epithelium is a narrow zone of nonciliated, microvilli-covered surface epithelium, which has been referred to as nasal, nonciliated, respiratory epithelium or nasal transitional epithelium. Common, distinctive features of this nasal epithelium in all laboratory ani-

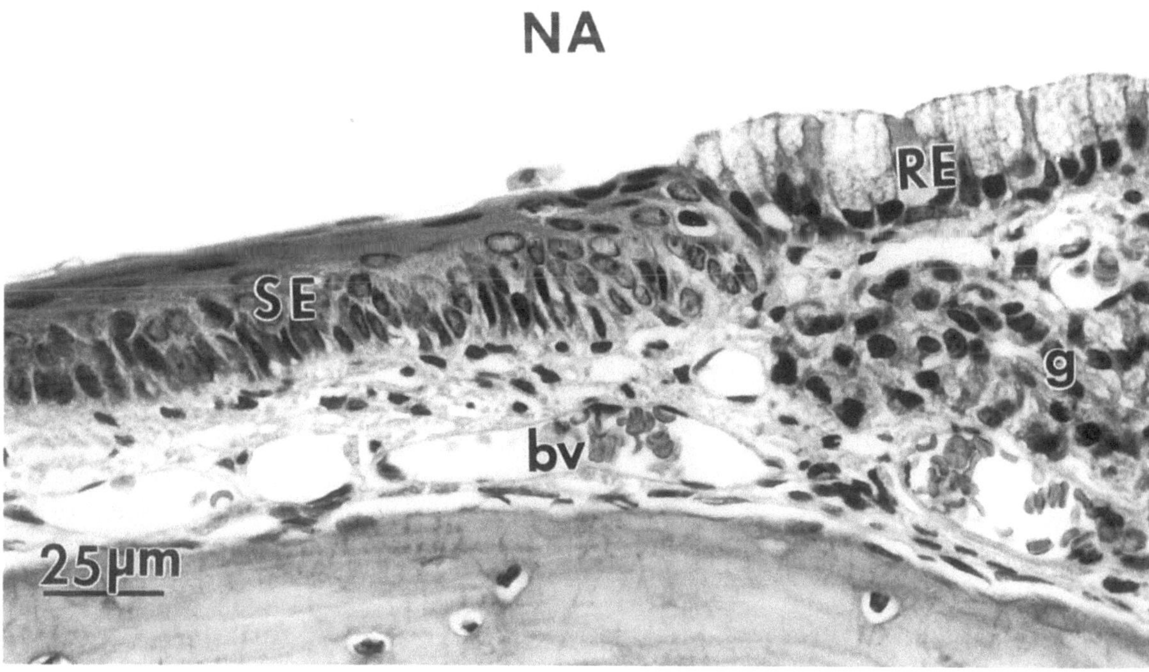


**Fig. 4.** Junction of squamous epithelium (*SE*) and respiratory epithelium (*RE*) lining the ventral meatus in the proximal nasal cavity of a F344 rat. *NA*, Nasal airway; *bv*, blood vessel in lamina propria; *g*, subepithelial gland in lamina propria. Alcian blue (pH 2.5), H&E

mal species and humans include: (a) anatomical location in the proximal aspect of the nasal cavity between the squamous epithelium and the respiratory epithelium, (b) the presence of nonciliated cuboidal or columnar surface cells and basal cells, (c) a scarcity of mucous (goblet) cells and a paucity of intraepithelial mucosubstances, and (d) an abrupt demarcation from squamous epithelium but a less abrupt border with respiratory epithelium.

In rats this nasal epithelium predominantly lines the lateral wall and lateral aspects of the nasoturbinates and maxilloturbinates that border the lateral meatus in the proximal aspect of the nasal cavity (Young's level I). In addition, the medial aspect of the maxilloturbinate in the proximal nasal airway is lined by transitional epithelium. This surface epithelium is thin (i.e., one or two cells thick), pseudostratified, and composed of three distinct cell types (basal, cuboidal, and columnar; Monteiro-Riviere and Popp 1984; Fig. 5). In contrast, transitional epithelium in monkeys is thick (i.e., four or five cells), stratified, and composed of at least five different cell types (Harkema et al. 1987). The luminal surfaces of transitional epithelial cells lining the nasal airway possess numerous microvilli. Luminal, nonciliated cells in the transitional epithelium of rodents have no secretory granules but do have abundant smooth endoplasmic reticulan (SER) in their apices (Monteiro-Riviere and Popp 1984; Fig. 6). SER has been shown to be an important intracellular site for xenobiotic-metabolizing enzymes, including cytochromes P450. The prominent presence of SER in these cells, as the sustentacular cells in the OE olfactory epithelium, suggests that they may have roles in the metabolism of certain inhaled xenobiotics.

The lamina propria beneath the transitional epithelium is a highly vascularized, loose, fibroelastic, connective tissue containing serous glands. Cavernous venous plexuses, referred to as "swell bodies," in the lamina propria are also present in distinct regions of the transitional epithelium that

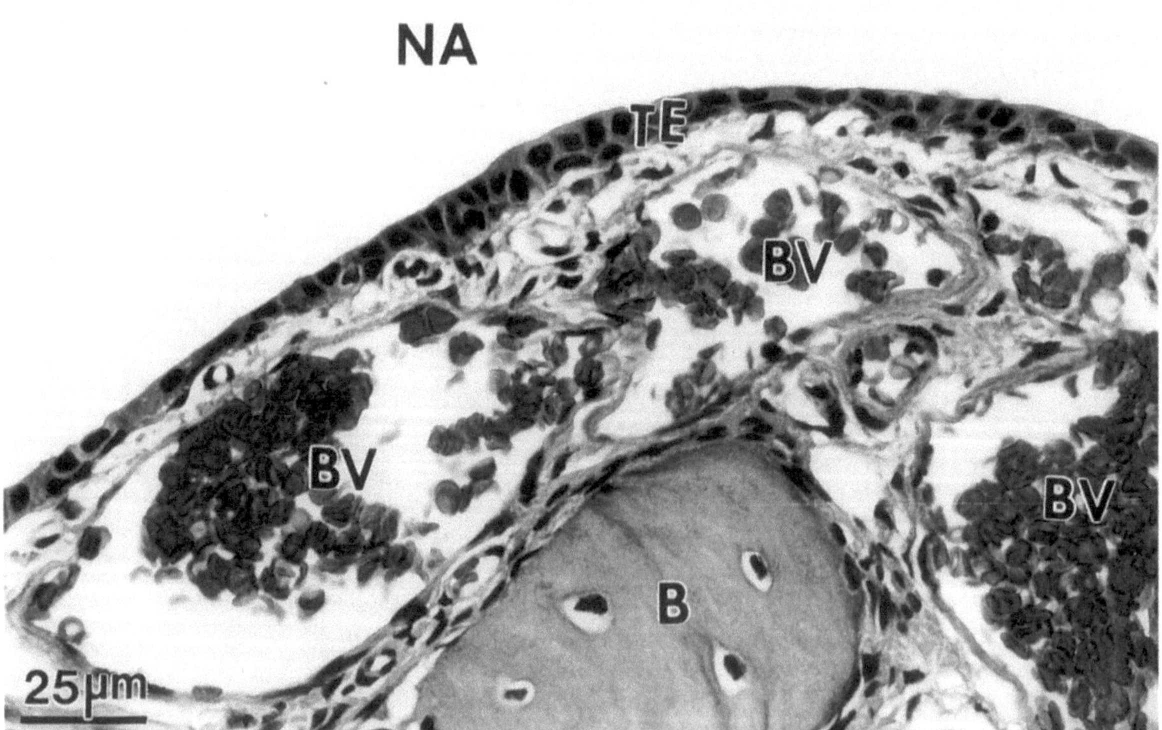


**Fig. 5.** Transitional epithelium (*TE*) lining the dorsolateral aspect of the maxilloturbinate in the nasal cavity of a F344 rat (Young's transverse section I). Large venous blood vessels (*BV*) in the lamina propria (known as "swell bodies"). *B*, Turbinate bone; *NA*, nasal airway. Alcian blue (pH 2.5), H&E

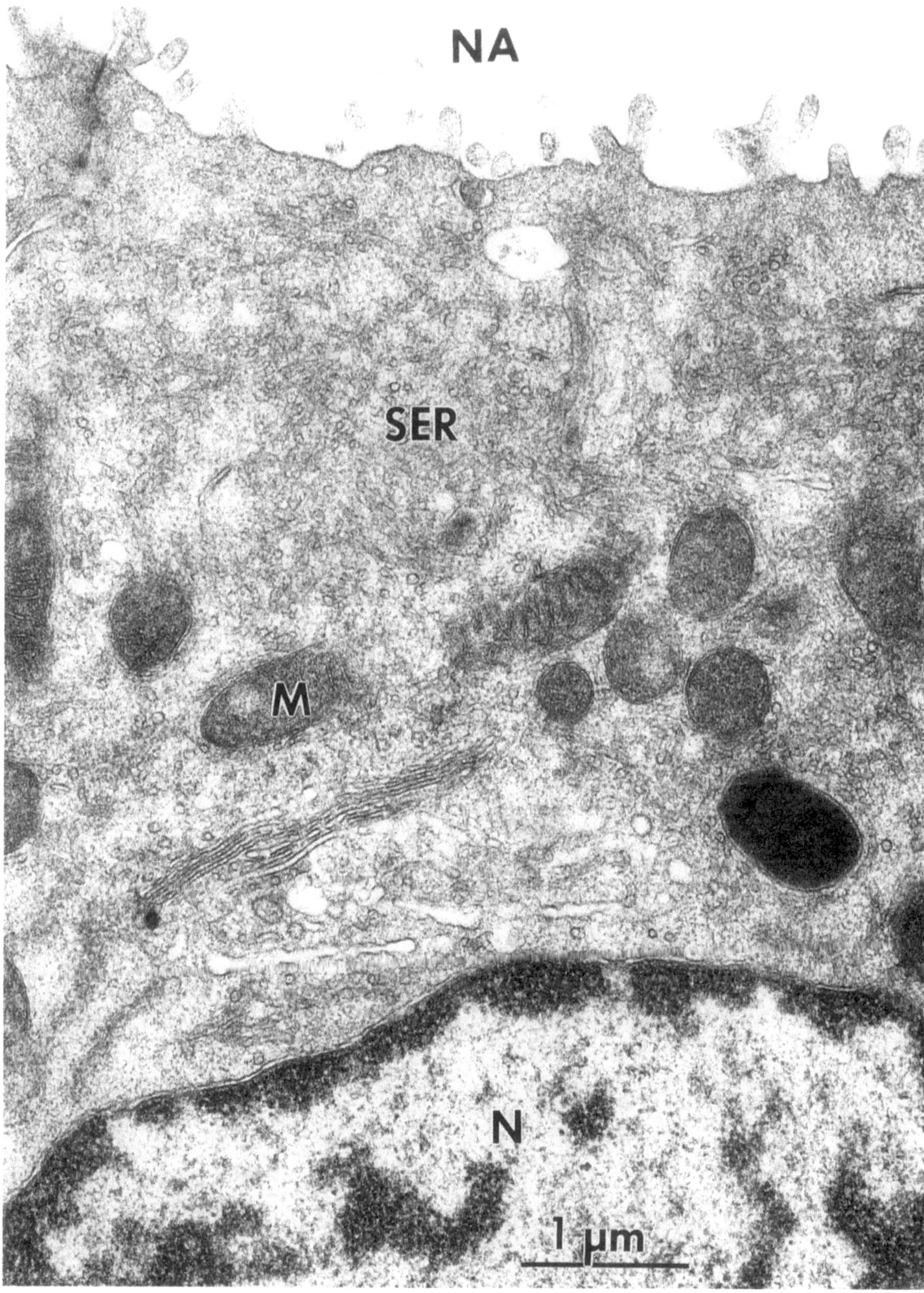


**Fig. 6.** Apical portion of a nonciliated cuboidal epithelial cell in the transitional epithelium of a F344 rat. *SER*, Abundant smooth endoplasmic reticulum in the apical cytoplasm; *M*, mitochondria; *N*, nucleus; *NA*, nasal airway lumen. TEM, ×30000

dilate to alter air flow in the nasal passage. The largest swell bodies in the rat are found in the lateral wall between the nasoturbinate and maxilloturbinate, with smaller swell bodies in the maxilloturbinate (Fig. 5). These swell bodies can cause variation in the air flow through the two nasal passages.

## Respiratory Epithelium

The majority of the nonolfactory nasal epithelium of laboratory animals and humans is ciliated respiratory epithelium (Fig. 2). Approximately 46% of the nasal cavity in a F344 rat is lined by respiratory epithelium (Gross et al. 1982; Young's transverse sections I–IV). This estimation includes the transitional epithelium, which probably contributes only a small fraction to this area. Although this pseudostratified nasal epithelium is similar to ciliated epithelium lining other proximal airways (i.e., trachea and bronchi), it also has unique features. Nasal respiratory epithelium in the rat is composed of six morphologically distinct cell types: mucous, ciliated, nonciliated columnar, cuboidal, brush, and basal (Monteiro-Riviere and Popp 1984). These cells are unevenly distributed along the rat mucosal surface. Using scanning electron microscopy, Popp and Martin (1984) demonstrated a proximal-to-distal increase in ciliated cells along the lateral walls of the rat. In the nasal septum of the rat ciliated cells are evenly distributed from proximal to distal.

As with the ciliated cell, the mucous cell is unevenly distributed in the respiratory epithelium of the nasal cavity. In the normal rat mucous cells are predominantly located in respiratory epithelium lining the proximal septum (Young's transverse section I) and lining the nasopharynx (Young's transverse section IV; Harkema et al. 1989; Fig. 7). Serous cells are the primary secretory cells in the remainder of the respiratory epithelium in rodents. Interestingly, secretory cells in the respiratory epithelium of both rats (Yamamoto and

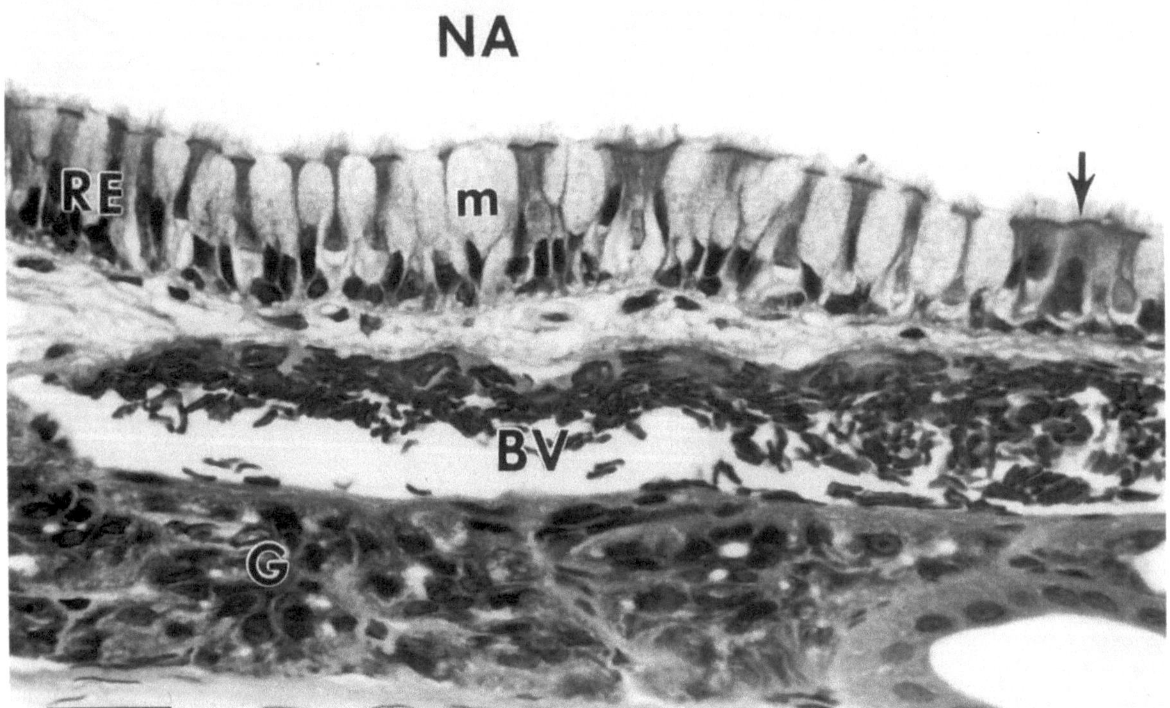


**Fig. 7.** Nasal respiratory epithelium (*RE*) lining the midseptum in the proximal nasal cavity of a F344 rat (Young's transverse section I). *BV*, Blood vessel; *G*, subepithelial gland in lamina propria; *m*, mucous cell; *arrow*, ciliated cell; *NA*, nasal airway lumen. Alcian blue (pH 2.5), Bar = 25 μm, H&E

Masudo 1982) and mice (Matulionis and Parks 1972) have abundant SER. This may suggest that these cells, as the nonciliated cell in the transitional epithelium, may have metabolic capacities for certain xenobiotics. Recent research in the area of xenobiotic metabolism in nasal respiratory and olfactory epithelium has demonstrated the presence of many enzymes previously described in other tissues (Bogdanffy 1990). In particular, carboxylesterase, aldehyde dehydrogenase, cytochrome P-450, epoxide hydrolase, and glutathione S transferases have been localized by histochemical techniques. The distribution of these enzymes appears to be cell type specific and the presence of the enzyme may predispose particular cell types to enhanced susceptibility or resistance to chemically induced injury.

Respiratory epithelium also lines the one pair of paranasal sinuses (the maxillary sinuses) located in the lateral wall of the nasal cavity. The respiratory epithelium of the maxillary sinuses is a pseudostratified, low-columnar epithelium composed of ciliated, serous, and basal cells. Few mucous cells are evident in the normal respiratory epithelium of the maxillary sinuses of rats or mice. Surrounding the maxillary sinuses are conspicuous lateral glands (Steno's glands) which extend deep into the connective tissue of the lateral wall to the ostium of the maxillary sinus (Warshawsky 1963; Moe and Boisen-Moller 1971). The ducts from Steno's glands open into the nasal vestibule. These glands also have extensive metabolic capacity and are specific targets for some chemicals that require metabolism to proximate carcinogens.

The lamina propria in the respiratory epithelial region is similar to that in the transitional epithelium, being characterized by a loose fibroelastic connective tissue containing numerous blood vessels and serous or mucous glands. The glands in the proximal half of the septum in the rat (anterior septal glands) are of the tubuloalveolar type consisting of numerous solitary acini and a single long duct which empties into the vestibule (Cuschieri and Bannister 1974; Kuijpers et al. 1983; Klaassen et al. 1981). These glands are primarily serous. In contrast, the more distal septal glands (posterior septal glands) located ventral to the junction between the respiratory epithelium and the olfactory organ of Masera and near the vomeronasal organ (see following), have a mucous secretion which empties into the vomeronasal organ (Klaassen et al. 1982; Tandler and Boisen-Moller 1978). Tubular and compound acinar glands, whose ducts open to the nasal lumen or maxillary sinus, are also present in the lamina propria of the turbinates and lateral wall.

## Olfactory Epithelium

The major difference in nasal epithelium among animal species is the percentage of the nasal airway that is covered by olfactory epithelium. A much greater percentage of nasal cavity is lined by olfactory epithelium in the rat than in monkeys or humans. Gross et al. (1982) determined morphometrically that approximately 50% of the nasal cavity surface area in F344 rats is lined by this sensory epithelium. Olfactory epithelium lines portions of the roof, septum, and turbinates (nasoturbinates or ethmoid turbinates) in Young's transverse section's II, III, and IV of the rat nose (Fig. 2). Although morphometric determinations have not been made for primates, the proportion of surface area covered by the olfactory epithelium is considerably less (Negus 1958). Mice, hamsters, rabbits, and dogs are much closer to rats than humans or monkeys with respect to the relative amount of olfactory epithelium within their nasal airways. For example, in B6C3Fl mice, 37% of the nasal cavity is lined by olfactory epithelium (Gross et al. 1982). Olfactory epithelium in humans is limited to an area of about 500 mm$^2$, which is only 3% of the total surface area of the nasal cavity (Sorokin 1988). This small focal area of the human nose is located in the middorsal aspect of the main nasal chamber (Negus 1958).

Three basic cell types compose the olfactory epithelium (sensory, sustentacular, and basal; Fig. 8) compared to six or seven epithelial cell types in respiratory epithelium. The olfactory sensory cells are bipolar neurons interposed between the sustentacular cells (Vollrath et al. 1985). The dendritic portion of this neuron extends above the epithelial surface and terminates into a bulbous olfactory knob from which protrude 12 or more immotile cilia. These cilia are enmeshed with each other and with microvilli in the surface fluid and provide an extensive surface area for reception of odorants. The axon of the olfactory sensory cell originates from the base of the cell and passes through the basal lamina to join axons from other sensory cells forming nonmyelinated nerves in the lamina propria. These axons perforate the cribriform plate to synapse with neurons in the olfactory bulb. Unlike other neurons in the

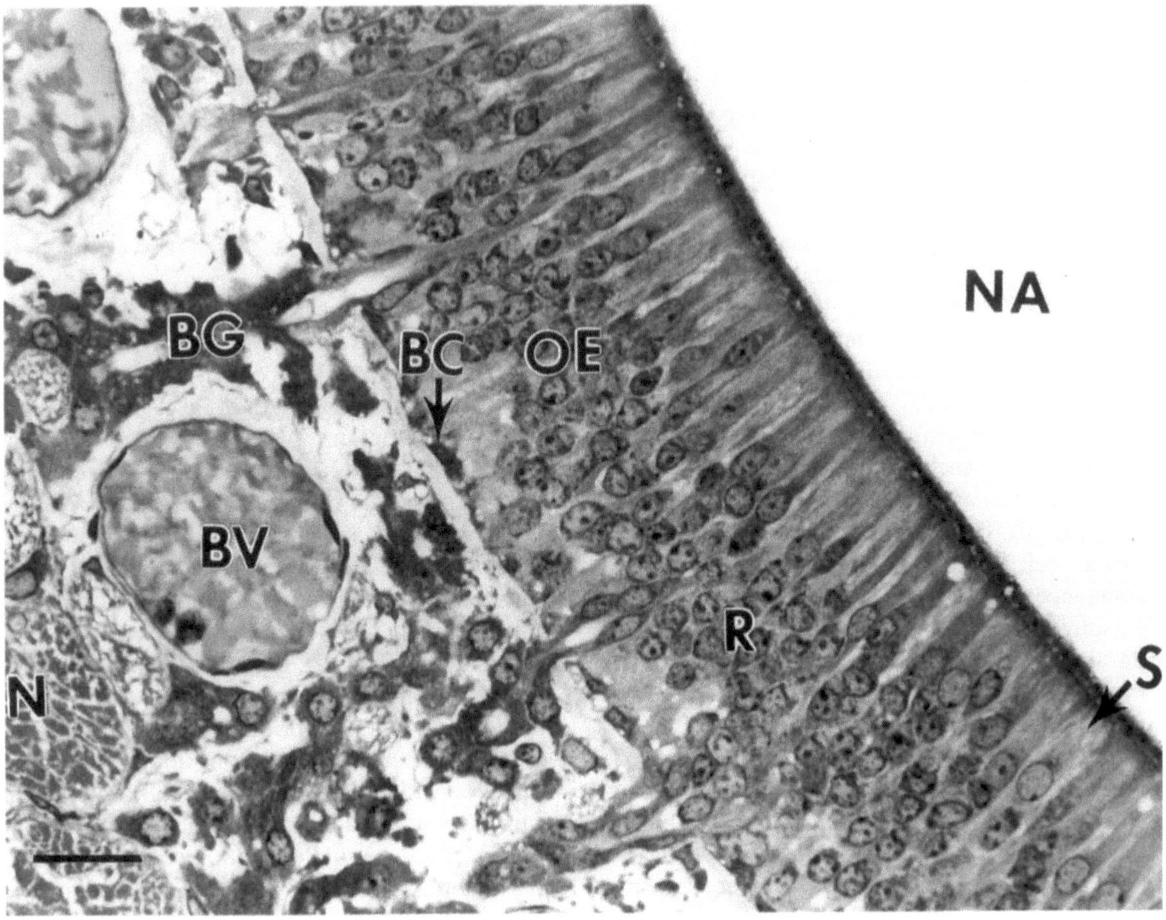


A

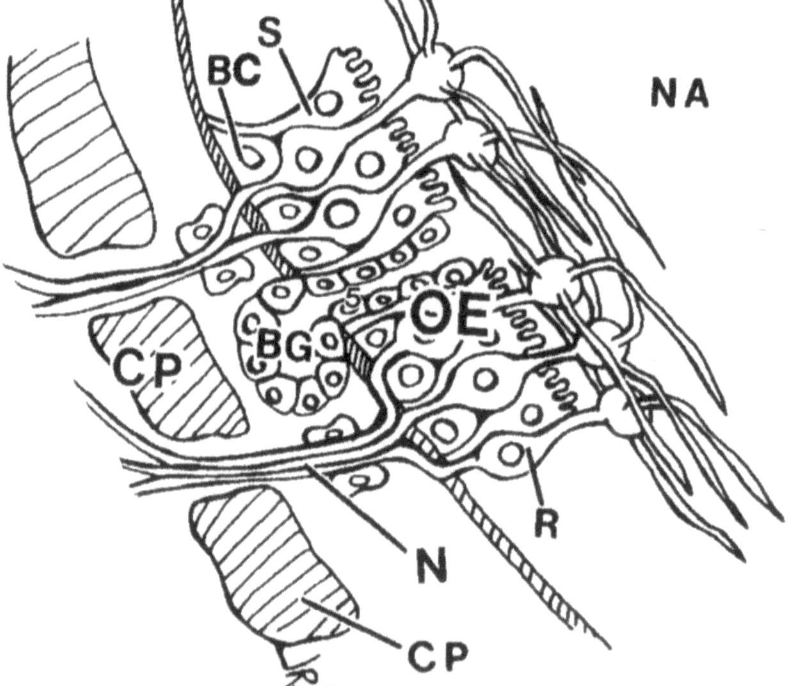


B

body, the olfactory sensory cell can regenerate, having a 28- to 30-day turnover rate in the rat (Graziadei and Monti Graziadei 1977). Basal cells are generally considered the stem cells for the regenerating olfactory epithelium. Regeneration of olfactory epithelium after experimental injury has been found to be an excellent model for the study of neurogenesis and axon regeneration in mammals (Graziadei and Monti Graziadei 1978). Sustentacular cells in olfactory epithelium have been considered as support cells for the sensory cells. These cells also have abundant SER and metabolizing enzymes (e.g., esterases, cytochrome P450). The enzyme activity in these cells may be important in metabolism of inhaled xenobiotics and in the function of smell (Dahl and Hadley 1991; Reed 1993).

Other important sites of xenobiotic metabolism associated with olfactory epithelium are the Bowman's glands (Fig. 8). These structures located in the underlying lamina propria and interspersed among the olfactory nerve bundles are simple tubular glands composed of small compact acini. Ducts from these glands transverse the basal lamina at regular intervals and extend through the olfactory epithelium to the luminal surface. Bowman's glands contain copious amounts of neutral and acidic mucosubstances that contribute to the mucous layer covering the luminal surface of the olfactory epithelium.

With few exceptions, the olfactory epithelium has greater xenobiotic metabolizing activity than does the respiratory epithelium in most animal species (Bond et al. 1988; Hadley and Dahl 1983). Immunohistochemical analyses suggest that sustentacular cells in the olfactory epithelium and Bowman's glands in the underlying lamina propria tend to have especially high concentrations of many xenobiotic-metabolizing enzymes. The presence of these enzymes in the olfactory epithelium readily explains numerous observations of nasal toxicity in animals exposed to certain inhaled toxicants (Dahl and Hadley 1991). With its generally higher enzyme activity, the olfactory mucosa is more sensitive to the toxic effects of many metabolizable materials.

In rodents the sense of smell is important for acquisition of food and for recognition of enemies, territory, and members of the same species for sexual and nonsexual interactions. Besides the olfactory epithelium, other structures in the rodent nose are thought to contribute to olfaction. The vomeronasal organ, sometimes referred to as the organ of Jacobson, is a paired tubular diverticulum located in the vomer bone in the ventral portion of the proximal nasal septum of most mammals (e.g., rodents, dogs, cats, and rabbits; Sorokin 1988; Uraih and Maronpot 1990; Fig. 1). It is poorly developed in higher primates. The lateral wall of each diverticulum is lined by a tall columnar epithelium, while the medial wall is lined by a neuroepithelium similar to that of the olfactory epithelium (Fig. 9). The sensory cells of the vomeronasal organ have long microvilli but lack the cilia found in neuronal cells in the olfactory epithelium. The sensory cells, however, do have axons that extend caudally to form the vomeronasal nerves, which connect with the accessory olfactory bulb. A small duct extends from each diverticulum to the proximal nasal airway lumen near the nasal opening of the nasopalatine canal that connects the nasal cavity with the oral cavity. Because of its neuroepithelium and gross anatomical location the vomeronasal organ has been proposed to function in the detection of pheromones and the determination of flavor of foods in the mouth by olfaction, as opposed to determination of taste by gustation on the tongue (Negus 1958).

Another unique olfactory structure in the rodent nose is the septal organ of Masera (Rodolfo-Masera 1943; Adams and McFarland 1971). It is a small isolated patch of neuroepithelium, resembling olfactory epithelium, lying near the base of the nasal septum at the entrances to the nasopalatine ducts (Young's transverse section II; Fig. 1). Masera's organ is part of the chemosensory system serving an alerting function. It is also thought to function in the detection of odors in the inhaled air (Marshall and Maruniak 1986).

◄
**Fig. 8. A** Olfactory epithelium (*OE*) in the nasal cavity of a F344 rat. **B** Diagrammatic illustration of OE and underlying lamina propria. *S*, sustentacular (support) cells; *R*, olfactory sensory receptor cells; *BC*, basal cells; *N*, olfactory nerve in lamina propria; *BG*, Bowman's gland; *CP*, cribiform plate between nasal and cranial cavities; *BV*, blood vessel; *NA*, nasal airway, Bar = 25 μm

## Lymphoepithelium

In addition to the four principal nasal epithelia already described, there is another specialized

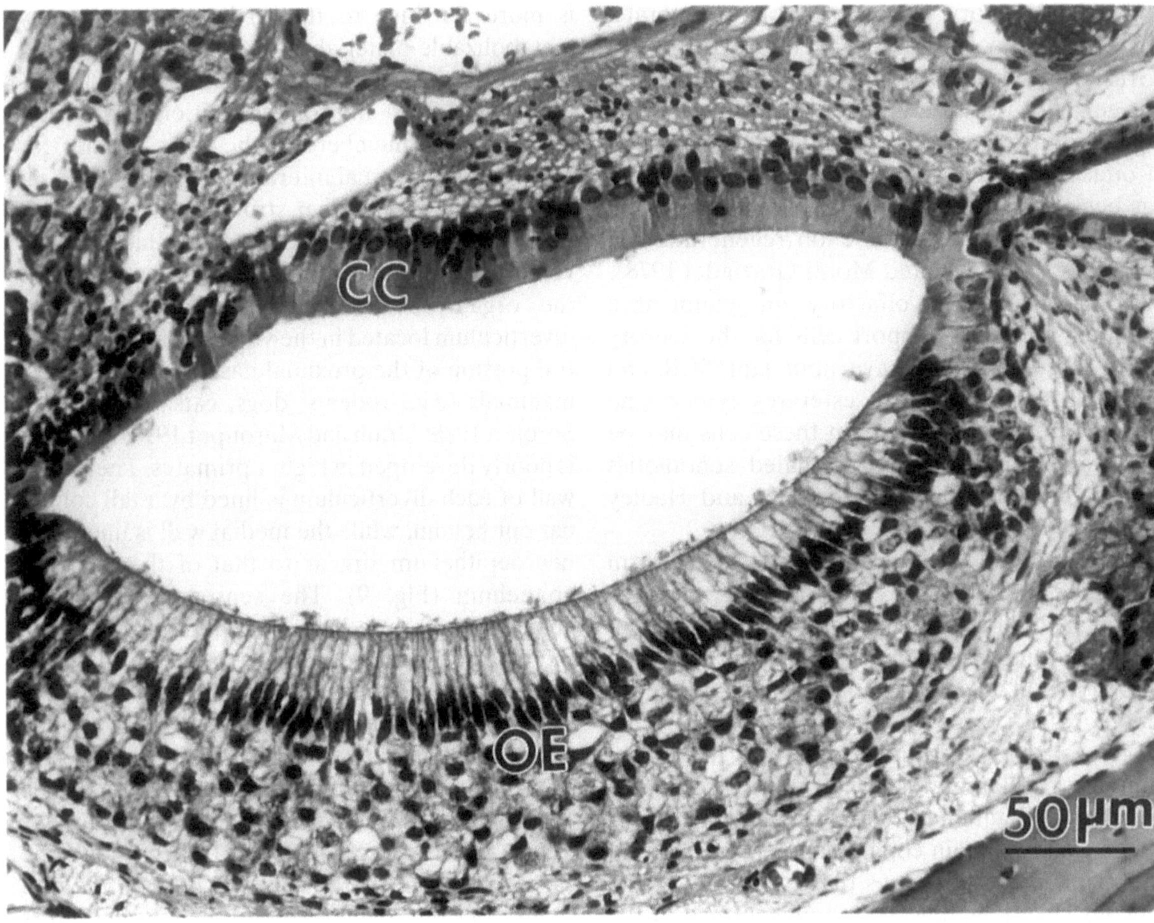


**Fig. 9.** Vomeronasal organ in the proximal-ventral nasal septum (Young's transverse section I) of a F344 rat. Ciliated columnar epithelium (*CC*) lining lateral wall and olfactory epithelium (*OE*) lining the medial wall of this septal structure

epithelium in the nasal airway that covers discrete focal aggregates of mucosal-associated lymphoid tissue in the underlying lamina propria (Fig. 10). In rats NALT with associated lymphoepithelium is restricted to the ventral aspects of the lateral walls at the opening of the nasopharyngeal duct (Spit et al. 1989; Fig. 1). The overlying lymphoepithelium is composed of cuboidal ciliated cells, a few mucous cells, and numerous nonciliated, cuboidal cells with luminal microvilli (membranous or M cells) similar to those in the gut- and bronchus-associated lymphoid tissues. Islands or patches of M cells cover focal areas of the rat lymphoid structures. These epithelial cells are thought to be involved in the uptake and translocation of inhaled antigen from the nasal lumen to the underlying lymphoid structures.

NALT, with its specialized lymphoepithelium, has a strategic position at the entrance of the nasopharyngeal duct since most of the nasal secretions and inhaled air, both presumably laden with antigenic material, pass over this area. Although the overall function of NALT and its place in the general mucosa-associated lymphoid system have not yet been determined, it may have an important function in regional immune defense of the upper airways.

## The Nasal Mucociliary Apparatus

When microscopically examining nasal passages, one must not forget that the luminal surface of the nasal mucosa in the live animal (with the exception of the most proximal regions of the nose lined by squamous epithelium) are covered by a watery, sticky material called mucus. This complex vis-

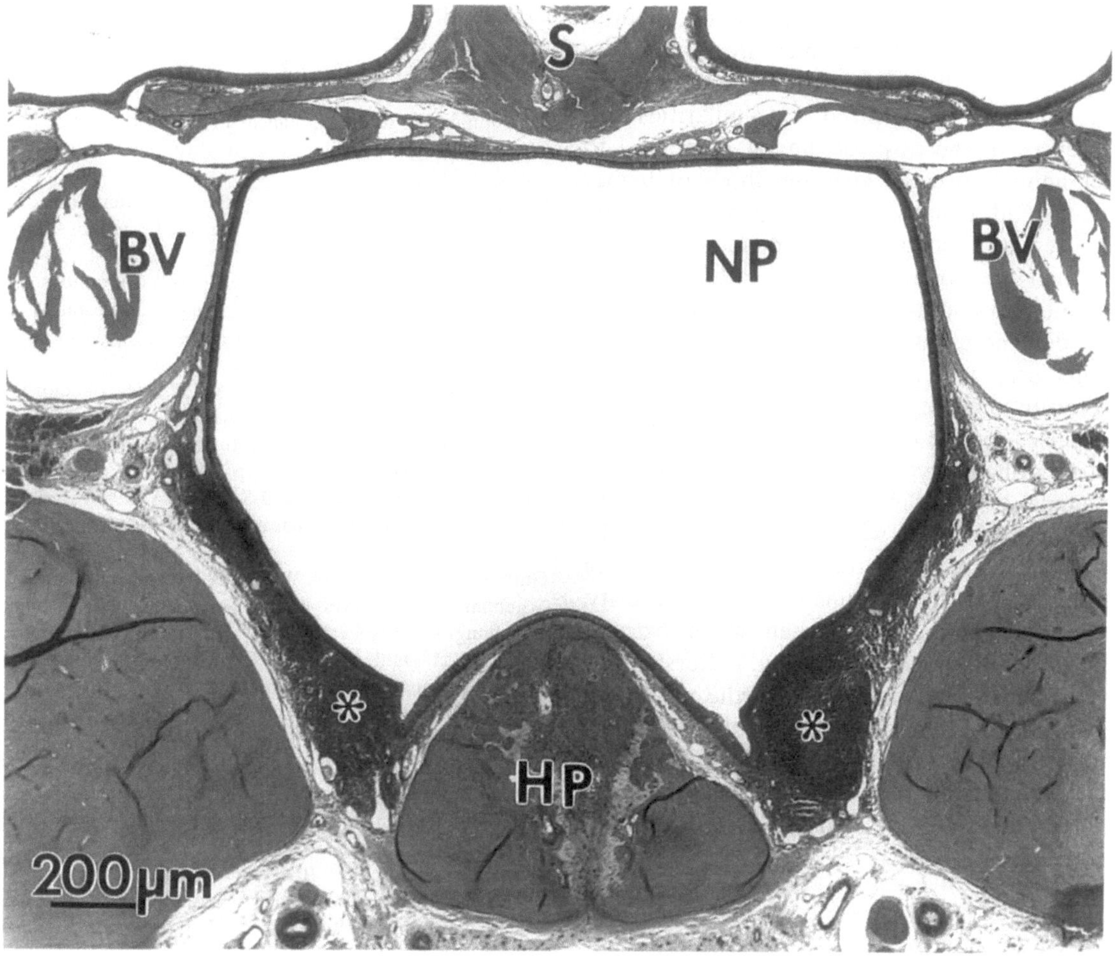


**Fig. 10.** Entrance of the nasopharyngeal duct (*NP*) of the nasal cavity of a F344 rat. The ventral aspects of the lateral walls contain NALT (*asterisk*) with an overlying lymphoepithelium. *BV*, Blood vessel; *HP*, hard palate; *S*, septum

coelastic fluid is often removed during routine tissue processing of the nasal tissues. Its physical and chemical properties are well suited for it role as an upper airway defense mechanism, i.e., filtering the inhaled air by trapping inhaled particles and possibly gases or vapors. The mucus is produced by secretory cells in the surface epithelium and subepithelial glands in the lamina propria. Synchronized beating of surface cilia propel the mucus at different speeds and directions depending on the intranasal location. Mucus covering the olfactory mucosa moves very slowly, with a turnover time of probably several days. In contrast, the mucous covering of the transitional and respiratory epithelium is driven along rapidly (1–30 mm/min) by the ciliary activity with an estimated turnover time of about 10 min in the rat (Morgan et al. 1984). The mucus with the entrapped materials ultimately is carried to the nasopharynx and is swallowed into the gastrointestinal tract. The nasal mucocilary apparatus (i.e., mucus and cilia) exhibits a range of responses to inhaled xenobiotics and can be a sensitive indicator of toxicity (Morgan et al. 1986). Since this upper airway apparatus is one of the first lines of defense against inhaled pathogens, dusts, and irritant gases, toxicant-induced compromises in its defense capabilities could lead to increased nasal infections and increased susceptibility to lower respiratory tract diseases.

## Summary

This chapter describes some of the important gross and microscopic features of the nasal passages in laboratory rodents. It is apparent that the nasal passages of rats and mice are structurally complex organs due to the varied functions of the nose. We have emphasized the similarities and differences of the nose of the rat compared to other animal species, especially those of higher primates and humans. Since rodents are obligate nose breathers and are more dependent on olfaction than are some oronasal-breathing species (e.g., monkeys, humans), it is not surprising that the rodent nose has a more elaborate intranasal architecture, with relatively more surface area covered by olfactory epithelium. Although there are species-specific differences in nasal structure, the four principal types of nasal epithelium in rats are similar to those in other mammalian species, including humans. A working knowledge of the normal structure of the rodent nose is crucial for the investigator to determine the nature, severity, distribution, and possible mechanisms of toxicant-induced nasal lesions. In addition, understanding the differences and similarities of the upper airways of rodents compared to those of humans and other laboratory animal species is critical in assessing the possible risks to human health of various nasal toxicants (DeSessio 1993).

## References

Adams DR, McFarland LZ (1971) Septal olfactory organ in Peromyscus. Comp Biochem Physiol A40:971–974

Aharonson EF, Menkes H, Gurtner G, Swift DL, Proctor DF (1974) Effect of respiratory airflow rate on the removal of soluble vapors by the nose. J Appl Physiol 37:654–657

Andersen I, Proctor DF (1982) The fate and effects of inhaled materials. In: Proctor DF, Andersen I (eds) The nose, upper airway physiology and the atmospheric environment. Elsevier Biomedical, Amsterdam, pp 423–455

Bogdanffy MS (1990) Biotransformation enzymes in the rodent nasal mucosa: the value of a histochemical approach. Environ Health Perspect 85:177–186

Bond JA, Harkema JR, Russell VI (1988) Regional distribution of xenobiotic metabolizing enzymes in airways of dogs. Drug Metab Dispos 16:116–124

Brain JD (1970) The uptake of inhaled gases by the nose. Ann Otol Rhinol Laryngol 79:529–539

Brain JD, Valberg PA (1979) Deposition of aerosol in the respiratory tract. Am Rev Respir Dis 120:1325–1373

Buckley LA, Jiang XZ, James RA, Morgan KT, Barrow CS (1984) Respiratory tract lesions induced by sensory irritants at the RD50 concentration. Toxicol Appl Pharmacol 74:417–429

Cuschieri A, Bannister LH (1974) Some histochemical observations on the mucosubstances of the nasal glands of the mouse. Histochem J 6:543–558

Dahl AR, Hadley WM (1991) Nasal cavity enzymes involved in xenobiotic metabolism: effects on the toxicity of inhalants. Crit Rev Toxicol 1:345–372

DeSesso JM (1993) The relevance to humans of animal models for inhalation studies of cancer in the nose and upper airways. Quality assurance: good practice, regulation, and law 21:345–372

Fowler BA, Kardish RM, Woods JS (1983) Alterations of hepatic microsomal structure and function by indium chloride. Lab Invest 48:471–478

Graziadei PPC, Monti Graziadei GA (1977) Continuous nerve cell renewal in the olfactory system. In: Jacobson M (ed) Handbook of sensory physiology, vol IX. Springer, Berlin Heidelberg New York, pp 55–82

Graziadei PPC, Monti Graziadei GA (1978) The olfactory system: a model for the study of neurogenesis and axon regeneration in mammals. In: Cotman CW (ed) Neuronal plasticity. Raven, New York, pp 131–153

Gross EA, Swenberg JA, Field S, Popp JA (1982) Comparative morphometry of the nasal cavity in rats and mice. J Anat 135:83–88

Guilmette RA, Wicks JD, Wolff RK (1989) Morphometry of human nasal airways in vivo using magnetic resonance imaging. J Aerosol 2:365–377

Hadley WM, Dahl AR (1983) Cytochrome P-450-dependent monooxygenases in nasal membranes of six species. Drug Metab Dispos 11:275–276

Harkema JR, Plopper CG, Hyde DM, Wilson DW, St. George JA, Wong VJ (1987) Nonolfactory surface epithelium of the nasal cavity of the bonnet monkey: a morphologic and morphometric study of the transitional and respiratory epithelium. Am J Anat 180:266–279

Harkema JR, Hotchkiss JR, Henderson RF (1989) Effects of 0.12 and 0.80 ppm ozone on rat nasal and nasopharyngeal epithelial mucosubstances: quantitative histochemistry. Toxicol Pathol 17:525–535

Hounam RF, Morgan A (1977) Particle deposition. In: Brain JD, Proctor DF, Reid LM (eds) Respiratory defense mechanisms. Dekker, New York, pp 125–126

Johnson NF, Hotchkiss JA, Harkema JR, Henderson RF (1990) Proliferative responses of rat nasal epithelia to ozone. Toxicol Appl Pharmacol 103:143–155

Kimbell JS, Gross EA, Joyner DR, Godo MN, Morgan KT (1993) Application of computational fluid dynamics to regional dosimetry of inhaled chemicals in the upper respiratory tract of the rat. Toxicol Appl Pharmacol 121:253–263

Klaassen AB, Kiujpers W, Denuce JM (1981) Morphological and histochemical aspects of the nasal glands in the rat. Anat Anz 149:51–63

Klaassen AB, Jap PH, Kuijpers W (1982) Ultrastructural aspects of the nasal glands in the rat. Anat Anz 191 (2):455–466

Kuijpers W, Klaassen ABM, Jap PHK, Tonnaer E (1983) Secretory characteristics of the rat nasal glands. Acta Otolaryngol (Stockh) 95:676–687

Lippmann M (1970) Deposition and clearance of inhaled particles in the human nose. Ann Otol Rhinol Laryngol 79:519–528

Marshall DA, Maruniak JA (1986) Masera's organ responds to odorants. Brain Res 366:329–332

Matulionis DH, Parks HR (1972) Ultrastructural morphology of the normal nasal respiratory epithelium of the mouse. Anat Rec 176:64–83

Mery S, Gross EA, Joyner DR, Godo M, Morgan KT (1994) Nasal diagrams: a tool for recording the distribution of nasal lesions in rats and mice. Toxicol Pathol 22:353–372

Moe H, Boisen-Moller F (1971) The fine structure of the lateral nasal gland (Steno's gland) of the rat. J Ultrastruct Res 36:127–148

Monteiro-Riviere NA, Popp JA (1984) Ultrastructural characterization of the nasal respiratory epithelium in the rat. Am J Anat 169:31–43

Monticello TM, Morgan KT, Everitt JI, Popp JA (1989) Effects of formaldehyde gas on the respiratory tract of rhesus monkeys. Pathology and cell proliferation. Am J Pathol 134:515–527

Monticello TM, Morgan KT, Uraih L (1990) Nonneoplastic nasal lesions in rats and mice. Environ Health Perspect 85:249–274

Morgan KT (1991) Approaches to the identification and recording of nasal lesions in toxicology studies. Toxicol Pathol 19:337–351

Morgan KT (1994) Nasal dosimetry, lesion distribution, and the toxicologic pathologist: a brief review. Inhal Toxicol 6:41–57

Morgan MS, Frank R (1977) Uptake of pollutant gases by the respiratory system. In: Respiratory defense mechanisms, Brain JD, Proctor DF, Reid LM (eds) Dekker, New York, pp 157–189

Morgan KT, Monticello TM (1990) Airflow, gas distribution, and lesion distribution in the nasal passages. Environ Health Perspect 88:209–218

Morgan KT, Jiang XZ, Patterson DL, Gross EA (1984) The nasal mucociliary apparatus: correlation of structure and function in the rat. Am Rev Respir Dis 130:275–281

Morgan KT, Patterson DL, Gross EA (1986) Response of the nasal mucociliary apparatus of F-344 rats to formaldehyde gas. Toxicol Appl Pharmacol 82:1–13

Morgan KT, Kimbell JS, Monticello TM, Patra AL, Fleishman A (1991) Studies in inspiratory airflow patterns in the nasal passages of the F344 rat and rhesus monkey using nasal molds: relevance to formaldehyde toxicity. Toxicol Appl Pharmacol 110:223–240

Negus VE (1958) The comparative anatomy and physiology of the nose and paranasal sinuses. Livingstone, Edinburgh

Patra AL, Gooya A, Menache MG (1986) A morphometric comparison of the nasopharyngeal airway of laboratory animals and humans. Anat Rec 215:42–50

Popp JA, Martin JT (1984) Surface topography and distribution of cell types in the rat nasal respiratory epithelium: scanning electron microscopic observations. Am J Anat 169:425–436

Proctor DF, Chang JCF (1983) Comparative anatomy and physiology of the nasal cavity. In: Reznik G, Stinson SF (eds) Nasal tumors in animals and man, vol I. CRC, Boca Raton, pp 1–33

Reed CJ (1993) Drug metabolism in the nasal cavity: relevance to toxicology. Drug Metab Rev 25:173–205

Rodolfo-Masera T (1943) Su l'esistenza di un particolare organo olfativo nel setto nasale della cavia e di altri roditori. Arch Hal Anat Embriol 48:157–212

Schreider JP, Raabe OG (1981) Anatomy of the nasal-pharyngeal airway of experimental animals. Anat Rec 200:195–205

Sorokin SP (1988) The respiratory system. In: Weiss L (ed) Cell and tissue biology: a textbook of histology. Urban and Schwarzenberg, Baltimore, pp 751–814

Spit BJ, Hendriksen EG, Bruijntjes JP, Kuper CF (1989) Nasal lymphoid tissue in the rat. Cell Tissue Res 255:193–198

Stott WT, McKenna MJ (1984) The comparative absorption and excretion of chemical vapors by the upper, lower, and intact respiratory tract of rats. Fundam Appl Toxicol 4:594–602

Swift DL (1981) Aerosol deposition and clearance in the human upper airways. Ann Biomed Engl 9:593–604

Tandler B, Boisen-Moller F (1978) Ultrastructure of the anterior medial glands of the rat nasal septum. Anat Rec 191 (2):147–167

Uraih LC, Maronpot RR (1990) Normal histology of the nasal cavity and application of special techniques. Environ Health Perspect 85:187–208

Vollrath M, Altmannsberger M, Weber K, Osborn M (1985) An ultrastructural and immunohistological study of the rat olfactory epithelium: unique properties of olfactory sensory cells. Differentiation 29:243–253

Walker D (1983) Histopathology of the nasal cavity in laboratory animals exposed to cigarette smoke and other irritants. In: Reznik G, Stinson SF (eds) Nasal tumors in animals and man, vol III. CRC, Boca Raton, pp 115–135

Warshawsky H (1963) Investigation of the lateral nasal glands of the rat. Anat Rec 147:443–455

Yamamoto T, Masuda H (1982) Some observation on the fine structure of the goblet cells in the nasal respiratory epithelium of the rat, with special reference to the well-developed agranular endoplasmic reticulum. Okajimas Folia Anat Jpn 58:583–594

Young JT (1981) Histopathologic examination of the rat nasal cavity. Fund Appl Toxicol 1:309–312

# Proliferative and Metaplastic Lesions in Nonolfactory Nasal Epithelia Induced by Inhaled Chemicals

Jack R. Harkema and Kevin T. Morgan

## Introduction

The nasal cavity is lined by surface epithelial cell populations that have specific roles in maintaining the normal functions of the nose. For example, the nasal respiratory epithelium, which lines approximately 50% of the rodent airway, is a pseudostratified, ciliated epithelium with numerous mucus-secreting cells that provide important nonolfactory functions. In this epithelium the ciliated cells with their motile cilia along with the mucus-secreting cells are the primary cellular components of the dynamic mucociliary apparatus. This apparatus is an important respiratory defense mechanism of the upper and lower respiratory tracts that protects the body from potentially injurious, inhaled, inorganic and organic particles and gases. These inhaled foreign agents deposit on the sticky mucous layer that is constantly being renewed by the underlying secretory cells and are propelled by the fast and synchronized beating of the cilia from the airway to the digestive tract where the agents are eliminated from the body. Because of this highly efficient defense mechanism the nasal airway has been described as a "scrubbing tower" that removes inhaled chemicals potentially harmful to the lower tracheobronchial airways and the delicate alveolar tissues in the lung where gas exchange occurs (Brain 1970). Although the nasal airways have important protective roles in the defense of the lower respiratory tract, their surface epithelial cells nonetheless are still vulnerable to injury from inhaled toxicants. The proximity of these surface epithelial cell populations to the inhaled airflow makes them prime targets for toxicant-induced damage. How these surface epithelial cells respond to toxic agents is predominantly dependent on the chemical makeup of the toxicant, the inherent sensitivity of the cell or tissue, and the dose of the xenobiotic to the cells.

Some examples are reviewed concerning how nasal surface epithelia, excluding the olfactory epithelium, can respond to inhaled chemical toxicants. The discussion focuses on structural (morphological) alterations that occur in the proximal nasal passages of laboratory animals after acute or chronic toxicant exposure. The wide range of nonneoplastic lesions observed in extraolfactory tissues of the nasal passages of rodents has been extensively reviewed (Boorman et al. 1990; Jiang et al. 1986; Monticello and Morgan 1994; Monticello et al. 1990; Sills et al. 1994; St. Clair and Morgan 1992). This chapter addresses the issue of interpretation of epithelial responses in the nose of laboratory animals after exposure to ozone or formaldehyde. These chemicals are chosen as examples because an extensive data base exists for the nasal lesions induced by these inhaled toxicants in both rodents and nonhuman primates. Cigarette smoke induced epithelial lesions in the nasal passages of laboratory rats are also discussed and compared to ozone- and formaldehyde-induced lesions.

The discussion is restricted to chemically induced responses (e.g., hyperplasia, metaplasia) of the three distinct nonolfactory epithelia that line the proximal nasal cavity of laboratory rodents: (a) the stratified squamous epithelium that lines the nasal vestibule and the floor of the ventral meatus, (b) the nonciliated, pseudostratified, transitional epithelium that lines the lateral meatus, and (c) the ciliated, respiratory epithelium that lines most of the remaining nonolfactory regions. The reader is referred to the first chapter in this monograph for detailed morphological descriptions of these nonolfactory nasal epithelia. Whenever possible we compare toxicant-induced responses in rodent epithelium to those observed in the nasal epithelium of nonhuman primates after similar exposure regimes. The anatomy of the monkey nose is more similar to human nasal anatomy than is that of the rodent nose (Negus 1958; Harkema 1991; DeSesso 1993). Comparative animal pathology is often useful in estimating the possible risk to human health of potentially harmful atmospheric agents. We conclude this chapter by examining the intranasal distribution of nonneoplastic lesions in the nose of rodents exposed to various xenobiotics to emphasize the importance of recording nasal lesion distribution for understanding the possible mechanisms involved in the pathogenesis of the chemical-induced injury.

### Chemical-Induced Lesions of Stratified Squamous and Transitional Epithelium

These two nasal epithelia are assumed to be exposed to near ambient concentrations of atmospheric pollutants and to be particularly vulnerable to inhaled irritants because of their proximal location in the nasal airways. Although many inhaled nasal toxicants cause lesions in the proximal nasal passages, only a few of these irritants have been shown to induce structural damage to the stratified epithelial lining the nasal vestibule or the ventral meatus in rodents. Therefore this epithelium is believed to be more resistant to injury than transitional or respiratory epithelium. A few irritants, such as diethylamine (Buckley et al. 1985), glutaraldehyde (Gross et al. 1994), ammonia (Bolon et al. 1991), and hydrogen chloride (Jiang et al. 1986) can, however, cause lesions. The caustic nature of these chemicals and the airflow driven, locally high dose to this tissue are the probable reasons for these chemical-induced lesions in the stratified squamous epithelium rather than cellular susceptibility. Acute alterations of this epithelium are usually erosion or ulceration, with or without accompanying inflammation. Lesions induced after long-term exposures may include hyperplasia or hyperkeratosis. The latter changes may represent defensive or adaptive responses to prolonged exposure to the irritant and/or early indicators of a subsequent neoplastic response.

The transitional epithelium is caudal to the stratified squamous epithelium and proximal to the ciliated respiratory epithelium, and lines the lateral meatus in the proximal aspect of the rodent nasal airway. It is a narrow zone of nonciliated, pseudostratified cuboidal/columnar epithelium with few mucous cells (see p. 7 this volume). This transitional epithelium is thought to be more sensitive than squamous epithelium to certain toxicant-induced injury. Exposure to less irritating oxidants, such as ozone (Harkema et al. 1987a,b, 1989; Johnson et al. 1990) and chlorine gas (Wolf et al. 1995) causes hyperplastic and/or metaplastic changes in this transitional epithelium in laboratory animals. These changes are often preceded by acute inflammation with an influx of neutrophils into the lamina propria, luminal epithelium, and airway lumen.

Ozone is a common, irritating, oxidant air pollutant that has been experimentally demonstrated to induce epithelial hyperplasia and secretory cell (mucous cell) hyperplasia/metaplasia in the transitional epithelium of both rats (Harkema et al. 1989) and monkeys (Harkema et al. 1987a,b). F344 rats exposed for 7 days to 0.8 ppm ozone, 6 h/day, developed mucous cell metaplasia in the transitional epithelium lining the maxilloturbinates (Fig. 11), lateral wall, and lateral aspects of the nasoturbinates in the proximal nasal passages (Harkema et al. 1989). The ozone-induced lesion in the rat resembled those that were experimentally induced in the nasal cavity of bonnet monkeys. There were, however, some noticeable differences. The increase in mucous cells in the rat nasal airway was restricted to the transitional epithelium that is normally devoid of mucous cells. Therefore the ozone-induced, nasal epithelial alteration in the rat was a true metaplastic response (transformation of an epithelium with no mucous cells into an epithelium with numerous mucous cells) which differed from the hyperplastic response (increase in the number of mucous cells in an epithelium that normally contains some mucous cells) that was induced in monkeys after ozone exposure. In addition, no epithelial alterations were evident in the respiratory epithelium in the proximal nasal airways of the rat, unlike in the monkey. The rats exposed to 0.8 ppm ozone did, however, have attenuation of cilia in the lateral walls of the nasopharynx. Finally, no metaplastic alterations were evident in the transitional epithelium of rats exposed to 0.12 ppm, 6 h/day for 7 days. This was in contrast to the conspicuous mucous cell hyperplasia that was induced in monkeys after a 6-day (8 h/day) exposure to 0.15 ppm ozone (Fig. 12). These observations suggest that the transitional epithelium of the rat may not be as sensitive to ozone-induced injury as the same tissue in the monkey.

The reasons for the induction of mucous cell metaplasia in transitional epithelium after ozone-exposure are unknown. An influx of neutrophils (Hotchkiss et al. 1989) and an increase in epithelial DNA synthesis (Hotchkiss and Harkema 1992; Johnson et al. 1990) have been shown to precede the mucous cell metaplasia induced by ozone. These inflammatory and proliferative responses decrease as the mucous cell metaplasia develops (Harkema and Hotchkiss 1994). Six hours after the start of an exposure to 0.8 ppm ozone an acute rhinitis occurs with an influx of neutrophils into the transitional epithelium of F344 rats. With repeated exposures of ozone (6 h/day, for 3 or 7 days) there is a gradual

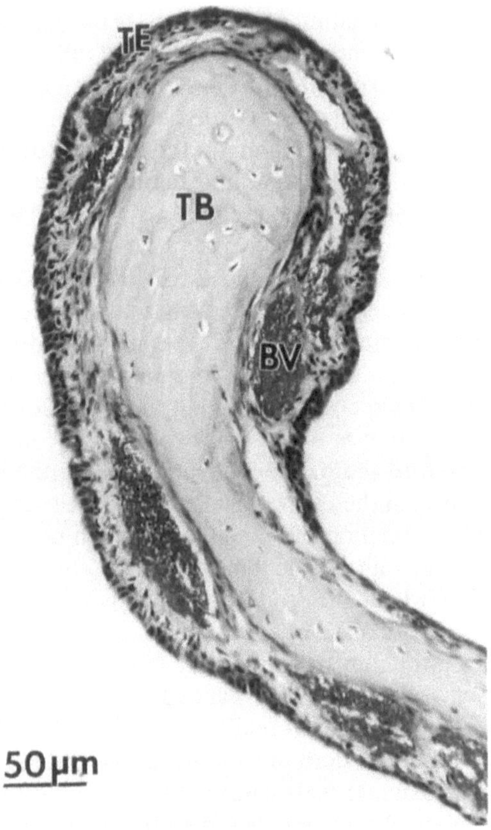


A

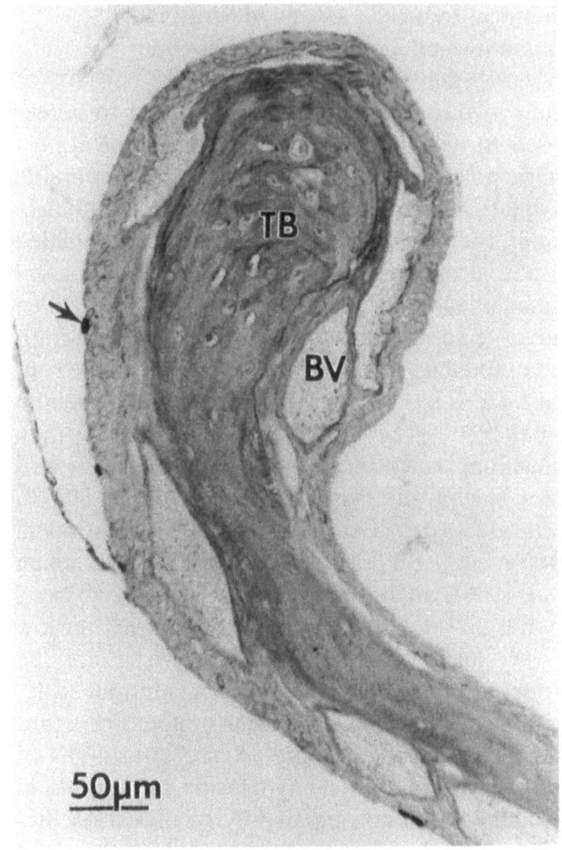


B

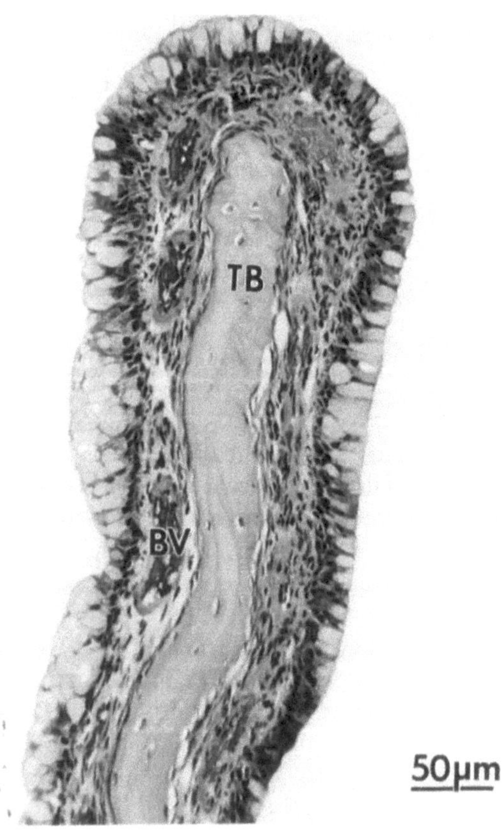


C

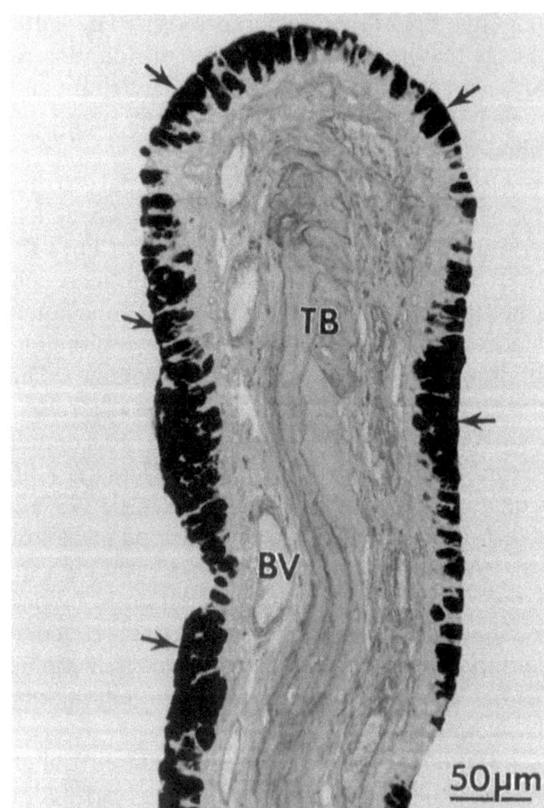


D

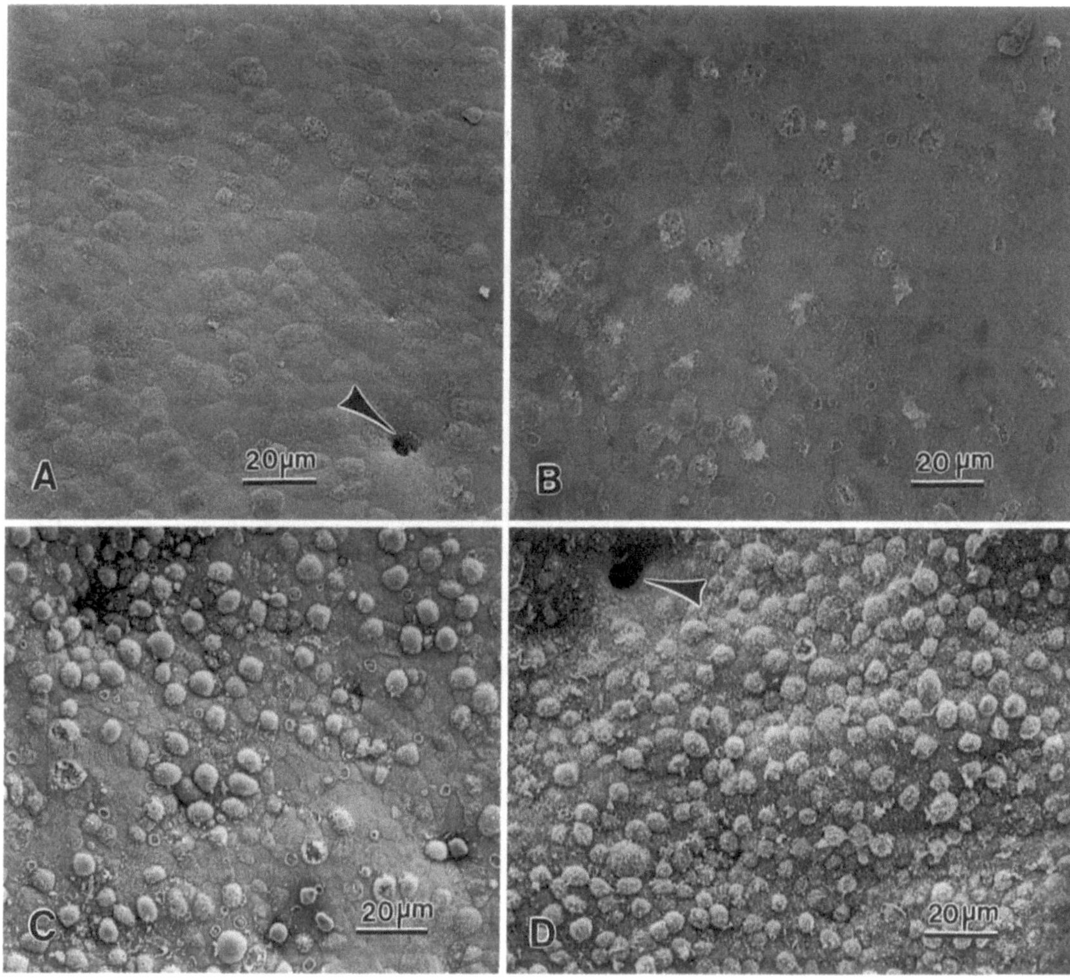


**Fig. 12A–D.** Luminal surfaces of the transitional epithelium from the nasal septum of monkeys exposed to 0 ppm ozone (**A**, control), 0.15 ppm ozone for 6 days (**B**), 0.15 ppm ozone for 90 days (**C**), and 0.30 ppm ozone for 90 days (**D**). **B,C,D** The dome-shaped protrusions are the apical aspects of mucous cells, indicating ozone-induced mucous cell metaplasia in these tissues. *Arrowheads*, openings of ducts from subepithelial gland. SEM. (From Harkema et al. 1987a by permission)

attenuation of this inflammatory response as measured by the number of intraepithelial neutrophils. The reason for this attenuation is unknown but may be due to an induction of mucosal antioxidants that protect the tissue from further ozone-induced injury. Interestingly, as the ozone-induced influx of neutrophils decrease, a concomitant increase in mucosubstances develops within the transitional. Since airway mucus is known to be a good antioxidant (Cross et al. 1984), it is plausible that these newly formed intraepithelial mucosubstances, with a corresponding increase in secreted mucins, act as a protective shield for the nasal epithelium and underlying lamina propria, preventing further injury by the continued ozone exposure. Therefore the reduction in surface injury would lead to the subsequent attenuation of the inflammatory response.

In addition to the acute inflammatory response to ozone exposure of transitional epithelium in the

◄

**Fig. 11A–D.** Maxilloturbinates from rats repeatedly exposed to 0 ppm ozone (control; **A,B**) or 0.5 ppm ozone (**C,D**). Staining of tissues: **A,C** H&E and Alcian blue (pH 2.5); **B,D** Alcian blue (pH 2.5)/periodic acid–Schiff (*AB/PAS*). **A,B** The nonciliated transitional epithelium (*TE*) lining the maxilloturbinate is thin with few mucous cells and little AB/PAS-stained mucosubstances (*arrows* in **B**). **C,D** The maxilloturbinate exposed to ozone is thick and metaplastic with numerous mucous cells and copious amounts of AB/PAS-stained mucosubstances (*arrows* in **D**). *TB*, Turbinate bone; *BV*, blood vessel in lamina propria

rat, there is also marked induction of DNA synthesis in this epithelium prior to the onset of the mucous cell metaplasia. In a study by Johnson et al. (1990), the effects of ozone exposure (3- or 7-day exposure, 6h/day, to 0, 0.12, or 0.8ppm ozone) on DNA synthesis in all four types of rat nasal epithelium were examined in vivo. DNA synthesis was monitored by immunohistochemical staining of epithelial cells that had incorporated bromodeoxyuridine (BrdU; an analog of thymidine) into their nuclei. Three of the nasal epithelia, respiratory, transitional and olfactory, in control rats (exposed to 0ppm ozone) were found to have low levels of DNA synthesis (one BrdU-labeled cell/mm basal lamina). In contrast, squamous epithelium had a high level of DNA synthesis (40 BrdU-labeled cells/mm basal lamina). Only rats exposed to 0.8ppm ozone had significantly greater DNA synthesis in nasal epithelia than air-exposed (0ppm) controls. Following exposure to 0.8ppm ozone a transient but marked increase in DNA synthesis (30 times more than controls) was evident in the transitional epithelium while in the respiratory and olfactory epithelium the transient increase was less marked (five and four times greater than controls). The number of S phase cells in the squamous epithelium was similar to controls after 3 or 7 days of ozone exposure. The ozone-induced increase in DNA synthesis was prominent after 3 days of exposure and absent by 7 days of exposure in the respiratory and olfactory epithelium. The ozone-induced increase in BrdU-labeled cells in the transitional epithelium was, however, markedly less at 7 days of exposure compared to 3 days of exposure (10- and 30-fold greater than controls, respectively). The transient nature of the DNA response in the transitional and respiratory epithelium to the week-long, repeated ozone exposure was similar to the transient nature of the inflammatory response in the nasal mucosa brought on by similar exposures to ozone that were mentioned above.

Recently the effects of chronic ozone exposures on the structure and function of the nasal epithelium of F344 rats exposed to 0, 0.12, 0.5, or 1ppm ozone for 20mo (6h/day, 5 days/week) have been examined (Harkema et al. 1992, 1994). Rats were killed 1 week after the end of the exposures. Immediately after death flow rates of mucus throughout the nasal passages were determined using in vitro video-motion analysis. Following assessment of mucociliary function the nasal tissues were processed for light microscopy and stained for detection of intraepithelial mucosubstances. Rats exposed to 0.5 and 1ppm ozone had markedly slower flow rates of mucus over the lateral walls and turbinates of the proximal third of the nasal passages than rats exposed to 0 and 0.12ppm ozone. Interestingly, these intranasal regions in the rats exposed to 0.5 and 1ppm ozone also had marked mucous cell metaplasia and 200 and 400 times greater amounts of intraepithelial mucosubstances than controls (0ppm ozone), respectively. No ozone-induced morphological alterations were present in the nasal epithelium of rats exposed to 0.12ppm ozone. This was the first study to demonstrate that the ozone-induced, mucous cell metaplasia in the rat transitional epithelium is associated with a functional alteration (i.e., decreased mucous flow rates). This alteration could significantly modify an important respiratory defense mechanism of the upper airways (i.e., mucociliary clearance) and leave the more distal pulmonary airways vulnerable to potentially injurious concentrations of inhaled xenobiotics or infectious agents.

Cigarette smoke is another irritant that can alter the transitional epithelium in rodents. Unlike ozone, which predominantly induces a mucous cell hyperplasia/metaplasia, cigarette smoke exposure results in squamous metaplasia (Fig. 13) along with epithelial cell proliferation (Walker 1983; Maples et al. 1993). Others have shown that irritants differ considerably in their ability to induce squamous metaplasia in laboratory rodents (Jiang et al. 1986). Formaldehyde is one irritant that has been demonstrated to induce squamous metaplasia in the nasal cavities of both rodents and nonhuman primates (Chang et al. 1983; Monticello et al. 1989).

It is important to remember that laboratory rodents exposed to highly water-soluble gaseous irritants most often have lesions in the surface epithelium lining the lateral meatus (lateral margins of the naso- and maxilloturbinates and on the adjacent lateral wall) in the proximal aspects of the nasal cavity, which are covered by transitional epithelium (Mery et al. 1994; Jiang et al. 1986; Harkema et al. 1989). This regional sensitivity to injury may be due to (a) greater exposure of the tissue to the toxicant compared to other intranasal regions or (b) to an inherently susceptible population of epithelial cells. With respect to ozone toxicity, Hotchkiss et al. (1994) have compared the regional differences in ozone-induced injury in

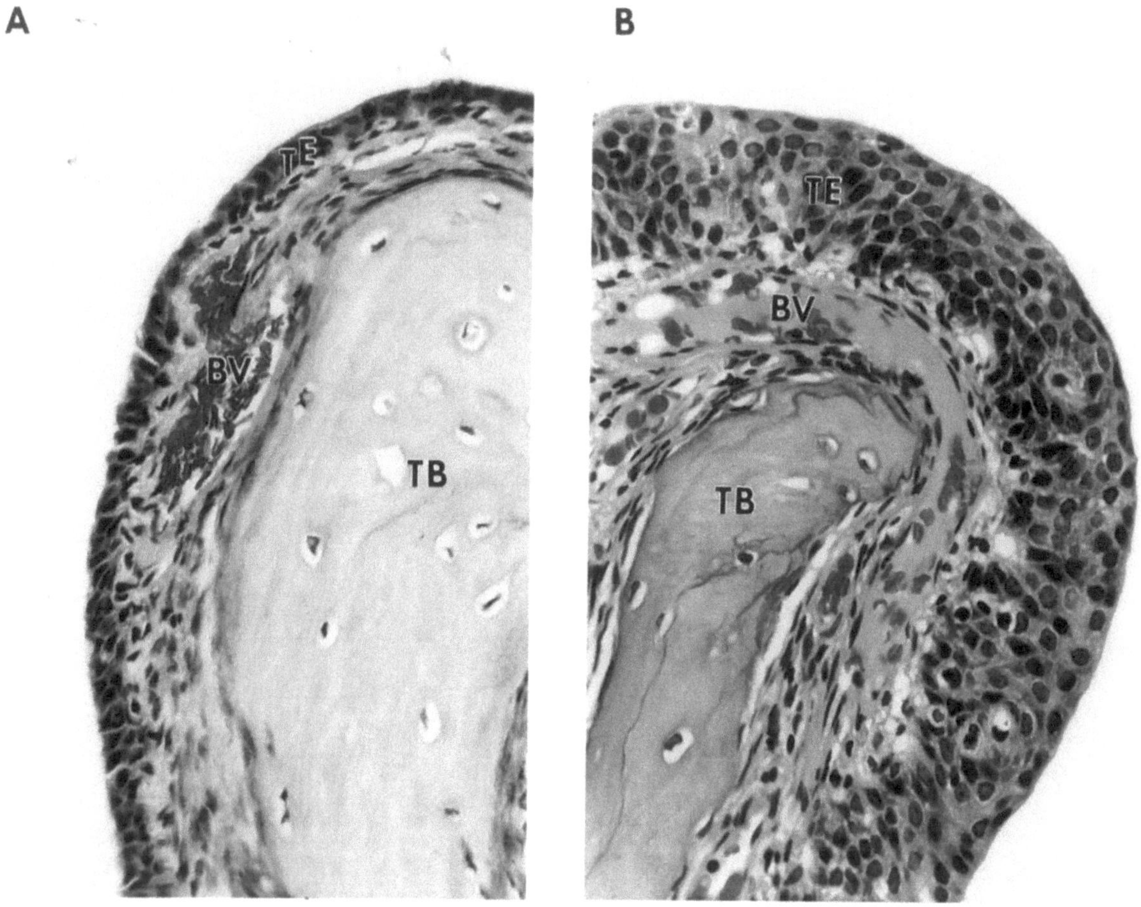


**Fig. 13.** Maxilloturbinates from rats repeatedly exposed to 0 (control; **A**) or 250 mg/m³ (**B**) of cigarette smoke. **B** The transitional epithelium (*TE*) is thick due to cigarette smoke induced squamous cell metaplasia. *BV*, Blood vessel in lamina propria; *TB*, turbinate bone. H&E, ×500

nasal epithelia of the proximal nasal airways of the rat with predicted ozone dosimetry based on computational airflow-driven mass flux patterns that were developed by Kimbell et al. (1993). The results of their study suggest that while dosimetry may play a role in the observed pattern of ozone-induced injury, much of the observed response must be due to inherent differences in epithelial susceptibility to ozone-induced injury. In contrast, nasal lesions induced by cigarette smoke or formaldehyde are probably driven by airflow rather than by tissue susceptibility.

## Chemical-Induced Lesions of Respiratory Epithelium

As in transitional epithelium, lesions in respiratory epithelium may be superficial or extend to the underlying lamina propria. A common superficial, and often reversible, effect of irritants on respiratory epithelium involves attenuation and/or loss of cilia along the luminal surface in the proximal nasal cavity. This effect was frequently seen in mice and rats exposed to chlorine gas (Jiang et al. 1983) and was a common alteration observed in monkeys exposed to 0.15 and 0.30 ppm ozone for 6 or 90 days (8 h/day; Harkema et al. 1987a; Fig. 14). Ciliated cell necrosis, mucous cell hyperplasia, and inflammatory cell influx (after 6 days of exposure only) were additional features of respiratory epithelia in monkeys exposed to ozone.

In contrast, rats exposed to approximately twice the concentrations of ozone as the nonhuman primates had no evidence of loss of cilia in the proximal nasal cavity, but they did have deciliation along the walls of the more distal nasopharyngeal meatus (Harkema et al. 1989). The reasons for

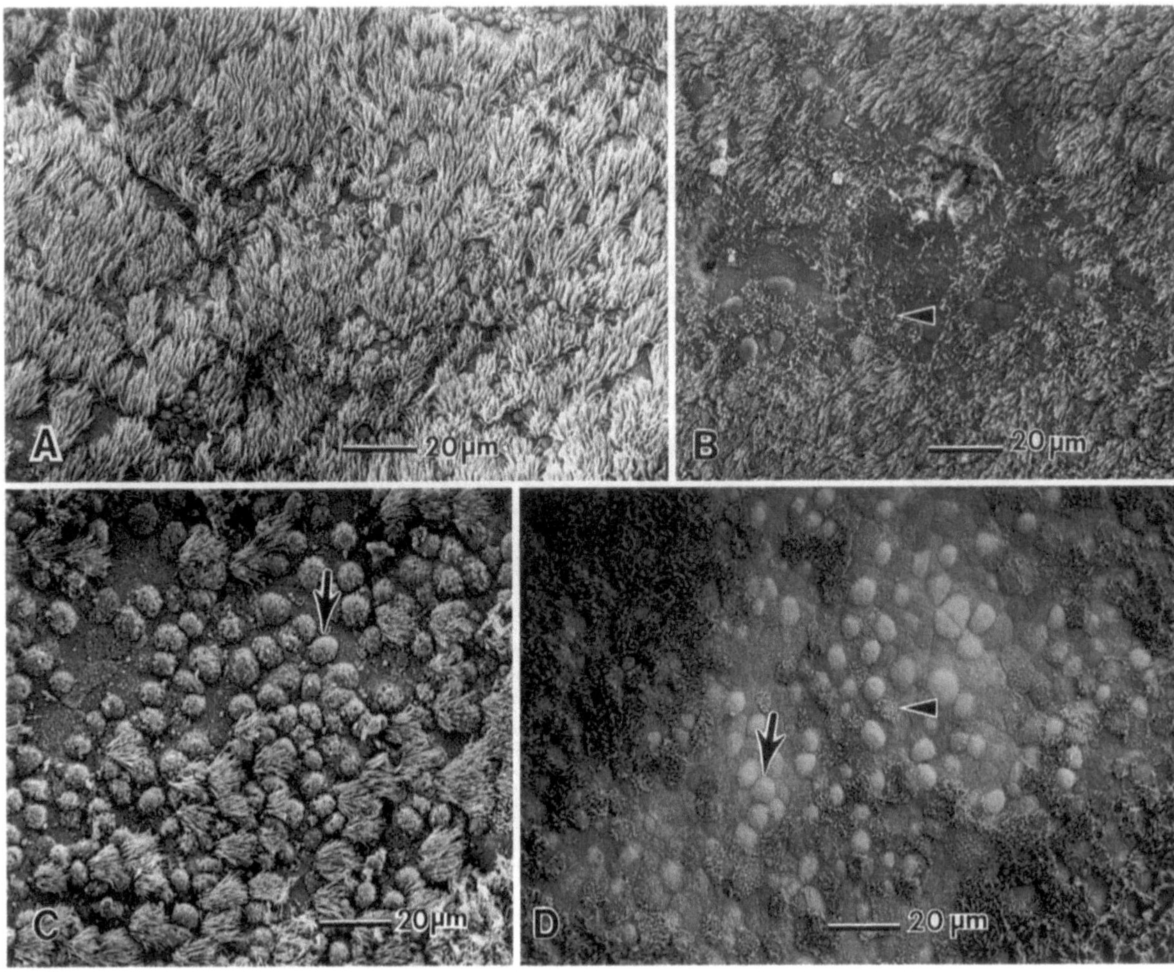


**Fig. 14.** Luminal surfaces of respiratory epithelium from the nasal septum of monkeys exposed to 0 ppm ozone (**A**; normal, control), and 0.15 ppm ozone for 6 days (**B**), 0.15 ppm ozone for 90 days (**C**), and 0.30 ppm ozone for 90 days (**D**). Surface exposed to 0.15 ppm and 0.30 ppm ozone had loss of cilia (*arrowheads*) and nonciliated cells with domed luminal surfaces (*arrows*; mucous cells). SEM (Used by permission from Harkema et al. 1987a)

these species differences are unknown, but they may be partially explained by differences in nasal airflow patterns, differing amounts of protective mucus overlying the nasal mucosa, and/or varying sensitivities of respiratory epithelial cells to ozone (DeSesso 1993). More elaborate studies must be specifically designed to investigate the mechanisms responsible for these species-specific differences in epithelial response.

Studies have demonstrated that the respiratory epithelium in both rodents and monkeys is susceptible to repeated exposures to formaldehyde, which result in loss of mucous cells and cilia, epithelial proliferation with or without squamous metaplasia, and an associated inflammatory response (Chang et al. 1983; Monticello et al. 1989). These nonneoplastic lesions in the proximal nasal cavity of rats occurred in the same regions in which formaldehyde-induced nasal tumors were identified after chronic exposures to this irritant (Morgan et al. 1986). The formaldehyde-induced squamous metaplasia of respiratory epithelium of the rat was not considered to be a preneoplastic lesion unless it was accompanied by dysplastic lesions (e.g., excess keratin production, cellular atypia, disrupted tissue organization).

Studies investigating formaldehyde-induced toxicity (Chang et al. 1983; Swenberg et al. 1986; Monticello et al. 1991) have shown that increases in cell proliferation occur following acute exposure, and that alterations in cell proliferation are sensitive indicators for formaldehyde-induced toxic insults. Formaldehyde-induced nasal carcinogenesis is probably related to these increases in cell proliferation which presumably result from formaldehyde-induced cytotoxicity (Swenberg et al. 1983) and attempts to repair.

Inflammation is also consistently observed in the nasal passages of rats exposed to cytotoxic or carcinogenic concentrations of formaldehyde gas. This inflammation ranges from minimal neutrophilic infiltration to severe rhinitis with purulent exudate. Harkema et al. (1988) demonstrated that transepithelial migration of neutrophils, a response commonly seen following exposure to formaldehyde, elicited a transient depletion of stored mucosubstances in nasal respiratory epithelium. It is conceivable that intraepithelial degranulation of neutrophils may also induce other epithelial responses, such as local cytotoxicity and the associated squamous metaplasia.

Hotchkiss et al. (1995) have examined the effect of mainstream cigarette smoke on the dorsal, middle, and ventral regions of the proximal nasal septum of rats exposed for 2 weeks (6 h/day) to 250 mg/m$^3$ of smoke. Interestingly, these investigators found that the character and severity of the alterations in the respiratory epithelium are dependent on the septal region examined. The cigarette smoke exposure induced a mucous cell hyperplasia with an increase in intraepithelial mucosubstances in the dorsal aspect of the septum and squamous cell metaplasia with a loss of intraepithelial mucosubstances in the respiratory epithelium of the midseptum. There was no histological alteration to the respiratory epithelium lining the ventral septum. Cigarette smoke exposure also caused a marked increase in DNA synthesis in the respiratory epithelium of the midseptum, a moderate increase in DNA synthesis in the respiratory epithelium of the ventral septum but no changes in DNA synthesis in the dorsal septum. Although this study was not specifically designed to determine the basis for the observed dorsoventral variation in response of the respiratory epithelium to cigarette smoke, Hotchkiss et al. (1995) presented some plausible explanations for this regional variability in response.

These investigators considered the regional differences in nasal airflow (Kimbell et al. 1993) and regional respiratory epithelial morphology, and interpreted the results of their study as follows: The dorsal septal region experiences the lowest airflow and thus receives the smallest total dose of cigarette smoke. The induced injury/irritation results in locally increased expression of airway mucins that are sufficient to protect the epithelium from further injury and subsequent increase in DNA synthesis and cell proliferation. The ventral septal epithelium receives a greater dose of cigarette smoke due to higher regional airflow patterns but also has significantly more intraepithelial mucosubstances prior to cigarette smoke exposure. The induced increase in DNA synthesis suggested that cigarette smoke-exposure results in injury to a sensitive cell population; however, the dose of cigarette smoke to this region was insufficient to alter the mucociliary phenotype of the epithelium. The midseptum was subjected to the highest airflow and the highest dose of cigarette smoke. They hypothesized that cigarette smoke induced toxicity in this region results in significant respiratory epithelial cell injury, death, and exfoliation, early in the 2-week exposure period. The normal mucociliary respiratory epithelium in this region of the nasal septum is replaced by a squamous epithelium (i.e., squamous metaplasia). The squamous epithelial cells may have been more resistant to cigarette smoke injury than respiratory epithelial cells, or the rate of cell proliferation may be sufficient to replace cells killed by cigarette smoke exposure at the luminal surface. In summary, the variability in type and magnitude of the epithelial results in the different regions of the rat septum may have reflected both site-specific differences in the dose of cigarette smoke associated toxicants delivered to the respiratory epithelium, due to intranasal airflow patterns, and regional differences in the susceptibility of this epithelium to cigarette smoke induced cytotoxicity. The results of this study underscore the necessity for consistent, systematic sampling of the nasal cavity when evaluating the toxicity of inhaled materials and the pathogenesis of toxicant-induced nasal lesions.

## Distribution of Nasal Lesions induced by Inhaled Chemicals

As illustrated above, knowledge of lesion distribution in the nose can provide insight into the relative roles played by regional tissue dose and local tissue susceptibility in toxic responses to xenobiotics. Site specificity of nasal lesions has been reported for the major epithelial types in the nose, including the nonolfactory regions (squamous, transitional, and respiratory epithelium). Therefore it is important to have a consistent approach for recording lesion distribution patterns in the complex nasal airways of rats and mice. Mery et al. (1994) have recently published a series of diagrams of the nasal passages of the F344 rat and the B6C3F1 mouse, designed for mapping nasal lesions.

Lesion distribution in the nose may be attributed to local dose, regional tissue susceptibility, or a combination of these factors (Morgan 1994). Mery et al. (1994) recorded the distribution of chemical-induced nasal lesions from previously reported studies on both transverse and longitudinal diagrams of the nose. These lesions were selected because they occur in diverse regions of the nose, have characteristic patterns of distribution, and exhibit clear concentration-response relationships. They concluded that some irritants, such as formaldehyde, induce lesions in the major inspiratory airways of the nose, especially in the nasal vestibule, and in the proximal regions of the lateral and middle medial meatuses, and in the dorsal medial meatus. This characteristic pattern is attributed to airflow-driven deposition. Similar factors could account for the proximal-distal severity gradient of nasal lesions induced by many inhaled sensory irritants (Buckley et al. 1984). The pattern of epithelial lesion distribution induced by other xenobiotics, such as ozone or chlorine, suggests that tissue or cellular susceptibility in addition to air flow are important in the pathogenesis of the specific lesions caused by these irritating, oxidant gases.

Although there is often a decrease in severity of irritant-induced nasal lesions from proximal to distal aspects of the nose, this does not exclude the possibility of irritant-induced lesions in the more distal pulmonary airways. Harkema et al. (1993) have demonstrated that ozone-induced lesions of nearly equal severity are evident in both the proximal nasal cavity and the terminal and respiratory bronchioles of bonnet monkeys. Interestingly, Monticello et al. (1989) demonstrated that the same formaldehyde exposure regime (6 ppm for 5 days/week for 1 or 6 weeks), which induced lesions only in the nasal cavity in rats, caused lesions in the nasal cavity, larynx, trachea, and carina of monkeys. Based on these results they suggested that the monkey is more sensitive than the rat to the acute and subacute effects of formaldehyde. The difference in the distribution of the lesions in the respiratory tract between the two species may have been related to physiological differences. For instance, rats are obligate nose breathers while monkeys are oronasal breathers.

## Summary

In this chapter we provide examples of the proliferative and metaplastic responses of the nonolfactory nasal epithelia to various inhaled xenobiotics. Because of the proximal location of the nose in the respiratory tract its surface epithelia are susceptible to injury to inhaled chemicals. The character, severity, and distribution of these induced lesions may be dependent on the nature of the toxicant, the regional cell or tissue susceptibility, the local dose of the xenobiotic to the epithelial cells or a combination of these factors. In addition, the type of animal species exposed may determine the character and distribution of the toxicant-induced epithelial injury in the nasal passages. Although the squamous epithelium in the nasal vestibule is often less vulnerable to chemical-induced injury than the more distal epithelia, certain caustic agents can induce ulcerative or hyperplastic lesions in this epithelium. The transitional epithelium lining the lateral meatus in rats and mice is often altered by inhaled irritants and can undergo adaptive responses that include mucous cell metaplasia (ozone) or squamous cell metaplasia (cigarette smoke, formaldehyde) depending on the inhaled toxicant. Several inhaled toxicants (e.g., cigarette smoke, formaldehyde, ozone) cause loss or attenuation of the surface cilia in the respiratory epithelium after acute exposures. The nasal respiratory epithelium can also be replaced by squamous epithelium (i.e., squamous metaplasia) after long-term exposures to inhaled irritants such as formaldehyde or cigarette smoke. Because chemical-induced lesions in the nasal passages of laboratory animals are usually site-specific, it is important that a systematic and thorough examination and recording of the proximal to distal aspects of the nose be made for each animal. Diagrams of transverse sections of the nose are useful in recording these lesions. Knowledge of the patterns of lesion distribution can provide insight into the relative roles played by regional tissue dose and local tissue susceptibility in the pathogenesis of nasal lesions. This information will assist in the assessment of a nasal toxicant's potential risk to human health.

## References

Boorman GA, Morgan KT, Uraih LC (1990) Nose, larynx, and trachea. In: Boorman GA, Eustis SL, Elwell MR, Montgomery CA, Mackenzie WF (eds) Pathology of the Fischer 344 rat. Academic, San Diego, pp 315–337

Bolon B, Bonnefoi MS, Roberts KC, Marshall MW, Morgan KT (1991) Toxic interactions in the rat nose: pollutants from soiled bedding and methyl bromide. Toxicol Pathol 19:571–579

Brain JD (1970) The uptake of inhaled gases by the nose. Ann Otol Rhinol Laryngol 79:529–539

Buckley LA, Jiang XZ, James RA, Morgan KT, Barrow CS (1984) Respiratory tract lesions induced by sensory irritants at the RD50 concentration. Toxicol Appl Pharmacol 74:417–429

Buckley LA, Morgan KT, Swenberg JA, James RA, Hamm TEJ, Barrow CS (1985) The toxicity of dimethylamine in F-344 rats and B6C3F1 mice following a 1 year inhalation exposure. Fundam Appl Toxicol 5:341–352

Chang JCF, Gross EA, Swenberg JA, Barrow CS (1983) Nasal cavity deposition, histopathology and cell proliferation after single or repeated formaldehyde exposure in B6C3F1 mice and F344 rats. Toxicol Appl Pharmacol 68:161–176

Cross CE, Halliwell B, Allen A (1984) Antioxidant protection: a function of tracheobronchial and gastrointestinal mucus. Lancet 1:1328–1330

DeSesso JM (1993) The relevance to humans of animal models for inhalation studies of cancer in the nose and upper airways. Qual Assur 2:213–231

Gross EA, Mellick PW, Kari FW, Miller FJ, Morgan KT (1994) Histopathology and cell replication responses in the respiratory tract of rats and mice exposed by inhalation to glutaraldehyde for up to thirteen weeks. Fundam Appl Toxicol 23:348–362

Harkema JR (1991) Comparative aspects of nasal airway anatomy: relevance to inhalation toxicology. Toxicol Pathol 19:321–336

Harkema JR, Hotchkiss JA (1994) Ozone-induced proliferative and metaplastic lesions in nasal transitional and respiratory epithelium: comparative pathology. Inhal Toxicol 6:187–204

Harkema JR, Plopper CG, Hyde DM, St George JA, Wilson DW, Dungworth DL (1987a) Response of the macaque nasal epithelium to ambient levels of ozone. A morphologic and morphometric study of the transitional and respiratory epithelium. Am J Pathol 128:29–44

Harkema JR, Plopper CG, Hyde DM, St George JA, Dungworth DL (1987b) Effects of an ambient level of ozone on primate nasal epithelial mucosubstances. Quantitative histochemistry. Am J Pathol 127:90–96

Harkema JR, Hotchkiss JA, Harmsen AG, Henderson RF (1988) In vivo effects of transient neutrophil influx on nasal respiratory epithelial mucosubstances. Am J Pathol 130:605–615

Harkema JR, Hotchkiss JR, Henderson RF (1989) Effects of 0.12 and 0.80 ppm ozone on rat nasal and nasopharyngeal epithelial mucosubstances: quantitative histochemistry. Toxicol Pathol 17:525–535

Harkema JR, Bermudez EG, Morgan KT, Mellick PW (1992) Effects of chronic ozone exposure on the nasal mucociliary apparatus in the rat. Am Rev Respir Dis 145:A98

Harkema JR, Plopper CG, Hyde DM, St. George JA, Wilson DW, Dungworth DL (1993) Respose of macaque bronchiolar epithelium to ambient concentrations of ozone. Am J Pathol 143:857–866

Harkema JR, Morgan Kt, Gross EA, Catalano PJ, Griffith WC (1994) Consequences of prolonged inhalation of ozone on F344/N rats: collaborative studies. VII. Effects on the nasal mucocilliary apparatus. Capital City, Montpelier (Health Effects Institute report 65)

Hotchkiss JA, Harkema JR (1992) Endotoxin or cytokins attenuate ozone-induced DNA synthesis in rat transitional epithelium. Toxicol Appl Pharmacol 114:182–187

Hotchkiss JA, Harkema JR, Sun JD, Henderson RF (1989) Comparison of acute ozone-induced nasal and pulmonary inflammatory responses in rats. Toxicol Appl Pharmacol 98:289–302

Hotchkiss JA, Kimbell JS, Herrera LK, Hatch GE, Morgan KT, Harkema JR (1994) Regional differences in ozone-induced nasal epithelial cell proliferation in F344 rats: comparison with computational mass flux predictions of ozone dosimetry. Inhal Toxicol 6:440–443

Hotchkiss JA, Evans WA, Chen BT, Finch GL, Harkema JR (1995) Regional differences in the effects of mainstream cigarette smoke on stored mucosubstances and DNA synthesis in F344 rat nasal respiratory epithelium. Toxicol Appl Pharmacol 131:316–324

Jiang XZ, Buckley LA, Morgan KT (1983) Histopathology of toxic responses to chlorine gas in the nasal passages of rats and mice. Toxicol Appl Pharmacol 71:225–236

Jiang XZ, Morgan KT, Beauchamp RO (1986) Histopathology of acute and subacute nasal toxicity. In: CS Barrow (ed) Toxicology of the nasal passages. Hemisphere, Washington, pp 51–66

Johnson NF, Hotchkiss JR, Harkema JA, Henderson RF (1990) Proliferative responses of rat nasal epithelia to ozone. Toxicol Appl Pharmacol 103:143–155

Kimbell JS, Gross EA, Joyner DR, Godo MN, Morgan KT (1993) Application of computational fluid dynamics to regional dosimetry of inhaled chemicals in the upper respiratory tract of the rat. Toxicol Appl Pharmacol 121:253–263

Maples KR, Harkema JR, Nikula KJ, Chen BT, Finch GL, Griffith WC Jr (1993) Effects of cigarette smoke on the glutathione status of the upper and lower respiratory tract of rats. Inhal Toxicol 5:389–401

Mery S, Gross EA, Joyner DR, Godo M, Morgan KT (1994) Nasal diagrams: a tool for recording the distribution of nasal lesions in rats and mice. Toxicol Pathol 22:353–372

Monticello TM, Morgan KT (1994) Nasal lesion distribution and toxicity in the squamous epithelial region. Inhal Toxicol 6:177–186

Monticello TM, Morgan KT, Everitt JI, Popp JA (1989) Effects of formaldehyde gas on the respiratory tract of rhesus monkeys: pathology and cell proliferation. Am J Pathol 134:515–527

Monticello TM, Morgan KT, Uraih L (1990) Nonneoplastic nasal lesions in rats and mice. Environ Health Perspect 85:249–274

Monticello TM, Miller FJ, Morgan KT (1991) Regional increases in rat nasal respiratory epithelial cell proliferation following acute and subchronic inhalation of formaldehyde. Toxicol Appl Pharmacol 111:409–421

Morgan KT (1994) Nasal dosimetry, lesion distribution, and the toxicologic pathologist: a brief review. Inhal Toxicol 6:41–57

Morgan KT, Jiang XZ, Starr TB, Kerns WD (1986) More precise localization of nasal tumors associated with chronic exposure of F-344 rats to formaldehyde gas. Toxicol Appl Pharmacol 82:264–271

Negus VE (ed) (1958) The comparative anatomy and physiology of the nose and paranasal sinuses. Livingstone, Edinburgh

Sills RC, Morgan KT, Boorman GA (1994) Accessory nasal structures in toxicology studies. Inhal Toxicol 6:221–248

St Clair MBG, Morgan KT (1992) Age-related changes in the upper respiratory tract of the rat. In: Mohr U, Dungworth DL, Capen CC (eds) Pathobiology of the aging rat. ILSI, Washington, pp 111–127

Swenberg JA, Barrow CS, Boreiko CJ, Heck HD, Levine RJ, Morgan KT, Starr TB (1983) Non-linear biological responses to formaldehyde and their implications for carcinogenic risk assessment. Carcinogenesis 4:945–952

Swenberg JA, Gross EA, Randall HW (1986) Localization and quantitation of cell proliferation following exposure to nasal irritants. In: Barrow CS (ed) Toxicology of the nasal passages. Hemisphere, Washington, pp 291–298

Walker D (1983) Histopathology of the nasal cavity in laboratory animals exposed to cigarette smoke and other irritants. In: Reznik G, Stinson SF (eds) Nasal tumors in animals and man. vol III. CRC, Boca Raton, pp 115–135

Wolf DC, Morgan KT, Gross EA, Barrow C, Moss OR, James RA, Popp JA (1995) Two-year inhalation exposure of female and male B6C3F1 mice and F344 rats to chlorine gas induces lesions confined to the nose. Fundam Appl Toxicol 24:111–131

# Nonneoplastic Lesions of the Olfactory Mucosa

Kevin T. Morgan and Jack R. Harkema

## Introduction

In recent years there has been a considerable increase in the number of reports on the histopathology of nasal olfactory mucosal responses to inhaled and parenterally administered chemicals (Bogdanffy 1990; Doty et al. 1991; Gaskell 1990; Mery et al. 1994a; Morgan and Monticello 1989). There has also been a concomitant increase in understanding of olfaction (Serby and Chobar 1992), including its role in such functions as memory and reproduction (Halász 1990). In toxicology, recent interest has focused on the role of olfactory mucosal metabolism in toxic processes in this target site (Bogdanffy 1990; Dahl and Hadley 1991; Reed 1993). Interest in the olfactory mucosa has also been spurred by the observations that inhaled materials may enter the central nervous system via the olfactory nerves (Hastings and Evans 1991), and early changes in the sense of smell are a feature of Alzheimer's disease in humans (Mann and Esiri 1988). Lesions in the olfactory bulb of the brain have been observed in association with olfactory mucosal destruction in laboratory animals (Genter et al. 1992), highlighting the close anatomical association between the brain and this region of the nose (Fig. 15). The neural nature of the olfactory mucosa, and its unique histological structure, combined with characteristic artifacts and toxic responses, justifies a separate description of the toxicology of this region of the nasal airway lining.

In addition to the olfactory mucosa, two other chemosensory structures in nose have olfactory or "olfactorylike" activity: the septal olfactory organ and the vomeronasal organ. The septal olfactory organ is histologically identical to other regions of the olfactory mucosa with which it is considered below. The vomeronasal organ is histologically and functionally distinct (Uraih and Maronpot 1990; Vaccarezza et al. 1981), but it has some similarities with the olfactory mucosa and is briefly addressed. This chapter focuses on rats, the species for which the most extensive data base is available, but the basic principles described apply to most mammalian species used in toxicology studies, including mice and hamsters, for which less information is available. The normal structure and function of the olfactory mucosa, septal olfactory organ, and vomeronasal organ have been reported extensively (Eccles et al. 1987; Greene 1963; Gross and Morgan 1992; Hebel and Stromberg 1986; Kuper et al. 1989; Negus 1958; Proctor and Chang 1983; Uraih and Maronpot 1990) and are addressed in a companion chapter (Harkema and Morgan, this volume; see p. 3).

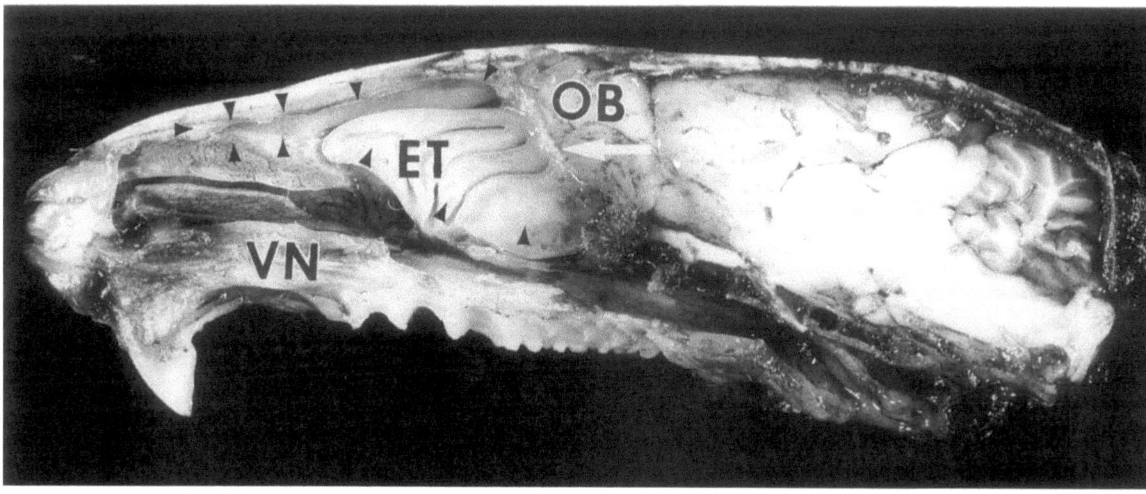


**Fig. 15.** Head of a F344 rat opened adjacent to the midline with the septum removed to show the limits of the olfactory mucosa (*arrowhead*), the ethmoid turbinates (*ET*), cribriform plate (*white arrow*), olfactory bulb (*OB*), and vomeronasal organ (*VN*) in a remnant of the ventral nasal septum. The olfactory mucosa in this young rat is pale yellowish green, but it becomes much more darkly pigmented with increasing age. ×6

## Clinical and Gross Pathology

Defective vision or hearing may be more readily apparent in humans than is a deficiency of the sense of smell, which could account, at least in part, for the relative paucity of data on olfactory function in rodent toxicology studies. A range of tests is available for the assessment of olfactory dysfunction (dysosmia) in human and nonhuman animals (Amoore 1986; Getchell et al. 1991; Halász 1990; Serby and Chobar 1992). A simple but time-consuming approach, the buried food pellet test, has been successfully applied in studies of olfactory function in rats exposed to methyl bromide (Hurtt et al. 1988). The latter study revealed treatment-induced loss of olfactory function associated with extensive olfactory epithelial damage. However, methyl bromide is also a neurotoxin, inducing severe damage to the central nervous system, with the potential for inability to find a pellet being attributable to defective function of the central nervous system. More complex procedures have been developed that can discriminate between olfactory deficits of nasal mucosal or central neural origin (Peele et al. 1990; Youngentob et al. 1991). These techniques, which are not generally available for routine toxicology studies, provided the first indication of an olfactory deficit induced by β,β′-iminodipropionitrile (IDPN; Genter et al. 1992). For further details of approaches to the study of olfactory function, see Getchell et al. (1991).

In routine toxicology studies less direct clinical evidence for lesions in the olfactory system include large masses that may be observed externally or may result in occlusion of the nasolachrymal duct, with subsequent chromodachryorhea (Morgan 1991). In the absence of post mortem nasal dissection, which is generally not advisable due to its effect on histological lesions, gross lesions in the olfactory region of the nose are most readily detected during tissue trimming following decalcification.

## Microscopic Features

Adequate characterization of olfactory mucosal histopathology requires (a) knowledge of the normal structure and physiology of the nose, (b) understanding of the anatomy of this region (Mery et al. 1994a; Negus 1958; Reznik 1983), and, (c) familiarity with fixation and other histological artifacts of the olfactory mucosa (Uraih and Maronpot 1990). The pathology narrative should ideally incorporate details of target cell populations, lesion progression and recovery, adaptive modifications of the mucosa, and lesion distribution (Mery et al. 1994a; Morgan 1991). This approach facilitates determination of the relative roles of regional dosimetry and tissue susceptibility in site specificity of lesions, provides indications of potential mechanisms of action, and permits more meaningful interspecies extrapolations.

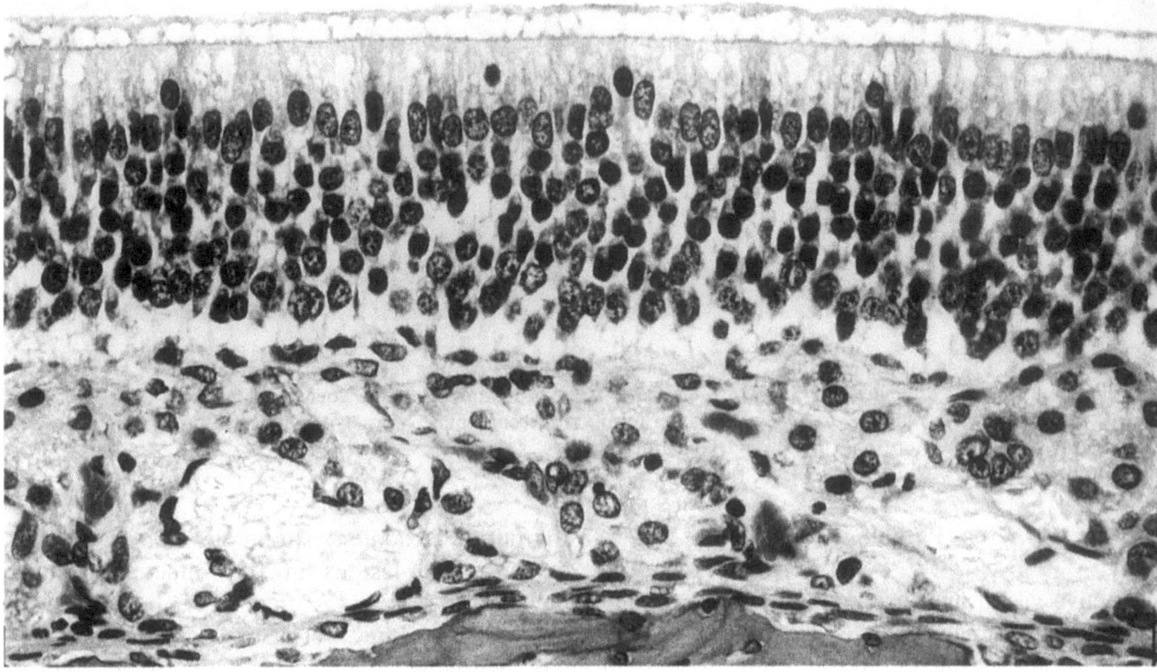

**Fig. 16.** Olfactory mucosa of a F344 rat, fixed by intra-airway infusion of neutral buffered formalin, to show the normal architecture of the epithelium and lamina propria. Note normal layers of sustentacular cell apical cytoplasm and sustentacular cell nuclei near the airway lumen, a central zone of variably mature sensory cells, immature sensory cells with larger nuclei, and artifactual vacuolation near the basement membrane due to postmortem swelling of sustentacular cell basal cytoplasm. H&E, ×560

*Olfactory Mucosal Artifacts.* The olfactory mucosa is prone to a range of fixation artifacts, including increased intercellular space and cellular shrinkage. Severe epithelial condensation, which may obscure most cellular details, has been observed with certain glutaraldehyde-based fixatives administered by airway or vascular routes. Even well-prepared olfactory mucosa exhibits variable degrees of swelling and vacuolation adjacent to the basal layer and in the olfactory nerves (Fig. 16). This vacuolation may be a consequence of the tendency of basal foot processes of sustentacular cells and olfactory neural Schwann's cells to swell after death. Perfusion fixation does not necessarily eliminate all of these problems, as vascular perfusion with neutral buffered formalin has been associated with considerable distortion of the sensory cell nuclei (Fig. 17) in studies of methyl bromide toxicity in rats (Hurtt et al. 1987). In our experience the best fixatives for light and electron microscopy are intranasally instilled neutral buffered formalin and intravascular perfusion of Fowler's fixative (Uraih and Maronpot 1990), respectively. Adequate examination of controls, identically fixed and processed, should minimize confusion of artifacts with treatment-induced olfactory lesions (Figs. 18, 19).

*Aging and Other Background Lesions.* A range of aging-associated changes occurs in the nasal passages of rats, and a number of these responses

▶

**Fig. 17.** (*above*) Olfactory mucosa of an untreated, young control rat from studies by Hurtt et al. (1988). Perfusion fixation with neutral buffered formalin results in considerable distortion of sensory cell nuclei. H&E, ×560

**Fig. 18.** (*below*) Dorsal scroll of the 2′-ectoturbinate of a F344 rat to show normal structure. Note clear airway lumen, even pattern of olfactory epithelium and underlying olfactory nerve bundles, and delicate compact bone supporting this turbinate scroll. H&E, ×140

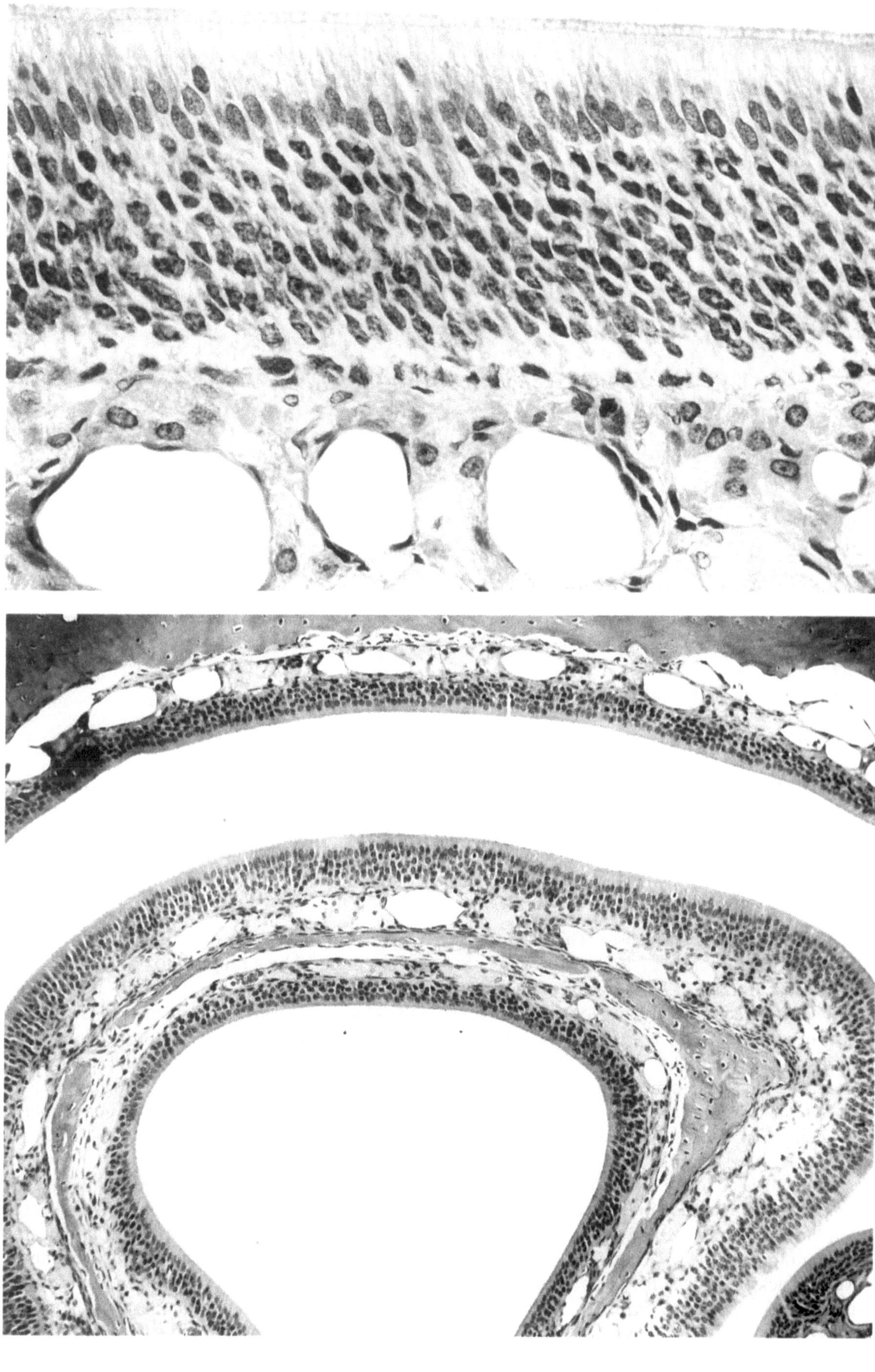

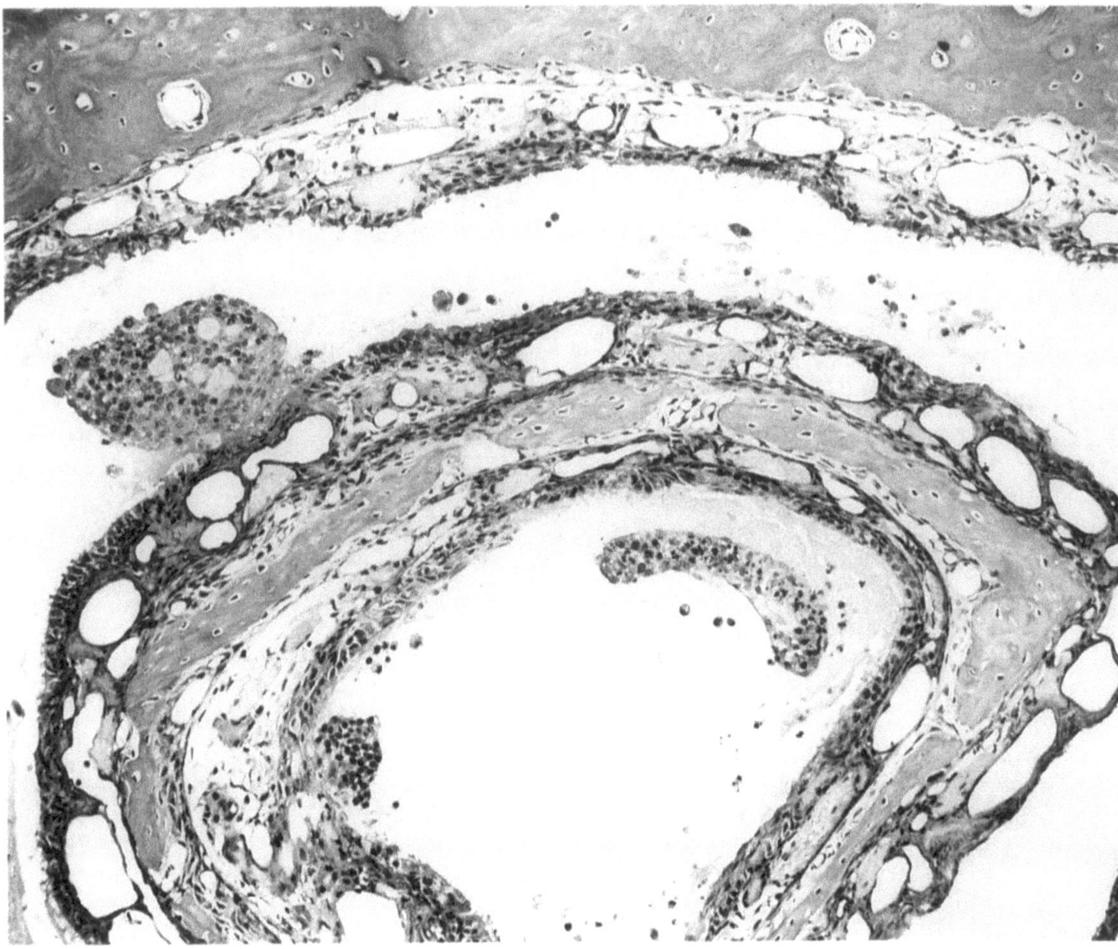

**Fig. 19.** Dorsal scroll of the 2′-ectoturbinate of a F344 rat following several days exposure to methyl bromide vapor (Hurtt et al. 1988). There is extensive loss of olfactory sensory cells and olfactory nerve bundles, with thickening of the ethmoid bone, and cellular debris with serous exudate in the nasal lumen. Note foci of basement membrane mineralization in the dorsal wall. This lesion is commonly seen in control animals; it increases in frequency with age and following exposure to a range of nasal irritants. H&E, ×140

involve the olfactory mucosa. These changes, which were the subject of a recent review (St. Clair and Morgan 1992), include increased amounts of olfactory pigment, loss of olfactory mucosa in specific regions of the nose, mineralization of the epithelial basement membrane (Fig. 19), increased amounts of eosinophilic intracellular deposits (Fig. 20), and focal respiratory metaplasia. Olfactory mucosal damage may also occur in association with inflammatory or dysplastic changes of the molar teeth (Monticello et al. 1990), inflammation induced by foreign bodies in the nose, or as a response to environmental cage contaminants (Fig. 21; Bolon et al. 1991). Severe olfactory damage may also occur as a feature of infectious disease processes, such as respiratory mycoplasmosis.

*Treatment-Induced Lesions.* Olfactory mucosal lesions induced by a range of toxic chemicals have been reported in rats (Gaskell 1990), mice (Buckley et al. 1984), and hamsters (Feron and Kruysse 1978), but the most extensive data base is available for rats. Reports of nasal lesions vary in the detail provided, and systematic approaches are needed for the classification of nonneoplastic responses in this location.

*Distribution of Olfactory Mucosal Responses.* The olfactory mucosa of the rat, a macrosmatic creature (Negus 1958), has a complex anatomy that reflects the convoluted structure of the ethmoid turbinates of this species (Hebel and Stromberg 1986; Reznik 1983). This complexity may present a challenge when attempting to determine the

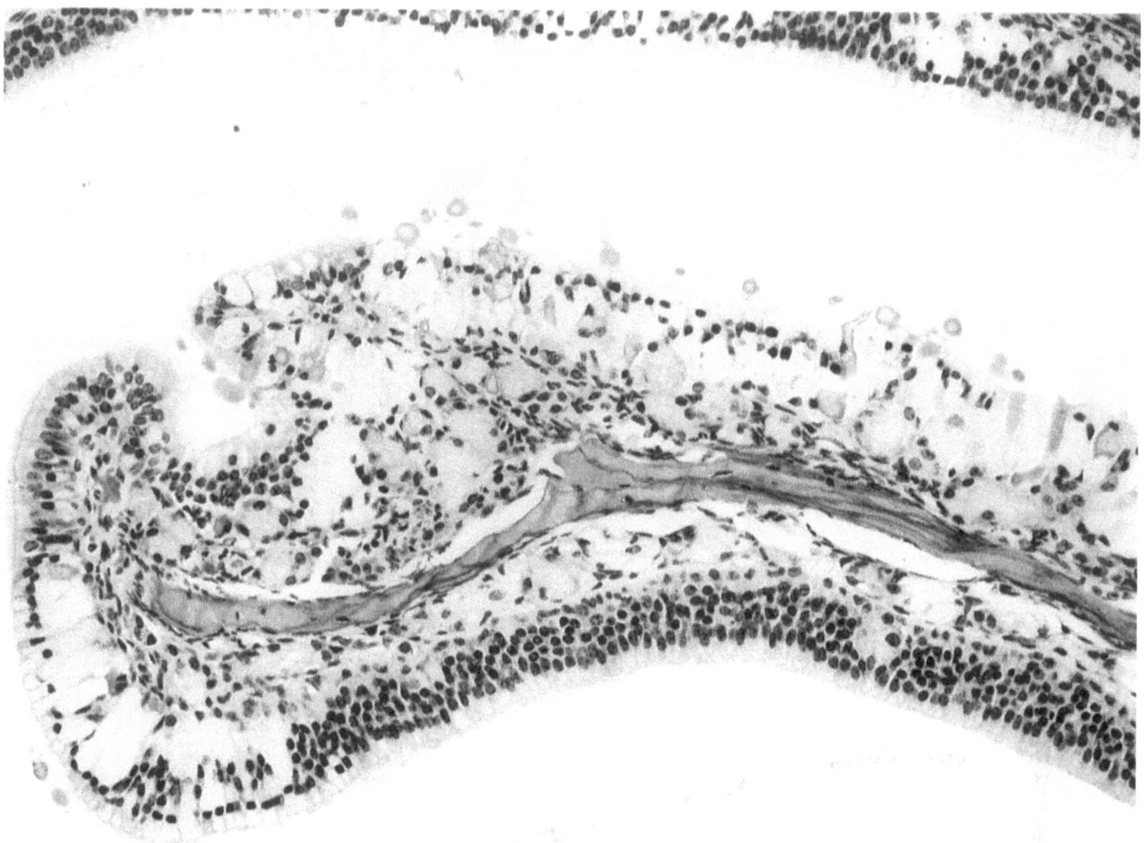

**Fig. 20.** Eosinophilic proteinaceous droplets filling cytoplasm of olfactory sustentacular cells in the lateral scroll of the first ectoturbinate. H&E, ×280

distribution pattern of olfactory mucosal lesions. If a single site is involved, which for many inhaled irritants (Buckley et al. 1984) is frequently the epithelial lining of the dorsal medial meatus (Morgan et al. 1991), this is a relatively simple task. However, certain materials induce more complex patterns of olfactory mucosal damage, whether exposure is by inhalation [e.g., 3-methyl furan (Morse et al. 1984), methyl isocyanate (Uraih et al. 1987), methyl bromide (Hurtt et al. 1988), dibasic esters (Lee et al. 1992), and chloroform (Mery et al. 1994b)] or by noninhalation routes [e.g., IDPN (Genter et al. 1992), 3-methyl indole (Peele et al. 1990), and a number of nitrosamines (Belinsky et al. 1987; Reznik-Schüller 1983)]. It may then be necessary to resort to the use of maps or diagrams of the nasal passages to record the distribution pattern of the lesions induced (Mery et al. 1994a). A number of basic patterns of nasal lesions have appeared during studies of olfactory mucosal lesions induced by chemical exposure (Fig. 22). These patterns are generally attributable to regional dosimetry of the material, local tissue metabolism, or other factors determining local tissue susceptibility (Mery et al. 1994a).

In addition to regional distribution of nasal lesions, specific patterns of damage may be apparent within the affected regions of the mucosa. For instance, IDPN induces degenerative changes in the olfactory epithelium and superficial Bowman's glands (Genter et al. 1992), while inhaled chloroform specifically targets the deep Bowman's glands and adjacent bones (Mery et al. 1994b), sparing the structures that are destroyed by IDPN. In contrast, dimethylamine (Buckley et al. 1985) and certain esters (Miller et al. 1984, 1985) induce loss of olfactory sensory cells. Ultrastructural

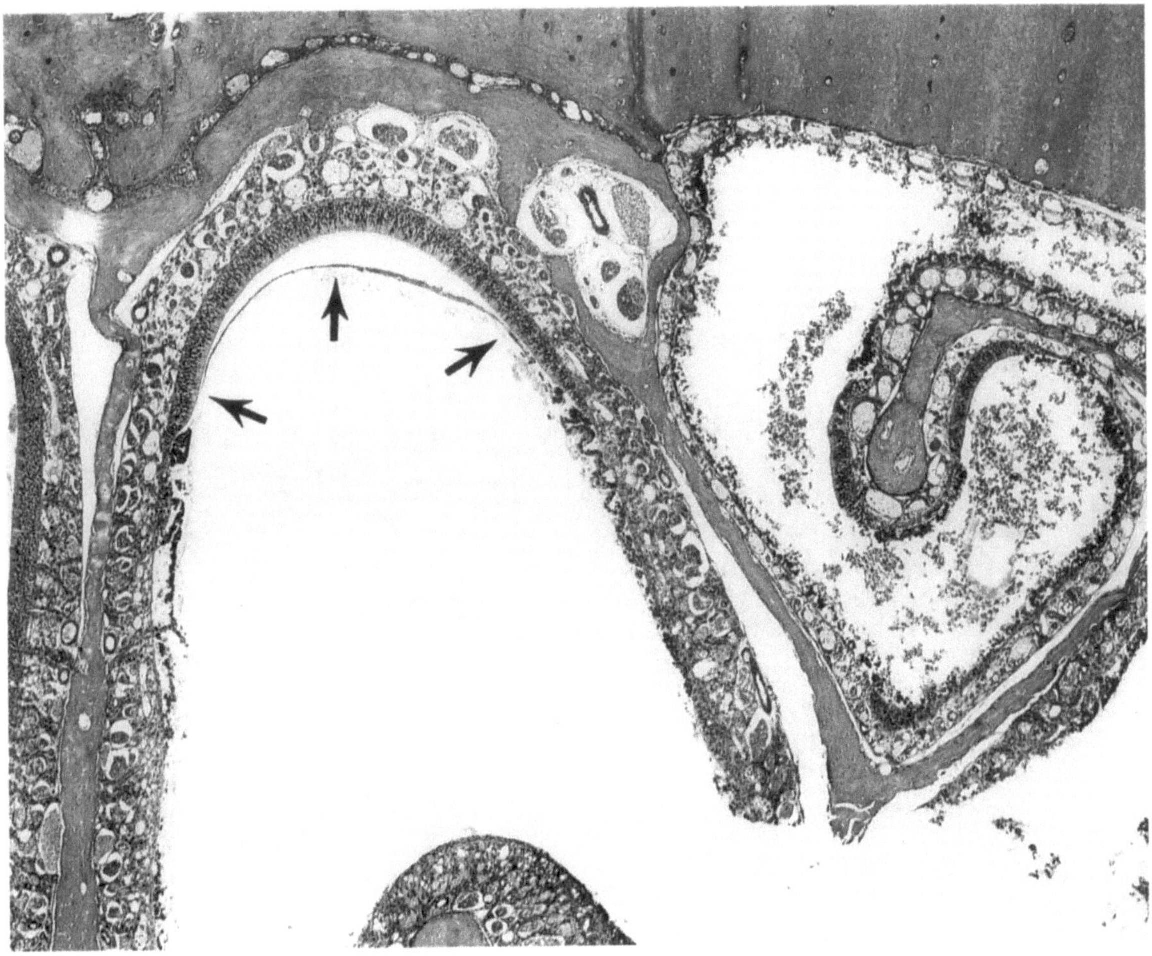

**Fig. 21.** Olfactory mucosa of a F344 rat exposed by inhalation to methyl bromide. Note extensive destruction of the olfactory mucosa of the septum and first ethmoid turbinate, while the olfactory epithelium lining the dorsal portion of the dorsal medial meatus is generally unaffected (*arrows*). This lesion pattern was attributed to concomitant effects of inhaled cage contaminants on the olfactory mucosa in this site (Bolon et al. 1991). H&E, ×70

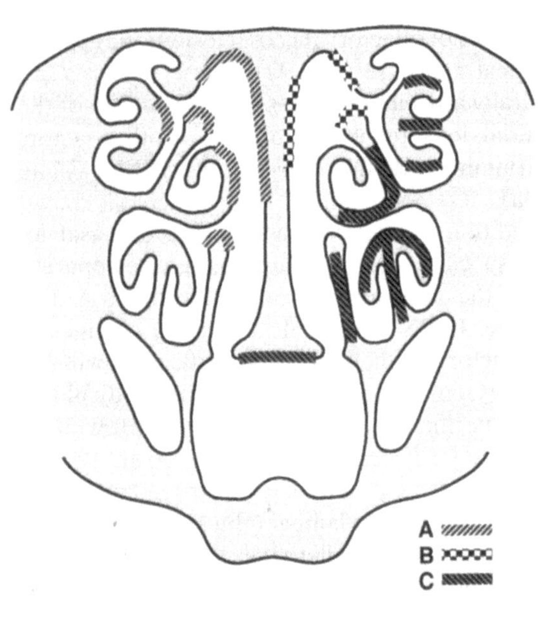


**Fig. 22.** Diagram developed for mapping of nasal lesions (Mery et al. 1994a) to show distribution of lesions induced by a number of olfactory mucosal toxicants. *A*, β, β′-iminodipropionitrile (*IDPN*; Genter et al. 1992); *B*, dibasic esters (Lee et al. 1992); *C*, chloroform (Mery et al. 1994b)

studies of nasal toxicity of the dibasic esters demonstrated that sensory cell loss may be secondary to a primary lesion of the olfactory sustentacular cell (Trela et al. 1992). The latter observation played a critical role in clarifying the role of cell type specific nasal esterases in toxic responses to these esters. Therefore a detailed description of lesion location in the nose, the cell types affected, and the sequence of events observed may each be of value when attempting to determine mechanisms responsible for these nasal lesions (Morgan 1994).

## Nature of Olfactory Mucosal Responses

It has been proposed that nonneoplastic olfactory mucosal lesions may be usefully classified as (a) degenerative, (b) inflammatory, (c) regenerative, (d) adaptive, and (e) proliferative (Morgan 1991). This approach is used below, but it should be remembered that not all responses fall neatly into such a scheme. Proliferative lesions of the olfactory mucosa are addressed separately in another chapter in this volume on nasal neoplasia (Morgan and Harkema).

*Degeneration.* Olfactory mucosal degeneration may be acute and dramatic or more subtle and slowly progressive. The first histological indication of exposure to an aggressive nasal toxicant may be extensive destruction of the olfactory epithelium (Fig. 23). A characteristic process has been observed by the authors for a number of such chemicals, including methyl bromide and IDPN, and is reported in the literature for certain herbicides (Brittebo et al. 1991; Fig. 23). During the acute phase of such a process the epithelium frequently

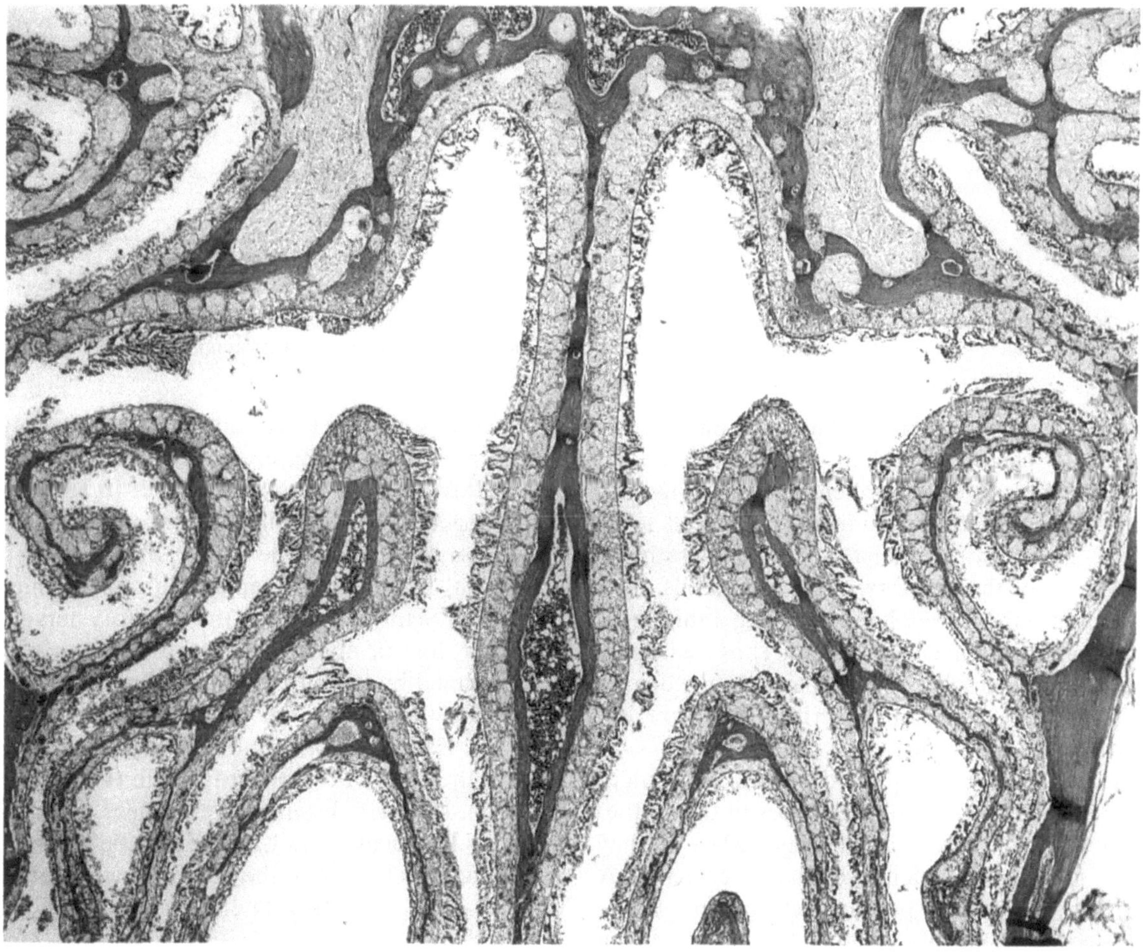

**Fig. 23.** Extensive destruction of the olfactory mucosa following i.p. administration of 300 mg/kg methimazole (an anti-hyperthyroid drug; kindly provided by Dr. Mary Beth Genter, North Carolina State University). H&E, ×28

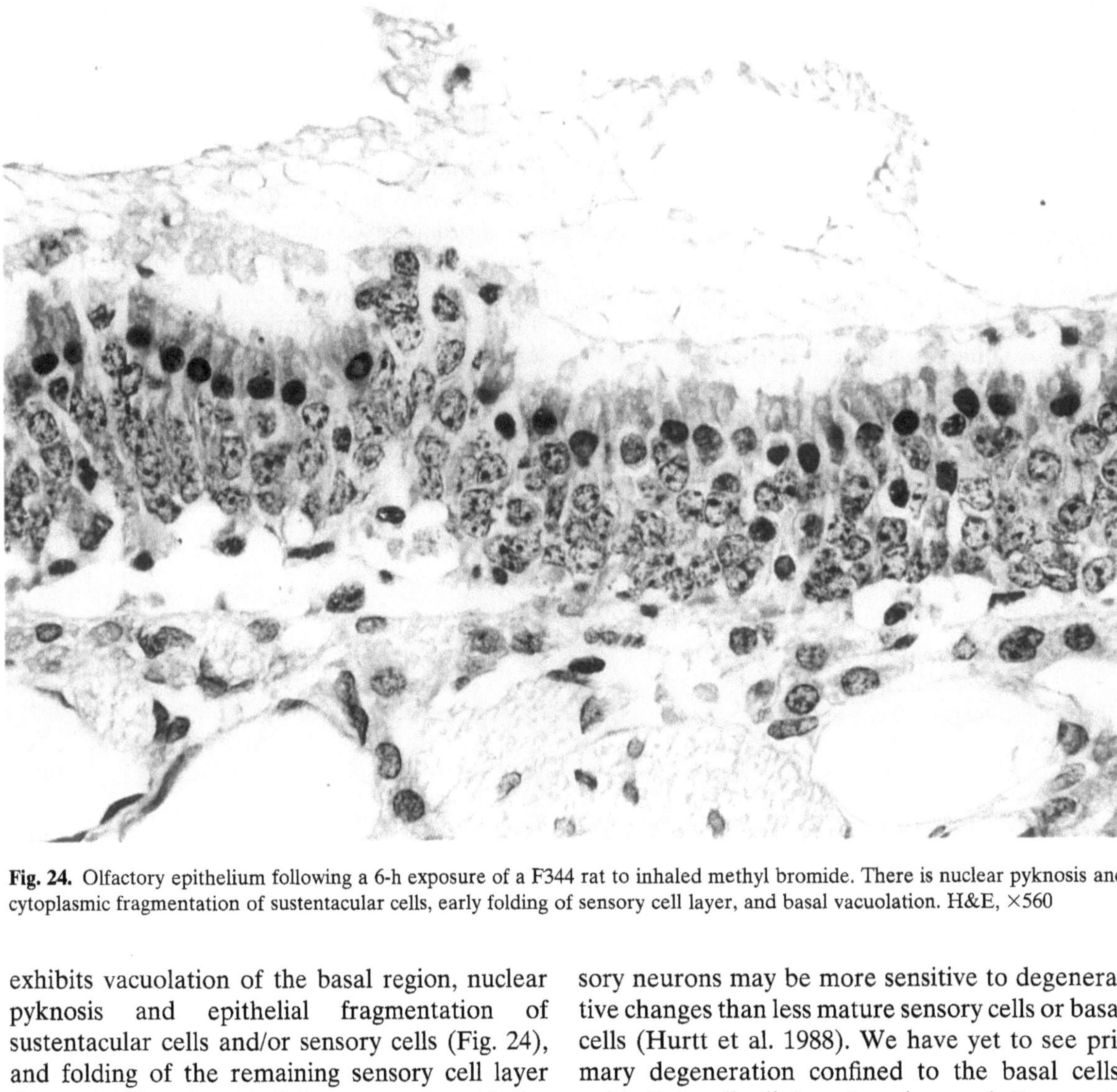

**Fig. 24.** Olfactory epithelium following a 6-h exposure of a F344 rat to inhaled methyl bromide. There is nuclear pyknosis and cytoplasmic fragmentation of sustentacular cells, early folding of sensory cell layer, and basal vacuolation. H&E, ×560

exhibits vacuolation of the basal region, nuclear pyknosis and epithelial fragmentation of sustentacular cells and/or sensory cells (Fig. 24), and folding of the remaining sensory cell layer (Figs. 24, 25). All epithelial components, with the exception of the majority of the basal cells, then slough into the airway lumen, leaving a thin layer of remaining basal cells (Fig. 26). These cells play a critical role in subsequent repair, and the degree of basal cell loss is probably critical during regeneration (see following).

For specific chemicals these degenerative changes may involve one or more cell types in the epithelium or lamina propria (Morgan 1994), or they may show no evident cellular specificity. A number of frequent primary cellular target sites include the epithelial sustentacular cells, epithelial sensory neurons, and the superficial and deep secretory cells of the Bowman's glands. Mature sensory neurons may be more sensitive to degenerative changes than less mature sensory cells or basal cells (Hurtt et al. 1988). We have yet to see primary degeneration confined to the basal cells, epithelial cells lining the ducts of Bowman's glands in the olfactory epithelium or lamina propria, or Schwann's cells of the olfactory nerves. However, loss of olfactory neurons is frequently accompanied by loss of the nonmyelinated axons of olfactory nerve bundles in the lamina propria (Fig. 21). Extensive loss of olfactory nerves is evident at the level of the olfactory bulb (Genter et al. 1992). If severe degenerative changes occur in the deep Bowman's glands, there may be an associated tissue response in the adjacent periosteum of the nasal turbinates or lateral nasal wall (Mery et al. 1994b).

Cell type specific or nonspecific degeneration or necrosis may be focal, multifocal, or diffuse, with a

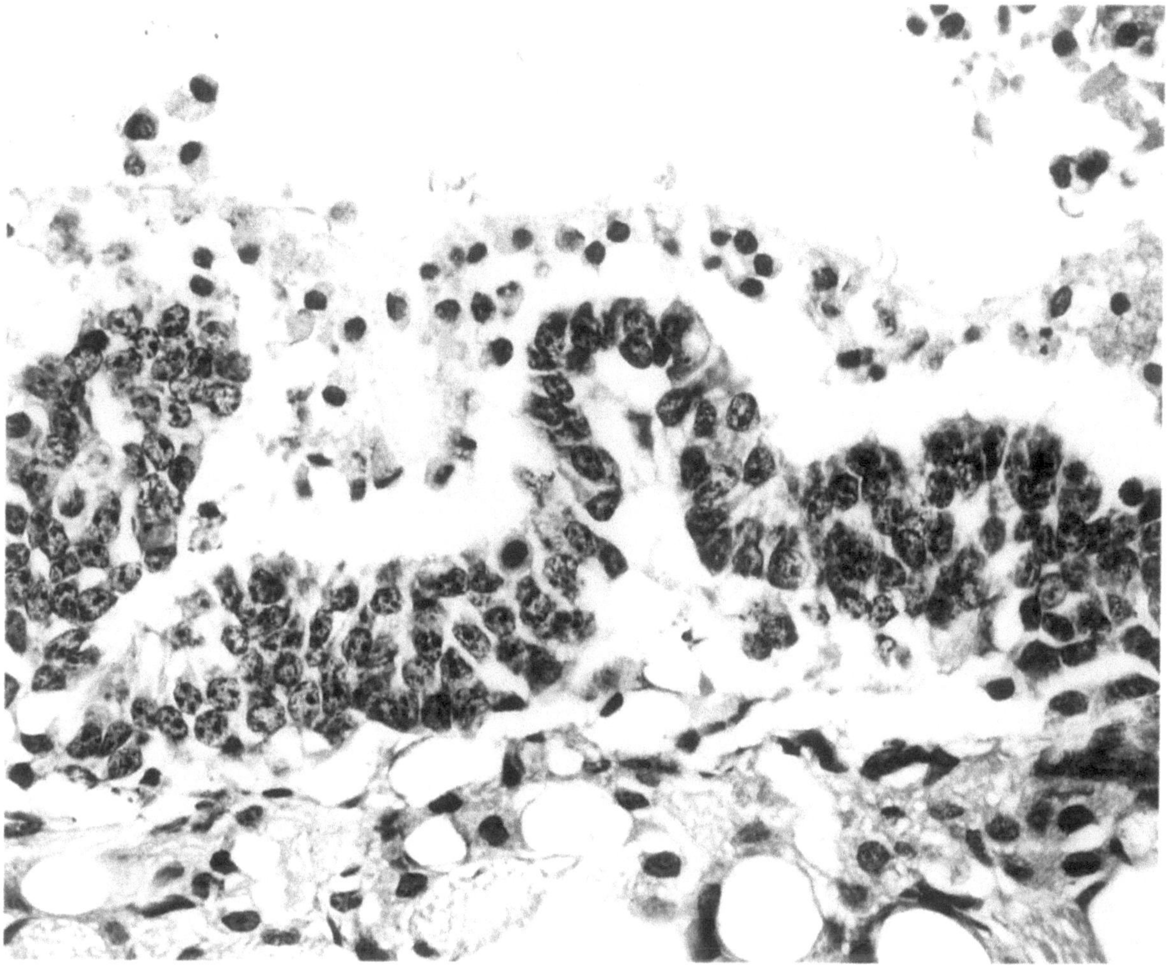

**Fig. 25.** Olfactory epithelium following a 6-h exposure of a F344 rat to inhaled methyl bromide. Olfactory degeneration with folding and fragmentation. Compare with Fig. 24. H&E, ×560

range of severity that extends to ulceration of the epithelium lining the airway. Degeneration of olfactory neurons may be associated with nuclear pyknosis, karyorrhexis, or apoptosis. The cytoplasm of sustentacular cells may exhibit coagulative necrosis with hyalinization and increased eosinophilia of the cytoplasm or cytoplasmic swelling and fragmentation. Bowman's glands are frequently a target for xenobiotics, and they may exhibit a range of degenerative changes, including extensive necrosis of ductular and acinar elements with coagulation or fragmentation of nuclei and cytoplasm. Olfactory nerves may also exhibit histological evidence of degeneration in the form of swelling of Schwann's cells, giving the nerve bundles a foamy appearance.

*Inflammation.* Olfactory epithelial degeneration frequently occurs in the absence of overt inflammatory changes (Hurtt et al. 1988). When inflammation is present, it may be suppurative, nonsuppurative, or mixed, with variable involvement of the epithelium and underlying lamina propria. In some cases inflammation is a prominent feature of the toxic response, being extensive and severe (Morse et al. 1984; Uraih et al. 1987), with an associated serous, serofibrinous, or cellular exudate filling the overlying airway. Complete occlusion of the ethmoid meatuses by inflammatory exudate and cellular debris may be associated with, and possibly account for, subsequent remodeling of this region of the nose observed following exposure to 3-methyl furan (Morse et al. 1984) and 3-methyl indole (Peele et al. 1990).

*Regeneration.* Following epithelial degeneration there may be rapid repair and a concomitant recovery of olfactory function. Histologically, regen-

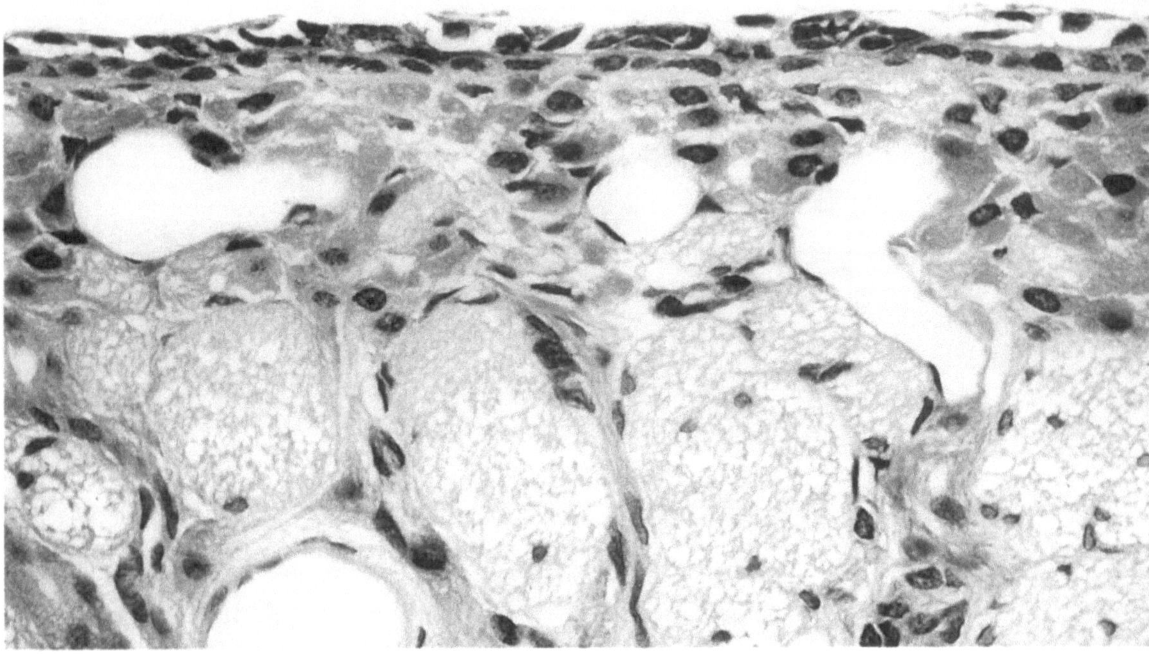

**Fig. 26.** Olfactory epithelium 48-h following a 6hr exposure of a F344 rat to inhaled methyl bromide. Only a thin layer of basal cells remains. H&E, ×560

eration of the olfactory epithelium may yield a complex and sometimes confusing pattern of changes as different regions of the mucosa reach different stages of the regenerative process. There is considerable variation in the morphology of this process, which has been described in detail by a number of workers (Cancalon 1982; Graziadei 1973; Hurtt et al. 1988). The rate of recovery depends, at least to some extent, on the degree of local damage, and severely affected regions may fail to return to normal, or exhibit modified histology (see following). Generally recovery is characterized by an initial phase of proliferation of residual basal cells that enlarge and develop increased amounts of basophilic cytoplasm and polyhedral outlines. Proliferating basal cells may accumulate at the margins of areas of complete epithelial denudation (Genter et al. 1992) and subsequently migrate to restore the epithelial barrier. Subsequent proliferation yields an increasingly thick layer of apparently randomly arranged cells, followed by gradual appearance of the olfactory epithelial features (Fig. 27), including a superficial zone of sustentacular cell apical cytoplasm with an underlying single layer of sustentacular cell nuclei, and a variably thick layer of sensory neuronal perikarya (one to ten cells deep) in varying stages of differentiation. The sensory cells during later stages of regeneration may be more numerous than normal, giving the regenerating epithelium a hypercellular appearance (Fig. 28). Finally, after a period of weeks to months the epithelium recovers its normal histological features, including

▶

**Fig. 27.** (*above*) Olfactory epithelium 4 weeks following a 6-h exposure of a F344 rat to inhaled methyl bromide. Considerable regeneration of olfactory epithelium which exhibits early stages of recovery of normal olfactory epithelial morphology. H&E, ×560

**Fig. 28.** (*below*) Olfactory epithelium 8 weeks following a 6-h exposure of a F344 rat to inhaled methyl bromide. Residual evidence of exposure to methyl bromide is confined to slight hypercellularity of the sensory cell layer. H&E, ×560

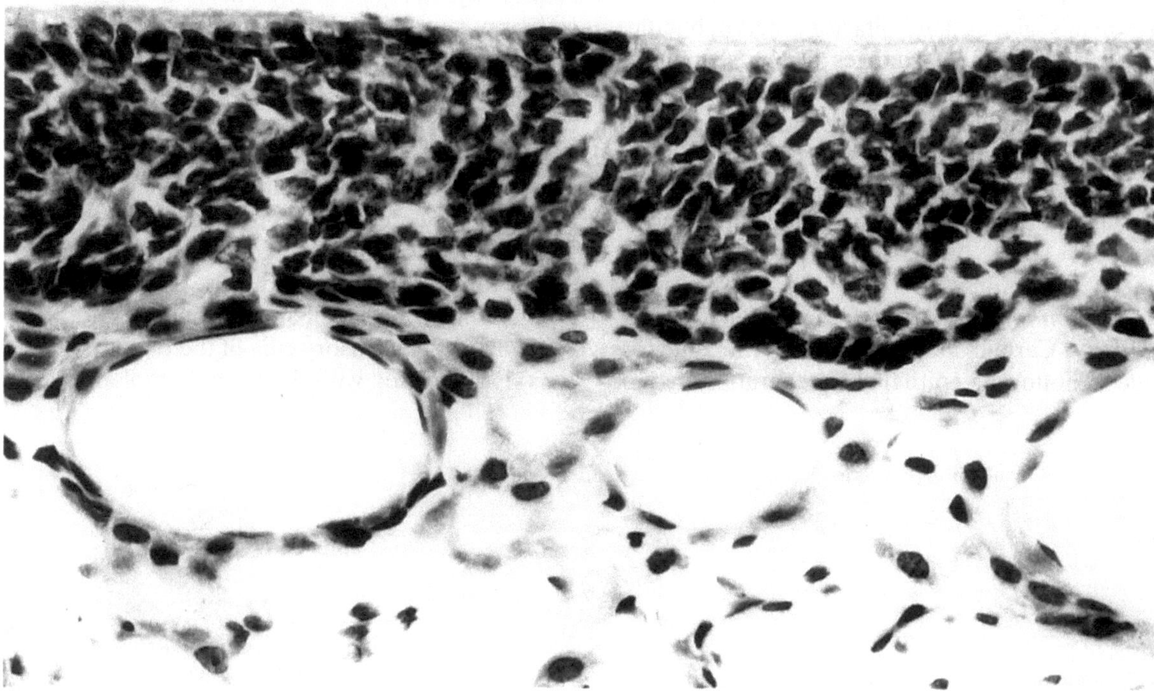

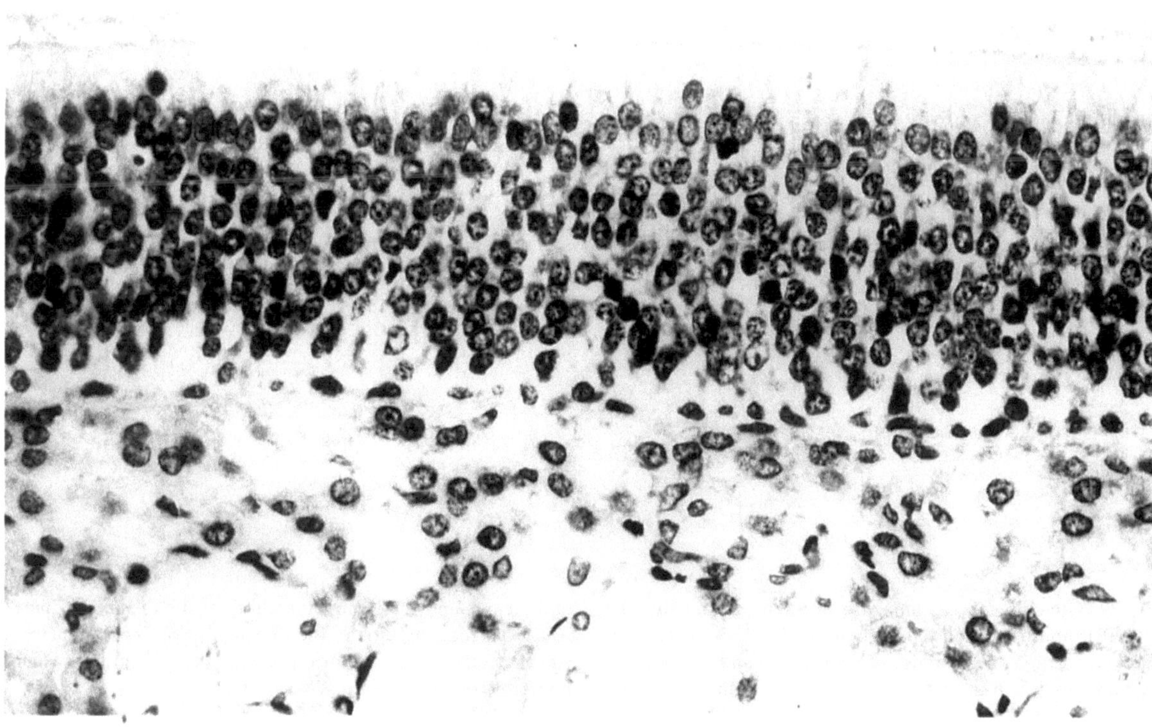

replacement of intraepithelial ducts of Bowman's glands.

During olfactory epithelial regeneration a wide range of changes may be observed in the underlying lamina propria, including regeneration of Bowman's glands and olfactory nerve bundles. The nature of these changes depends upon the extent of degeneration of the overlying epithelium, associated inflammation, and the severity of degenerative changes that occurred in the lamina propria. However, the process of regeneration of the lamina propria has been less well characterized.

*Adaptation or Modification of Epithelial Morphology.* Certain modifications of the olfactory mucosa following epithelial degeneration may be adaptive in nature, leading to the development of a modified and possibly more resistant (or less susceptible) epithelial barrier to inhaled xenobiotics. These changes include squamous and respiratory metaplasia. Squamous metaplasia is a common response following injury of the transitional and respiratory epithelia, but it occurs more rarely in the olfactory region. Respiratory metaplasia, a more common response of the olfactory epithelium to injury, leads to the development of an epithelial type that morphologically resembles pseudostratified respiratory epithelium (Fig. 29), with a paucity of goblet cells but numerous ciliated and nonciliated cells. Ciliation of the epithelium by motile cilia (replacing the morphologically distinct sensory cilia of the olfactory neurons) is associated with the formation of an active

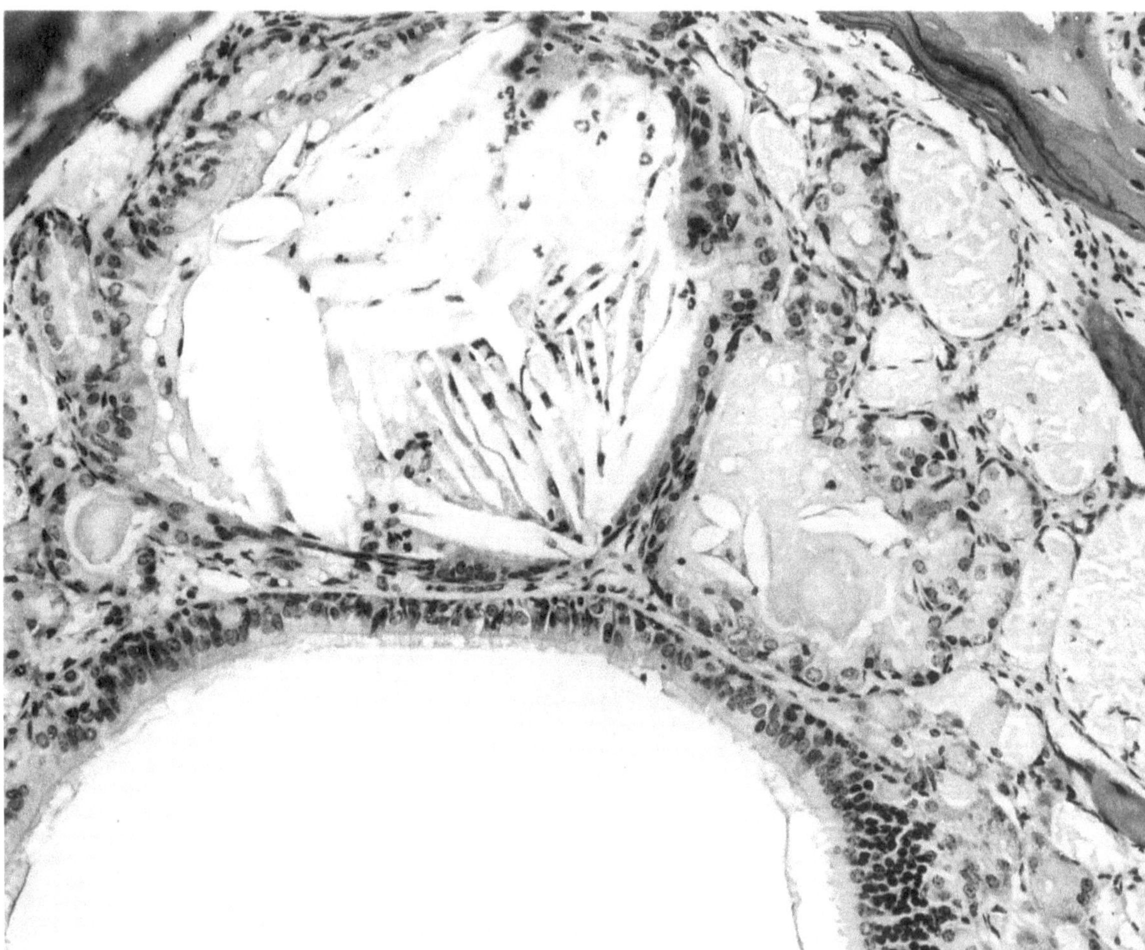

**Fig. 29.** Olfactory mucosa lining the dorsal medial meatus of a B6C3F1 mouse exposed to nitrobenzene for 2 years. There is marked ectasia of glands of Bowman and respiratory metaplasia of both the olfactory epithelium of the dorsal medial meatus and the lining epithelium of the distended ducts. Yellowish pigmentation of the Bowman's glands and olfactory sustentacular cells is not apparent in this monochrome photomicrograph. H&E, ×280

mucociliary apparatus and mucus flow rates characteristic of respiratory mucosa (Gross et al. 1987). Whether respiratory metaplasia of the olfactory epithelium is adaptive in nature, providing a degree of protection against subsequent exposures, remains to be determined. However, this response would clearly be associated with loss of olfactory function in the affected areas.

*Other Olfactory Mucosal Lesions.* A wide range of olfactory mucosal lesions has been reported; however, a complete review of such changes is not possible here. Such changes include olfactory pigments, ectasia and other lesions of the Bowman's glands and their ductular system (Fig. 29), and a range of proliferative or "preneoplastic" lesions which are addressed elsewhere (Morgan and Harkema, this volume). There is a clear need for a systematic approach to the classification of such nasal lesions.

## Ultrastructure

Electron microscopy can provide a valuable adjunct to light microscopy when assessing olfactory mucosal damage. Scanning electron microscopy permits detection of subtle damage to the surface of the olfactory epithium, such as loss of sensory cilia (Jiang et al. 1983). Recently, ultrastructural studies demonstrated primary damage to olfactory sustentacular cells following exposure to dibasic esters (Trela et al. 1992), indicating the nature of the primary target cell population and clarifying the significance of previous studies of nasal carboxyl esterases using enzyme histochemistry (Bogdanffy et al. 1987). However, successful application of electron microscopy requires careful attention to tissue fixation and sampling (Uraih and Maronpot 1990).

## Etiology and Frequency

Olfactory dysfunction, with or without demonstrated olfactory mucosal defects, may have a genetic basis or be attributable to viral infections, physical trauma, or exposure to a range of chemical agents (Getchell et al. 1991). However, in the majority of rodent toxicology studies olfactory function is rarely assessed. In light of the wide range of chemicals that have demonstrated effects on human olfaction (Amoore 1986), such assessments might provide a valuable addition to rodent toxicology studies.

## Interpretation

A wide range of lesions has been reported in the olfactory mucosa, with new reports occurring with increasing frequency as the nose is examined in greater detail in routine toxicology studies. The nose is one of the first tissues exposed to inhaled air, making the olfactory mucosa a possible target for chemicals delivered to the nose by this route. Furthermore, the olfactory mucosa has considerable metabolic capacity, which competes with that of the liver on the basis of activity per unit tissue weight (Dahl and Hadley 1991; Reed 1993). This metabolic activity probably accounts for many lesions induced in the olfactory mucosa by chemicals delivered by both the inhalation and noninhalation routes. A recent review of the role of dosimetry in these toxic processes (Morgan 1994) noted that the toxicological pathologist has an important role to play in the determination of mechanisms of nasal toxicity through detection of patterns of responses at the tissue and cellular levels. Determination of such patterns is essential for human risk assessment, as detection of critical events focuses research efforts on relevant endpoints for interspecies extrapolation.

Another important role for the pathologist reading rodent toxicology studies is interpretation of the relevance of the observations. For responses in the olfactory mucosa a number of human diseases are of concern, with loss of the sense of smell (anosmia) or a defective sense of smell (dysosmia, hyposmia) being primary concerns. Whenever functional endpoints can be correlated with histopathological changes, such interpretations are facilitated. Examples of detailed mechanistic research on the olfactory mucosa were the subject of a recent review of the role of the toxicological pathologist in studies of nasal toxicity (Morgan 1994). These examples, which incorporate histopathology as an endpoint, may provide insight when olfactory lesions are encountered, and the relevant human disease risk needs to be determined.

## Comparison with Other Species

Olfactory mucosal lesions have been reported in companion animals (Mattix et al. 1994), but this region of the respiratory tract is apparently rarely studied in farm animals. Fairly extensive research has also been conducted on the olfactory system using fish and amphibians (Getchell et al. 1991). There is also a large database on defects of human olfactory function. We have been unable to find literature on environmental effects on the olfactory system of feral animals. The olfactory sense is a primitive one and the morphology of the olfactory mucosa appears to be highly conserved in the majority of mammalian species studied to date (Negus 1958). However, there is little information available on differences in the toxicological pathology of the olfactory mucosa across these species.

## References


Amoore JE (1986) Effects of chemical exposure on olfaction in humans. In: Barrow CS (ed) Toxicology of the nasal passages. Hemisphere, Washington DC

Belinsky SA, Walker VE, Maronpot RR, Swenberg JA, Anderson MW (1987) Molecular dosimetry of DNA adduct formation and cell toxicity in rat nasal mucosa following exposure to the tobacco specific nitrosamine 4-(N-methyl-N-nitrosamino)-1-(3-pyridyl)-1-butanone and their relationship to induction of neoplasia. Cancer Res 47:6058–6065

Bogdanffy MS (1990) Biotransformation enzymes in the rodent nasal mucosa: the value of a histochemical approach. Environ Health Perspect 85:177–186

Bogdanffy MS, Randall HW, Morgan KT (1987) Biochemical quantitation and histochemical localization of carboxylesterase in the nasal passages of the Fischer-344 rat and B6C3F1 mouse. Toxicol Appl Pharmacol 88:183–194

Bolon B, Bonnefoi MS, Roberts KC, Marshall MW, Morgan KT (1991) Toxic interactions in the rat nose: pollutants from soiled bedding and methyl bromide. Toxicol Pathol 19:571–579

Brittebo EB, Eriksson C, Feil V, Bakke J, Brandt I (1991) Toxicity of 2,6-dichlorothiobenzamide (chlorthiamid) and 2,6-dichlorobenzamide in the olfactory nasal mucosa of mice. Fundam Appl Toxicol 17:92–102

Buckley LA, Jiang XZ, James RA, Morgan KT, Barrow CS (1984) Respiratory tract lesions induced by sensory irritants at the RD50 concentration. Toxicol Appl Pharmacol 74:417–429

Buckley LA, Morgan KT, Swenberg JA, James RA, Hamm TEJ, Barrow CS (1985) The toxicity of dimethylamine in F-344 rats and B6C3F1 mice following a 1 year inhalation exposure. Fundam Appl Toxicol 5:341–352

Cancalon P (1982) Degeneration and regeneration of olfactory cells induced by ZnSO4 and other chemicals. Tissue Cell 14:717–733

Dahl AR, Hadley WH (1991) Nasal cavity enzymes involved in xenobiotic metabolism: effects on the toxicity of inhalants. Crit Rev Toxicol 21:345–372

Doty RL, Bartoshuk LM, Snow JBJ (1991) Causes of olfactory and gustatory disorders. In: Getchell TV, Doty RL, Bartoshuk LM, Snow JBJ (eds) Smell and taste in health and disease. Raven, New York, pp 449–462

Eccles R, Bende M, Widdicombe JG (1987) Nasal blood vessels. In: Mygind N, Pipkor U (eds) Allergic and vasomotor rhinitis: pathophysiological aspects, 1st edn. Munksgaard, Copenhagen, pp 63–76

Feron VJ, Kruysse A (1978) Effects of exposure to furfural vapor in hamsters simultaneously treated with benzo[a]pyrene or diethylnitrosamine. Toxicology 11:127–144

Gaskell BA (1990) Nonneoplastic changes in the olfactory epithelium – experimental studies. Environ Health Perspect 85:275–289

Genter MB, Llorens J, O'Callaghan JP, Peele DB, Morgan KT, Crofton KM (1992) Olfactory toxicity of β,β′-iminodipropionitrile (IDPN) in the rat. J Pharmacol Exp Ther 263:1432–1439

Getchell TV, Doty RL, Bartoshuk LM, Snow JBJ (1991) Smell and taste in health and disease. Raven, New York

Graziadei PPC (1973) Cell dynamics in the olfactory mucosa. Tissue Cell 5:113–131

Greene EC (1963) Anatomy of the rat. Hafner, New York

Gross EA, Morgan KT (1992) Architecture of nasal passages and larynx. In: Parent RA (ed) Treatise on pulmonary toxicology. CRC, Boca Raton

Gross EA, Patterson DL, Morgan KT (1987) Effects of acute and chronic dimethylamine exposure on the nasal mucociliary apparatus of F-344 rats. Toxicol Appl Pharmacol 90:359–376

Halász N (1990) The vertebrate olfactory system, chemical neuroanatomy, function and development. Akadémiai Kiadó, Budapest

Hastings L, Evans JE (1991) Olfactory primary neurons as a route of entry for toxic agents in the CNS. Neurotoxicology 12:707–714

Hebel R, Stromberg MW (1986) Anatomy and embryology of the laboratory rat. Williams and Wilkins, Baltimore

Hurtt ME, Morgan KT, Working PK (1987) Histopathology of acute toxic responses in selected tissues from rats exposed by inhalation to methyl bromide. Fundam Appl Toxicol 9:352–365

Hurtt ME, Thomas DA, Working PK, Monticello TM, Morgan KT (1988) Degeneration and regeneration of the olfactory epithelium following inhalation exposure to methyl bromide: pathology, cell kinetics, and olfactory function. Toxicol Appl Pharmacol 94:311–328

Jiang XZ, Buckley LA, Morgan KT (1983) Pathology of toxic responses to the RD50 concentration of chlorine gas in the nasal passages of rats and mice. Toxicol Appl Pharmacol 71:225–236

Kuper CF, Spit BJ, Bruijntjes JP, Hendriksen EGJ, Hameleers DMH (1989) Nasal lymphoid tissue, its specialized position in the upper respiratory tract. In: Feron VJ, Bosland MC (eds) Nasal carcinogenesis in rodents: relevance to human health risk. Pudoc, Wageningen, pp 30–35

Lee KP, Valentine R, Bogdanffy MS (1992) Nasal lesion development and reversibility in rats exposed to aerosols of dibasic esters. Toxicol Pathol 20:376–393

Mann DMA, Esiri MM (1988) The site of the earliest lesions of Alzheimer's disease. N Engl J Med 318:789–790

Mattix ME, Mattix RJ, Williams BH, Ribas JL, Wilhelmsen CL (1994) Olfactory ganglioneuroblastoma in a dog: a light, ultrastructural, and immunohistochemical study. Vet Pathol 31:262–265

Mery S, Gross EA, Joyner DR, Godo M, Morgan KT (1994a) Nasal diagrams: a tool for recording the distribution of nasal lesions in rats and mice. Toxicol Pathol 22:353–372
Mery S, Larson JL, Butterworth BE, Wolf DC, Harden R, Morgan KT (1994b) Nasal toxicity of chloroform in male F-344 rats and female B6C3F1 mice following a 1-week inhalation exposure. Toxicol Appl Pharmacol 125:214–227
Miller RR, Hermann EA, Young JT, Calhoun LL, Kastl PE (1984) Propylene glycol monomethyl ether acetate (PGMEA) metabolism, disposition, and short-term vapor inhalation toxicity studies. Toxicol Appl Pharmacol 75:521–530
Miller RR, Young JT, Kociba RJ, Keyes DG, Bodner KM, Calhoun LL, Ayres JA (1985) Chronic toxicity and oncogenicity bioassay of inhaled ethyl acrylate in Fischer 344 rats and B6C3F1 mice. Drug Chem Toxicol 8:1–42
Monticello TM, Morgan KT, Uraih C (1990) Nonneoplastic nasal lesions in rats and mice. Environ Health Perspect 85:249–274
Morgan KT (1991) Approaches to the identification and recording of nasal lesions in toxicology studies. Toxicol Pathol 19:337–351
Morgan KT (1994) Nasal dosimetry, lesion distribution, and the toxicologic pathologist: a brief review. Inhal Toxicol 6:41–57
Morgan KT, Monticello TM (1989) Airflow, mucociliary clearance, and lesion distribution in the nasal passages of experimental animals. In: Feron VJ, Bosland MC (eds) Nasal carcinogenesis in rodents: relevance to human health risk. Pudoc, Veldhoven, pp 36–41
Morgan KT, Kimbell JS, Monticello TM, Patra AL, Fleishman A (1991) Studies of inspiratory airflow patterns in the nasal passages of the F344 rat and rhesus monkey using nasal molds: relevance to formaldehyde toxicity. Toxicol Appl Pharmacol 110:223–240
Morse CC, Boyd MR, Witschi H (1984) The effect of 3-methylfuran inhalation exposure on the rat nasal cavity. Toxicology 30:195–204
Negus V (1958) The comparative anatomy and physiology of the nose and paranasal sinuses. Livingstone, Edinburgh
Peele DB, Allison SD, Bolon B, Prah JD, Jensen KF, Morgan KT (1990) Functional deficits produced by 3-methylindole-induced olfactory mucosal damage revealed by a simple olfactory learning task. Toxicol Appl Pharmacol 107:191–202
Proctor DF, Chang JCF (1983) Comparative anatomy and physiology of the nasal cavity. In: Reznik G, Stinson SF (eds) Nasal tumors in animals and man, vol 1. CRC, Boca Raton, pp 1–33
Reed CJ (1993) Drug metabolism in the nasal cavity: relevance to toxicology. Drug Metab Rev 25:173–205
Reznik G (1983) Comparative anatomy and histomorphology of the nasal and paranasal cavities in rodents. In: Reznik G, Stinson SF (eds) Nasal tumors in animals and man, vol 1. CRC, Boca Raton, pp 35–44
Reznik-Schüller HM (1983) Nitrosamine-induced nasal cavity carcinogenesis. In: Reznik G, Stinson SF (eds) Nasal tumors in animals and man, vol 3. CRC, Boca Raton, pp 47–77
Serby MJ, Chobar KL (1992) Science of olfaction. Springer, Berlin Heidelberg New York
St Clair MBG, Morgan KT (1992) Age-related changes in the upper respiratory tract of the rat. In: Mohr U, Dungworth DL, Capen CC (eds) Pathobiology of the aging rat, vol 1. ILSI, Washington DC, pp 111–127
Trela BA, Frame SR, Bogdanffy MS (1992) A microscopic and ultrastructural evaluation of dibasic esters (DBE) toxicity in rat nasal explants. Exp Mol Pathol 56:208–218
Uraih LC, Maronpot RR (1990) Normal histology of the nasal cavity and application of special techniques. Environ Health Perspect 85:187–208
Uraih LC, Talley FA, Mitsumori K, Gupta BN, Bucher JR, Boorman GA (1987) Ultrastructural changes in the nasal mucosa of Fischer 344 rats and B6C3F1 mice following an acute exposure to methyl isocyanate. Environ Health Perspect 72:77–88
Vaccarezza OL, Sepich LN, Tramezzani JH (1981) The vomeronasal organ of the rat. J Anat 132:167–185
Youngentob SL, Markert LM, Hill TW, Matyas EP, Mozell MM (1991) Odorant identification in rats: an update. Physiol Behav 49:1293–1296

# Microscopic Anatomy of Toxicologically Important Regions of the Larynx of the Rat, Mouse, and Hamster

Roger A. Renne and Rodney A. Miller

## Introduction

Laboratory rats, mice, and hamsters are the species most frequently used for subchronic and lifetime inhalation toxicity studies. The relatively high incidence of exposure-induced lesions in the upper respiratory tract in these species has generated considerable interest in the microscopic anatomy and histopathology of the nasal cavity (Brown et al. 1991; Harkema 1991; Morgan 1991) and the larynx (Brockmeyer et al. 1989; Gopinath et al. 1987; Lewis and Prentice 1980; Lewis 1981a,b; Lewis 1991; Nakano and Muto 1987; Renne et al. 1992a, 1994; Sagartz et al. 1992). Although the anatomy of the rodent larynx is less complex than the nose, the distribution of the

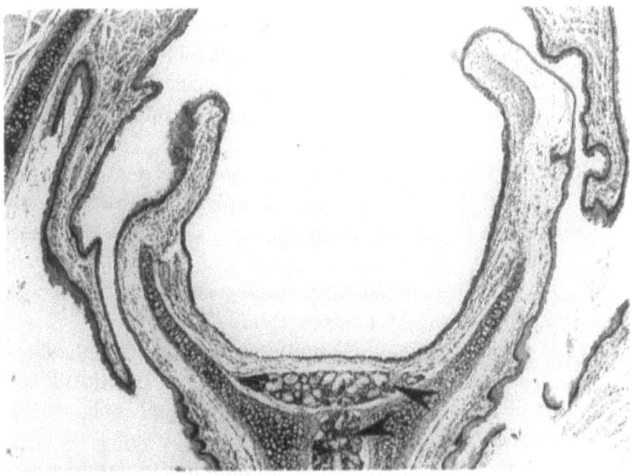

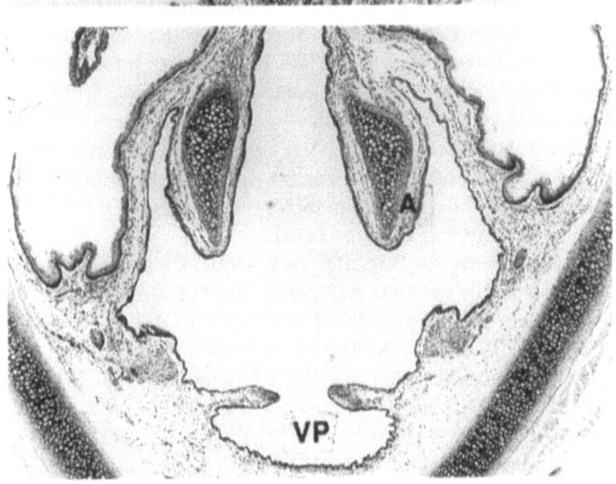


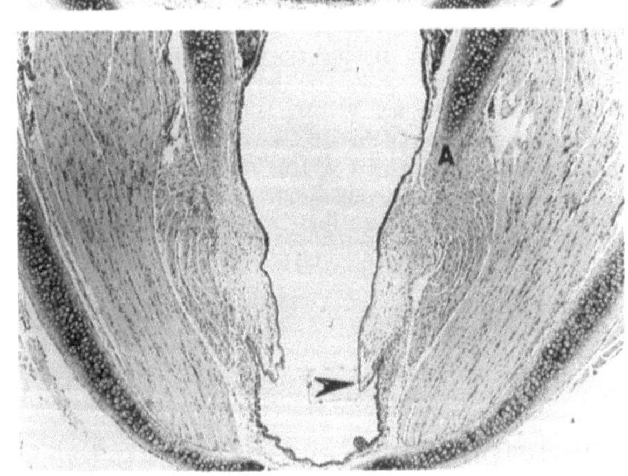


**Fig. 30.** (*above*) Transverse section through rat larynx at the level of the base of the epiglottis. Submucosal seromucous glands are visible (*arrowheads*). H&E, ×10

**Fig. 31.** (*middle*) Transverse section through rat larynx at the level of the ventral pouch (*VP*) and the vocal processes of the arytenoid cartilages (*A*). H&E, ×10

**Fig. 32.** (*below*) Transverse section through rat larynx at the level of the vocal folds (*arrowhead*), extending ventromedially into lumen from vocal processes of arytenoid cartilages (*A*). H&E, ×20

types of epithelium lining the laryngeal lumen is similar to the nasal airway in that the mucosal epithelium changes from stratified squamous cranially to pseudostratified ciliated columnar (respiratory) epithelium caudally. These areas of transition from stratified squamous to respiratory epithelium are the most sensitive sites for cellular changes such as degeneration, squamous metaplasia, or hyperplasia in response to inhaled xenobiotics (Gopinath et al. 1987; Lewis 1991). As in the nose, the predilection of these sites for lesions in rodents is probably due to airflow characteristics and regional epithelial sensitivity (Chevalier and Dontenwill 1972; Gopinath et al. 1987; Lewis 1981b, 1991).

This chapter compares the normal histology of areas of the rat, mouse, and hamster larynx most likely to contain lesions induced by inhalation of xenobiotics, and discusses the possible role of these interspecies anatomic variations in the location and morphology of laryngeal lesions induced in rats and hamsters by the inhalation of xenobiotics.

Similar but not identical methods were used to provide transverse sections of larynx from rats, mice, and hamsters for microscopic examination (Coggins et al. 1989; Coggins et al. 1990; Renne et al. 1992a,b, 1994; Sagartz et al. 1992; Wehner et al. 1990). Emphasis was placed on the preparation of sections through the base of the epiglottis (Fig. 30), ventral pouch and the vocal processes of the arytenoid cartilages (Fig. 31), and the vocal folds (Fig. 32).

Multiple sections of each of the above areas of the larynx from animals were routinely examined microscopically on a number of inhalation studies. Serial transverse or longitudinal (midsagittal) sections of larynges from additional rats and hamsters of the same strain, source, and approximate age were prepared and examined histologically to study normal laryngeal histology.

## Histology of Rat Larynx (5 Months of Age)

The stratified squamous epithelium covering the anterior and middle portions of the laryngeal surface of the epiglottis is composed of a layer of oval, vertically oriented basal cells with oval to round nuclei, several layers of round to oval cells, and a surface layer of squamous cells, the majority of which are not keratinized (Fig. 33). In the caudal portion of the epiglottis there is a gradual transition to round or cuboidal cells, with fewer surface squamous and occasional columnar ciliated cells. At the base of the epiglottis the surface epithelium is a mixture of cell types, predominantly cuboidal, with smaller numbers of ciliated columnar and oval to flattened squamoid cells (Fig. 34). Figure 35 is a schematic diagram of a midsagittal section through the base of the epiglottis and ventral pouch of a rat larynx. A consistent point of reference for the transition from stratified squamous to mixed type of epithelium at the base of the epiglottis in rats is the submucosal seromucous glands on the ventral midline. In most rats these glands extended anteriorly to the point where the surface epithelium changes from mixed type to stratified squamous (Fig. 36). In a few rats the surface epithelium on the ventral midline covering the most anterior extension of the seromucous glands is composed of two to three layers of squamous cells; however, this epithelium is thinner than the stratified squamous epithelium lining the anterior epiglottis and does not have a prominent basal cell layer typical of stratified squamous epithelium.

Ciliated columnar epithelial cells frequently line the openings of the ducts of seromucous glands and the adjacent surface of the base of the epiglottis. The number of ciliated cells in the epithelium covering the laryngeal surface of the base of the epiglottis gradually decreases caudally from the anterior extension of the mixed type of epithelium. Ciliated cells are rarely present in sections through the junction of the epiglottal and thyroid cartilages. The surface epithelium covering the caudal epiglottis is composed of three or four layers of round or cuboidal cells and gradually becomes thinner caudally as it covers the base of the U-shaped cartilage supporting the ventral pouch (Fig. 37).

The submucosal seromucous glands extend caudally and ventrally to the junction of the epiglottal and thyroid cartilages (Fig. 37). The epithelium covering the laryngeal surface of the base of the U-shaped cartilage is only one or two cells thick, with no discernible basal cell layer (Fig. 38). Sections through this area also include the anterior extension of the ventral pouch, which is lined by cuboidal or round epithelial cells two to four cells thick, depending on its degree of distension (Fig. 38). At the point where the ventral pouch opens into the laryngeal lumen the mucosa covering the wings of the U-shaped cartilages is squamoid epithelium two cells thick.

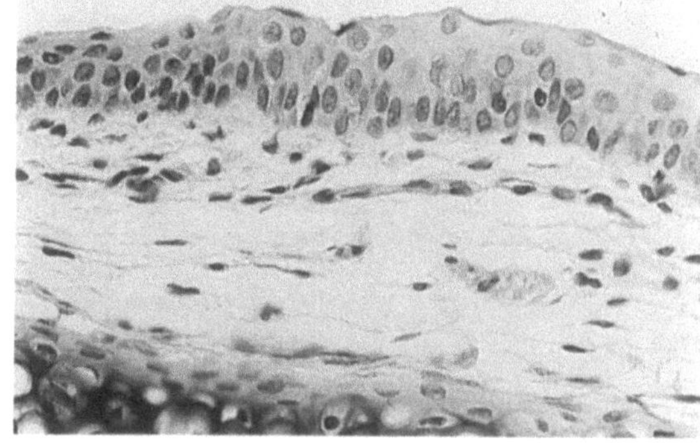

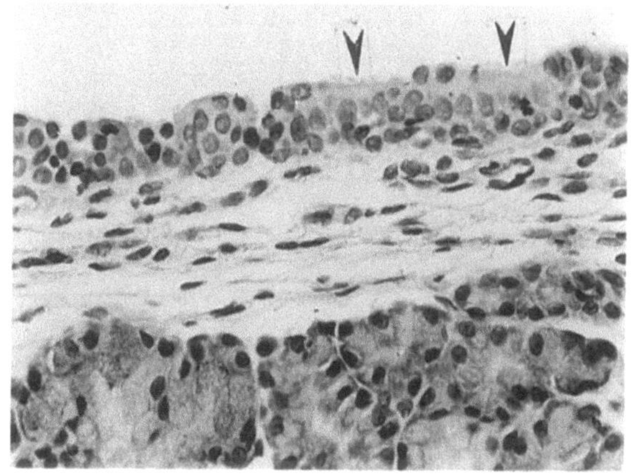

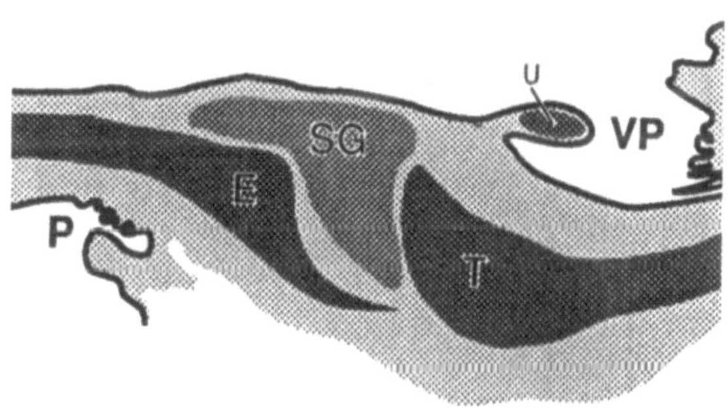


**Fig. 33.** (*above*) Transverse section through epithelium covering the anterior epiglottis of rat. Vertically oriented basal cells with oval or round nuclei, several layers of round or oval cells, and surface layer of unkeratinized squamous cells. H&E, ×100

**Fig. 34.** (*middle*) Transverse section through epithelium covering the base of the epiglottis of 5-month old rat. Poorly defined basal cell layer covered by a mixture of round, oval, cuboidal, and columnar ciliated cells (*arrowheads*). H&E, ×100

**Fig. 35.** (*below*) Schematic diagram of a midsagittal section through the base of the epiglottis and the ventral pouch of a rat larynx. *E*, Epiglottal cartilage; *P*, pharyngeal lumen; *T*, thyroid cartilage; *U*, U-shaped cartilage; *VP*, ventral pouch; *SG*, seromucous glands

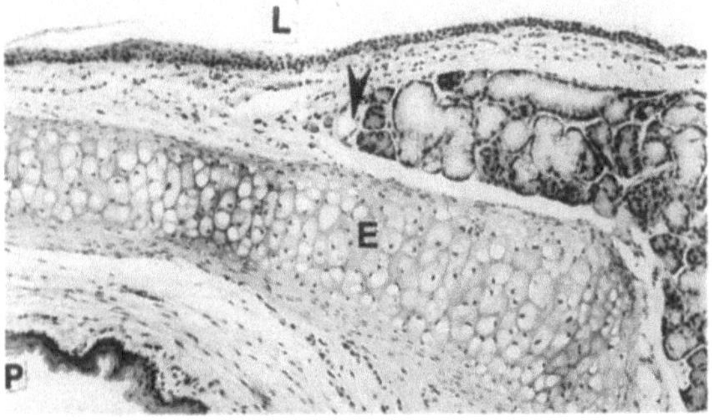


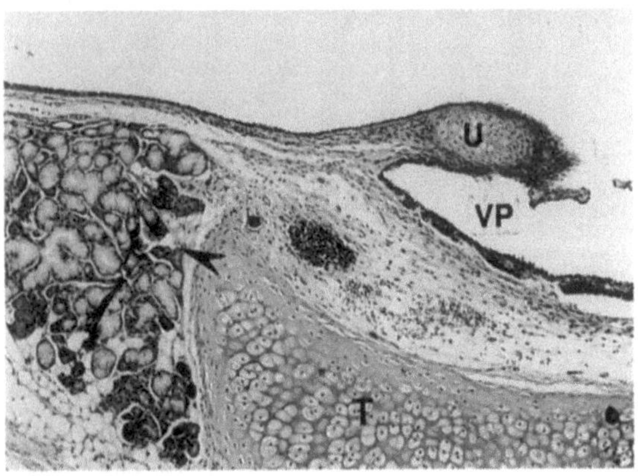


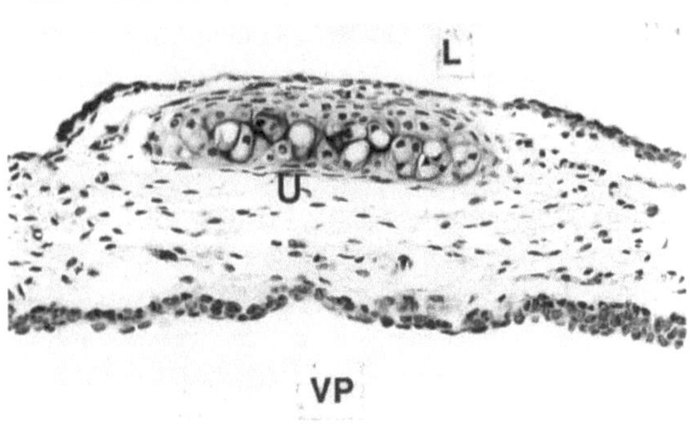


**Fig. 36.** (*above*) Midsagittal section through base of rat epiglottis. Surface epithelium changes from stratified squamous to intermediate type of epithelium at the level of the anterior extension of the submucosal glands (*arrowhead*). *E*, Epiglottal cartilage; *L*, laryngeal lumen; *P*, pharyngeal lumen. H&E, ×25

**Fig. 37.** (*middle*) Midsagittal section through rat larynx at the level of the caudal extent of the seromucous glands (*arrowhead*), the anterior aspect of the thyroid cartilage (*T*), the base of the U-shaped cartilage (*U*), and the anterior aspect of the ventral pouch (*VP*). H&E, ×25

**Fig. 38.** (*below*) Transverse section of rat larynx through the anterior aspect of the ventral pouch (*VP*) and the base of the U-shaped cartilage (*U*). *L*, Laryngeal lumen; *T*, thyroid cartilage. H&E, ×25

In sections through the larynx at the level of the ventral pouch the vocal processes of the arytenoid cartilages are visible protruding ventrally into the laryngeal lumen (Fig. 39). In the most anterior sections through the vocal processes the ventral portions of their medial surfaces are covered with unkeratinized squamous epithelium two to three cells thick, while the dorsal portions are covered with slightly thicker, keratinized squamous epithelium. In sections taken further caudally the degree of keratinization of the epithelium on the medial surfaces of the vocal processes gradually decreases.

In sections through the caudal larynx the roof of the ventral pouch recedes laterally, and the larynx is elongated dorsoventrally. The vocal processes

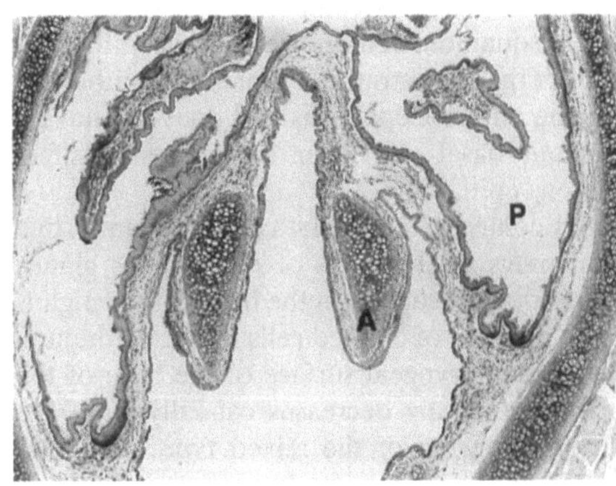


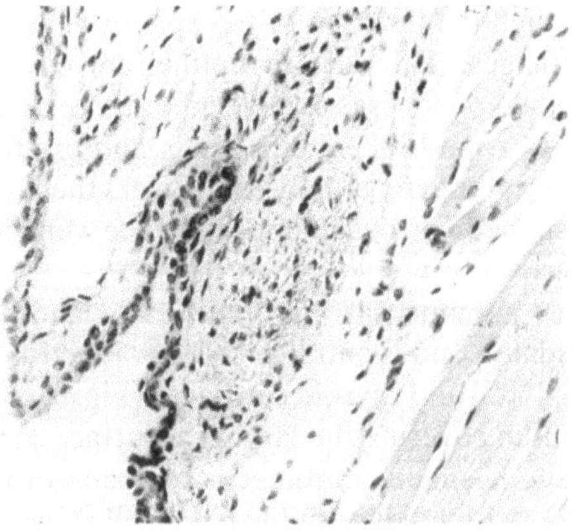

**Fig. 39.** (*above*) Transverse section of rat larynx through vocal processes of arytenoid cartilages (*A*) at the level of the ventral pouch (*P*). The stratified squamous epithelium covering the distal aspect of the medial surfaces of the arytenoids is sparsely keratinized, gradually becomes more keratinized proximally. H&E, ×10

**Fig. 40.** (*below*) Transverse section through vocal folds in caudal rat larynx. Vocal folds are covered by a low cuboidal or squamoid epithelium two or three cells thick. H&E, ×25

of the arytenoid cartilages are visible extended ventromedially in the lateral walls (Fig. 32). It is difficult consistently to obtain sections through the protrusion of the vocal folds into the lumen. When present in sections, the vocal folds are visible as narrow folds of connective tissue covered by flattened to cuboidal epithelium two or three cells thick (Fig. 40) and extending ventromedially from the vocal processes into the lumen of the ventral larynx. The surface epithelium of the dorsal half of the larynx in this area is predominantly ciliated columnar cells.

## Mouse Larynx

Microscopic examination of laryngeal sections from mice reveal differences in normal laryngeal anatomy between rats and mice. As in rats, the seromucous glands beneath the surface epithelium are a consistent point of reference for the transition from stratified squamous to mixed epithelium at the base of the epiglottis. However, ciliated columnar cells are much more numerous than in rats. The epithelium covering the submucosal glands at the base of the epiglottis of the mouse is composed almost entirely of ciliated columnar cells (Fig. 41), with fewer round to oval cells than seen in this area of the epiglottis in rats. In mice the epithelium covering the laryngeal surface from the base of the epiglottis to the anterior edge of the ventral pouch is predominantly low columnar or cuboidal, with many ciliated cells (Fig. 42; compare with Fig. 37). The ventral pouch of mice does not extend anteriorly from its opening into the laryngeal lumen as it does in rats. The base of the U shaped cartilage is much less prominent in mice than in rats, and the overlying epithelium is not as flattened. (Fig. 42; compare with Fig. 37). The epithelium lining the ventral pouch of mice is a mixture of ciliated columnar and cuboidal cells. The ventral surface of the pouch is covered almost completely by ciliated cells (Fig. 42). The epithelium covering the wings of the U-shaped cartilage at the junction of the ventral pouch with the laryngeal lumen is somewhat flattened, similar to this area in rats.

The vocal folds of mice are covered with low cuboidal or squamoid epithelium. The remaining laryngeal lumen in sections containing the vocal folds is lined by ciliated epithelium dorsally and a mixture of ciliated and nonciliated cuboidal cells ventrally.

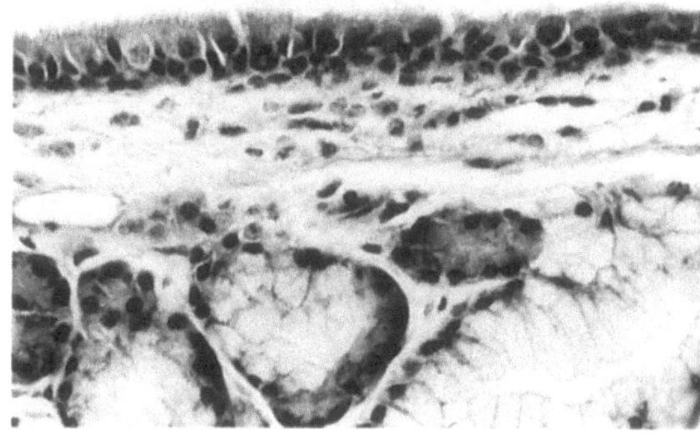

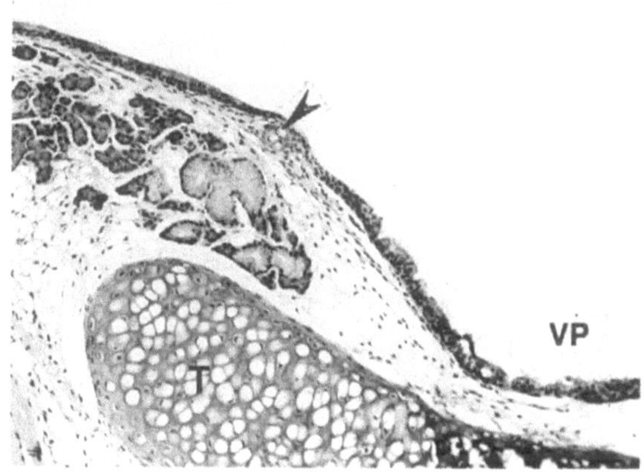


**Fig. 41.** (*above*) Transverse section through the base of the epiglottis of mouse. Surface epithelium is composed predominantly of ciliated columnar cells. H&E, ×100

**Fig. 42.** (*below*) Midsagittal section through mouse larynx at the level of the seromucous glands at the base of the epiglottis, the anterior aspect of the thyroid cartilage (*T*), the base of the U shaped cartilage (*arrowhead*) and the anterior aspect of the ventral pouch (*VP*). H&E, ×25

## Hamster Larynx

Figure 43 includes a longitudinal section through the larynx of a hamster, identifying the location of sections in Figs. 44–50. The mucosa of the cranial and middle portions of the laryngeal surface of the epiglottis is similar to that in rats (Fig. 44). In all three species transition occurs in the caudal epiglottis from stratified squamous epithelium to a mixed type of epithelium, consisting of several cell types. However, there are notable interspecies differences in the morphology of this epithelium, and in the relationship between the location of this transitional zone and the presence of underlying seromucous glands.

In a midsagittal section through the cranial epiglottis of a hamster, (Fig. 45) the seromucous

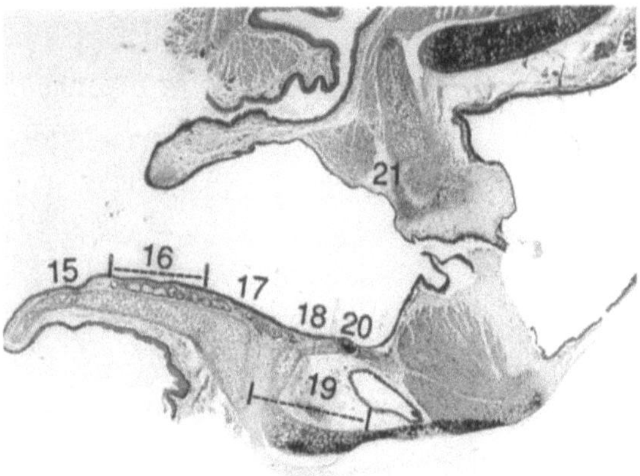


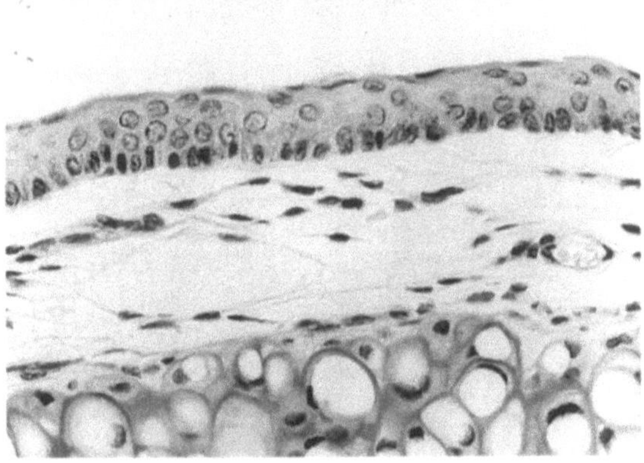

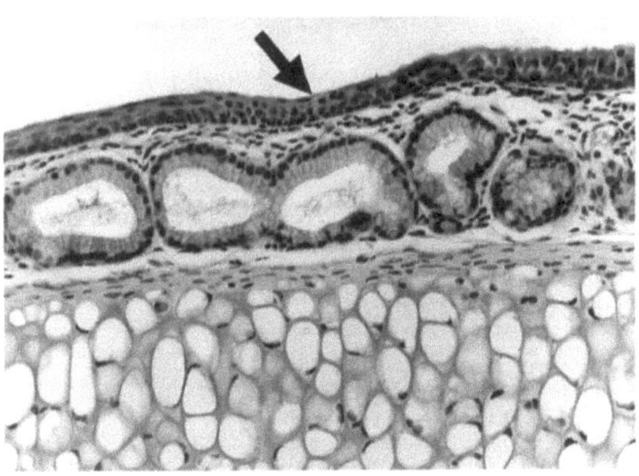

**Fig. 43.** (*above*) Midsagittal section through the larynx of a Syrian golden hamster illustrating location of sections in Figs. 44(15)–50(21). H&E, ×5

**Fig. 44.** (*middle*) Transverse section through the surface epithelium and cartilage of cranial epiglottis of hamster (15 in Fig. 43). Vertically oriented basal cells with oval or round nuclei, several layers of round to oval cells, and a surface layer of usually unkeratinized squamous cells. H&E, ×100

**Fig. 45.** (*below*) Midsagittal section through hamster epiglottis (16 in Fig. 43), note submucosal glands underlying stratified squamous surface epithelium cranial to transition zone, which begins at arrow. H&E, ×50

glands of the epiglottis extend cranially beneath the stratified squamous surface epithelium. Thus these glands do not indicate the cranial border of the zone of transition in hamsters as they do in rats and mice.

In this zone of transition from stratified squamous epithelium in hamsters the basal cells and the middle layers of epithelium gradually become more elongated vertically, increasing the total depth of the mucosal epithelium. Further caudally, squamous cells are absent, and the mucosa is a mixture of ciliated columnar, spherical, and cuboidal surface cells and a layer of basal cells with round or vertically oriented oval nuclei (Fig. 46). The mucosa of the caudal epiglottis is made up almost entirely of tall columnar ciliated epithelium, which extends downward into the openings of the ducts of submucosal glands (Fig. 47). The

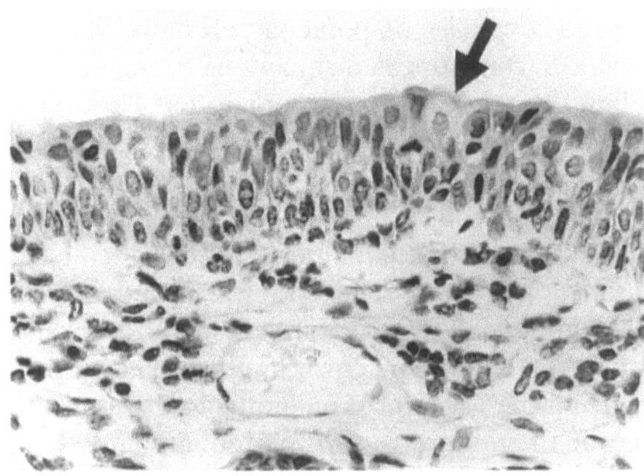

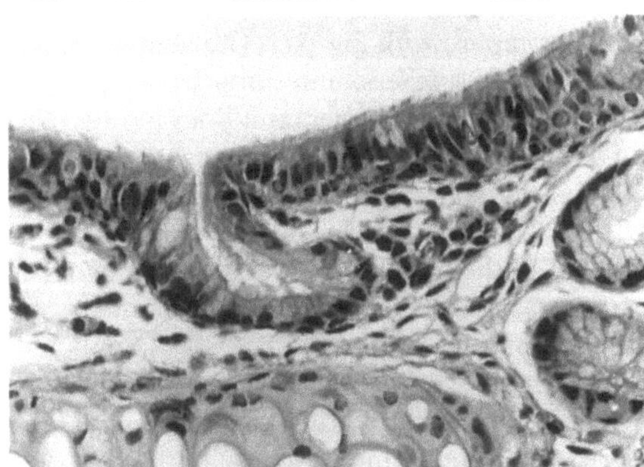

**Fig. 46.** (*above*) Transverse section through mucosa in transitional zone at base of epiglottis of hamster. Surface cells are cuboidal, round, or columnar; some are ciliated (*arrow*) (17 in Fig. 43). H&E, ×100

**Fig. 47.** (*below*) Transverse section caudal to area shown in Fig. 46 (18 in Fig. 43). Surface epithelium is entirely tall columnar ciliated cells, extending downward into submucosal gland ducts. H&E, ×100

epithelium in this part of the larynx of the hamster is much thicker than in rats, due in part to the more vertically elongated cells. In this respect it more closely resembles the mucosal epithelium covering this area in mice (Renne et al. 1992a, 1994).

In hamsters the U-shaped cartilage supporting the cranial rim of the ventral pouch has a broad base (Fig. 48), which forms a distinct protrusion of the overlying mucosa into the laryngeal lumen (Fig. 49). In rats this protrusion is not nearly as prominent as in hamsters (compare Fig. 49 with Fig. 37). At the highest point of this protuberance in hamsters, the surface cells on its apex are rounded, oval, or flattened, with few or no ciliated cells (Fig. 49), while the surface cells on the sides of the protuberance are tall columnar with abundant cilia.

The ventral pouch does not usually extend cranially in Syrian hamsters as it does in rats (compare Fig. 48 with Fig. 37), thus is not usually present in transverse sections through the protuberance. The mucosal epithelium lining the ventral pouch of hamsters is predominantly flattened, made up of oval or cuboidal cells similar to those in rats (Renne et al. 1992a, 1994). However, this epithelium is less convoluted in hamsters than in rats, suggesting less variability in the size of the pouch in hamsters.

In transverse sections through the hamster larynx at the level of the ventral pouch the vocal processes of the arytenoid cartilages protrude ventrally into the laryngeal lumen (Fig. 50). These processes are not as prominent in hamsters as in rats (compare Fig. 50 with Fig. 39). This interspecies difference has been described previously (Lewis 1981b). The squamous epithelium lining the medial surfaces of the vocal processes is similar to that in rats.

In sections through the caudal larynx in hamsters the larynx appears gradually elongated dorsoventrally, and the vocal processes of the arytenoid cartilages are visible extending ventromedially in the lateral walls. The vocal folds are similar histologically to those in rats and mice (Renne et al. 1992a, 1994).

We have described a number of differences among rats, mice, and hamsters in the microscopic anatomy of the larynx, some of which may have toxicological significance. Our studies (Coggins et al. 1989, 1990; Renne 1992a,b, 1994; Sagartz et al. 1992; Wehner et al. 1990) support the conclusion of Lewis (1981b, 1991) and Gopinath et al. (1987)

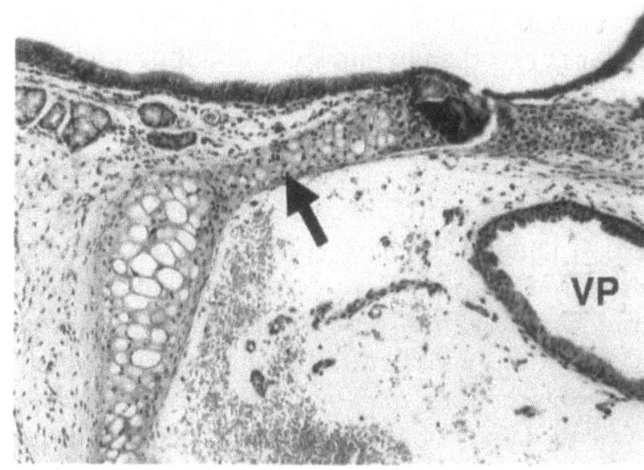


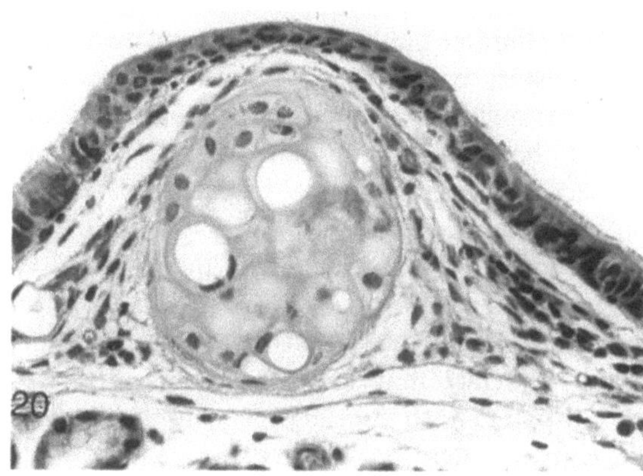


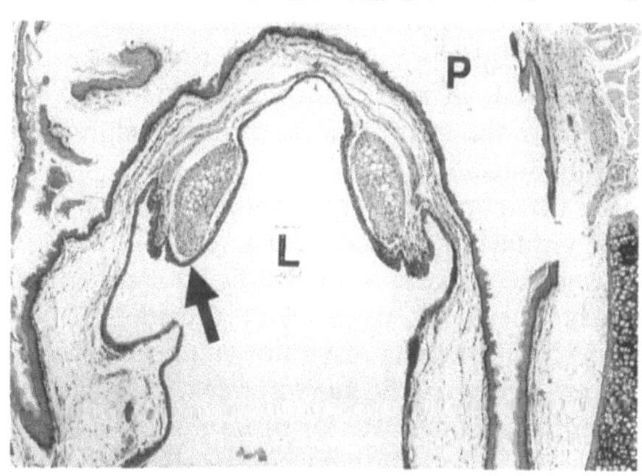


**Fig. 48.** (*above*) Midsagittal section through U-shaped cartilage and ventral pouch (*VP*) of hamster (19 in Fig. 43), showing attachment of U-shaped cartilage to thyroid cartilage (*arrow*). H&E, ×25

**Fig. 49.** (*middle*) Transverse section of hamster larynx through highest point of protuberance (20 in Fig. 43). Cells covering apex of protuberance are round, oval, or flattened with no cilia; tall columnar ciliated cells cover sides of protuberance. H&E, ×100

**Fig. 50.** (*below*) Transverse section of hamster larynx at level of vocal processes of arytenoid cartilages (*arrow*) (21 in Fig. 43). *L*, Laryngeal lumen; *P*, pharyngeal lumen. H&E, ×10

that the epithelium lining the base of the epiglottis is the part of the laryngeal mucosa in laboratory rodents most susceptible to changes induced by inhaled irritants. The epithelium covering this key target area at the base of the epiglottis is much thinner in rats than in hamsters, and thus might be more susceptible to injury from inhaled irritants. However, in hamsters the increased thickness of this epithelium is due in part to a large number of vertically elongated cells, most of which are ciliated. Ciliated columnar epithelium is generally considered to be more vulnerable to damage than cuboidal or squamous epithelium (Glaister 1986). This site in hamsters, although covered by a thicker epithelium, may be more susceptible than in rats to damage by inhaled materials.

Lewis (1981b) described squamous metaplasia of the epithelium at the base of the epiglottis in rats and hamsters exposed to cigarette smoke. The squamous metaplasia extended caudally from the base of the epiglottis into the ventral pouch in exposed hamsters; whereas in rats the ventral pouch was not affected. Lewis (1981b) also described smoke-induced lesions in the vocal processes of the arytenoid cartilages of rats, but not hamsters, and attributed this interspecies difference to the fact that these arytenoid processes extend further into the laryngeal lumen in rats. The converse may be true for the protuberance cranial to the ventral pouch in the hamster, i.e., it is more likely to be an important site for exposure-induced lesions in the hamster larynx than in the rat, due to the fact that it protrudes much further into the lumen.

Since the ultimate intent of most inhalation toxicology studies is to assess the potential toxicity of the subject material if inhaled by humans, an important question is which species provides the best model for the human respiratory tract. The cranial (upper) portion of the human larynx, including the upper half of the posterior surface of the epiglottis, is lined by stratified squamous epithelium (Stevens and Lowe 1992). The lower half of the posterior surface of the human epiglottis and most of the caudal larynx is lined by ciliated pseudostratified columnar epithelium, except for the vocal folds, which are lined with stratified squamous epithelium. Thus the distribution of epithelial types in the rodent epiglottis is more similar to the human larynx than is that of domestic animals such as dogs, in which the entire cranial portion of the larynx, including the entire laryngeal surface of the epiglottis is covered with stratified squamous epithelium. However, the epithelium covering the vocal folds of rodents is a thin cuboidal to squamoid epithelium (Renne et al. 1992a, 1994), much thinner than the stratified squamous epithelium covering the vocal folds of the human larynx. This is an important point because the vast majority of proliferative and inflammatory laryngeal lesions in humans occur on the vocal folds, which are adjacent to an area of transition from squamous to respiratory epithelium (Robbins 1974). Although the most frequent site of induced lesions in rodent larynges is in a different area of the larynx than in humans, there is a similarity in that this site in both rodents and humans is in or near an area of transition from squamous to respiratory epithelium.

Laryngeal lesions have been induced in rodents by a number of different inhaled materials, and the larynx is considered an important site to examine for evidence of exposure-induced changes in inhalation studies (Gopinath et al. 1987). We have described a number of rather subtle interspecies differences in the normal anatomy of the rat, mouse, and hamster larynx that should be taken into account when examining this important tissue for exposure-induced changes.

## References


Brockmeyer C, Thiedmann KU, Heinrich U, Mohr U (1989) Light and scanning electron microscopic investigation of the laryngeal mucosa of Syrian golden hamsters. Exp Pathol 36:237–245

Brown HR, Monticello TM, Maronpot RR, Randall HW, Hotchkiss JR, Morgan KT (1991) Proliferative and neoplastic lesions in the rodent nasal cavity. Toxicol Pathol 19:358–372

Chevalier HJ, Dontenwill W (1972) Experimental studies on deposition of inhaled particles in the larynxes of Syrian golden hamsters. Z Versuchstierkd 14:271–276

Coggins CR, Ayres PH, Mosberg AT, Sagartz JW, Burger GT, Hayes AW (1989) Ninety-day inhalation study in rats, comparing smoke from cigarettes that heat tobacco with those that burn tobacco. Fundam Appl Toxicol 13:460–483

Coggins CRE, Ayres PH, Mosberg AT, Burger GT, Sagartz JW, Hayes AW (1990) Comparative inhalation study in rats, using a second prototype of a cigarette that heats rather than burns tobacco. Inhal Toxicol 1:197–226

Glaister JR (1986) Principles of toxicologic pathology. Taylor and Francis, London

Gopinath C, Prentice DE, Lewis DJ (1987) The respiratory system. In: Gresham GA (ed) Atlas of experimental toxicologic pathology. MTP Press, Norwell, pp 22–42 (Current Histopathology, vol 13)

Harkema JR (1991) Comparative aspects of nasal airway anatomy: relevance to inhalation toxicology. Toxicol Pathol 19:321–336

Lewis DJ (1981a) Mitotic indices of rat laryngeal epithelia. J Anat 132:419–428

Lewis DJ (1981b) Factors affecting the distribution of tobacco smoke-induced lesions in the rodent larynx. Toxicol Lett 9:189–194

Lewis DJ (1991) Morphological assessment of pathological changes within the rat larynx. Toxicol Pathol 19:352–357
Lewis DJ, Prentice DE (1980) The ultrastructure of rat laryngeal epithelia. J Anat 130:617–632
Morgan KT (1991) Approaches to the identification and recording of nasal lesions in toxicology studies. Toxicol Pathol 19:337–351
Nakano T, Muto H (1987) The transitional zone in the epithelium lining the mouse epiglottis. Acta Anat 130:285–290
Renne RA, Gideon KM, Miller RA, Mellick PM, Grumbein SL (1992a). Histologic methods and interspecies variations in the laryngeal histology of F344/N rats and B6C3F1 mice. Toxicol Pathol 20:44–51
Renne RA, Wehner AP, Greenspan BJ, DeFord HS, Ragan HA, Westerberg RB, Buschbom RL, Burger GT, Hayes AW, Suber RL, Mosberg AT (1992b) 2-week and 13-week inhalation studies of aerosolized glycerol in rats. Inhal Toxicol 4:95–111
Renne RA, Sagartz JW, Burger GT (1994) Interspecies variation in the histology of toxicologically important areas in the larynges of CRL:CD rats and Syrian golden hamsters. Toxicol Pathol 21:542–546
Robbins SL (1974) Pathologic basis of disease. Saunders, Philadelphia
Sagartz JW, Madarasz AJ, Forsell MA, Burger GT, Ayres PH, Coggins CRE (1992) Histological sectioning of the rodent larynx for inhalation toxicity testing. Toxicol Pathol 20:118–121
Stevens A, Lowe SJ (1992) Histology. Gower Medical, London
Wehner AP, Renne RA, Greenspan BJ, DeFord HS, Ragan HA, Westerberg BW, Wright CW, Buschbom RL, Burger GT, Hayes AW, Coggins CRE, Mosberg AT (1990) Comparative subchronic inhalation bioassay in hamsters of a cigarette that only heats tobacco. Inhal Toxicol 2:255–284

# Effects of Xenobiotics on the Larynx of the Rat, Mouse and Hamster

Rodney A. Miller and Roger A. Renne

## Introduction

The larynx as a common site for lesions caused by inhaled xenobiotics has largely been ignored until recently (Gopinath et al. 1987; Lewis 1991; Renne et al. 1992). Laryngeal lesions tend to occur selectively at specific anatomic sites. Proper evaluation of the larynx requires a thorough knowledge of normal gross and microscopic anatomy of this organ and the availability of consistent histologic samples of specific small areas of the larynx (Renne et al. 1992).

## Spontaneous Lesions and Aging Changes

Spontaneous laryngeal lesions are rare in SPF barrier maintained rats and are limited to a few foci of inflammation at the base of the epiglottis, an inflammatory reaction in the ventral pouch due to an accumulation of hair and minimal squamous metaplasia (less than 1%; Lewis 1991). At the base of the epiglottis of aged rats and mice squamous metaplasia is also rare (less than 1%). Cystic dilatation of the submucosal glands, often containing mineralized and inflammatory debris and sometimes plant material, is common in the ventral pouch of rats and mice. Rats necropsied at 26 months of age have a higher percentage of ciliated columnar cells at the transitional zone near the base of the epiglottis than rats necropsied at 5 months of age (Renne et al. 1992). Some aged control B6C3Fl mice (24–30 months old) may have minimal hyperplasia of the squamous epithelium lining the medial aspects of the arytenoid cartilages with or without small foci of ulceration and neutrophil infiltration (Fig. 51). The base of the epiglottis remains normal. At 24 months the frequency of this finding in two chronic studies was 4% and 10%, respectively. In one 30-month study the incidence in control females was of 24% while in males only 6% were affected (R.A. Miller, personal observation).

## General Considerations

The larynx is not an unusual site for induced changes in inhalation studies. Xenobiotic-induced lesions are relatively nonspecific and of limited variety. The type of lesion is generally a function of dose rather than the nature of the chemical inhaled (Lewis 1991). Areas involved by lesions may be very small, and the abnormalities are often metaplastic lesions and resemble normal tissue in an abnormal location. Sites of predisposition for

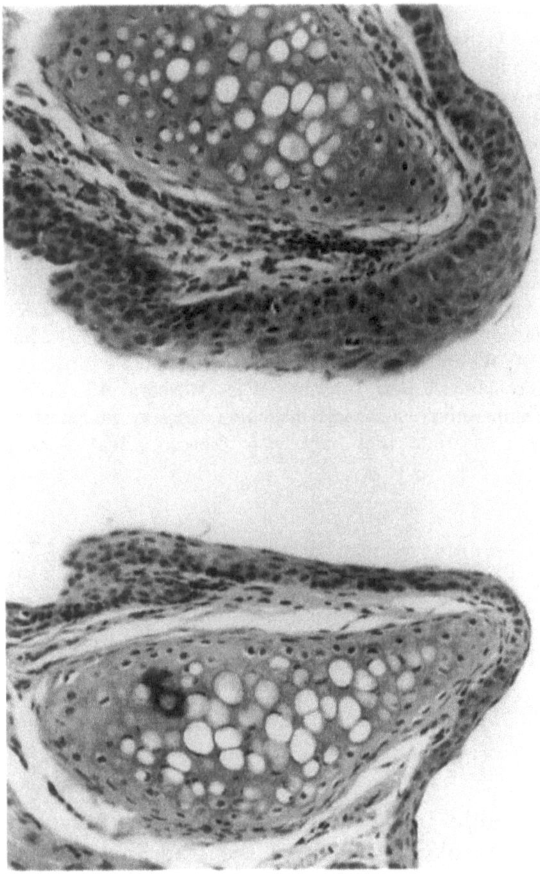

**Fig. 51.** Medial aspect of the arytenoid cartilage of a 24-month-old control mouse demonstrating (*top*) a thickened stratified squamous epithelium and focal infiltrate of inflammatory cells. H&E, ×160

development of lesions are: the (a) columnar, mostly ciliated epithelial cells at the base of the epiglottis overlying small submucosal glands, (b) medial aspect of the arytenoid cartilage (normally covered by squamous epithelium), and (c) areas anterior and lateral to the ventral pouch which is normally covered by cuboidal epithelium. In areas of cuboidal and ciliated epithelium the most common changes are necrosis, hyperplasia, and squamous metaplasia. Lesions may develop rapidly; necrosis can occur within hours, and hyperplasia and metaplasia can occur within a few days. Usually these are accompanied by an influx of neutrophils. In rats globule leukocytes disappear (Lewis 1991). In areas of squamous epithelium such as the median aspect of the arytenoid cartilage the reaction to injury is usually hyperplasia, resulting in a thickening of the squamous epithelium and rounding up of increased numbers of squamous cells. Hyperkeratosis may or may not be present.

The reasons for the susceptibility of a specific laryngeal site are generally unknown but are likely related to airflow patterns and sensitive cell types in seemingly vulnerable locations. For example, distribution of smoke-induced laryngeal lesions (hyperplasia and squamous metaplasia) differ in rats and hamsters, a point which stimulated investigations as to the causes (Lewis 1981b). Anatomically, the arytenoid cartilages of hamsters project into the laryngeal lumen less than those of rats and thus do not infringe on the airway as much. This reduces access of the tissue over the arytenoid cartilage to toxic materials in hamsters. These animals do not have arytenoid epithelial hyperplasia, as seen in rats. Also the larynx is a major constriction of the respiratory tract, and particles tend to impact on surfaces at sites of directional flow change. Squamous epithelium is considered more resistant to toxic change than respiratory epithelial cells, and cuboidal cells are intermediate in sensitivity. The more resistant squamous epithelium is generally more cranial, and the more sensitive respiratory epithelium is more caudal, except for the base of the epiglottis where respiratory epithelial cells can be found. Thus a more sensitive cell type appears in a vulnerable site (Lewis 1981b). Raab et al. (1977) investigated the larynx of rats and hamsters and found smaller amounts of particulate retention in the larynx than in the lung but higher values than in the trachea. Few chemicals result in specific lesions, however, somewhat specific lesions can be observed. An agrochemical is reported to cause an ulcerative lesion on the lateral aspects of the arytenoid cartilages rather than the medial portion and an aqueous silane solution caused granulomas (Lewis 1991). Inhalation exposures to rats, conducted in our laboratory, indicate that cobalt sulfate causes inflammatory laryngeal polyps. Although much of the literature on laryngeal lesions are described in rats, hamsters, and mice respond similarly in regard to types and location of non-neoplastic lesions (Lewis 1991; Renne et al. 1992). Some investigators report that laryngeal lesions are rarely seen with exposures to dusts (Gopinath et al. 1987); however, in studies for the National Toxicology Program, our laboratory has identified a few chemical aerosols that cause laryngeal lesions in rats and mice.

## Basic Lesion Types

In our laboratory we have induced numerous lesions in the larynx of rats, mice, and hamsters by using a variety of xenobiotics. Most lesions can be grouped into the following general categories; of course, they may coexist.

*Degeneration, Epithelial.* Frequently when laryngeal effects wane at the lower exposure levels of a study or a minimal irritant is operant, the laryngeal lesions can be subtle. Often there is only a loss of cilia, the presence of one or two cell layers at the base of the epiglottis, and a slight rounding up of those cells (Fig. 52).

*Edema.* The larynx can be an important site to evaluate in inhalation exposures when animals die during or shortly after an exposure (Fig. 53). Rats exposed to red phosphorous smoke and rats, mice, and guinea pigs exposed to the combustion products of sodium and lithium for 1–2 h die during exposure and at varying time periods after. Most of the rats that die during exposure to the highest concentration of red phosphorous smoke do not have laryngeal edema but rather a heavy fibrin-like coat to the laryngeal and tracheal surface giving it a dry "cooked" appearance (Burton et al. 1982). Other animals, exposed to lower concentrations of red phosphorous smoke or the sodium and lithium combustion products, that die during or immediately after exposure have marked laryngeal/epiglottal edema. Vesiculation and mucus accumulation results in occlusion of the laryngeal orifice (Fig. 54; Burton et al. 1982; Busch et al. 1981; Zwicker et al. 1979). Rats that survive 7–14 days after exposure to red phosphorous smoke have blunting/erosion of the epiglottis; some appear to be completely missing (Fig. 55; Burton et al. 1982).

*Acute Inflammation/Necrosis/Ulceration.* This is a severe reaction and can occur in survivors as a sequel to edema and vesiculation. The epithelium is necrotic, ulcerated, and accompanied by marked exudation (Fig. 56). There can be an ex-

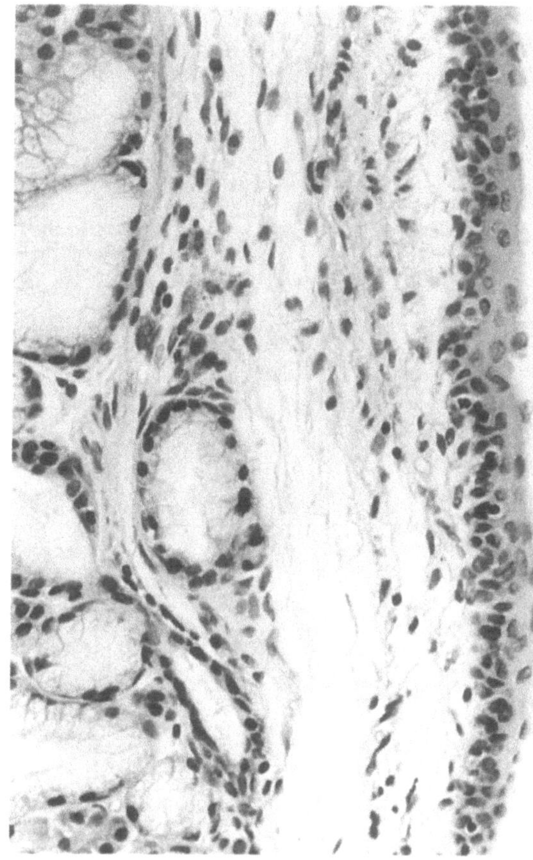

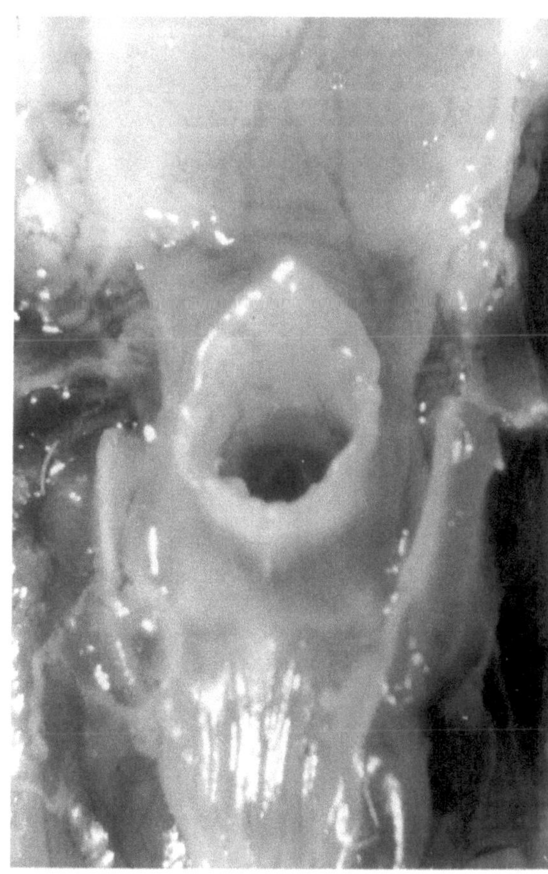

▶

**Fig. 52.** (*above*) Base of the epiglottis of a rat with degeneration of the epithelium characterized by loss of cilia and rounding up of superficial epithelial cells. H&E, ×160

**Fig. 53.** (*below*) Normal rat larynx. ×20

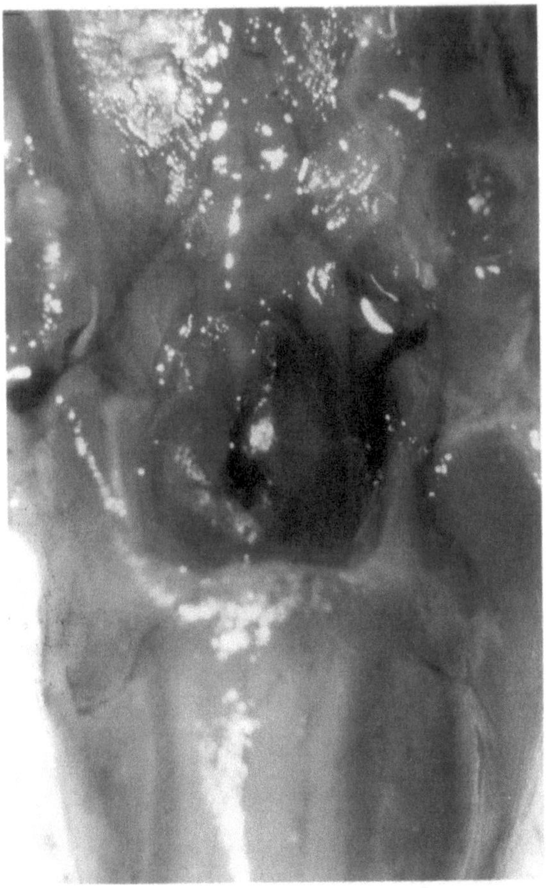

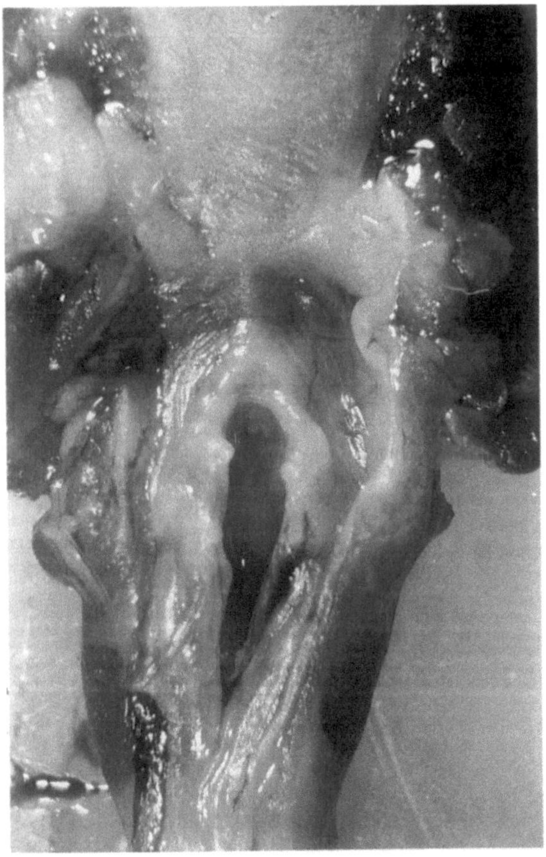

tension of inflammation into the laryngeal musculature and submucosal vascular thrombosis as in sodium and lithium combustion product exposures (Busch et al. 1981; Rebar et al. 1986). Bacterial contamination may occur in these lesions, and if severe enough, cartilage necrosis and mineralization are possible. Cartilage may protrude through epithelial defects (Lewis 1991).

*Hyperplasia.* Cell proliferation subsequent to injury may lead to an increased thickness of the laryngeal epithelium. If it occurs on the median aspect of the arytenoid cartilages, the hyperplastic epithelium is of course squamous, with underlying cells being plumper than normal and displaying some degree of karyomegaly. If the hyperplasia occurs at the base of the epiglottis, the epithelial cells of the luminal layer are oval to round, and often mitotic figures and karyomegaly of underlying cells are present.

*Inflammation Chronic/inflammatory Polyps.* Some chemicals induce changes resulting in formation of chronic inflammatory tissue/fibrosis in the submucosa and sometimes projection of this tissue into the laryngeal lumen. Cobalt sulfate exposure in rats results in the formation of inflammatory polyps projecting into the lumen of the larynx at the level of the base of the epiglottis (Fig. 57; Bucher et al. 1990). Formaldehyde exposure in mice results in submucosal fibrosis (Maronpot et al. 1986).

*Squamous Metaplasia.* In a relatively short period of time many types of compounds can induce squamous metaplasia of the laryngeal epithelium. In our experience, the base of the epiglottis is by far the most sensitive area to be affected; however, lesions are not limited to that area (Maronpot et al. 1986; Wehner et al. 1990). Squamous metaplasia is characterized by the replacement of cuboidal, ciliated, or squamoid cells by squamous epithelial cells that are usually multilayered (over three cells thick, but usually not over six or seven

◀

**Fig. 54.** (*above*) Larynx of rat that died sometime during 4-h exposure to red phosphorus smoke. Severe epiglottal and laryngeal edema occlude the laryngeal orifice. (From Burton et al. 1982). ×20

**Fig. 55.** (*below*) Rat larynx 14 days after a 1-h exposure to red phosphorus smoke. Note the absence of the epiglottis. (From Burton et al. 1982). ×20

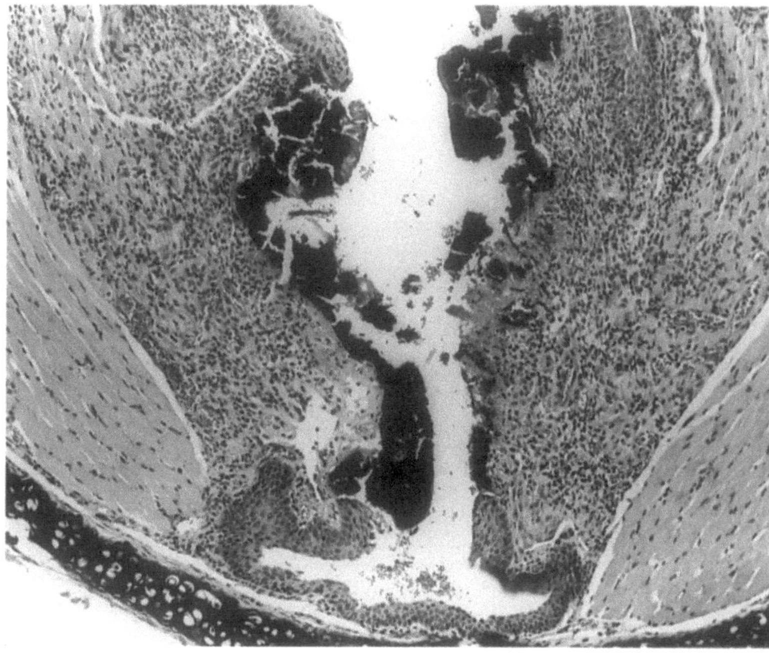

**Fig. 56.** Larynx of a mouse exposed to a strong irritant showing necrosis of the epithelium at many sites in this cross-section. Inflammatory cells infiltrate the submucosa and muscles, and inflammatory cells and necrotic debris spill into the lumen of the larynx. Note marked squamous metaplasia above and below the necrotic lesions. H&E, ×80

cell layers thick; Fig. 58). A well-defined basal cell layer may or may not be present, and the luminal layer or two of epithelial cells is horizontally oriented. Keratinization may be prominent. Typically, the squamous cells are well differentiated, but occasionally prominent focal cellular atypia occurs as in formaldehyde-exposed mice (Maronpot et al. 1986).

*Submucosal Gland Degeneration.* Rarely distention and acinar atrophy of the submucosal glands at the base of the epiglottis is observed due to obstruction of the duct by ulceration and exudation or squamous metaplasia, especially if keratinized (Lewis 1991). More frequently only squamous metaplasia of the ducts of the submucosal gland extends as a continuation of the squamous metaplasia at the base of the epiglottis.

*Laryngeal Granuloma.* Granulomas of the larynx as a response to exposure to aqueous silane solution has been reported (Lewis 1991).

### Neoplasms of the Larynx

Spontaneous tumors of the larynx of rats and mice are unreported. Polyoma virus has been reported to cause benign epithelial tumors of the submucosal glands but not those of the surface epithelial cells of the larynx of mice (Stewart et al. 1979). Few tumors of the larynx have been reported as spontaneous lesions in hamsters. Hamsters are reported to rarely (less than 1%) develop adenocarcinomas of the larynx as a spontaneous disease (Pour et al. 1976). Clear cell carcinomas of undetermined origin have been described to occur at an incidence of 1%–3% in some groups of Syrian hamsters and are more common in males than females (Pour 1985).

Studies of experimental carcinogenesis of the larynx use the hamster as the model of choice. The popularity of the hamster is due to the rarity of spontaneous tumors, its resistance to respiratory infections, and susceptibility to induction of respiratory tract cancer. Three categories of carcinogens have generally been employed: polyaromatic hydrocarbons, *N*-nitroso-compounds, and tobacco smoke (Stinson and Saffiotti 1985). Various polyaromatic hydrocarbons have generally been adsorbed to a variety of particulates (usually ferric oxide) and administered by intratracheal instillation, resulting in respiratory tract tumors including laryngeal cancers and mostly squamous cell carcinomas (Stinson and Saffiotti 1985). Many nitrosamines and nitrosamides are strong carcinogens in animals and induce a wide spectrum of tumors often independent of the exposure route. Diethylnitrosamine preferentially affects the respiratory tract, including the larynx where it can

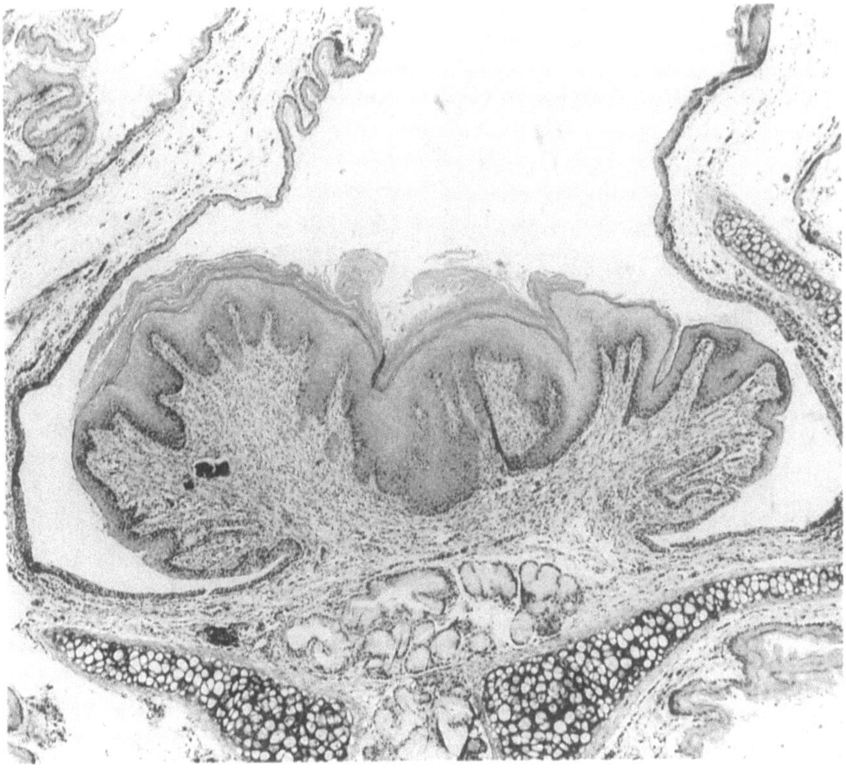

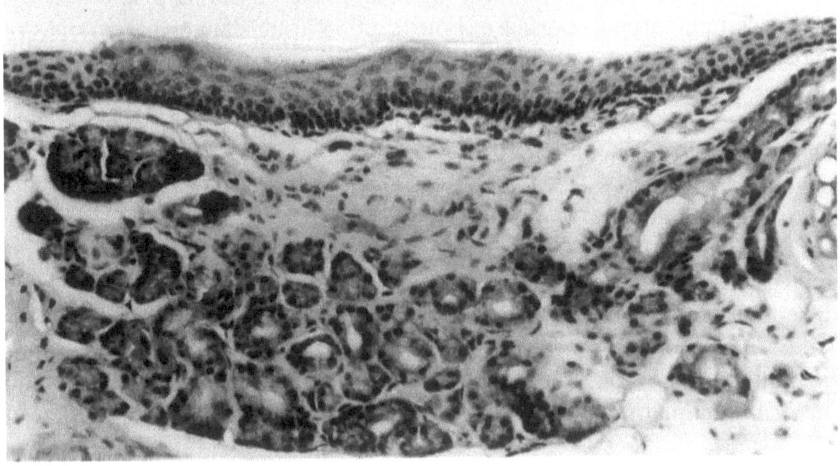

**Fig. 57.** (*above*) Larynx of rat, exposed to cobalt sulfate in a subchronic study. Note inflammatory polyp. The polyp was clearly restricted to the base of the epiglottis. H&E, ×33

**Fig. 58.** (*below*) Mouse larynx, base of epiglottis. Note well-developed squamous metaplasia. The epithelium is thicker than normal and has changed from a ciliated columnar to a squamous epithelium. H&E, ×160

cause a high incidence of papillomas regardless of the route of exposure. *N*-Methyl-*N*-nitrosourea causes squamous cell carcinomas of the larynx only when instilled intratracheally (Stinson and Saffiotti 1985). Exposure of hamsters to cigarette smoke can result in hyperplastic and squamous metaplastic lesions and squamous cell carcinomas of the larynx very similar to those found in the larynx of human smokers (Bernfeld et al. 1979). The squamous cell carcinomas may be endophytic or exophytic. F344 rats are resistant to developing laryngeal cancers after being exposed to cigarette smoke, although they do develop the nonneoplastic laryngeal lesions of hyperplasia and squamous metaplasia (Dalbey et al. 1980).

## Special Techniques to Detect and Characterize Laryngeal Changes

In rats the mitotic indices using cholchicine techniques have been determined to define the relative mitotic activity of different cell populations; 5.6% for squamous epithelium, 2.4% for squamoid epithelium of the vocal folds, 2.2% for cuboidal epithelium of the ventral lateral region at the base of the epiglottis, 1.6% for the cuboidal epithelium of the ventral pouch, and 0.6% in respiratory epithelium (Lewis 1981a). Evaluation of mitotic activity after colchicine administration following injury demonstrates increased activity by 24 h; this activity peaks in 3 days and subsides after 7 days (Lewis 1991).

Horseradish peroxidase has been used to label injured laryngeal cells in rats exposed to tobacco smoke (Lewis 1981c). Cells at the base of the epiglottis had intensely stained cytoplasm and nuclei. Staining of the cell was considered in the study to be an indication of cell membrane damage and increased permeability (cell injury).

Proliferating cell nuclear antigen and 5-bromo-2′-deoxyuridine have been used in our laboratory to measure cell turnover in the larynx after exposure to inhaled materials (personal communication).

## References


Bernfeld P, Hamburger F, Russfield AB (1979) Cigarette smoke-induced cancer in the larynx in hamsters (CINCH): a method to assay the carcinogenicity of cigarette smoke. In: Hamburger F (ed) Progress in experimental tumor research; the Syrian hamster. Karger, Basel, pp 315–319 (Toxicology and carcinogenesis research, vol 24)

Bucher JR, Elwell MR, Thompson MB, Chou BJ, Renne RA, Ragan HA (1990) Inhalation toxicity studies of cobalt sulfate in F344/N rats and B6C3Fl mice. Fundam Appl Toxicol 15:357–372

Burton FG, Clark ML, Miller RA, Schirmer RE (1982) Generation and characterization of red phosphorous smoke aerosols for inhalation exposure of laboratory animals. Am Ind Hyg Assoc J 43(10):767–772

Busch RH, McDonald KE, Briant JK (1981) Toxicology of sodium and lithium. In: Pacific northwest laboratory annual report for 1980 to the DOE assistant secretary for environment, part 1, biomedical sciences, PNL-3700. NTIS, Springfield, VA, pp 124–126

Dalbey WE, Nettesheim P, Griesemer R, Caton JE, Guerin MR (1980) Chronic inhalation of cigarette smoke by F344 rats. J Natl Cancer Inst 64(2):383–390

Gopinath C, Prentice DE, Lewis DJ (1987) The respiratory system. In: Gresham GA (ed) Atlas of experimental toxicologic pathology. MTP Press, Norwell, pp 22–42 (Current histopathology, vol 13)

Lewis DJ (1981a) Mitotic indices of rat laryngeal epithelia. J Anat 132(3):419–428

Lewis DJ (1981b) Factors affecting the distribution of tobacco smoke-induced lesions in the rodent larynx. Toxicol Lett 9:189–194

Lewis DJ (1981c) The use of horseradish peroxidase to demonstrate degenerate cells in rat larynx after acute tobacco smoke exposure. Toxicol Lett 9:195–199

Lewis DJ (1991) Morphological assessment of pathological changes within the rat larynx. Toxicol Pathol 19:352–357

Maronpot RR, Miller RA, Clarke WJ, Westerberg RB, Decker JR, Moss OR (1986) Toxicity of formaldehyde vapor in B6C3FI mice exposed for 13 weeks. Toxicology 41:253–266

Pour PM (1985) Clear cell carcinoma, larynx, Syrian hamster. Respiratory system. In: Jones TC, Mohr U, Hunt RD (eds) Monographs on pathology of laboratory animals. Springer, Berlin Heidelberg New York, pp 75–77

Pour P, Mohr U, Cardesa A, Afthoff J, Kmoch N (1976) Spontaneous tumors and common diseases in two colonies of Syrian hamsters. II. Respiratory tract and digestive system. J Natl Cancer Inst 56(5):937–948

Raab OG, Yeh HC, Newton GJ, Phalem RF, Valesquez DH (1977) Deposition of inhaled monodisperse aerosols in small rodents. In: Wafton WH (ed) Inhaled particles, vol IV. Pergamon, Oxford, pp 3–22

Rebar AH, Greenspan BJ, Allen MD (1986) Acute inhalation toxicopathology of lithium combustion aerosols in rats. Fundam Appl Toxicol 7:58–67

Renne RA, Gideon KM, Miller RA, Mellick PW, Grumbein SL (1992) Histologic methods and interspecies variations in the laryngeal histology of F344/N rats and B6C3Fl mice. Toxicol Pathol 20(1):44–50

Stewart HL, Dunn TB, Snell C, Deringer MK (1979) Tumours of the respiratory tract. In: Turusov VS (ed) Pathology of tumours in laboratory animals, vol II. Tumours of the mouse. International Agency for Research on Cancer, Lyons, pp 251–288

Stinson SR, Saffiotti U (1985) Experimental laryngeal carcinogenesis. In: Ferlito A (ed) Cancer of the larynx. CRC, Boca Raton, pp 36–51

Wehner AP, Renne RA, Greenspan BJ, DeFord HS, Ragan HA, Westerberg RB, Wright CW, Buschbom RL, Burger GT, Hayes AW, Coggins CRE, Mosberg AT (1990) Comparative subchronic inhalation bioassay in hamsters of a cigarette that only heats tobacco. Inhal Toxicol 2:255–284

Zwicker GM, Allen MD, Stevens DL (1979) Toxicity of aerosols of sodium reaction products. J Environ Pathol Toxicol 2:1139–1150

# Development of Syrian Golden Hamster Tracheal Epithelium During Prenatal and Immediate Postnatal Stages

Makito Emura

## Introduction

The Syrian golden hamster (*Mesocricetus auratus*) makes an excellent model for studies on chemical carcinogenesis of the respiratory tract, in particular the trachea (Wynder and Hecht 1976). This organ is particularly sensitive to *N*-nitroso compounds, among others. It is also possible using these compounds to induce tumors transplacentally (Mohr 1973; Mohr et al. 1979). Recent studies have shown that in both pre- and postnatal hamster trachea not only squamous cell papillomas but also neuroendocrine cell tumors can be developed chemically, and the latter in particular also spontaneously (Mohr et al. 1994). The anlage of the trachea in the fetus cannot be easily distinguished until after the 9th day of pregnancy, but only a few days later signs of rapid growth and differentiation are clearly recognizable. Because of the great importance of this tissue at perinatal stages this chapter incorporates the more recent findings (McDowell et al. 1985a,b, 1994a,b) and attempts to assist in exploring new insights into the relationship between carcinogen susceptibility and cellular differentiation.

## Predifferentiation Stage

*Light Microscopy.* The tracheobronchial rudiments of the Syrian hamster become independent of the early esophageal ducts (Fig. 59) between the 9th and 10th gestational days. The next stage, extending from the 10th to 11th gestational days, can be regarded as the predifferentiation stage, since no marked sign of differentiation is detected in the epithelium either by light or electron microscopy. At this stage the tracheal epithelium is composed mainly of one layer of tall and narrow columnar cells (Fig. 60); the nuclei are elongated, ovoid, or round and basally situated. At the luminal surfaces the epithelium also contains a few ellipsoid or polygonal cells. Several cells possess cytoplasmic vacuoles. In a relatively few epithelial cells the luminal portion of the cytoplasm is PAS positive. When pretreated with diastase, very few cells subsequently react to PAS and none stain with Alcian blue.

*Electron Microscopy.* At this stage no signs of differentiation can be detected in the cells, and no particular cell types are discernible (Fig. 61). The

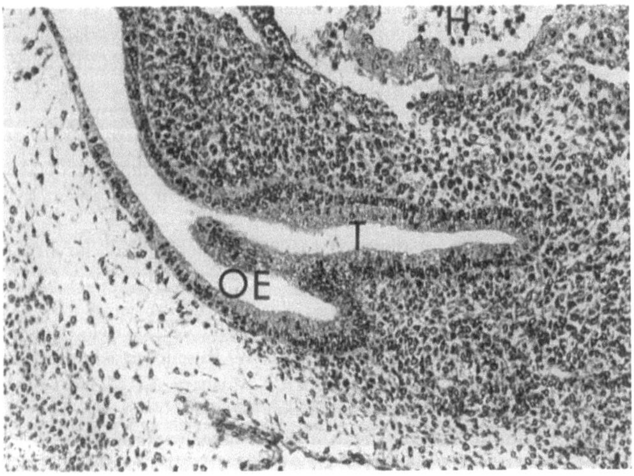


**Fig. 59.** (*left*) Longitudinal sections of tracheal epithelium, Syrian hamster on the 10th gestational day. *T*, Trachea; *OE*, esophagus; *H*, heart; *top*, ventral epithelium; *bottom*, dorsal epithelium. H&E, ×43

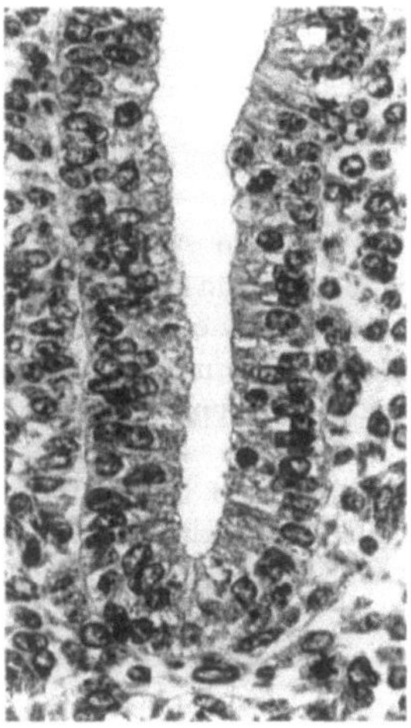

**Fig. 60.** (*right*) Trachea at higher magnification. H&E, ×106

irregular luminal surface usually possesses sparse cytoplasmic projections or microvilli of various lengths (Figs. 62, 63). The nuclei are round to ovoid, and their contours are mostly smooth and usually contain two to four nucleoli. The nuclear chromatin fibrils are uniformly dispersed in the nucleoplasm of epithelial cells, and none of the chromatin condensations of the type seen in maturing cell types are recognizable until the 12th day. In the stromal fibroblasts, however, such chromatin condensations are already beginning to occur. Glycogen granules are either scattered throughout the cytoplasm or accumulate in a small part of it (Fig. 62). Some cells possess one or two cilia (Fig. 64). In the luminal part of the cytoplasm a few centrioles are occasionally observed (Figs. 61, 64) and peculiar, tightly bound intercellular junctions are formed directly against the lumen (Figs. 61, 62). The mitochondria are round to elongated, frequently club-shaped, and their matrices contain dense or sparse fine fibrillar or granular materials. Free polyribosomes prevail.

Distinct but not well-developed Golgi apparatus assumes mainly lamellar structures with some vesicles, mostly located near the nuclei (Fig. 62). The basement membrane is distinct and further deposition of fibrillar material progresses.

On the 10th gestational day the smooth and rough endoplasmic reticulum (ER) of the epithelial cells seems poorly developed and in most cases flattened sac or saccule forms are found. The outer nuclear membrane in these cells very frequently has widely distributed extranuclear protrusions (Emura 1978) and often contains membranous structures.

On the 11th gestational day the smooth and rough ER increases only slightly (Fig. 62), and the frequency and size of the protrusions extending from the outer nuclear membrane decrease remarkably. The rough and smooth membrane bound vacuoles and vesicles also notably decrease in number. Around the periphery of the nuclei peculiar intranuclear membranous inclusions appear at intervals, and their frequency increases as time progresses.

The possibility that these vacuoles and vesicles contribute to the formation of ER cannot be excluded since in vertebrate and invertebrate oocytes (Wischnitzer 1974) and in embryonic epithelium of chick choroidal plexus (Birge and Doolin 1974) the rough ER has been demonstrated to originate in vesicles derived from the outer nuclear membrane.

## Early Morphological Indication of Differentiation

*Light Microscopy.* On the 12th gestational day the epithelial cells are somewhat flatter than those seen on previous days. No distinct cell types are detected by light microscopy except a cell type constituting neuroepithelial bodies (NEB; McDowell et al. 1994a). While NEB can sometimes, though not always, be recognized in H&E sections (Fig. 97), singly existing endocrine cells are difficult to identify without immunohistochemical staining (McDowell et al. 1994a). At an early stage of differentiation NEB are distributed more densely in the larynx and cranial part of the trachea than in the caudal part. On the 13th gestational day approximately 20 horseshoe-shaped cartilaginous condensates consisting of mesenchymal cells are formed in the trachea (Fig. 65). In the epithelium three cell types can be distinguished. These are tentatively designated as type I, type II, and type III cells in this report.

Type I cells feature a hemispherical luminal apex protruding into the lumen and are characterized by a somewhat basophilic or less eosinophilic cytoplasm (Fig. 65). Flat luminal surfaces and somewhat eosinophilic or less basophilic cytoplasm characterize type II cells (Fig. 66). Cells of this type are most prominent in the dorsal epithelium and are not positive to PAS. Type III cells are basally situated without reaching the lumen and have oblong, triangular, or polygonal shapes (Fig. 65). The presence of type I and type III cells causes the epithelium to assume a double-layered appearance in parts, i.e., a luminal and basal layer. These observations have been confirmed by a detailed study (McDowell et al. 1985a). Several epithelial cells react positively to PAS, but after pretreatment with diastase practically no cell has a positive reaction to PAS, suggesting the presence of glycogen in the cytoplasm.

*Electron Microscopy.* On the 12th gestational day the luminal apices in most epithelial cells protrude slightly into the lumen, although their luminal surfaces are still irregular. The scattered glycogen granules have diminished in many of the cells; the ER is not well developed, possesses rough surfaces, and assumes flattened saclike forms.

The outer nuclear membrane again starts to form circumscribed extensions, which are small but similar to those observed on the 10th gestational

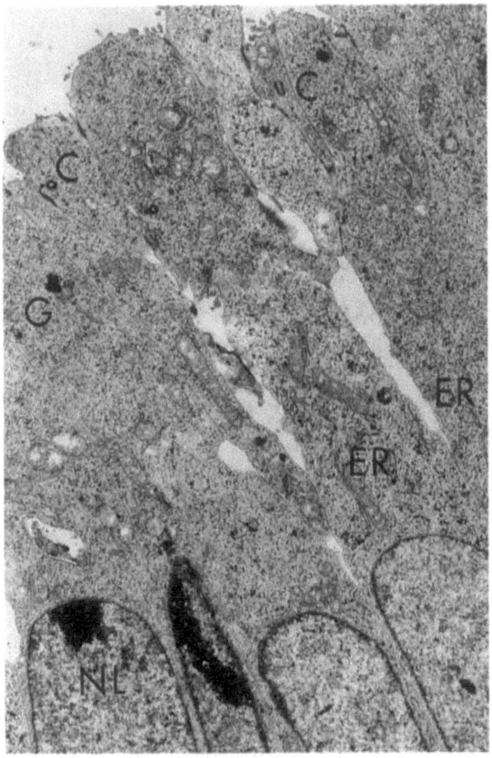


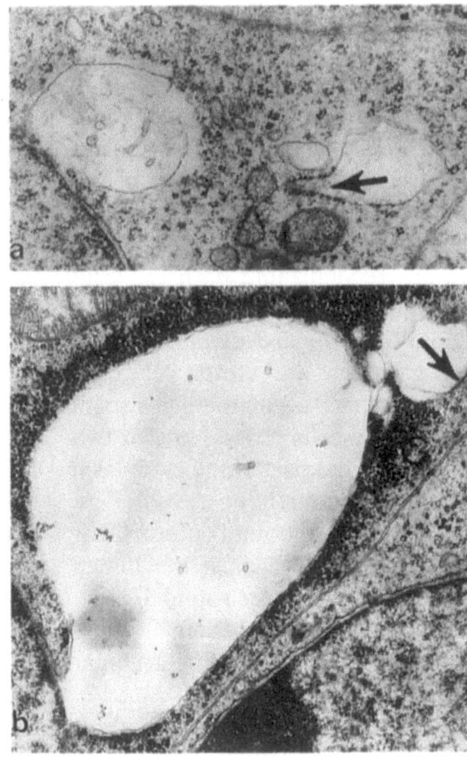


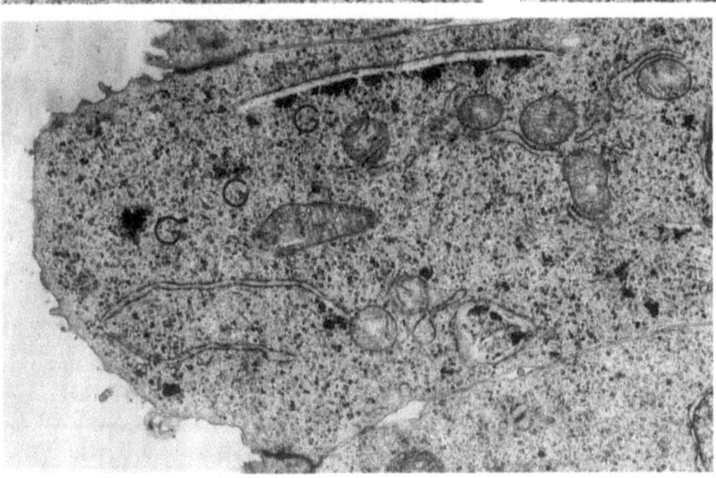


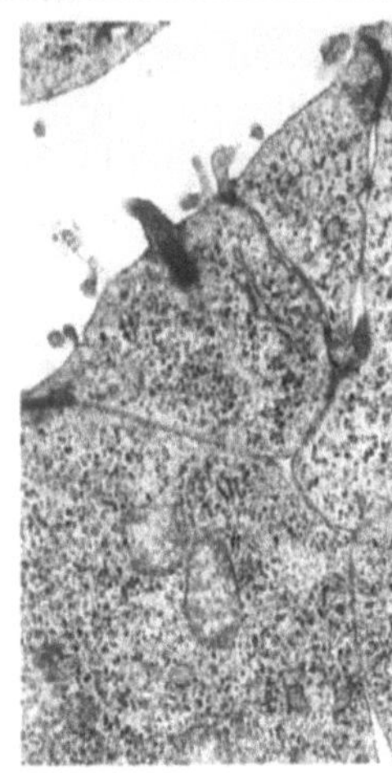

**Fig. 61.** (*upper left*) Epithelial cells on the 11th gestational day. Note sparse endoplasmic reticulum (*ER*), abundance of free polyribosomes and glycogen granules (*G*), uniformly diffuse nuclear chromatin fibrils, smooth contours of nuclei, distinct nucleolonemas of the nucleoli (*NL*), and intercellular spaces. In comparison with the 10th gestational day, the only difference is the absence of cytoplasmic vacuoles and vesicles. Centrioles (*C*) and small cytoplasmic projections can be seen. Uranyl acetate and lead citrate, TEM, ×5070

**Fig. 62.** (*lower left*) Epithelial cell on the 11th gestational day. Note the small amount of ER and glycogen (*G*). Uranyl acetate and lead citrate, TEM, ×11 640

**Fig. 63.** (*upper right*) **a** Vesicles in the epithelial cells on the 10th gestational day. Note relatively large polyribosomes in the cytoplasm and vesicles (*arrow*), which begin to resemble ER. Uranyl acetate and lead citrate, TEM, ×19 890. **b** Accumulation of glycogen (*G*) can be observed around the protrusions and vesicle membrane. *Arrow*, ribosomes attached to membrane. Uranyl acetate and lead citrate, TEM, ×14 230

**Fig. 64.** (*lower right*) A solitary immature cilium projecting from the luminal surface. Uranyl acetate and lead citrate, TEM, ×11 640

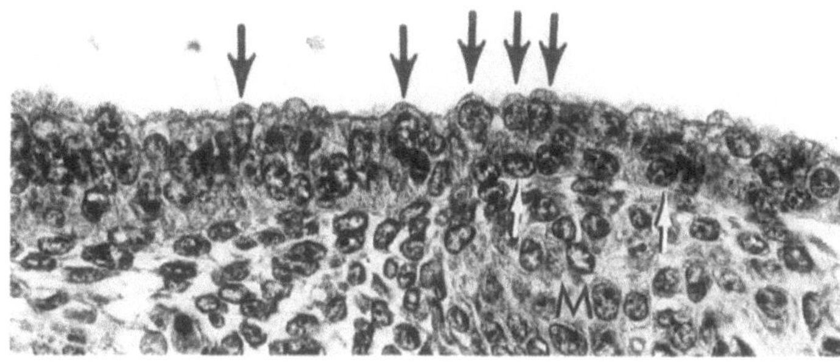


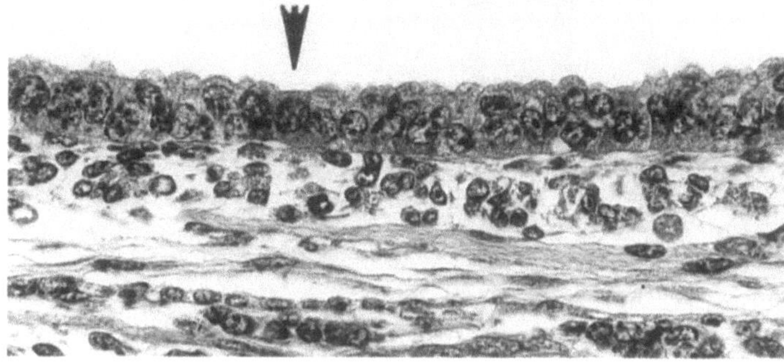

**Fig. 65.** (*above*) Longitudinal section of tracheal epithelium. Cranial ventral section. A cartilaginous mesenchyme condensate (*M*), cells with hemispherical luminal apices and basophilic cytoplasm (*black arrows*), and basally situated cells (*white arrows*) are shown. H&E, ×170

**Fig. 66.** (*below*) Longitudinal section of tracheal epithelium. Caudal, dorsal section. Note cell with flat luminal surface and eosinophilic cytoplasm (*thick arrow*). H&E, ×170

day. Membranous and vesicular intranuclear inclusions at the nuclear periphery occur more frequently than on the 11th gestational day. The rough- and smooth membrane bound vacuoles and vesicles seen as early as the 10th gestational day occur again, although only occasionally.

The nuclei are still round to ovoid in shape with smooth contours. Distinct condensations of nuclear chromatin fibrils occur in 20%–30% of epithelial cells along the nuclear envelope as well as in the inner area of the nuclei, although this is much less extensive than in maturing fetal mucous cells.

On the 13th gestational day three cell types can be distinguished in the epithelium. The first type (I) is composed of cells with smooth hemispherical luminal surfaces protruding into the lumen (Fig. 67). The second type (II) consists of cells with flat luminal surfaces, on which several short microvilli or cytoplasmic projections can be observed (Figs. 67, 68). The ventral and lateral epithelial cells are largely composed of type I cells. In the dorsal epithelium type II cells seldom occur; type I cells still predominate. Cells of both types often contain one or two regional accumulations of a considerable amount of vesicular and tubular smooth ER in the luminal apices (Figs. 67, 69).

In the luminal cytoplasm, the rough ER and free polyribosomes are frequently more abundant in type I than in type II cells. However, the basal cytoplasm of both cell types apparently contains the same amount of rough ER. In a small number of type I cells fairly numerous ER vesicles surrounded by a partly rough membrane can be observed. Generally in both types of cells rough ER increases only fractionally in comparison with previous days of development. Connection of smooth ER with Golgi (or dictyosome) cisternae is occasionally encountered.

Located near the smooth ER accumulations and dictyosomes sometimes found in type II cells are small areas of fine fibrillar material, often interspersed with a few dark granules, ranging from 21 × 21 to 87 × 114 nm (average 49 × 65 nm) in size. These are identified as structures similar to "proliferative elements" (Dirksen and Crocker 1966; Figs. 68, 69), and they also occur in the luminal cytoplasm of type I cells, although much less frequently. The inner sections of this fibrillar material are usually devoid of ribosomes.

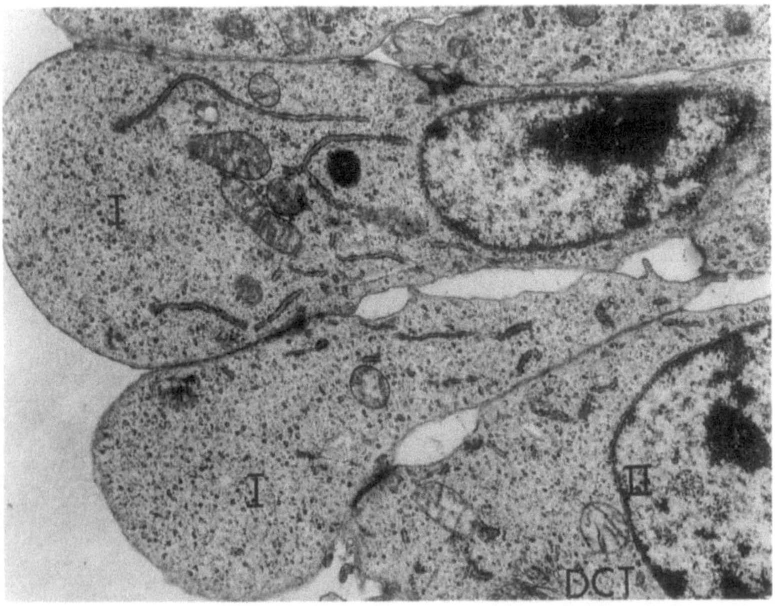


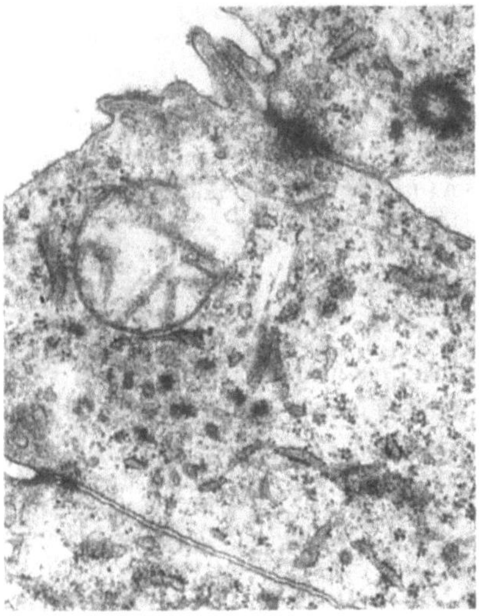

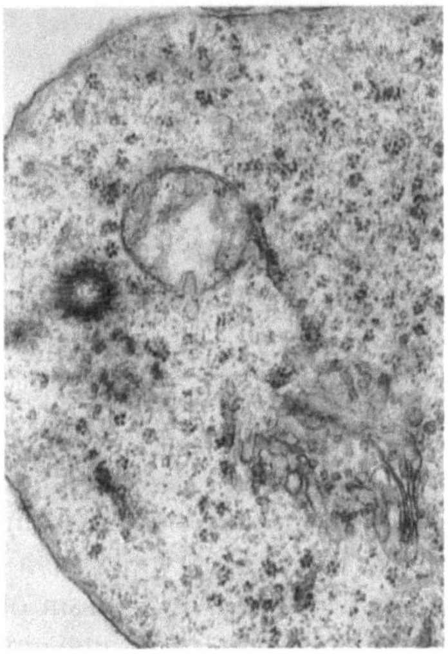

**Fig. 67.** (*above*) Luminal cytoplasm of cells with hemispherical surfaces (type I) and cells with flat luminal surfaces (type II). Note the abundance of rough ER. DCT, Dictyosome. Uranyl acetate, lead citrate, TEM, ×11640

**Fig. 68.** (*lower left*) Luminal part of a type II cell on the 13th gestational day. Note fibrillar material interspersed with dark granules, 21 × 21 to 87 × 114nm in size. Uranyl acetate and lead citrate, TEM, ×22770

**Fig. 69.** (*lower right*) Luminal part of a cell resembling type I on the 13th gestational day. Fibrillar material interspersed with dark granules can be seen (26 × 53 to 42 × 65nm). Note the proximity of the fibrillar material to existing centriole. Uranyl acetate and lead citrate, TEM, ×22770

The third type (III) of cells are basally situated in the epithelium and resemble type I cells except that they have no free luminal surfaces. Thus, the type I, II, and III cells are consistent with presecretory, preciliated, and prebasal cells, respectively (McDowell et al. 1985a). In cells of all three types, as well as stromal fibroblasts, a few immature-looking cilia and centrioles occasionally occur.

On the 13th gestational day the circumscribed extensions of outer nuclear membrane in the trachea, also encountered in the three epithelial cell types and in stromal fibroblasts, are more frequent and more conspicuous than on the previous day. Their frequency and size are similar to those of the 10th gestational day.

The vesicular and tubular intranuclear inclusions are also more frequent and more conspicuous than on the 11th and 12th days. However, the rough and smooth membrane bound vacuoles and vesicles, which persistently occur, are not as fre-

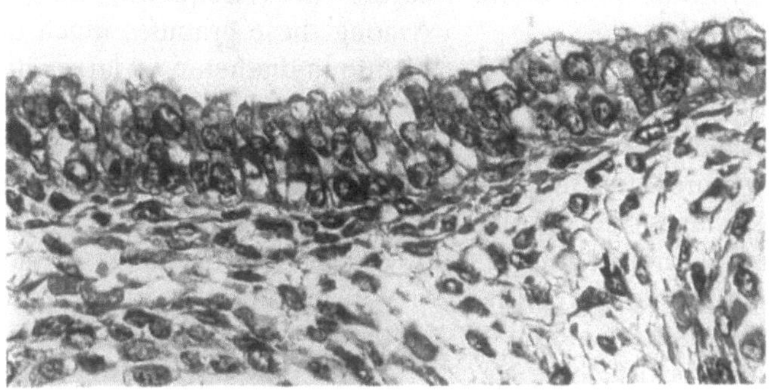

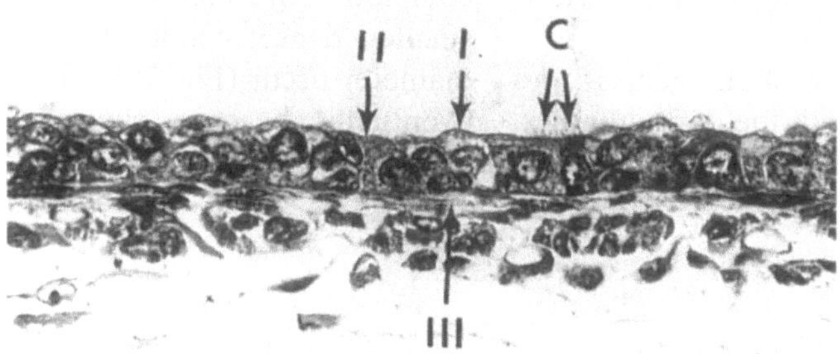


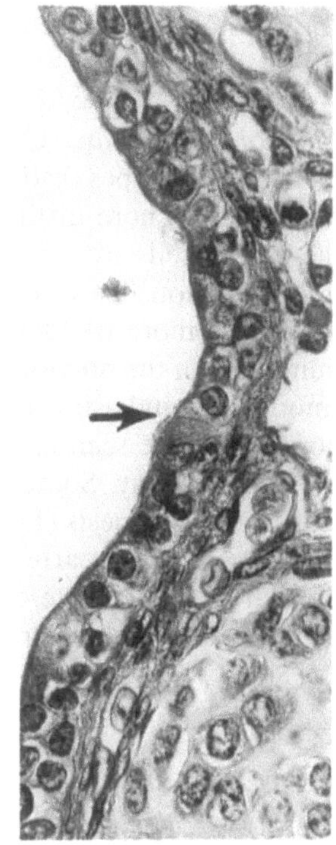

**Fig. 70.** (*upper left*) Longitudinal section of the ventral epithelium (pars cartilaginea). No ciliated cells are seen. Cytoplasmic vesicles are prominent. H&E, ×170

**Fig. 71.** (*lower left*) Longitudinal section of dorsal epithelium (pars membranacea). A few obviously ciliated cells (*C*), type I cells (*I*), type II cells (*II*), and type III cells (*III*) classified on the 14th gestational day. H&E, ×170

**Fig. 72.** (*right*) Longitudinal section of cranial part of the ventral tracheal epithelium on the 16th gestational day. Note ciliated cell (*arrow*). H&E, ×170

quent as in the differentiating type II cells on the 14th gestational day. These vacuoles and vesicles appear to fuse occasionally with the preexisting rough ER.

Golgi cisternae are sometimes connected to the nuclear envelope. Condensation of nuclear chromatin occurs more extensively on the 13th gestational day in 80%–90% of cells of all types, including the stromal fibroblast.

## Differentiation of Ciliated Cells

Electron microscopy reveals that the primary stage of ciliogenesis takes place on the 13th gestational day in some of the type II cells. However, the first ciliated cells can be detected on the 14th gestational day in the dorsal epithelium (pars membranacea) by both light and electron microscopy. Quantitative data on the various perinatally differentiating cell types are now available (McDowell et al. 1985a,b).

*Light Microscopy.* The epithelium on the 14th gestational and following days of development also has a double-layered appearance. The ciliated cells possess granular eosinophilic cytoplasm and flat luminal surfaces (Figs. 70, 71), which are features similar to those of the type II cells of the 13th gestational day. At the caudal part of the dorsal epithelium these cells are usually cylindrical or cuboidal, sometimes oblong, and extend from the basement membrane to the lumen. In the cranial part of the epithelium they often assume either conchoidal or bell shapes. Ciliated cells are sparse in the ventral and lateral epithelium (pars cartilaginea). In most of the trachea the cilia are often longer in the cranial part than in the caudal part of the epithelium.

The type II cells observed on the 13th gestational day (Fig. 66) are still encountered frequently on the 14th gestational day, particularly in the middle to caudal part of the dorsal epithelium. On the 15th and 16th gestational days ciliated cells are found only sporadically in the ventral and lateral epithelium (Fig. 72). On the last gestational day the cells are well developed in the dorsal epithelium but occur less frequently in the ventral and lateral epithelium.

*Electron Microscopy.* On the 14th gestational day the three cell types distinguished on the previous day develop more distinct features. On this day the type II cells are at various stages of organellic differentiation. They possess flat luminal surfaces and occur more frequently in the dorsal epithelium than on the previous day. A small amount of smooth ER and a few ribosomes exist; these can occasionally be seen in cells of the same type on the previous day. Some cells are seen in various stages of ciliogenesis (Figs. 73–80).

In the cells at an early stage of ciliogenesis, the fibrillar material alone or with the dark granules, 39 × 42 to 73 × 96 nm (average 53 × 66 nm), occurs more frequently than on the 13th day. Among these granules much darker bodies, 63–148 nm in diameter, or larger hollow bodies, 148–208 nm and 63–104 nm in outer and inner diameters, respectively, are often identified as "condensation forms" (Dirksen and Crocker 1966; Figs. 73–78). Tubular and vesicular structures are often located near areas of dark granules (Figs. 76–79). In cells at a different stage of ciliogenesis several precentrioles, measuring between 116 × 127 and 158 × 180 nm are associated with the condensation forms. In more advanced cells almost complete centrioles measuring 180–380 nm and smaller, denser condensation forms 48–95 nm in diameter occur (Fig. 78). These centrioles, which eventually become ciliary basal bodies, are formed by a process which Anderson and Brenner

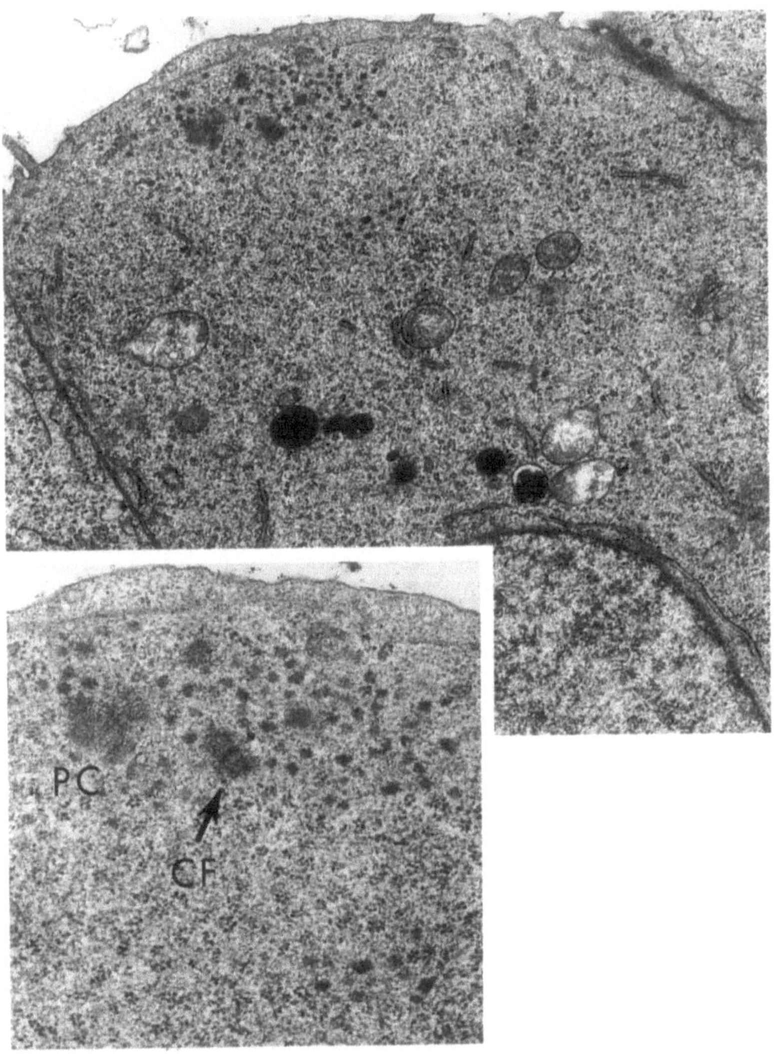


**Fig. 73.** (*above*) Type II (ciliated) cell on the 14th gestational day. Note absence of rough ER. Uranyl acetate and lead citrate, TEM, ×16640

**Fig. 74.** (*below*) Higher magnification of Fig. 73. *PC*, Precentrioles; *CR*, "condensation forms." Uranyl acetate and lead citrate, TEM, ×31590

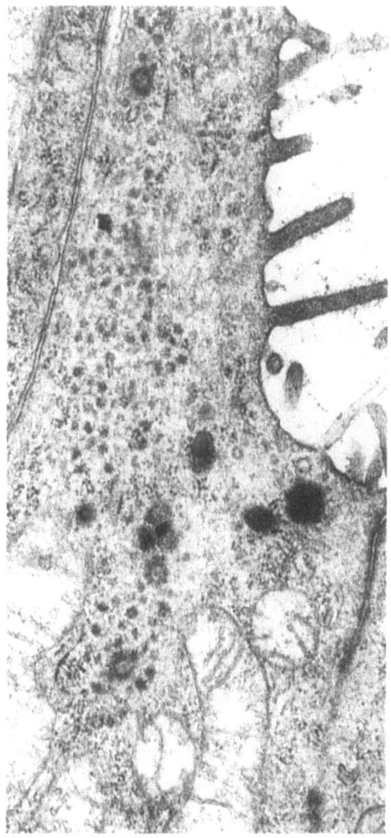

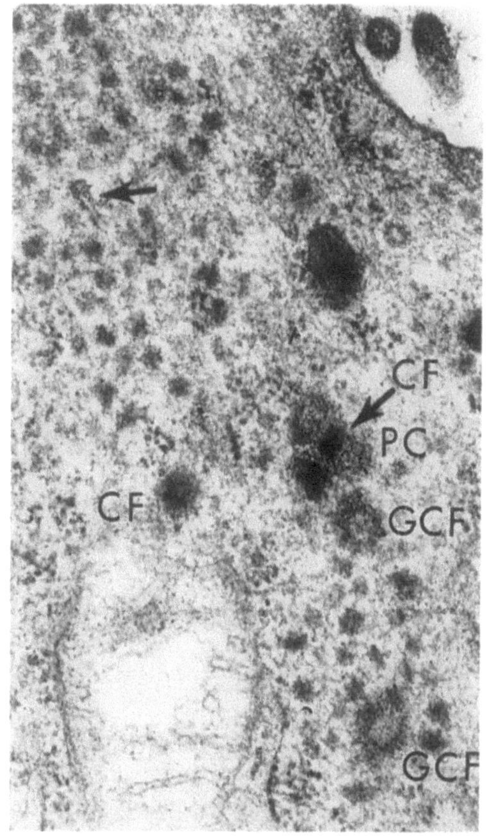


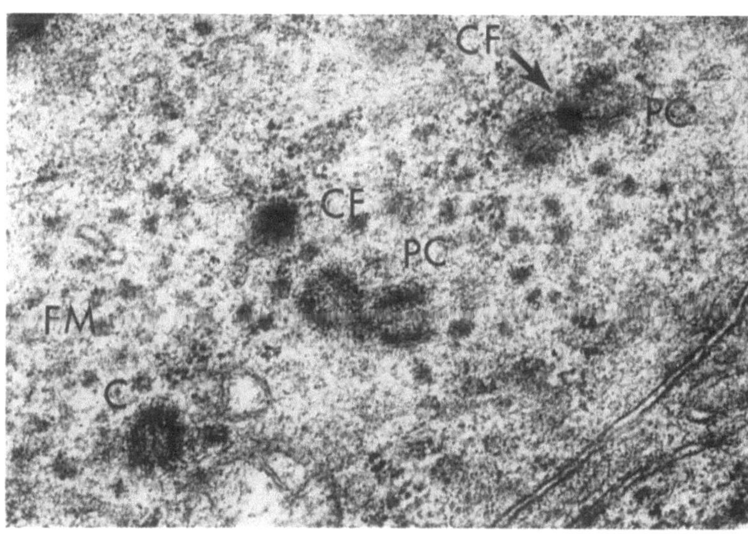


**Fig. 75.** (*upper left*) Type II (ciliated) cell on the 14th gestational day. Uranyl acetate and lead citrate. ×22770

**Fig. 76.** (*upper right*) Higher magnification of Fig. 75. *GCF*, "Growing condensation forms" with hollow center; *CF*, a solitary condensation form; *PC*, precentriole; *arrow*, ciliary bud-like tubule. Uranyl acetate and lead citrate, TEM, ×47320

**Fig. 77.** (*below*) Type II (ciliated) cell on the 14th gestational day. Various structures related to ciliogenesis: *FM*, fibrogranular material; *C*, centriole; *CF*, condensation forms; *PC*, precentrioles. Uranyl acetate and lead citrate, TEM, ×47320

(1971) termed "acentriolar basal body formation," in which the centrioles develop together with structures which bear no resemblance to centrioles.

The process of ciliogenesis described here seems to correspond to this theory. In developing fetal rats (Stockinger and Cireli 1965; Dirksen and Crocker 1966) and mice (Frisch and Farbman 1968) such fibrogranular material has been reported. Stockinger and Cireli (1965) suggested

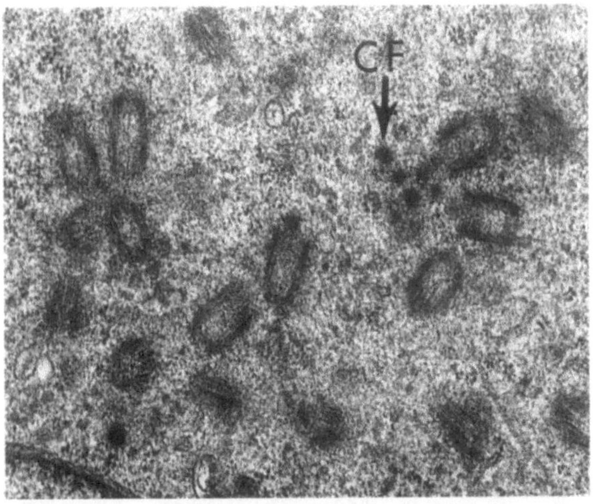


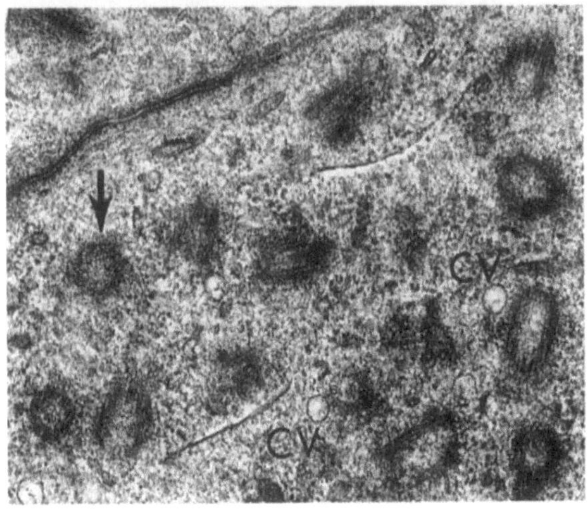


**Fig. 78.** (*above*) Type II cell. Centrioles near maturation and condensation forms (*CF*). Uranyl acetate and lead citrate, TEM, ×31590

**Fig. 79.** (*below*) Type II cell. Almost mature centrioles. Note the microtubule triplets in one cross-section (*arrow*) and the centriole-associated vesicles (*CV*). Uranyl acetate and lead citrate, TEM, ×31590

that this fibrogranular material is formed de novo without any influence of preexisting mature centrioles, and that the granular materials which were considered to be precentrioles develop through various intermediate stages into mature centrioles. Dirksen and Crocker (1966) found a direct link between mature centrioles and this fibrogranular material and termed them "proliferative elements." In the fetal rat Sorokin (1968) suggested a similar process in which "deuterosomes" seem to correspond to the condensation forms. Another possibility is that the preexisting centrioles are decondensed into the fibrillar material which would function later as templates for new microtubule proteins (Dirksen and Crocker 1966; Staprans and Dirksen 1974). In cells at a somewhat later stage of ciliogenesis complete centrioles possessing nine triplets of microtubules accumulate in the luminal apices (Fig. 79). The cells undergoing ciliogenesis usually possess well-developed microvilli. Glycogen granules are often absent from the type II and ciliated cells. In the developing Syrian hamster trachea the fibrillar material with dense granules can first be detected on the 13th gestational day, and only on the following day do ciliated cells occur. Therefore it can be supposed that a period of 1 day is sufficient for completion of the successive stages preceding ciliogenesis.

From the 14th gestational day onward, ciliogenesis occurs in an increasing number of type II cells. Preciliated and ciliated cells are more prevalent caudally (McDowell et al. 1985a). On the 1st postnatal day typical mature ciliated cells are frequently observed (Fig. 81). However, ciliogenesis on the 14th and subsequent gestational days is not always restricted to type II cells but also occurs in cells apparently of type I at various stages of differentiation of secretory systems, although much less frequently. Similar observations have been confirmed by other authors (Keenan et al. 1983).

## Differentiation of Non-endocrine Secretory Cells

*Light Microscopy.* On the 14th gestational day type I and type II cells are prominent in the epithelium (Figs. 70, 71). Their cytoplasm often appears vacuolated. The epithelium of the 15th and 16th gestational days resembles that of the 14th gestational day. However, the luminal apices of the type I cells are no longer hemispherical but slightly protruded and round. Although occurring at a low frequency, cells with pale cytoplasm between the luminal surface and nucleus appear in the cranial part of the epithelium (Fig. 82). On the last gestational day the epithelial cells with pale cytoplasm (Fig. 82) are more numerous, and the first mature mucous cells are observed (Fig. 83). The number of cells that react positively to PAS increases sharply around the 14th gestational day (Emura and Mohr 1975) and continues to increase during the next 4 weeks of the postnatal period. Notably, even the type III cells react positively to PAS, particularly around the nuclei. After dia-

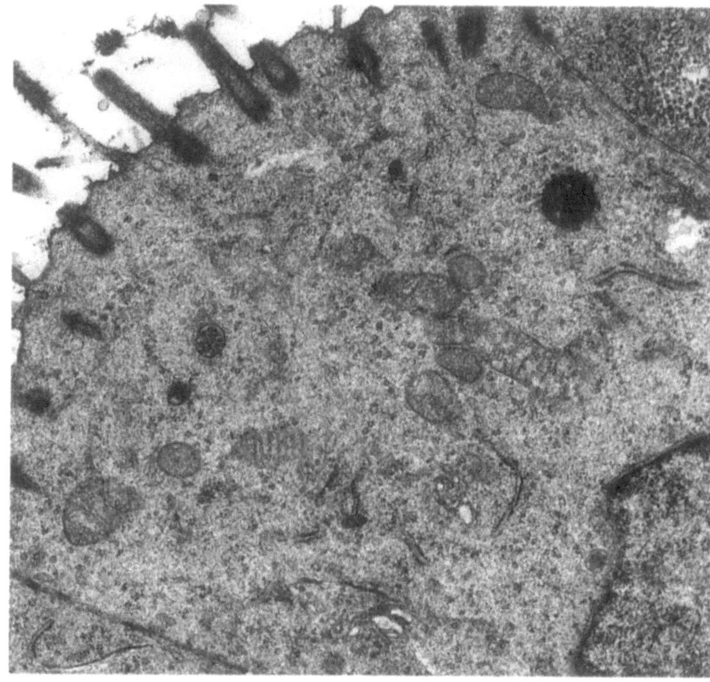

**Fig. 80.** Cilia growing from centrioles in type II cells on the 14th gestational day. Uranyl acetate and lead citrate. ×16640

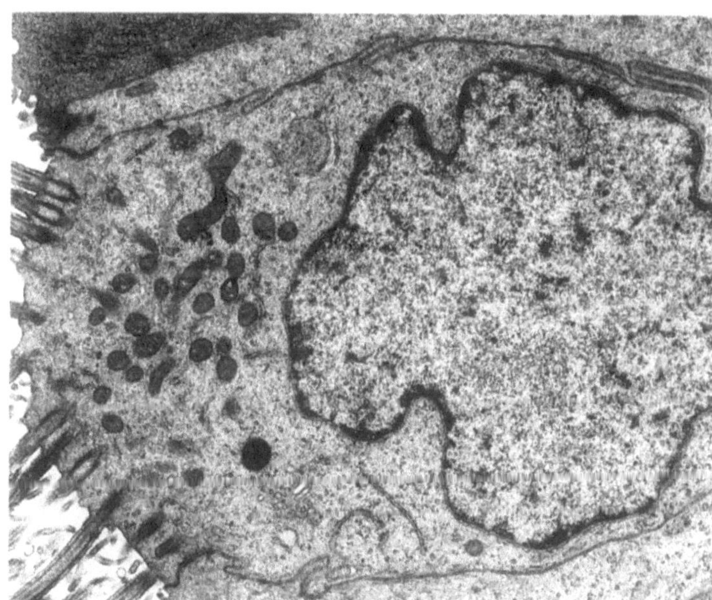

**Fig. 81.** Mature ciliated cell on the 1st postnatal day. Uranyl acetate and lead citrate, TEM, ×11640

stase pretreatment, however, the positive PAS reaction disappears from around the nuclei of many cells, especially from those of the basal layer (type III).

On the 14th gestational day very few cells react to PAS following diastase, but around the 16th gestational or 1st neonatal day the frequency of such cells increases (Emura and Mohr 1975). In these cells only the cytoplasmic portion between the luminal surface and nucleus reacts positively to PAS. With progressive development these areas acquire more and larger granules, expand, and finally occupy the entire cytoplasm above the nucleus. Many differentiating type I cells contain PAS-positive material in the cytoplasm above the nucleus. Such material greatly diminishes in cells toward the caudal part of the epithelium (Fig. 84). Few cells stain with Alcian blue until the 14th gestational day. From this day onward they remain at an average level of 13% of epithelial cells,

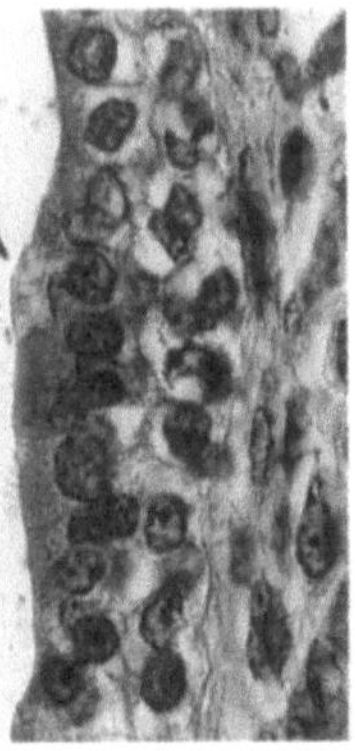

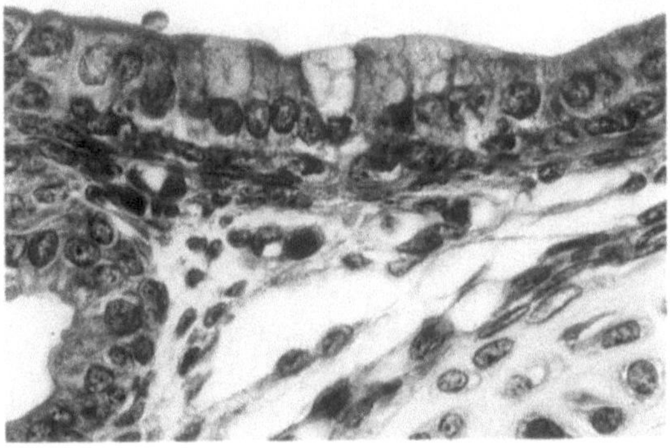

**Fig. 82.** (*left*) Dorsal epithelium on the 15th gestational day. Note cell with pale cytoplasm (*arrow*). H&E, ×170

**Fig. 83.** (*right*) Ventral epithelium, 15th gestational day. A few secretory cells with pale cytoplasm. H&E, ×170

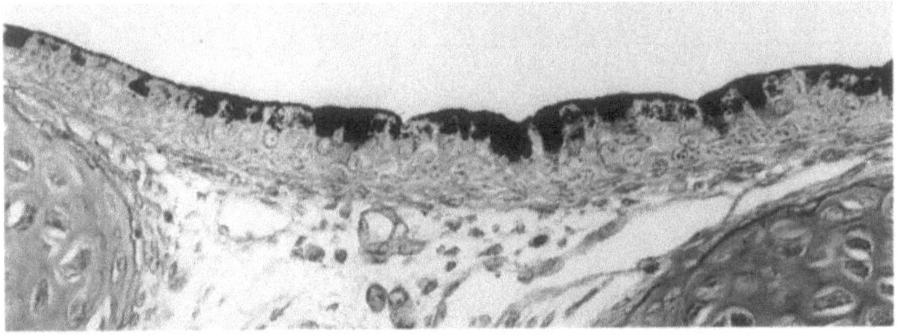

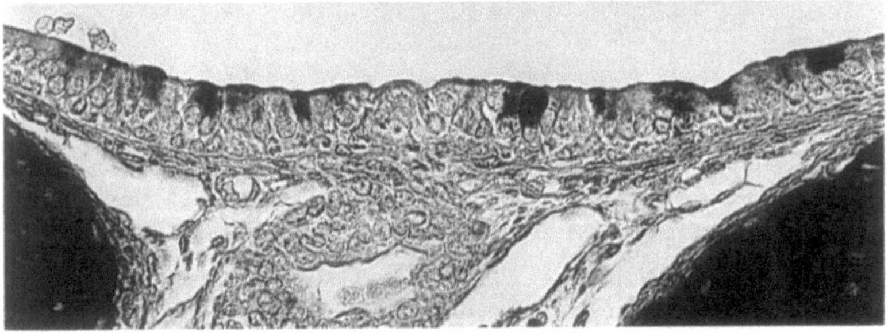

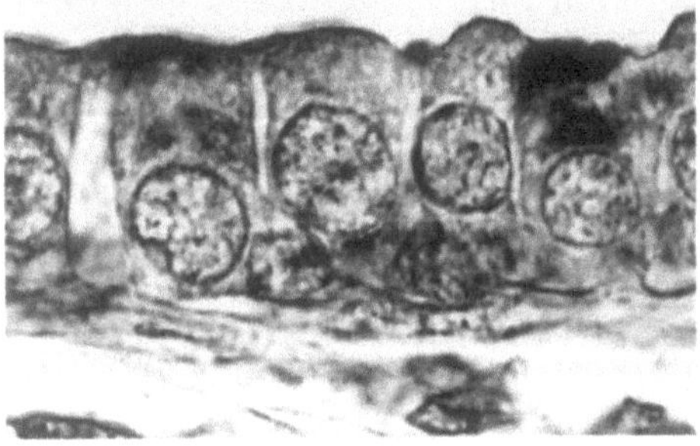

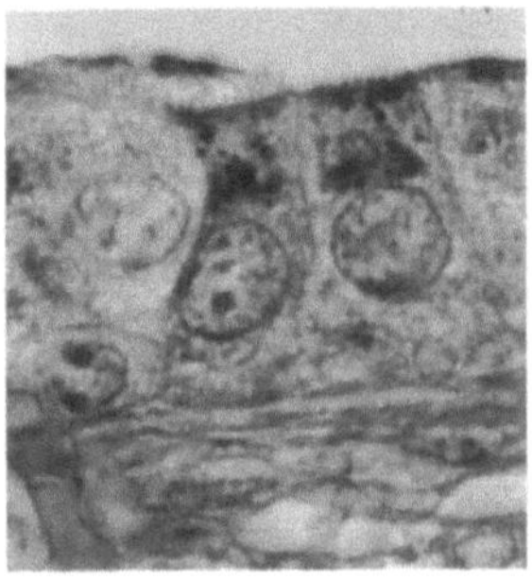

**Fig. 84.** (*above*) Ventral epithelium on the 1st postnatal day. Diastase and PAS, ×106

**Fig. 85.** (*middle*) Epithelium on the 1st postnatal day, ventral surfaçe. *Dark*, cells positive to Alcian blue. Alcian blue, ×105

**Fig. 86.** (*lower left*) Dorsal epithelial cells on the 1st postnatal day. Cytoplasm near lumen stains with alcian blue. Alcian blue and nuclear red, ×425

**Fig. 87.** (*lower right*) Tracheal epithelium on the 1st postnatal day. *Left*, a ciliated cell; in the center are two cells which, following diastase, have PAS-positive material in their cytoplasm. The cell in the center is ciliated; the two on the right have spiny processes on the luminal side. PAS and hematoxylin, ×425

which is approximately half the average frequency of PAS-positive cells that resist diastase treatment. Throughout these developmental stages the majority of cells that stain with Alcian blue also react to PAS after diastase, but the reverse is not true (Emura and Mohr 1975).

On the 14th and 15th gestational days the cytoplasm of some cells stains with Alcian blue around the nucleus and just beneath the luminal surface. These cells occur more frequently in the cranial to middle parts of the dorsal epithelium on the 16th gestational to the 1st postnatal day (Figs. 84, 85). At these stages cells stain with Alcian blue, mainly in the cytoplasmic portion between the luminal surface and the nuclei (Figs. 85, 86).

No marked difference can be detected in the frequency of cells reacting to PAS and Alcian blue between the prenatal and the neonatal epithelium on the 16th day. Some ciliated cells on the 16th gestational and the 1st postnatal days clearly react to PAS even after diastase pretreatment (Fig. 87). A few also stain with Alcian blue.

*Electron Microscopy.* In type I cells rough ER noticeably increases on the 14th–16th gestational days. It can therefore be presumed that type I cells eventually become secretory cells. However, the ultrastructure of the rough ER has several different aspects, depending on the stage of differentiation of the cells. In some of the primitive type I cells at the primary stage (Figs. 88, 90), the vacuoles and vesicles possessing both smooth and rough areas begin to resemble ER. These structures are found in blastic nerve cells (Pannese 1968), in developing pancreatic cells (Wessells and Evans 1968), and in embryonic choroidal epithelial cells (Birge and Doolin 1974).

The nuclear envelope of these primitive type I cells usually undergoes local cisternal dilation and/or circumscribed extensions of the outer membrane. This is most frequent and prominent on the 14th gestational day. In differentiating type I cells at advanced stages, almost all of the ER is rough, and its flattened winding cisternae are extended and contain electron dense, fibrillar, and amorphous material (Fig. 89). In these type I cells at more advanced stages rough and smooth vesicular ER occur in addition to the flattened, winding ER. The cisternae of this vesicular ER usually contain fibrillar or amorphous material. Thus, in time an increasing number of type I cells with cisternae of rough ER and/or vesicles limited by smooth and rough ER membranes, all containing electron dense, fibrillar, and amorphous material, fill the entire cytoplasm (Fig. 89). At the same time, dictyosomes of Golgi apparatus develop extensively (Fig. 90). Finally, on the 1st postnatal day maturing secretory (type I) cells appear (Figs. 91, 92). In these cells the nuclear chromatin is more condensed than that of the mature ciliated cell (Fig. 81).

The cisternae of the nuclear envelope are usually locally dilated in many areas (Fig. 92) and the outer nuclear membrane frequently comes into contact with the cytoplasmic vesicles. Some vesicles contain less electron-dense material than others. Both types of vesicles frequently fuse together in the luminal cytoplasm (Fig. 92). This kind of secretory cell is presumably of the neonatal type since it occurs only during the neonatal period and is not found in the adult epithelium. On the 1st postnatal day cells with well-developed rough ER and Golgi apparatus at various stages of differentiation are still abundant (Fig. 93).

From the 14th gestational until the 1st postnatal day many of the epithelial cells, including basal cells, contain glycogen granules (Fig. 90). Frequent association of glycogen granules with protrusions of the outer nuclear membrane suggests that some of these membranes play a part in glycogen metabolism similar to the function of smooth ER of liver parenchymal cells (Coimbra and Leblond 1966).

After the 15th gestational day another type of cell which appears to be secretory in nature occurs (Fig. 91), although its origin is unclear. The cells lack the typical rough ER that synthesizes secretory protein. Instead, they contain vacuoles and vesicles surrounded by smooth and rough membranes. From around postnatal day 10 onwards two ultrastructurally distinct secretory cell types can be identified. The detection techniques have been described previously (Hopwood et al. 1977). One type demonstrates the secretory vesicles containing neutral glycoconjugates, which build fine granular dark precipitates (Fig. 94) by reacting with silver methenamine after periodic acid preoxidation. This cell type contains practically no glycogen granules in the cytoplasm.

The other type reveals secretory vesicles containing materials that form only a small amount of such dark precipitates after reacting with silver methenamine (Fig. 95). Instead, the cytoplasm contains abundant glycogen granules which make fine dark precipitates in reaction with silver. The

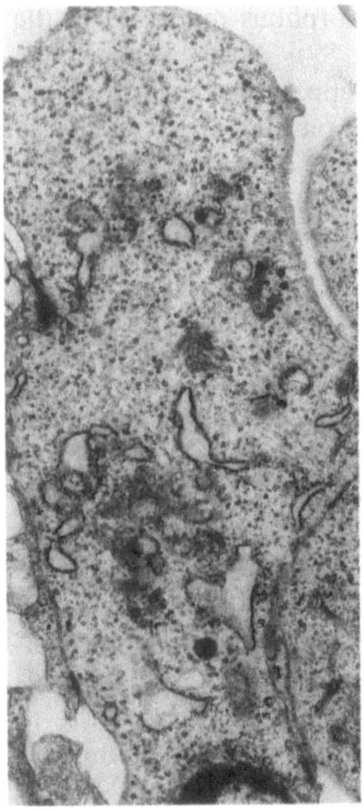

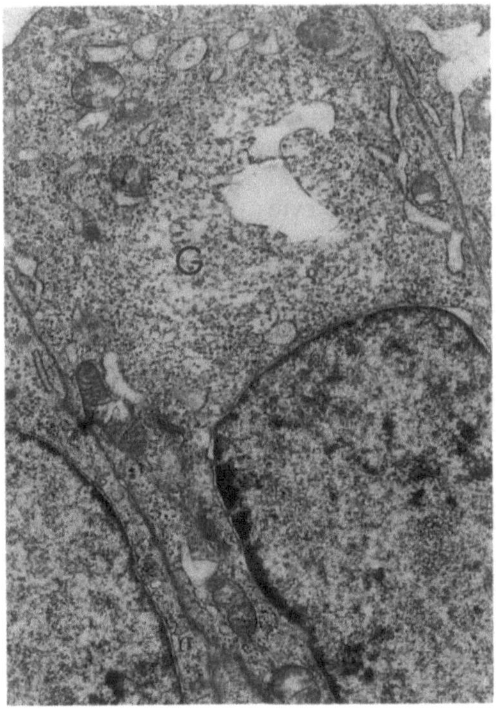


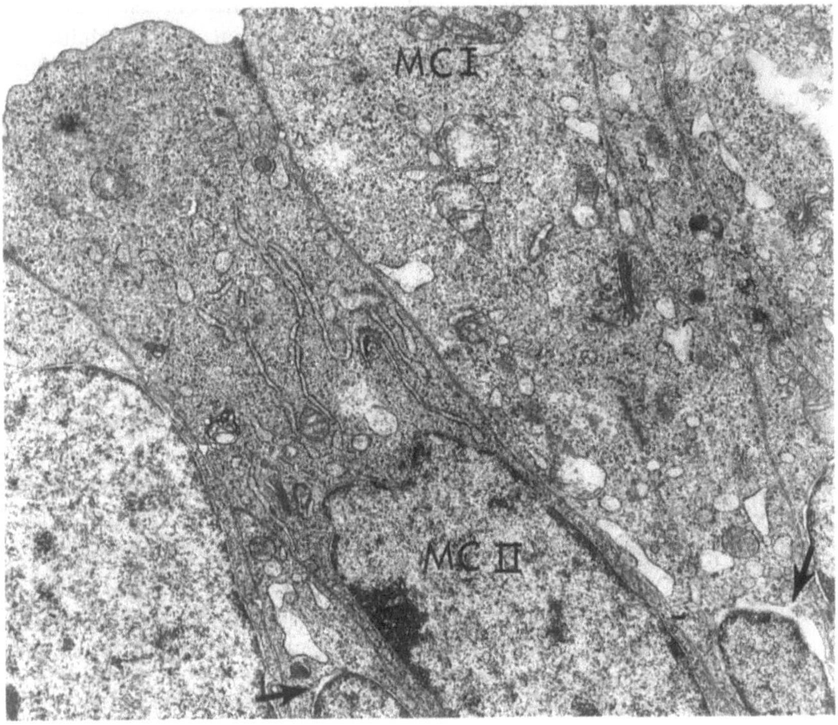


**Fig. 88.** (*upper left*) Hamster trachea, 13th gestational day. Type I epithelial cell with partly rough vesicles resembling ER. Uranyl acetate and lead citrate, TEM, ×11 640

**Fig. 89.** (*below*) Differentiating type I cells on the 14th gestational day. Cells at two different stages of differentiation. In the cell MCII the winding cisternae of rough ER containing dense material are prominent. There already exists a small amount of vesicular ER. The cells MCI seem to be at the same stage as those in Fig. 90. The extensions and the local cisternal dilation of the nuclear envelope are no longer detectable in the cell MCII, while in MCI they are both conspicuous (*arrows*). Note the partly rough membrane portion of the vesicles in MCI. The cell MCII appears to be at a later stage of differentiation than the cell MCI. Uranyl acetate and lead citrate, TEM, ×11 640

**Fig. 90.** (*upper right*) Type I (presecretory) cells on the 14th gestational day. Vesicles are enclosed by a partially granular membrane. Note chromatin condensation, focal cisternal dilation of the nuclear envelope, and glycogen granules (*G*). Uranyl acetate and lead citrate, TEM, ×11 640

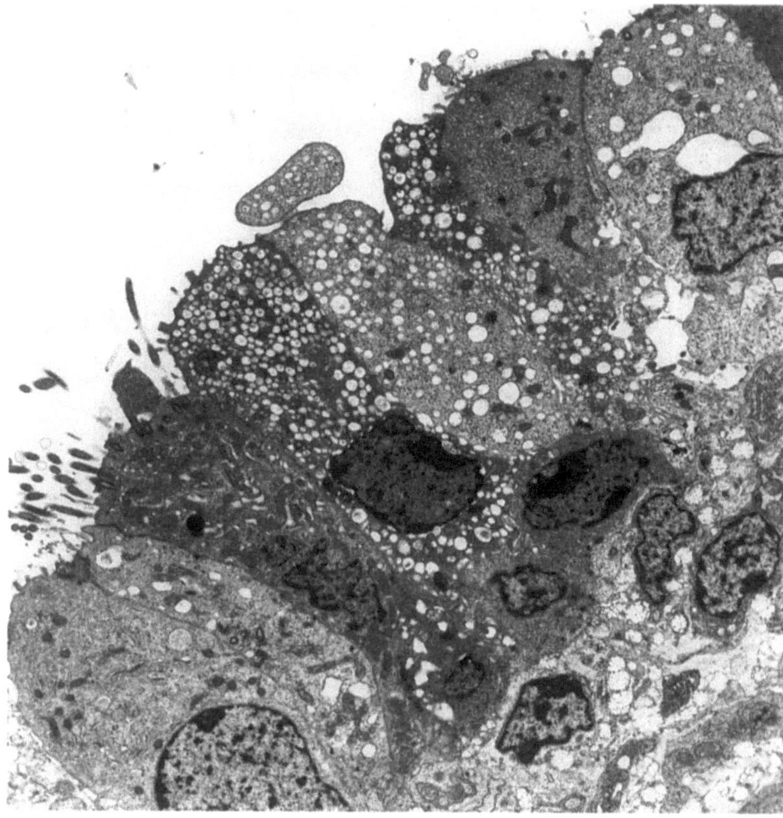

**Fig. 91.** Epithelium, 1st postnatal day, dorsal aspect. Cells in various stages of differentiation. Uranyl acetate and lead citrate, TEM, ×5070

secretory materials of this cell type are therefore considered to be mainly acidic glycoconjugates. Since both cell types appear to be mature, each may be a discretely differentiated cell type. However, precursor stages of each cell type have not been identified.

As observed by light microscopy, after the 14th gestational day cells frequently undergo ciliogenesis (type II) and produce secretory materials (type I). In prospective secretory cells rough and smooth membrane bound vesicles exist, together with proliferating centrioles. Other such cells possess several cilia, Golgi apparatus, and rough ER, which develop to a considerable extent (Fig. 96). Cells containing both secretory granules and cilia have been reported in the respiratory epithelium of neonatal rats (Stockinger and Cireli 1965), adult Syrian hamsters in regeneration (McDowell et al. 1979), and adult humans (McDowell et al. 1978).

## Neuroendocrine Cells

Respiratory neuroendocrine cells belong to a group of amine precursor uptake and decarboxylation (APUD) cells. They are known to produce bombesin and gastrin-releasing peptide, calcitonin and calcitonin gene-related peptide, and serotonin supposedly responsible for the regulation of cell proliferation in a paracrine and autocrine manner (Polak et al. 1993). The investigation of developing hamster trachea by McDowell et al. (1994a) revealed that there are morphologically two types of endocrine cells, one representing such cells as those growing in groups, forming a NEB (Figs. 97, 98), and the other the solitary cells. Earlier in the organogenesis of the trachea NEB is primarily distributed in the larynx and more cranial part of the trachea. With ontogenesis progressing the wave of its distribution spreads towards the caudal part, and in the

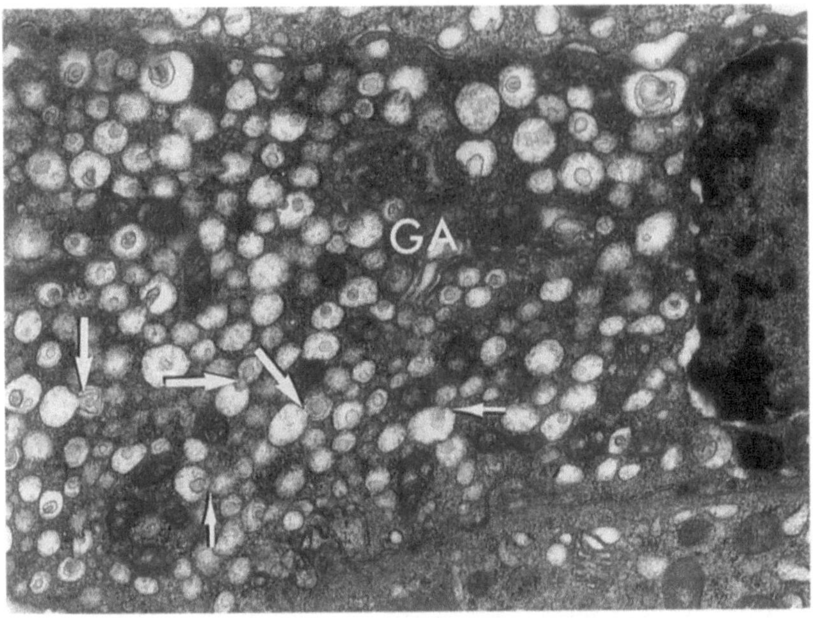


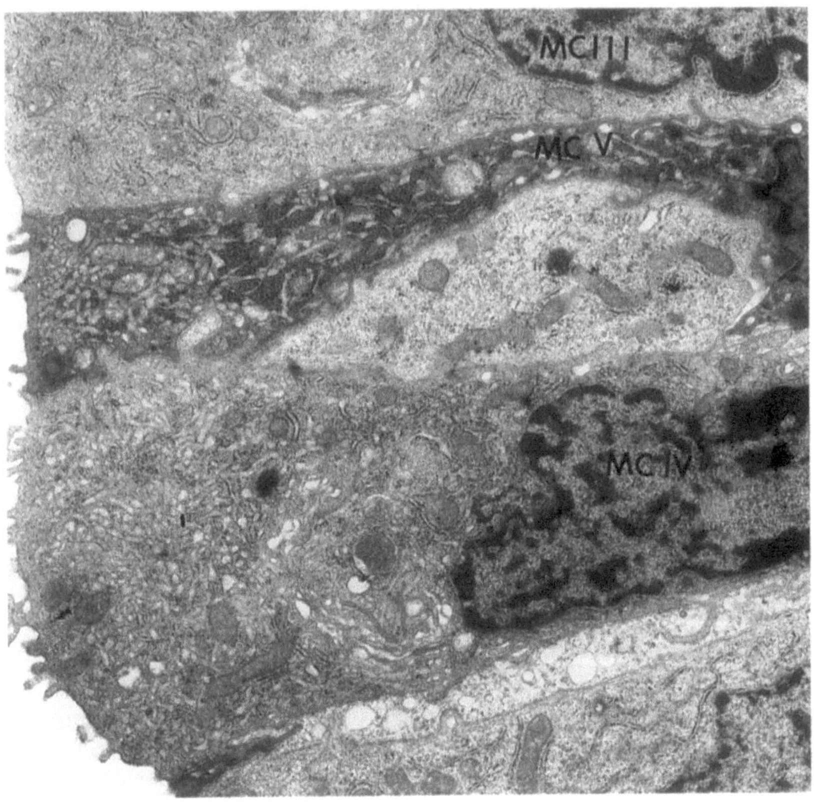


**Fig. 92.** (*above*) Type I cell on 1st postnatal day. Nearly mature secretory cell with vesicles of low and high density. In vesicles of high density the limiting membrane is difficult to distinguish. Note the fusion of the two different types of vesicles (*arrows*). Golgi apparatus (*GA*). Uranyl acetate and lead citrate, TEM, ×16640

**Fig. 93.** (*below*) Type I cells in dorsal cranial epithelium on 1st postnatal day. The cell MCIII seems to be at a slightly more advanced stage than the cell MCII in Fig. 89, and MCIV more advanced than MCIII. The cell MCV appears to be developing into the cell shown in Fig. 92. Uranyl acetate and lead citrate, TEM, ×11640

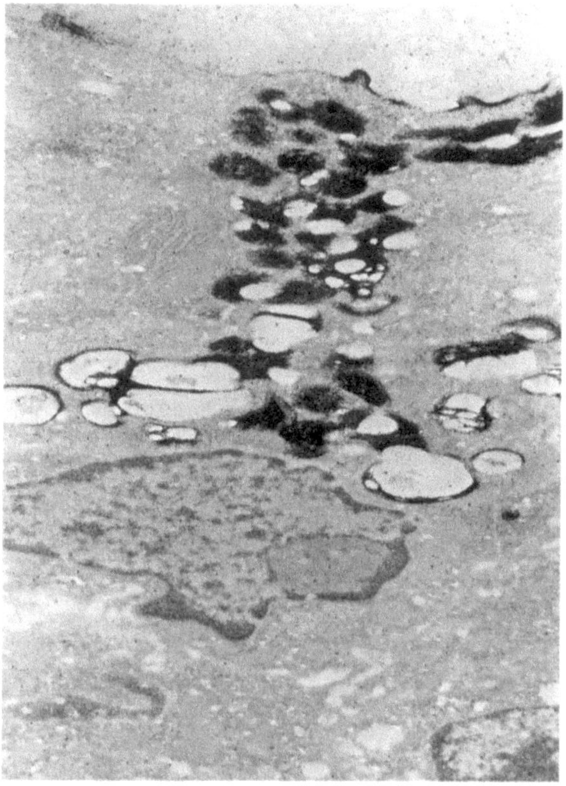

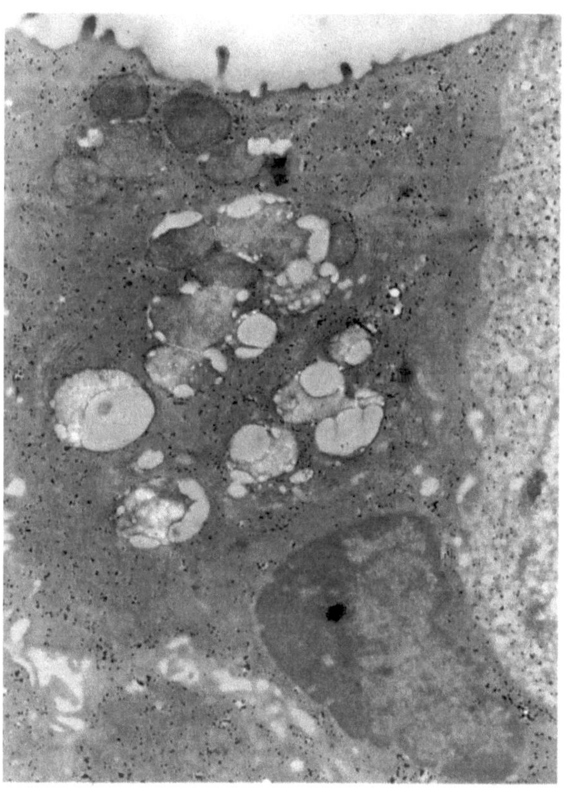

**Fig. 94.** (*above*) An epithelial cell containing neutral secretory glycoconjugates in the trachea of a Syrian hamster on the 10th postnatal day. Note the dark precipitates stained with silver methenamine in the secretory vesicles and on the luminal surface. There are no glycogen granules (dark precipitates, see Fig. 95) in the cytoplasm. Glycol methacrylate section, TEM, ×11 000

**Fig. 95.** (*below*) An epithelial cell containing secretory vesicles with acidic glycoconjugates and small granular glycogens scattered in the cytoplasm. Only a small amount of silver methenamine precipitates are seen in the secretory vesicles. Glycol methacrylate section, TEM, ×11 000

◀

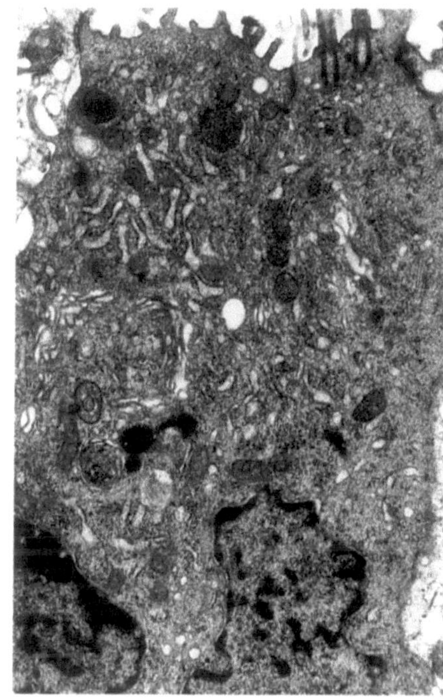

**Fig. 96.** A differentiating type I cell (*left*) and a cell between a secretory and ciliated cell (*right*), on the 1st postnatal day. Note that the state of the chromatin condensation of the cell on the right appears to be at a stage between the ciliated and the type I cell. Uranyl acetate and lead citrate, TEM, ×11 640

postnatal period further into the intrapulmonary bronchiolar region. In parallel, the NEBs in the larynx and trachea decrease in number and in adults are replaced by solitary endocrine cells.

*Changes in Mitotic Activity.* In the longitudinally cut hamster tracheal epithelium the mitotic indices are counted in percentages (see Emura and Mohr 1975). The tracheas are all fixed between 9 A.M. and 11 A.M. to exclude the effect of the diurnal rhythm on mitotic activity. The highest percentage of 4.5% is seen on the 11th gestational day during

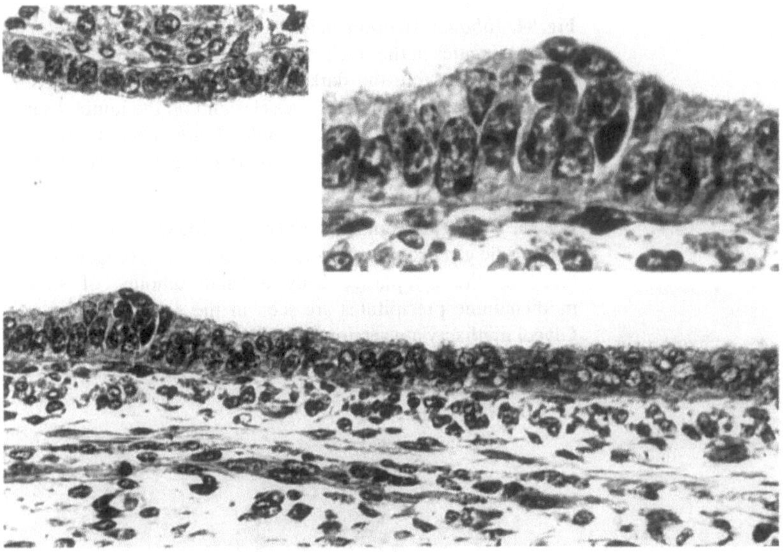

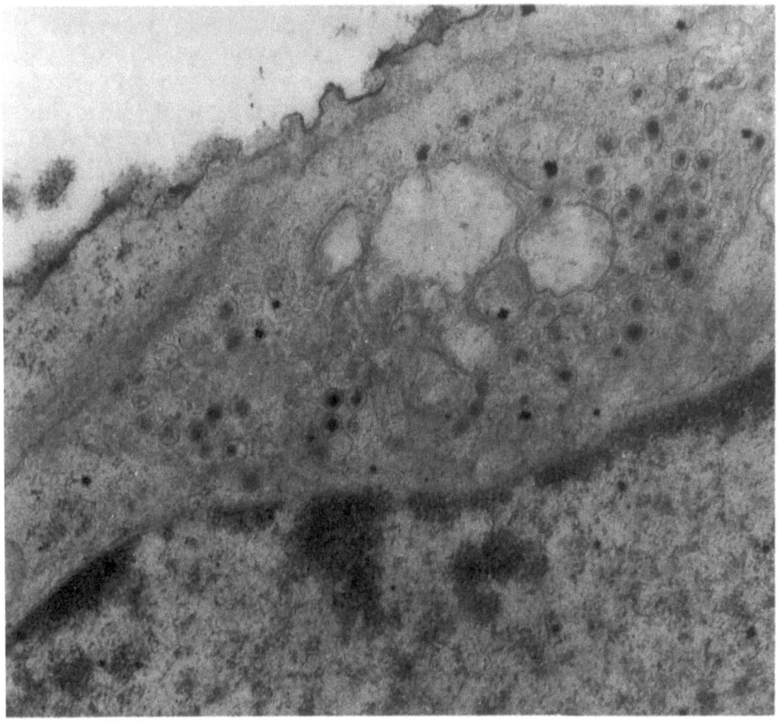

**Fig. 97.** (*above*) Longitudinal section of the dorsal tracheal epithelium (more caudal) of a fetal trachea on day 13 of gestation with a neuroepithelial body (*NEB*). No innervation is seen. H&E, ×140. *Insert*, NEB, ×220

**Fig. 98.** (*below*) Part of a cross-section of neuroepithelial body (*NEB*) of a fetal trachea on day 14 of gestation. Note numerous dense-cored granules in the cytoplasm of a cell located adjacent to the lumen. Uranyl acetate and lead citrate, TEM, ×18200

the predifferentiation stage. The index sharply declines on the 12th gestational day (2.5%) and then continues to decline until the 14th gestational day (1.8%), when the first ciliated cells can be observed. Following this a more gradual decrease is noticed on the 1st postnatal day (0.3%) when mature secretory cells are first observed. These observations were virtually confirmed by a later study (McDowell et al. 1985b).

*Uneven Differentiation Pattern of Ciliated and Secretory Cells.* The first ciliated cells occur in the dorsal epithelium (pars membranacea) of the trachea on the 14th gestational day. Ciliated cells are virtually absent in the ventral and lateral epithelium (pars cartilaginea) and at this stage occur more frequently and are longer in the cranial than in the caudal part of the dorsal epithelium. On the 15th gestational day the cells also appear in the ventral and lateral epithelium and thereafter increase gradually in number. Even on the 1st postnatal day they are seen more frequently in the dorsal than in the ventral and lateral epithelium.

The cells which are resistant to diastase treatment and react positively to PAS and those cells that stain with Alcian blue are unevenly distributed along the ventral and dorsal epithelium during the developmental stages (Figs. 84, 85). Both of these cell types occur primarily in the cranial part of the epithelium. As development progresses, they gradually appear in the caudal part of the epithelium. From the 14th to 16th gestational days they occur more frequently in the dorsal than in the ventral epithelium. On the 1st postnatal day this difference is no longer evident.

## Conclusion

The epithelium of trachea in mature Syrian hamsters consists of various differentiated cell types, which can be grouped into secretory and nonsecretory cell types. The former includes at least three distinct cell types different from each other not only morphologically but also functionally. Of these, the neuroendocrine cell (NEC) type is vastly different from the other two that mainly secrete neutral or acidic glycoconjugates. Nevertheless, the data so far available (McDowell et al. 1994b; Emura p. 71, this volume) strongly indicate that the neuroendocrine cells, if not all of them, also develop from a single common precursor (stem) cell type (endodermal) that also gives rise to other secretory, ciliated and basal cells of respiratory epithelium. The induction of laryngotracheal papillomas by diethylnitrosamine (DEN) is a well-established example of organotropic tumorigenesis in the laryngotracheal epithelium. The mechanisms involved have been proposed to be closely related to the state of cellular differentiation in this epithelium (Emura et al. 1980; Strum et al. 1990). Spontaneous occurrence of the papillomas in this species has very seldom been reported (Mohr et al. 1994). In contrast, NEC tumors (malignant/benign) occur spontaneously with an incidence of up to 9%, depending on the strain (Mohr et al. 1994), although the incidence can be significantly elevated by transplacental DEN exposure of prenatal hamsters (Mohr et al., in preparation).

Therefore, some intriguing questions are: What factors determine the differentiation of NECs from the common stem cells? What mechanisms are responsible for the differential development of papillomas on the one hand, and NEC tumors on the other?

Although these questions are not easy to answer immediately, any approaches attempting to do so will provide valuable clues for exploring the relationship between tissue differentiation and cancer causation.

## References


Anderson RGW, Brenner RM (1971) The formation of basal bodies (centrioles) in the rhesus monkey oviduct. J Cell Biol 50:10–34

Birge WJ, Doolin PF (1974) The ultrastructural differentiation of the endoplasmic reticulum in choroidal epithelial cells of the chick embryo. Tissue Cell 6:335–360

Coimbra A, Leblond CP (1966) Sites of glycogen synthesis in rat liver cells as shown by electron microscope radioautography after administration of glucose-H[3]. J Cell Biol 30:151–175

Dirksen ER, Crocker TT (1966) Centriole replication in differentiating ciliated cells of mammalian respiratory epithelium. An electron microscopic study. J Microscop 5:629–644

Emura M (1978) Morphological studies on the development of tracheal epithelium in the Syrian golden hamster. IV. Electron microscopy: blebbing of nuclear membrane. Z Versuchstierkd 20:163–170

Emura M, Mohr U (1975) Morphological studies on the development of tracheal epithelium in the Syrian golden hamster I. Light microscopy. Z Versuchstierkd 17:14–26

Emura M, Richter-Reichhelm HB, Mohr U (1980) Some aspects of prenatal risk of N-nitrosodiethylamine carcinogenesis. IARC Sci Publ 31:767–777

Frisch D, Farbman AI (1968) Development of order during ciliogenesis. Anat Rec 162:221–232

Hopwood D, Logan KR, Milne G (1977) Mucosubstances in the normal human oesophageal epithelium. A comparison of periodic acid-silver and phosphotungstic acid techniques. Histochemistry 54:67–74

Keenan KP, Wilson TS, McDowell EM (1983) Regeneration of hamster tracheal epithelium after mechanical injury. IV. Histochemical, immunocytochemical and ultrastructural studies. Virchows Arch [B] Cell Pathol/Mol Pathol 43:213–240

McDowell EM, Barrett LA, Glavin F, Harris CC, Trump BF (1978) The respiratory epithelium. I. Human bronchus. JNCI 61:539–549

McDowell EM, Becci PJ, Schürch W, Trump BF (1979) The respiratory epithelium. VII. Epidermoid metaplasia of ham-

ster tracheal epithelium during regeneration following mechanical injury. JNCI 62:995–1008
McDowell EM, Newkirk C, Coleman B (1985a) Development of hamster tracheal epithelium. I. A quantitative morphologic study in the fetus. Anat Rec 213:429–447
McDowell EM, Newkirk C, Coleman B (1985b) Development of hamster tracheal epithelium. II. Cell proliferation in the fetus. Anat Rec 213:448–456
McDowell EM, Sorokin SP, Hoyt RF Jr (1994a) Ontogeny of endocrine cells in the respiratory system of Syrian golden hamsters. I. Larynx and trachea. Cell Tissue Res 275:143–156
McDowell EM, Hoyt RF Jr, Sorokin SP (1994b) Ontogeny of endocrine cells in the respiratory system of Syrian golden hamsters. II. Intrapulmonary airways and alveoli. Cell Tissue Res 275:157–167
Mohr U (1973) Effects of diethylnitrosamine on fetal and suckling Syrian golden hamsters. IARC Sci Publ 4:65–70
Mohr U, Reznik-Schüller H, Emura M (1979) Tissue differentiation as a prerequisite for transplacental carcinogenesis in the hamster respiratory system, with specific respect to the trachea. Natl Cancer Inst Monogr 51:117–122
Mohr U, Emura M, Dungworth DL, Ernst H (1994) Tumours of the lower respiratory tract. In: Pathology of tumours in laboratory animals, vol 3: tumours of the hamster. IARC Sci Publ (in press)
Pannese E (1968) Developmental changes of the endoplasmic reticulum and ribosomes in nerve cells of the spinal ganglia of the domestic fowl. J Comp Neurol 132:331–364
Polak JM, Becker KL, Cutz E, Gail DB, Goniakowska-Witalinska L, Gosney JR, Lauweryns JM, Linnoila I, McDowell EM, Miller YE, Scheuermann DW, Springall DR, Sunday ME, Zaccone G (1993) Lung endocrine cell markers, peptides, and amines. Anat Rec 236:169–171
Sorokin SP (1968) Reconstructions of centriole formation and ciliogenesis in mammalian lungs. J Cell Sci 3:207–230
Staprans I, Dirksen ER (1974) Microtubule protein during ciliogenesis in the mouse oviduct. J Cell Biol 62:164–174
Stockinger L, Cireli E (1965) Eine bisher unbekannte Art der Zentriolenvermehrung. Z Zellforsch 68:733–740
Strum JM, Ito T, Philpot RM, DeSanti AM, McDowell EM (1990) The immunocytochemical detection of cytochrome P-450 monooxygenase in the lungs of fetal, neonatal, and adult hamsters. Am J Respir Cell Mol Biol 2:493–501
Wessells NK, Evans J (1968) Ultrastructural studies of early morphogenesis and cytodifferentiation in the embryonic mammalian pancreas. Dev Biol 17:413–446
Wischnitzer S (1974) Die Kernhülle: ihre Ultrastruktur und funktionelle Bedeutung. Endeavour 33:137–142
Wynder EL, Hecht S (eds) (1976) Lung cancer. International Union Against Cancer, Geneva, pp 95–101 (UICC technical report series, vol 25)

# Morphological Response of Respiratory Epithelium to Carcinogens, Syrian Hamster (*Mesocricetus auratus* W.)

H.-B. Richter-Reichhelm, A. Schulte, and Jürgen Althoff

## Gross Appearance

Early morphological changes of the respiratory epithelium in the larynx, trachea, and stem bronchi that may lead to or are associated with the occurrence of neoplasia cannot be easily observed and diagnosed macroscopically. Exophytic papillary tumors, regardless of whether they fill the airway lumen, are detectable under a magnifying glass, a stereo microscope (Fig. 99), or even by the naked eye. In addition to their typical form and shape (sessile or pedunculated), the tumors are soft and reddish gray, clearly distinguishable from the surrounding normal respiratory epithelium. Small tumors are often indicated by focally increased vascularization at the site of origin. After perfusion of the tissues with fixative these neoplasms become a yellowish gray contrasting with the whitish adjacent epithelium. Macroscopically, invasive tumors and masses outside of the airways are usually found during necropsy, tissue trimming, and dissection.

## Microscopic Features

*Nonneoplastic Alterations and Neoplastic Precursor Lesions.* Since differentiation of the pseudostratified respiratory epithelium in the Syrian golden hamster is not complete at birth, lack of ciliated cells at an early stage of the animals life may represent a physiological status rather than pathological change. In terms of surface characteristics of the neonatal epithelium, proliferative patterns prevail during the first 10 days of postpartum life. Less differentiated cells (probably

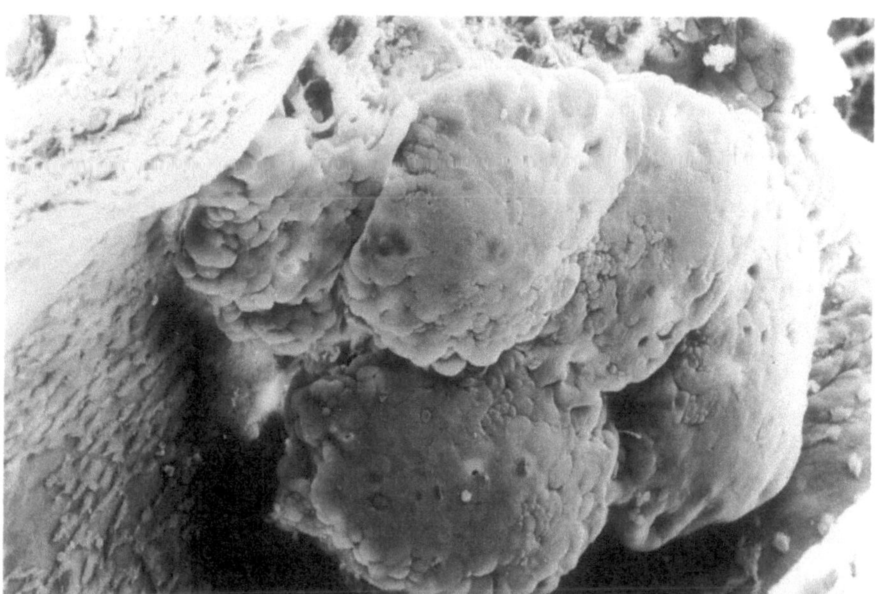

**Fig. 99.** Papillary mucoepidermoid tumor, trachea of Syrian golden hamster, filling almost 50% of the lumen. This neoplasm was easily detectable with a dissecting microscope. SEM, ×240

precursors of mucous cells) and mucus-producing cells outnumber ciliated cells for the first 20 days after birth. Time of maturation of the epithelium in the trachea may vary among different topographical sites such as the pars membranacea, intercartilaginea, and cartilaginea. Differentiation of the respiratory epithelium in the trachea appears to be complete approximately 30 days postpartum (Richter-Reichhelm et al. 1980). Early neoplastic alterations or tumor precursor lesions are not specific; toxic and non-compound-related degenerative and regenerative changes of the respiratory epithelium may have similar characteristics. These factors need to be considered in making a diagnosis (McDowell et al. 1979; Althoff et al. 1981). Common changes such as focal cell death are usually followed by regeneration from remaining basal cells. The number of mucous cells may increase in the tracheobronchial epithelium due to treatment-related injury (Becci et al. 1978c;

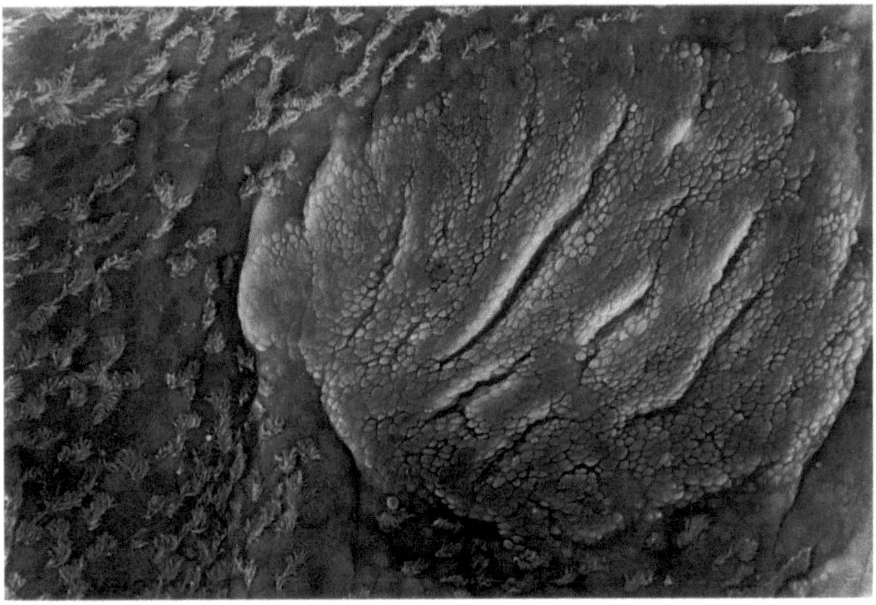

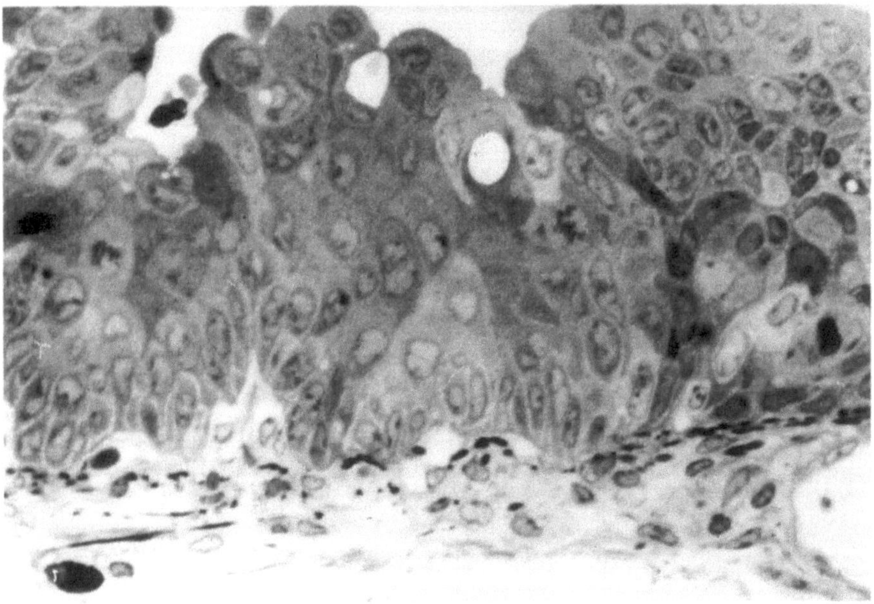

**Fig. 100.** (*above*) Circumscribed area of trachea consisting of cell surfaces varying in shape and form indicating hyperplasia and dysplasia. Note folds and slight projection into the tracheal lumen. SEM, ×320

**Fig. 101.** (*below*) Dysplastic alteration (carcinoma in situ) of the respiratory epithelium, trachea. Note multilayered atypical cell arrangement with vacuoles and epidermal cells in the uppermost layer. Semithin section, toluidine blue, ×350

Boutet et al. 1987) leading to mucous cell hyperplasia, a frequent toxic lesion. Loss of cilia from the surface of the respiratory epithelium (simple metaplasia) develops regularly due to inflammatory stimuli. Local treatment with chemicals including carcinogenic agents may cause traumatic injury at the site of application. Metaplasia together with slight atypia and hyperplasia may result in a multilayered epithelium. Since these changes may appear in the process of regeneration and early neoplastic growth, it may be difficult or impossible to determine morphologically the eventual nature of the lesion. These metaplastic and hyperplastic changes may be disseminated, focal, or multifocal.

*Simple Metaplasia.* This alteration of the normally pseudostratified ciliated epithelium lining the airways is recognized by loss of cilia, persisting presence of cells containing intracytoplasmic mucous granules, and flattening of the epithelium. In the now cuboidal unilayered epithelium cell nuclei are round or oval and mitotic activity is usually slightly increased.

*Hyperplasia.* The lesions may develop a multilayered pattern by an increase in the number of basal cells (so-called basal cell hyperplasia in light microscopy). Less differentiated cells constitute the intermediate layer between the line of basal cells and cells lining the epithelial surface. These cells may be either indifferent or highly differentiated (e.g., usually mucous cell hyperplasia).

*Squamous Cell Metaplasia.* Surface cells become flattened, have nuclei parallel to the basal lamina, may be nonkeratinized, or contain keratohyalin granules. This resulting squamous epithelium may undergo acanthosis, parakeratosis, hyperkeratosis, or dyskeratosis. Desquamation of surface cells is often observed. The cells in the surface layers may provide evidence for tight connections (spinae, desmosomes) and the cytoplasm may stain poorly or is eosinophilic. In this multilayered squamous epithelium a basal cell row is well defined.

*Dysplasia; Carcinoma In Situ.* Circumscribed areas in the respiratory epithelium with a slightly elevated, dome-shaped surface are composed of cells with irregular shapes and sizes that proliferate toward the lumen (Fig. 100). In profile they are irregular in shape and size and are folded. By light microscopy the lesion consists of one or two layers of basal cells covered by four or five layers of less differentiated (intermediate) cells, sometimes with increased mitotic activity and atypism. Loss of orientation and organization of cells is evident. In cross-sections of the epithelium varying cell shapes, forms, and sizes are seen; folds appear as or correspond to papillary projections into the lumen. The uppermost luminal layer is made up either of flat squamous or mucus-producing cells. Irregularly and apparently normally ciliated cells (single or in small clusters) occur in multifocal or disseminated sites of the lesion. The pleomorphism of the cells and the irregularity in cell surface patterns as well as on cross-section are indicative of dysplasia (Fig. 101) and/or carcinoma in situ (Becci et al. 1978a); angiogenesis and connective tissue stroma formation are absent.

**Papillary Tumors**

Exophytic papillary neoplastic alterations of the respiratory epithelium have largely the same cell surface pattern, i.e., epidermoid, less differentiated mucus-producing, and ciliated cells as those seen in dysplasia (Fig. 102). The hyperplastic and dysplastic portion of the tumors is supported by a delicate vascularized stroma (Fig. 103). Secondary inflammatory changes are frequent in the form of slight edema and inflammatory cells. The basal lamina continues into all branches of the papillary exophytic growth and is generally not disrupted. If the epithelium of such a papillary neoplasm is composed solely of squamous and precursor cells, it is regarded as an epidermoid or squamous papillary tumor. Sections reveal layers of flattened cells parallel to the basal membrane. Keratin may be formed in some instances.

A papillary mucoepidermoid tumor consisting of both mucus-producing and epidermoid cells (Fig. 104) is easily distinguished by applying Kreyberg's stain (green, mucus; red, keratin; Kreyberg 1967). In addition to the presence of differentiated mucus-producing cells at the surface and in the lining of intraepithelial cysts, cells containing mucous granules are found in the intermediate zone. Mitoses are seen in all cell layers, although they are not as frequent as expected in a malignant neoplasm. Subepithelial mucous glands may also undergo metaplastic and proliferative changes, a feature which could be falsely interpreted as

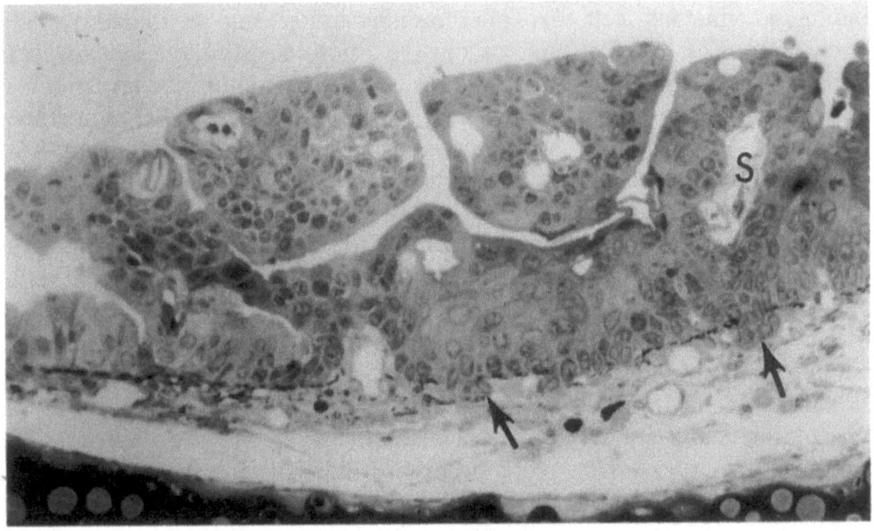


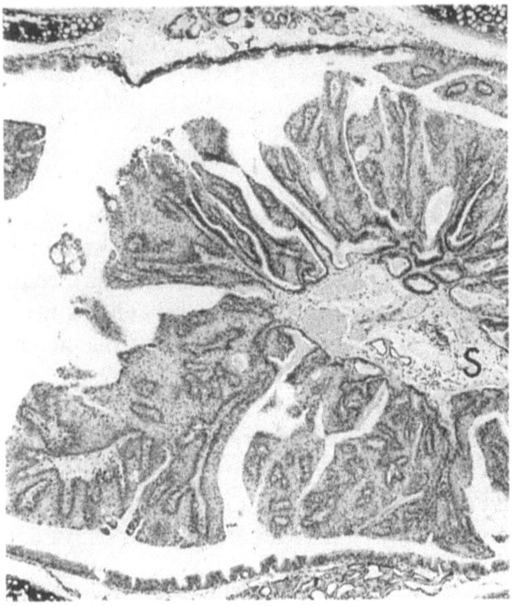


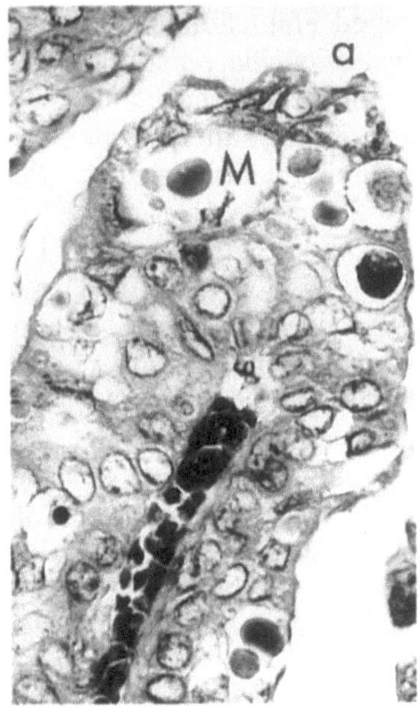


**Fig. 102.** (*above*) Early mucoepidermoid papillary tumor, trachea, with intraepithelial cysts and focal squamous metaplasia. Note the delicate vascularized connective tissue stalk (*S*). In some areas under the basal lamina early tumor growth seems to interrupt the basement membrane (*arrow*). Semithin section, toluidine blue, ×150

**Fig. 103.** (*lower left*) Mucoepidermoid papillary tumor of the respiratory epithelium filling the tracheal lumen. Note delicate mesenchymal stroma with capillaries (*S*). H&E, ×80

**Fig. 104.** (*lower right*) Epithelial cells, trachea, containing mucus (*M*; *green* in Kreyberg's stain). At the apex (*a*), flattened cells with reddish cytoplasm indicate nonkeratinized squamous cells. Kreyberg's stain, ×440

invasive growth. Papillary tumors may also originate in the cystic ducts of the subepithelial glands and be mistaken for carcinomas or inverted papillomas.

At the base of papillary exophytic tumor growth disruption of the basal membrane and invasion into the subepithelial connective tissue may indicate malignancy. An initially benign neoplasm (in terms of morphological criteria) has transformed into a carcinoma. Small or large mucous granules and keratinization patterns may be observed only focally. Malignant growth may occur in areas not going through benign papillary growth or any other precursor lesion. Carcinomas may invade the intercartilaginous and membranous portion of larynx, trachea, or stem bronchi and spread into the mediastinum. Metastases into the local lymph nodes are rare, although the primary tumor mass may reach considerable size.

## Ultrastructure: Nonneoplastic and Neoplastic Precursor Lesions

*Simple Metaplasia.* In this alteration of the respiratory epithelium cells are marked by the loss of cilia, and intracytoplasmic ciliary bodies disappear. In some cells few scattered cilia may occur, and occasionally cells with cytoplasmic protrusions contain small numbers of irregular cilia. In cross-sections of these cilia, microfilamentous patterns appear to be normal, with nine doublets around the periphery and two in the center. In some instances degenerative cell changes such as swelling of mitochondria and multivesiculated and laminated bodies (secondary lysosomes) are be found. In other cells mucous granules of varying size are found. At the luminal surface of the epithelium cells bear short and numerous microvilli; cell borders are clearly distinguishable by the slightly elevated cell membrane and increased density of cytoplasmic protrusions. Generally all cells have a similar shape and size and nuclei are oval and uniform.

*Squamous Cell Metaplasia.* In this lesion of the respiratory epithelium the alignment of cellular and nuclear axes parallel to the basal membrane is easily recognizable. Many cells in the multilayered epithelium contain numerous dense bundles of tonofilaments. Keratin granules are not always detectable. The number of desmosomes has increased, and interdigitation of cell membranes is pronounced. In the surface areas of epidermoid metaplasia nuclei are flat and deeply invaginated.

*Hyperplasia.* In this type of multilayered epithelium ciliogenesis may be disturbed as cells appear to produce premature intracytoplasmatic cilia. These cilia may be found even at intranuclear sites close to the basal layers. In other areas less differentiated and highly differentiated mucous cells may compose the majority of cells in focal lesions (mucous cell hyperplasia). These cells have highly developed and conspicuous endoplasmatic reticulum as well as Golgi complexes. Large mucous granules may not be present in all cells.

*Dysplasia.* Ultrastructural features of epithelial cells in sites of cellular atypia include empty vacuoles, intraepithelial cysts filled with mucus, and occasionally structurally intact cilia in addition to variously differentiated cell types. These features lead to the diagnosis of dysplasia or carcinoma in situ. In some cells numerous dense core intracytoplasmic granules are present as seen in neurosecretory cells or amine precursor uptake and decarboxylation cells. Areas are observed which contain squamous cells as evidenced by the irregularly folded luminal surface of the epithelium and microfolds and microridges on the cell surface. As observed in cross-sections, the content of cell organelles may vary considerably from cell to cell; cell nuclei vary in size and form deep invaginations. Atypical mitoses may occur.

## Papillary Tumors

In electron microscopy some papillary tumors have features of polymorphism similar to those seen in dysplasia, in terms of surface structure. In addition to the less differentiated areas consisting of cells with varying numbers of microvilli, groups of well-differentiated cells with cilia and mucus are found (Fig. 105). Ciliogenesis and mucogenesis may not be restricted to the surface layer (Figs. 106, 107). In other parts of the same tumor numerous desmosomes may be found, and some cells contain increased numbers of bundled tonofilaments. Cell boundaries are digitated; nuclei are flat and invaginated (Fig. 108). Keratohyalin granules are found occasionally, and some cells situated in the intermediate layer may contain high numbers of neurosecretory granules (amine precursor uptake and decarboxylation cells). Intracytoplasmic vacuoles and intraepithelial cysts are frequent. Usually the basal lamina is intact throughout the entire tumor stalk. Mitotic figures may be greater in number than in dysplasia.
The epithelial cell clusters in malignant tumors generally are less differentiated than in the benign counterpart, and characteristics of epidermoid or mucoepidermoid carcinomas may be easily distinguished. As in benign papillary tumors, a vascularized delicate stroma supports the malignant neoplastic growth.

## Differential Diagnosis

Papillary tumors originating in the epithelium of the larynx, trachea, and bronchi are classified according to their epithelial component. Neoplasms with squamous cell differentiation on their surface (nonkeratinizing or keratinizing) are classified as epidermoid (or squamous) papillary tumors. Exophytic neoplasms which contain goblet cells,

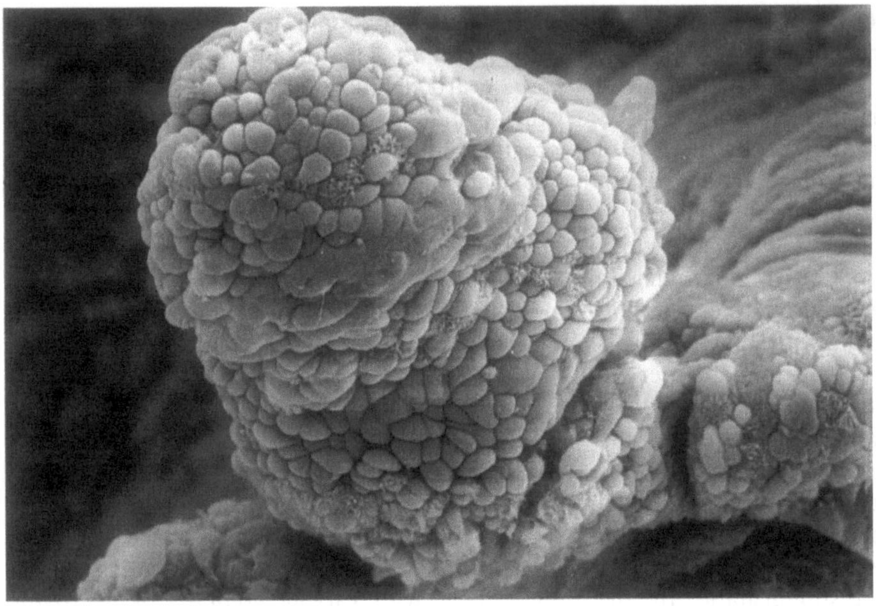

**Fig. 105.** Early papillary tumor, trachea. The surface of the mass consists of squamous mucus-producing and ciliated cells. SEM, ×420

an occasional ciliated cell, and squamous cells fulfill the criteria for mucoepidermoid papillary tumors. Routine histology (hematoxylin-eosin stain of paraffin sections or toluidine blue stain of plastic sections) may render sufficient information in terms of kind and type of neoplastic growth; however, special stains such as PAS reaction, Alcian blue, high-iron diamone, keratin, and/or Kreyberg's method allow further cytological identification of cell status, differentiation, and function (Herrold 1964a; Herrold and Dunham 1963; Dontenwill and Mohr 1961, 1962; Kreyberg 1967; Mohr 1970; Becci et al. 1978c; Cardesa et al. 1990). Transmission electron microscopy and scanning electron microscopy preparations may provide confirming evidence.

Nonneoplastic alterations and their changes associated with regeneration are difficult to differentiate from neoplastic precursor lesions since they have similar morphological characteristics. It may be that the induction of nonneoplastic alterations in the respiratory epithelium contribute to neoplastic transformation. Treatment procedure and route of exposure may need to be considered in diagnosis especially when the tissue is less differentiated (Marshall et al. 1987). Nonneoplastic structures caused by focal contraction and folding represent artifacts although they may appear as polypoid patterns on cross-sections.

## Biological Features

Papillary tumors of the larynx, trachea, and large bronchi develop as single or multiple neoplasms. They often originate in the epithelium of the membranaceous portion of airway. The tumors sometimes occlude the lumen of the involved airduct, leading to death by suffocation. Neoplasms that partially close the airway lumen can cause noisy and/or irregular breathing. Distal portions of the respiratory tract may undergo atelectases and emphysema, and infections of the lung are enhanced by hampered clearance and defense mechanisms. Papillary tumors arising in the respiratory epithelium of the larynx, trachea, and large bronchi may be torn from their site of origin and implanted into the lung after aspiration

▶

**Fig. 106.** (*above*) Mucus-producing cell from a mucoepidermoid respiratory tumor, bronchus, hamster. Note the Golgi complex (*G*) and mucous granules (*M*). ×47500

**Fig. 107.** (*middle*) Mucoepidermoid respiratory tumor, bronchus, revealing multiple ciliary bodies (*C*) in a cell attached to the basal lamina. TEM, ×9500

**Fig. 108.** (*below*) Portion of a respiratory mucoepidermoid tumor, bronchus, in a flattened cell layer. Nuclei are digitated (*N*); cytoplasm contains bundled tonofilaments (*E*). Note abundant desmosomes (*D*). TEM, ×6900

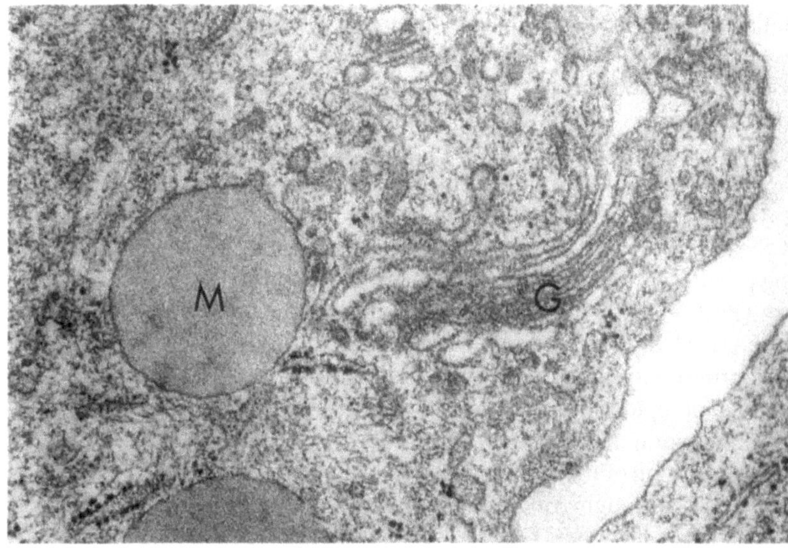
M
G

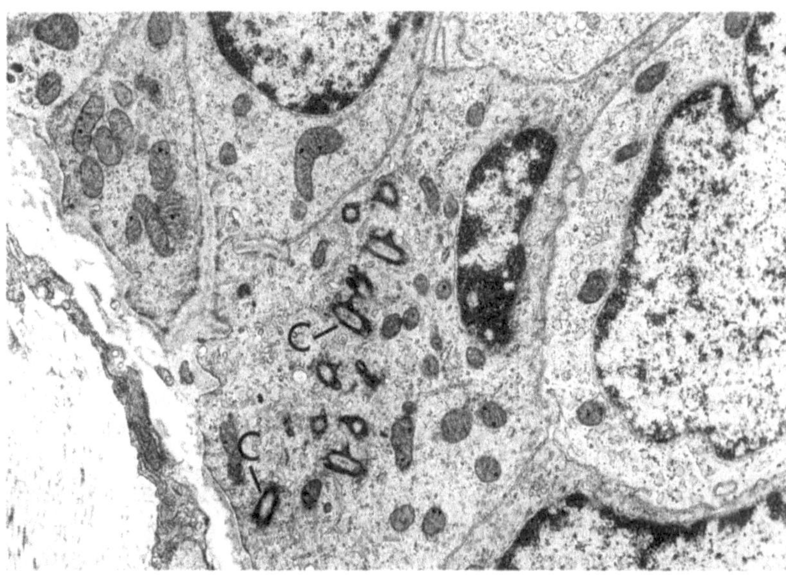
C
C

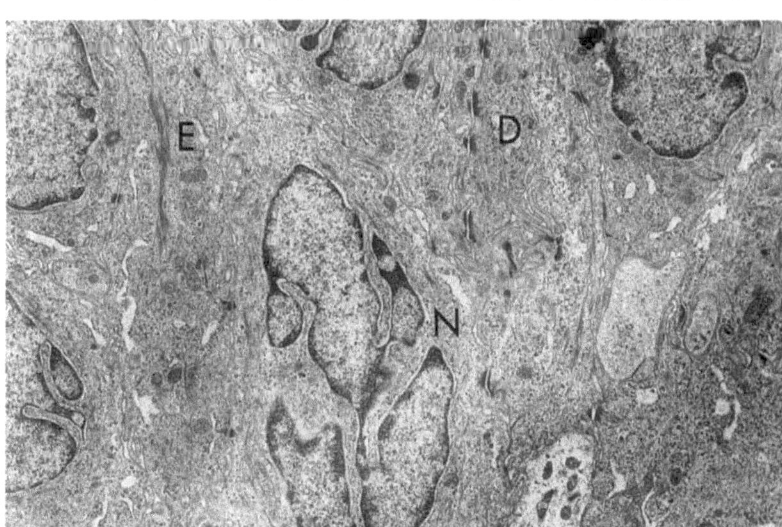
E
D
N

(Sellakumar et al. 1976). This could easily be the case if the neoplasms are pedunculated and dislodged by intralaryngeal and intratracheal instillation techniques. Metaplasia, hyperplasia, and dysplasia suspected of being preneoplastic lesions may be present simultaneously with tumor growth.

In Syrian golden hamsters spontaneously occurring papillary tumors of the airways are extremely rare (Pour et al. 1976a; Pour 1983; Homburger et al. 1983). Most induced tumors are benign; malignant progression is observed combining varying degrees of epidermoid and mucous differentiation. In general, metastasis of these tumors of the epithelial lining of the respiratory tract is not often observed, although invasive growth into the mediastinum has been reported (Herrold 1964b; Althoff et al. 1977a). Papillary tumors also arise in the ducts of subepithelial glands, and the epithelium of these glands also undergoes metaplastic changes; difficulty may occur in recognizing true invasive growth. The transplantability of papillary tumors originating in the respiratory epithelium indicates, however, their malignant potential.

**Table 1.** Carcinogens to Respiratory Epithelium

| Chemical Carcinogen | Reference |
|---|---|
| Diethylnitrosamine | Ishinishi et al. (1988)<br>Karube et al. (1991)<br>Mohr et al. (1975)<br>Schüller et al. (1990)<br>Wasito and Sleight (1989)<br>Yamamoto et al. (1985) |
| Dipropyinitrosamine | Althoff et al. (1977b) |
| *N*-Ethyl-*N*-nitrosourea | Grubbs et al. (1981) |
| Nitrosodi-*n*-propylamine | Ishinishi et al. (1988) |
| Nitroso-2-methylmorpholine | Lijinsky et al. (1984) |
| Nitrosomorpholine | Lijinsky et al. (1984)<br>Ishinishi et al. (1988)<br>Cardesa et al. (1990) |
| *N'*-Nitrosononicotine | Hecht et al. (1983) |
| 4-(*N*-nitrosomethylamino)-1-(3-pyridyl)-1-butanone | Boutet et al. (1987) |
| *N*-Methyl-*N*-nitrosourea | Grubbs et al. (1981)<br>Stinson et al. (1983) |
| Nitrosopiperidine | Cardesa et al. (1990) |
| *N*-Nitrosopyrolidine | McCoy et al. (1986) |
| Vinylethyinitrosamine | Althoff et al. (1977a) |

The respiratory epithelium of the Syrian golden hamster is highly sensitive to the adverse effects of systemically acting compounds as well as to locally applied or inhaled agents. Papillary tumors develop after a single exposure to a carcinogen or after exposure via the placenta or milk. Many experimental studies have been conducted with nitroso compounds (Table 1) and polycyclic aromatic hydrocarbons (Becci et al. 1978b; Yamamoto et al. 1985). Mucoepidermoid papillary tumors are seen exclusively after chronic administration of nitrosomorpholine and nitrosopiperidine in the trachea and subglottic larynx (Cardesa et al. 1990). Malignant progression and multiple carcinomas occur after treatment with *N*-methyl-*n*-nitrosourea (Grubbs et al. 1981) and vinylethylnitrosamine (Althoff et al. 1977a). Similar data are available from studies using two-stage initiation and promotion models. The incidence of tracheal neoplasms initiated by a single dose of a systemic carcinogen (nitrosodi-*n*-ethylamine) is increased after feeding polybrominated biphenyl (Wasito and Sleight 1989) and inhalation of nebulized sodium chloride solution (Karube et al. 1991).

In vitro models have been developed to identify mechanisms associated with the effects of carcinogens on the airways (Everitt et al. 1990). Tracheal explants from the Syrian golden hamster cultured in medium with benzo(a)pyrene mimic part of the in vivo local effect by undergoing squamous metaplasia. Epithelial proliferation with hyperplasia of atypical cells is evident as small nodular protrusions into the tracheal lumen after several weeks of exposure (He et al. 1987). Alterations in cell surface carbohydrates are interpreted as indicators for preneoplastic/neoplastic transformation (Chopra and Joiakim 1991). Exposure of fetal hamster tracheal explant with different polycyclic aromatic hydrocarbons for few days induces morphological changes of the epithelium as well as disturbances and retardation of differentiation (Richter-Reichhelm 1986). Metaplastic and hyperplastic changes in trachea explants are seen after treatment by the nitroso compounds diethylnitrosamine and *N*-methyl-*N*-nitronitrosoguanidine, but the aromatic amines such as acetylaminofluorene and aminoflourene fail to produce treatment related effects (Nowak et al. 1993). Responses to some naturally occurring and synthetic fibrous materials are of proliferative and metaplastic nature in hamster trachea cultures (Woodworth et al. 1983).

Data from in vitro experiments with tissue homogenate indicate that the trachea has a considerable capacity to metabolize polyaromatic hydrocarbonss. This metabolizing capacity of tracheal cells is higher per gram of tissue than that of lung tissue partially explaining the specific susceptibility of the hamster trachea to develop neoplasms (Dahl et al. 1985).

## Comparison with Other Species

Spontaneous pathological alterations and neoplastic changes in the upper respiratory epithelium in Syrian golden hamsters and other laboratory rodent species are infrequent (Nettesheim 1972; Pour et al. 1976a; Mohr and Richter-Reichheim 1982; Feron et al. 1990). Nonneoplastic epithelial alterations are caused mainly by infections and are found in all species. Sites where metaplasia occurs most frequently have been described also in man (Auerbach et al. 1962), pigs, dogs, and rabbits (Wang et al. 1972). Metaplasia of squamous epithelium is very common around ductal openings of subepithelial glands and the bifurcations of the tracheobronchial tree. This condition has been attributed to an increased disposition of particles at these sites resulting in prolonged alterations of mucociliary clearance and slow elimination of compounds.

If the results of experimental respiratory tract carcinogenesis are to be interpreted accurately, data from rat studies should be considered with some caution, taking into account chronic endemic bronchitis, which results in severe regenerative and dysplastic alterations, progressing to overt bronchiectasis (Pour et al. 1976b). In addition, the rat may differ significantly in the sensitivity of its respiratory epithelium to develop neoplasia after exposure to chemicals. In vitro studies on benzo(a)pyrene metabolism have indicated significant differences in hamster and rat tracheal epithelium (Mass and Kaufman 1983). Very little is known about spontaneous lesions in the main airways of mice.

Certain differences in distribution and preferential site exist between tumors of the upper respiratory system (larynx, trachea, bronchi) in hamsters and humans. In man papillary tumors of the larynx are more frequent than those of the trachea; in hamsters tracheal neoplasms predominate. Tumors which mainly occur in young human patients may be multiple, involving the entire tracheobronchial tree. Single papillary tumors have been described as developing predominately in the stem bronchi and carina, and occasionally in the main and segmental bronchi (Liebow 1952). From the histogenetic point of view the induced epithelial changes described in the respiratory tract of the Syrian golden hamster are quite comparable to findings in human bronchi (McDowell et al. 1982; Melamed and Zaman 1982).

Other hamster species, such as the European hamster (*Cricetus cricetus* L.) and the Chinese hamster (*Cricetulus griseus* M.E.) have been investigated in studies of respiratory tract carcinogenesis. Although the incidence of spontaneous tumors of the respiratory tract of European hamsters is also reported to be very low (Ernst et al. 1989), the Syrian golden hamster (*Mesocricetus auratus* W.) offers an appropriate model because of the accumulated knowledge in the physiology and pathology of lesions of this species (Mohr and Reznik 1982).

## References


Althoff J, Grandjean C, Russell L, Pour P (1977a) Vinylethylnitrosamine: potent respiratory carcinogen in Syrian hamsters. JNCI 58:439–442

Althoff J, Pour P, Grandjean C, Marsh S (1977b) Transplacental effects of nitrosamines in Syrian hamsters. Z Krebsforsch Klin Onkol Cancer 90:79–86

Althoff J, Richter-Reichhelm H-B, Green U, Kracke D (1981) Scanning electron microscopical investigations on the respiratory epithelium of the Syrian golden hamster. III. Regeneration after traumatic injury. Zentralbl Bakteriol Mikrobiol Hyg [B] 174:249–259

Auerbach O, Stout AP, Hammond EC, Garfinkel L (1962) Bronchial epithelium in former smokers. N Engl J Med 267:119–125

Becci PJ, McDowell EM, Trump BF (1978a) The respiratory epithelium. IV. Histogenesis of epidermoid metaplasia and carcinoma in situ in the hamster. JNCI 61:577–586

Becci PJ, McDowell EM, Trump BF (1978b) The respiratory epithelium. VI. Histogenesis of lung tumors induced by Benzo(a)pyrene-ferric oxid in the hamster. JNCI 61:607–618

Becci PJ, McDowell EM, Trump BF (1978c) The respiratory epithelium. II. Hamster trachea, bronchus, and bronchioles. JNCI 61:551–561

Boutet M, Montminy L, Castonguay A (1987) Cellular changes by the tobacco-specific carcinogen 4-(N-nitrosomethylamino)-1-(-3-pyridyl)-1-butanone in the respiratory tract of the Syrian golden hamsters. IARC Sci Publ 84:438–442

Cardesa A, Garcia-Bragado F, Ramirez J, Ernst H (1990) Histological types of laryngotracheal tumors induced in Syrian golden hamsters by nitrosomorpholine and nitrospiperidine. Exp Pathol 40:267–281

Chopra DP, Joiakim AP (1991) Cell-specific alterations in glycoconjugates in the development of squamous metaplasia induced by Benzo(a)pyrene in hamster tracheal explants. Toxicol Appl Pharmacol 109:529–537

Dahl AR, Coslett DS, Bond JA, Hesseltine GR (1985) Metabolism of Benzo(a)pyrene on the nasal mucosa of Syrian hamsters: comparison to metabolism by other extrahepatic tissues and possible role of nasally produced metabolites in carcinogenesis. JNCI 75:135–139

Dontenwill W, Mohr U (1961) Carcinome des Respirationstractus nach Behandlung von Goldenhamstern mit Diäthylnitrosamin. Z Krebsforsch 64:305–312

Dontenwill W, Mohr U (1962) Vergleichende Untersuchungen an metaplastischen und malignen Epithelveränfinderungen des Respirationstraktes im Tierexperiment. Z Krebsforsch 65:168–170

Ernst H, Kunstyr I, Rittinghausen S, Mohr U (1989) Spontaneous tumours of the European hamster (Cricetus cricetus L.). Z Versuchstierkd 32:87–96

Everitt JI, Hesterberg TW, Boreiko CJ (1990) The use of tracheal implants in toxicology and carcinogenesis research. Toxicology 60:27–40

Feron VJ, Woutersen RA, van Garderen-Hoetmer A, Dreef-van der Meulen HC (1990) Upper respiratory tract tumors in Cpb:WU (Wistar random) rats. Environ Health Perspect 85:305–315

Grubbs CJ, Becci PJ, Thompson HJ, Moon RC (1981) Carcinogenicity of N-methyl-N-nitrosourea and N-ethyl-N-nitrosourea when applied to a localized area of the hamster trachea. JNCI 66:961–965

He M, Hun S, Zhang L, Lian C (1987) In vitro alterations of tracheal epithelium of hamsters by carcinogens in organ cultures. Tohoku J Exp Med 152:87–100

Hecht SS, Young R, Maeura Y (1903) Comparative carcinogenicity in F344 Rats and Syrian golden hamsters of N'-nitrosonornicotine and N'-nitrosonornicotine-1-n-oxide. Cancer Lett 20:333–340

Herrold KM (1964a) Epithelial papillomas of the nasal cavity. Arch Pathol 78:189–195

Herrold KM (1964b) Effect of route of administration on the carcinogenic action of diethylnitrosamine (N-nitrosodiethylamine). Br J Cancer 18:763–767

Herrold KM, Dunham LJ (1963) Induction of tumors in the Syrian hamster with diethylnitrosamine (N-nitrosodiethylamine). Cancer Res 23:773–777

Homburger F, van Dongen CG, Adams R, Soto E (1983) Standardizing Syrian hamsters for toxicology. In: Homburger F (ed) Safety evaluation and regulation of chemicals. Karger, Basel, pp 225–232

Ishinishi N, Tanaka A, Hisanaga A, Inamasu T, Hirata M (1988) Comparative study on the carcinogenicity of N-nitrosodiethylamine, N-nitrosodimethylamine, N-nitrosomorpholine, N-nitrosopyrrolidine and N-nitrosodi-n-propylamine to the lung of Syrian golden hamsters following intermittent instillations to the trachea. Carcinogenesis 9:947–950

Karube T, Katayama H, Takemoto K, Watanabe S (1991) Promoting effect of sodium chloride solution mist on the induction of papillomas on Syrian hamster tracheal mucosa following administration of diethylnitrosamine. Jpn J Cancer Res 82:638–641

Kreyberg L (1967) International histological classification of tumours. No 1: histological typing of lung tumours. WHO, Geneva

Lijinsky W, Kovatch RM, Knutsen GL (1984) Carcinogenesis by nitrosomorpholines, nitrosooxazolidines and nitrosoazetidine given by gavage to Syrian golden hamsters. Carcinogenesis 5:875–878

Liebow AA (1952) Tumors of the lower respiratory tract. In: Atlas of tumor pathology, 1st series, fasicle 17, sect 5. Armed Forces Institute of Pathology, Washington DC

Marshall HE III, Keenan KP, McDowell EM (1987) The stathmokinetic and morphological response of the hamster respiratory epithelium to intralaryngeal instillations of saline and ferric oxide in saline. Fund Appl Toxicol 9:705–714

Mass MJ, Kaufman DG (1983) A comparison between the activation of benzo(a)pyrene in organ cultures and microsomes from the tracheal epithelium of rats and hamsters. Carcinogenesis 4:297–303

McCoy GD, Hecht SS, Furuya K (1986) The effect of chronic ethanol consumption of N-nitrosopyrrolidine in male Syrian golden hamsters. Cancer Lett 33:151–159

McDowell EM, Becci PJ, Schürch W, Trump BF (1979) The respiratory epithelium. VII. Epidermoid metaplasia of hamster tracheal epithelium during regeneration following mechanical injury. JNCI 62:995–1008

McDowell EM, Harris CC, Trump BF (1982) Histogenesis and morphogenesis of bronchial neoplasms. In: Shimosato Y, Melamed MR, Nettesheim P (eds) Morphogenesis of lung cancer, vol 1. CRC Press, Boca Raton, pp 1–36

Melamed MR, Zaman MB (1982) Pathogenesis of epidermoid carcinoma of the lung. In: Shimosato Y, Melamed MR, Nettesheim P (eds) Morphogenesis of lung cancer, vol 1. CRC, Boca Raton, pp 37–64

Mohr U (1970) Effects of diethylnitrosamine in the respiratory system of Syrian golden hamsters. In: Nettesheim P, Hanna MG, Deatherage JW (eds) Morphology of experimental respiratory carcinogenesis. USAEC, Division of Technical Information, Oak Ridge, pp 255–265 (AEC symposium series no 21)

Mohr U, Reznik G (1982) Three hamster species as models in cancer research. In: Turusov VS (ed) Pathology of tumours in laboratory animals, vol III. Tumours of the hamster. IARC Sci Publ 34:437–442

Mohr U, Richter-Reichhelm HB (1982) The impact of spontaneous pathology on the quality of animals for toxicological studies. In: Bartosek I, Guaitani A, Pacei E (eds) Animals in toxicological research. Raven, New York, pp 65–70

Mohr U, Reznik-Schüller H, Reznik G, Hilfrich J (1975) Transplacental effects of diethylnitrosamine (DEN) in Syrian hamsters as related to different days of administration during pregnancy. JNCI 55:681–683

Nettesheim P (1972) Respiratory carcinogenesis studies with the Syrian golden hamster: a review. Prog Exp Tumor Res 16:185–200

Nowak C, Gleier K, Christ M, Gorzelniak K, Richter-Reichhelm H-B (1993) Effects of nitroso compounds and aromatic amines on fetal tracheal explants. Exp Pathol Toxicol 45:81–86

Pour P (1983) Spontaneous respiratory tract tumors in Syrian hamsters. In: Reznik-Schüller HM (ed) Comparative respiratory tract carcinogenesis, vol 1. Spontaneous respiratory tract carcinogenesis. CRC, Boca Raton, pp 131–170

Pour P, Mohr U, Cardesa A, Althoff J, Kmoch N (1976a) Spontaneous tumors and common diseases in two colonies of Syrian hamsters. II. Respiratory tract and digestive system. JNCI 56:937–948

Pour P, Stanton MF, Kuschner M, Laskin S, Shabad LM (1976b) Tumours of the respiratory tract. In: Turusov VS (ed) Pathology of tumours in laboratory animals, vol I. Tumours of the rat, part 2. IARC Sci Publ 6:1–61

Richter-Reichhelm HB (1986) Perinatal induction of alterations in the respiratory epithelium. In vivo–in vitro comparison. In: Grosdanoff P, König W, Müller D, Otto H, Reznik GK, Ulmer WT (eds) Drug-related damage to the respiratory tract. Schriftenreihe des Bundesgesundheitsamtes, Medizin Verlag Munich, pp 587–594 (AMI-Berichte, vol 4)

Richter-Reichhelm HB, Emura M, Althoff J (1980) Scanning electron microscopical investigations on the respiratory epithelium of the Syrian golden hamster. I. Postnatal differentiation. Zentralbl Bakteriol Mikrobiol Hyg [B] 171:424-432

Schüller HM, Correa E, Orloff M, Reznik GK (1990) Successful chemotherapy of experimental neuroendocrine lung tumors in hamsters with an antagonist of Ca2+/calmodulin. Cancer Res 50:1645–1649

Sellakumar A, Stenback F, Rowland J (1976) Effects of different dusts on respiratory carcinogenesis in hamsters induced by benzo(a)pyrene and diethylnitrosamine. Eur J Cancer 12:313–319

Stinson SF, Reznik-Schüller HM, Reznik G, Donahoe R (1983) Spindle cell carcinoma of the hamster trachea induced by n-methyl-n-nitrosourea. Am J Pathol 111:21–26

Wang N-S, Huang S-N, Thurlbeck WM (1972) Squamous metaplasia of the opening of bronchial glands. Am J Pathol 67:571–582

Wasito, Sleight SD (1989) Promoting effect of polybrominated biphenyls on tracheal papillomas in Syrian golden hamsters. J Toxicol Environ Health 27:173–187

Woodworth CD, Mossman BT, Craighead JE (1983) Induction of squamous metaplasia in organ cultures of hamster trachea by naturally occurring and synthetic fibers. Cancer Res 43:4906–4912

Yamamoto A, Hisanga A, Ishinishi N (1985) Comparative study on the carcinogenicity of N-nitrosodiethylamine and benzo(a)pyrene to the lung of Syrian golden hamsters induced by intermittent instillations to the trachea. Cancer Lett 25:271–276

# Nasal Neoplasia

Kevin T. Morgan and Jack R. Harkema

## Introduction

The pathological features of nasal neoplasia in rats, mice, and hamsters has been extensively reviewed (Brown et al. 1991; Feron and Bosland 1989; Feron et al. 1990; Reznik and Stinson 1983). Tumors have been recorded for each of the major nasal epithelial types and a number of accessory structures, and some of these neoplasms are the subject of recent research on mechanisms of carcinogenesis. Toxicological pathology may contribute in a major way to this research through (a) determination of the site of origin of nasal tumors, (b) identification of the tissue or cell type from which they were derived, and (c) characterization of tumor progression from the earliest stages of the process. This paper outlines diagnostic issues of importance for nasal tumors, using selected examples. More detailed information is available in the literature cited. Throughout this text the anatomical identifiers are derived from classic anatomical texts (Hebel and Stromberg 1976; Negus 1958; Reznik 1983; Sorokin 1983), while the classification of the nasal meatuses and ethmoid turbinates are those proposed by Morgan et al. (1991) and Mery et al. (1994), respectively. No attempt is made to provide an exhaustive review of the extensive literature on nasal neoplasia in rodents. A number of critical reviews are cited and selected details of the major tumor types are presented.

## Classification of Nasal Neoplasms in Rodents

A number of classification schemes have been proposed for nasal neoplasms in rodents, including a fairly complex approach (Brown 1990). The latter classification, with our modifications to incorporate transitional epithelial neoplasms and other minor changes, is shown in Table 2. Classification systems such as this are largely based on light microscopic identification of the tissue or cell type of origin, with limited supportive evidence derived from cell type specific markers. For the squamous, transitional, and respiratory regions the morphogenesis of the majority of neoplasms is fairly distinct, though not necessarily well defined. Morphological studies indicate that polypoid adenomas (Kerns 1985) and squamous cell carcinomas (Morgan et al. 1986) induced by formaldehyde were derived from the airway lining epithelium. In contrast, squamous cell carcinomas and adenocarcinomas induced by nitrosomethylpiperazine in the respiratory portion of the nose were considered to originate from

**Table 2.** Provisional outline for classification of nasal neoplasms in the nasal passages of rats and mice (modified from Brown 1960)

| |
|---|
| Squamous epithelium |
| Squamous cell papilloma |
| Squamous cell carcinoma (not reported) |
| Transitional epithelium |
| Transitional (polypoid) adenoma |
| Transitional carcinoma |
| Squamous cell papilloma |
| Squamous cell carcinoma |
| Adenosquamous carcinoma |
| Respiratory Epithelium |
| Adenoma |
| Carcinoma |
| Squamous cell papilloma |
| Squamous cell carcinoma |
| Olfactory Epithelium |
| Neuroepithelial carcinoma |
| Sustentacular cell |
| Basal cell (neuroblastoma) |
| Solid |
| Neuroendocrine mixed |
| Bowman's gland carcinoma |
| Adenosquamous carcinoma |
| Squamous cell carcinoma |
| Epidermoid (inverted) papilloma |
| Mesenchymal tumors (selected examples) |
| Rhabdomyoma/rhabdomyosarcoma |
| Hemangioma/hemangiosarcoma |
| Chondroma/chondrosarcoma |
| Fibroma/fibrosarcoma |
| Malignant schwannoma |
| Nasal glands |
| Adenoma/adenocarcinoma of septal and mural nasal seromucous glands |
| Adenoma/adenocarcinoma of maxillary sinus (Steno's) glands |
| Tumors of Accesory and Paranasal Structures |
| Nasolacrymal duct squamous cell papilloma/carcinoma |
| Periodontal squamous cell carcinomas |

acinar cells of the submucous glands (Schüller 1989). In the olfactory region the issue of tumor histogenesis is more problematic due to the relative complexity of the olfactory mucosa. On the basis of immunocytochemical and ultrastructural approaches using serial sacrifices it has been proposed that many olfactory mucosal neoplasms induced in the nose by nitrosamines may be derived from neuroendocrine cells (Schüller 1989). Feron et al. (1990) have discussed evidence supporting the proposal that olfactory epithelial neoplasms induced by certain chemicals are derived from olfactory epithelial basal cells. The latter workers supported the view that all types of tumors derived from the olfactory epithelium be classified as neuroepitheliomas. As stated by Schüller (1989), these "diagnostic difficulties are reflected in the lack of an internationally applied tumor classification for this organ system, as well as vague descriptions rather than precise tumor classification."

## Background Incidence

Limited information is available on background incidence rates in rodents. Feron et al. (1990) reviewed nasal neoplasms in untreated control Cpb:WU (Wistar random) rats and found an incidence of 1.1% in males and 0% in females. These neoplasms were invariably squamous cell carcinomas, and a number of them were attributable to dental problems, such as the malocclusion syndrome. Another common paranasal site of squamous cell carcinomas in these rats was the nasolachrymal duct (Schoevera et al. 1994). Brown et al. (1991) reviewed the spontaneous nasal tumor incidence in Fischer 344 rats and B6C3Fl mice in the National Toxicology Program archives and found an incidence "usually far less than 0.5% for any tumor type in any location." Of these neoplasms squamous cell carcinoma occurred most frequently, with a slight excess in males. In mice spontaneous nasal tumor incidence was much lower than in rats, with the few tumors observed, hemangioma and adenoma, occurring in females.

## Gross Appearance

The first indication of nasal neoplasia may be seen as respiratory distress from airway obstruction or discoloration of periorbital skin due to occlusion of the nasolacrimal ducts. Larger locally invasive tumors may penetrate the subcutis and create a distinct mass. Anterior nasal neoplasms, generally squamous cell carcinomas, frequently produce a distinct protuberance over the anterior snout (Kerns et al. 1983). Neoplasms of the more posterior olfactory region lead to doming of the skull at the level of the eyes (Feron et al. 1990; Woutersen et al. 1986). Small neoplasms in critical regions of the upper airways, such as the nasopharyngeal meatus, may lead to the death of an animal by asphyxiation long before it exhibits evidence of true malignancy. Smaller nasal neoplasms are frequently identifiable during trimming of tissues following decalcification prior to histological processing. It is not recommended that nasal passages be dissected to find nasal neoplasms during routine toxicology studies, as this leads to serious impairment of histological preparations.

## Microscopic Features

Each of the major, or most frequently encountered, tumor types reported ia described below in the order presented in Table 2. The examples provided are somewhat biased toward those for which cases are available to the authors for photography.

### Squamous Epithelium

Squamous papillomas may arise from the squamous epithelium of the nasal vestibule, the ventral meatus, or the nasopalatine duct. Such neoplasms, unless present in the most anterior region of the vestibule, are difficult to distinguish from polypoid adenomas (see following) exhibiting squamous differentiation (Figs. 109, 111). In either case these squamous papillomas are comprised of fronds of well differentiated squamous epithelium, with variable degrees of keratinization, supported by a fibrovascular connective tissue core (Fig. 111). It is unlikely that neoplasms of the squamous lining of the nasal vestibule progress to overt malignancy before occlusion of the nasal airways results in severe respiratory difficulty.

### Transitional Epithelium

*Transitional (Polypoid) Adenoma/Carcinoma.* Kerns (1985) have described transitional adenomas in detail at both the light microscopic and ultrastructural levels. These neoplasms arise as small areas of transitional epithelial hyperplasia in the lateral meatus and on the free margins of

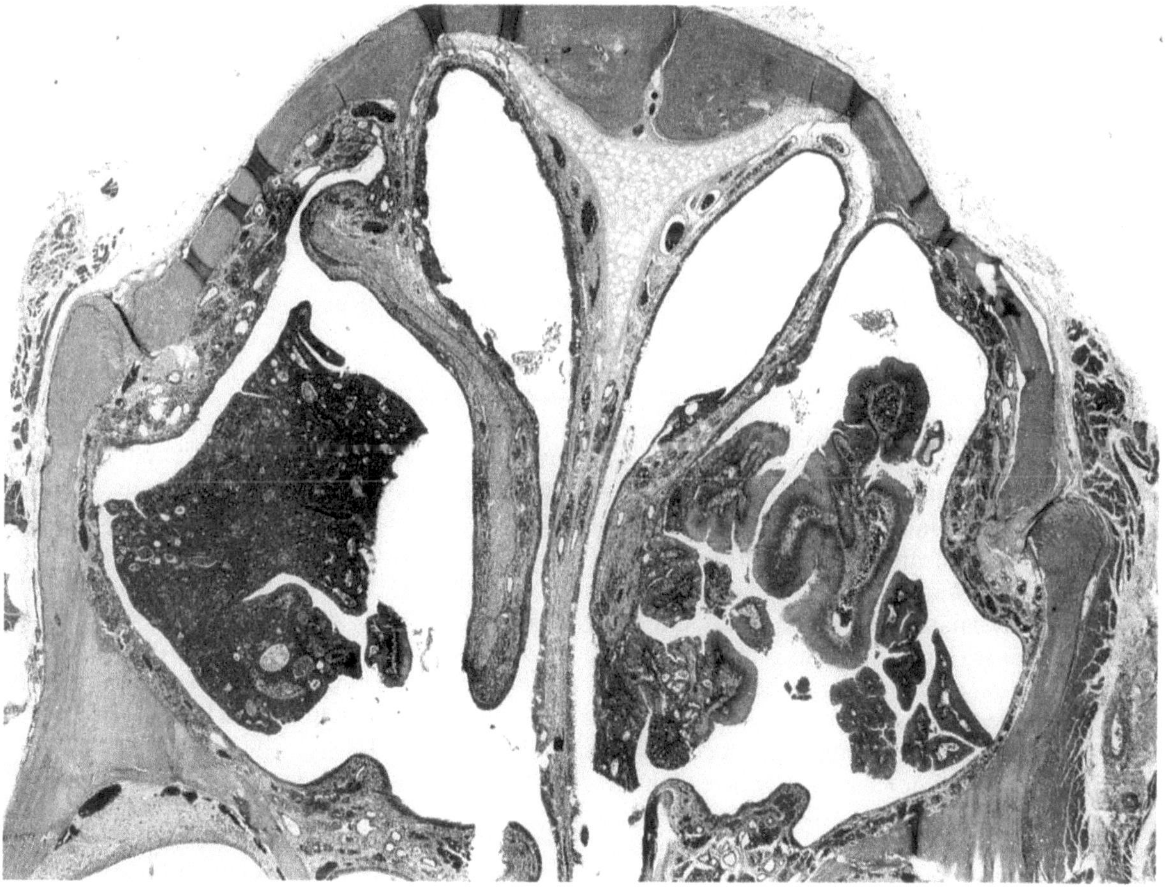

**Fig. 109.** Anterior nasal passages of a rat exposed to nitrosodiethylamine exhibiting bilateral neoplasia, with a transitional (polypoid) adenoma on one side (*left*) and a squamous papilloma on the other. Portions of these neoplasms are shown in Figs. 110 and 111, respectively. H&E, ×28

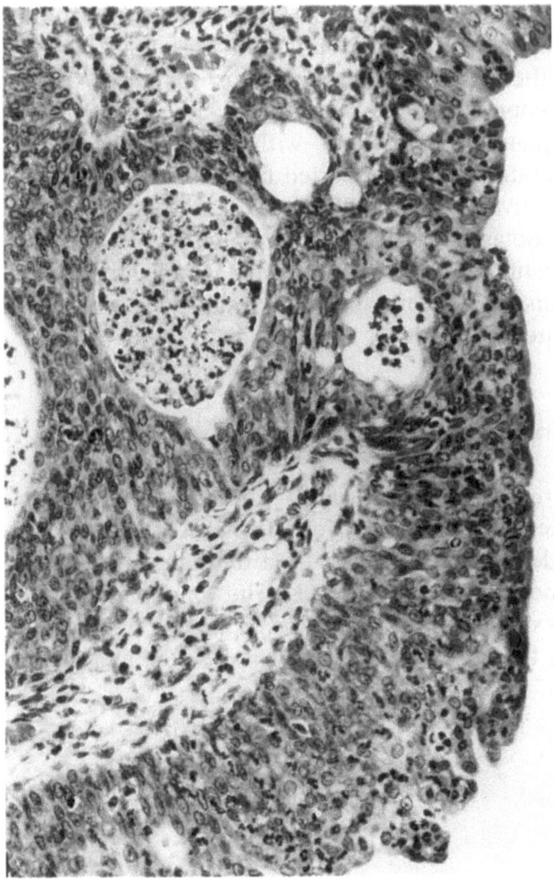

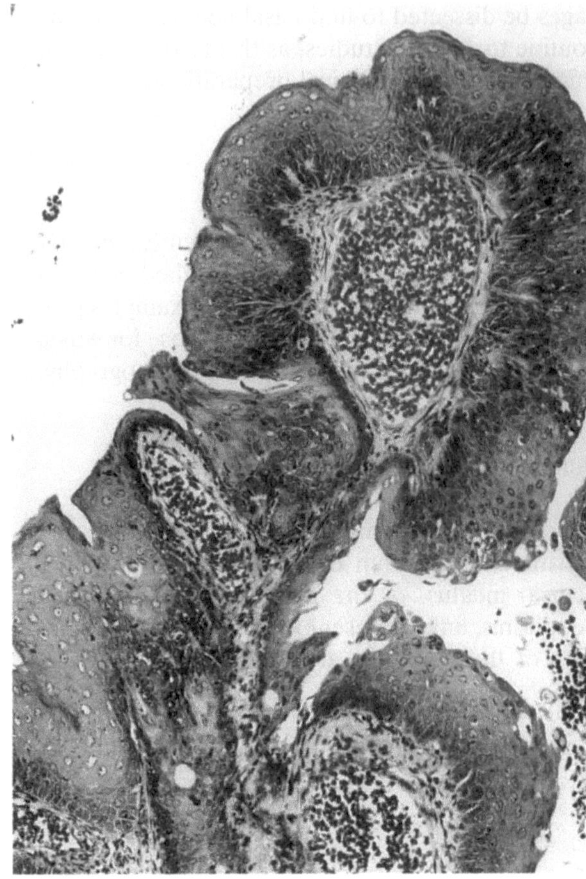

**Fig. 110.** *(left)* Transitional polypoid adenoma with thickened transitional epithelial exhibiting inflammatory cell infiltration, and microcysts containing cellular debris. H&E, ×140

**Fig. 111.** *(right)* Squamous papilloma with well-differentiated squamous epithelium supported by a highly vascular connective tissue core. H&E, ×140

the naso- and maxilloturbinates in the anterior nose. Transitional adenomas are typically comprised of masses or fronds of hyperplastic transitional epithelium which is rarely ciliated and is supported by a delicate fibrous or fibrovascular stroma. As a consequence of a small peduncle these neoplasms may appear to be free floating in the nasal lumen (Fig. 110). The tumor cells are cuboidal to low columnar, and they form solid sheets or microcysts containing large numbers of neutrophils or cellular fragments of uncertain origin (Fig. 110). These neoplasms may be exophytic or endophytic, may occasionally exhibit areas of epidermoid differentiation, and have been reported to progress to carcinomas.

*Squamous Cell Papilloma/Carcinoma/Adenosquamous Carcinoma.* These neoplasms of the transitional epithelium resemble morphologically their counterparts in the respiratory epithelial region described below.

## Respiratory Epithelium

*Respiratory Epithelial Adenoma.* Papillary adenomas of the respiratory epithelium occur throughout the nose, even arising occasionally in the posterior ethmoid region at the respiratory/olfactory epithelial junction. These neoplasms are comprised of small clusters or fronds of well-differentiated ciliated respiratory epithelium with variable numbers of goblet cells. These neoplasms are generally rare, and we are not aware of the relative preponderance of endophytic versus exophytic types.

*Respiratory Epithelial Carcinoma.* Adenocarcinomas of the respiratory epithelium are reportedly most common in the anterior nose (Brown et al. 1991) arising from regions of folding or invagination of the surface epithelium of the air-

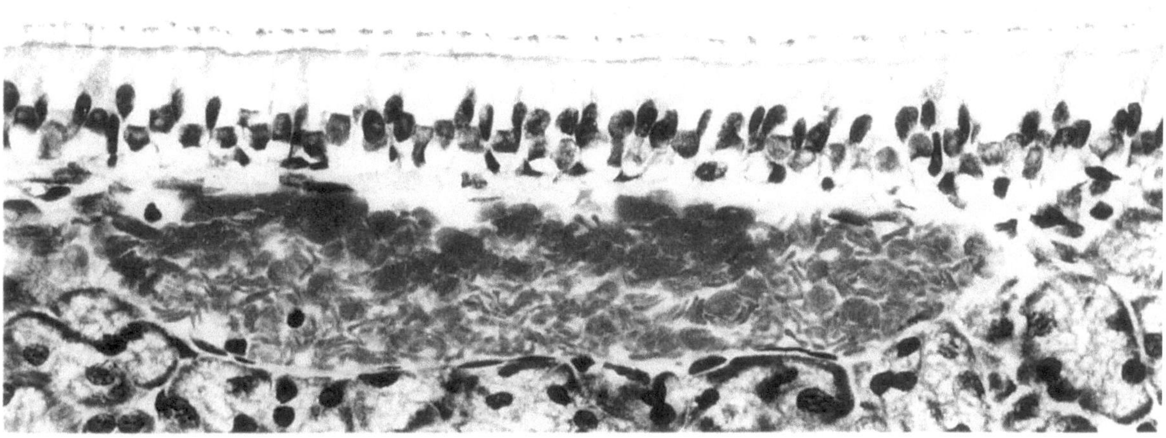

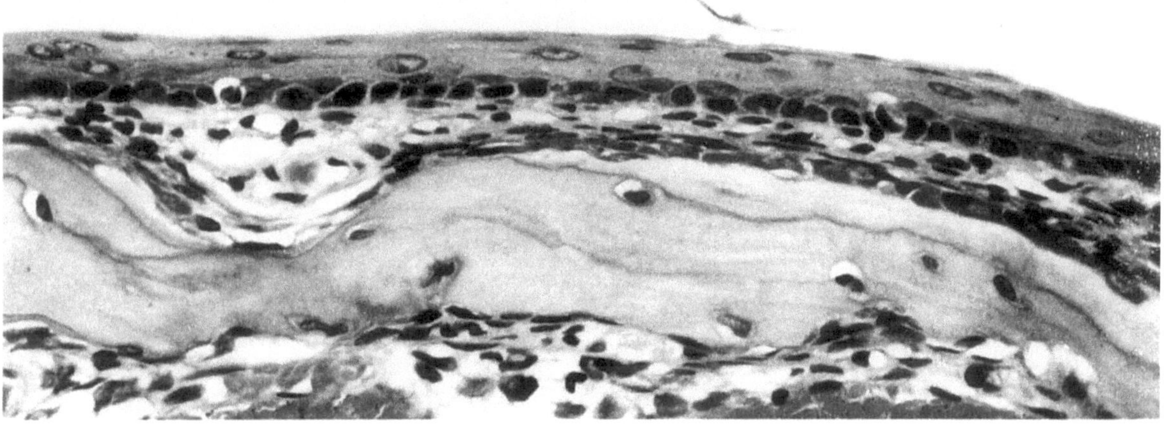

**Fig. 112.** (*above*) Normal ciliated respiratory epithelium of the nasal septum of an untreated control male F344 rat. H&E, ×280

**Fig. 113.** (*below*) Squamous metaplasia of the respiratory epithelium of the nasoturbinate induced by 1-week exposure to 15 ppm formaldehyde. H&E, ×280

way. Basal growth of these neoplasms leads to the formation of parallel columns or solid sheets of cells. Distinction of adenocarcinomas arising from respiratory versus transitional epithelium may be challenging in the anterior nose. Tumor location provides a valuable guide, with transitional epithelial tumors being confined to the anterior half of the lateral meatus. However, in the absence of adequate material from respiratory epithelial neoplasms distinctive criteria for their differentiation could not be developed by the authors. Such neoplasms also need to be distinguished from adenocarcinomas arising in the subepithelial glands. Respiratory epithelial adenocarcinomas of the maxillary sinus have been observed invading adjacent tooth structures. The latter neoplasms have been reported to form serous glands with poorly organized acini (Brown et al. 1991). These adenocarcinomas are generally rare, and little material was available to us for a detailed review of their morphology.

*Squamous Cell Papilloma/Carcinoma of the Respiratory Epithelium.* Squamous cell neoplasms of the transitional and respiratory regions of the nose are induced by a number of chemicals, including formaldehyde, hexamethylphosphoramide, hydrazine, and 1,4-dioxane. The morphogenesis of these neoplasms includes the appearance of keratinizing squamous lesions. However, the role of "adaptive" squamous metaplasia in this process, if any, remains to be determined. Squamous metaplasia is a common response to many nasal irritants, the majority of which are noncarcinogenic in this site. [The distinction of such "nonneoplastic" squamous metaplasia (Figs. 112, 113) from keratinizing squamous epithelial lesions is an important task during the interpretation of nasal responses.] Squamous

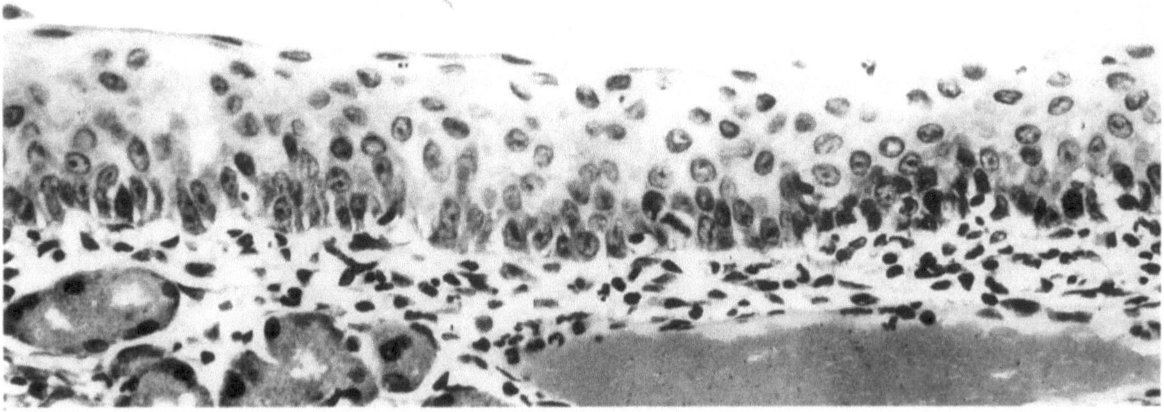

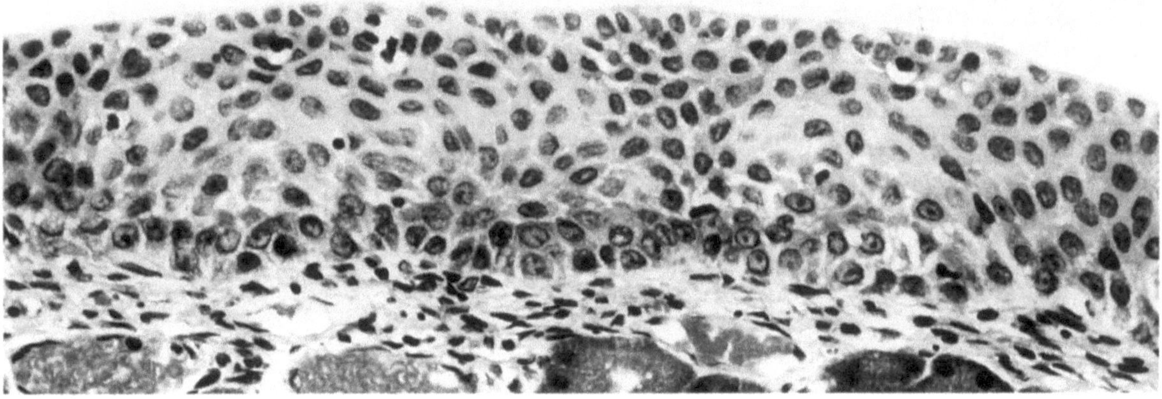

**Fig. 114.** (*above*) Nonkeratinizing epithelial hyperplasia with evidence of squame formation on the surface. Early "preneoplastic" lesion induced by 15 ppm formaldehyde inhalation in a male F344 rat. H&E, ×280

**Fig. 115.** (*below*) Severe epithelial hyperplasia with clusters of large polyhedral epithelial cells with prominent cytoplasm and considerable basal proliferation in a "putative preneoplastic" lesion induced by formaldehyde in the transitional epithelium of a male F344 rat. H&E, ×280

metaplasia induced by chemicals that are noncarcinogenic in the nose characteristically undergoes minimal keratization. In contrast, certain preneoplastic lesions (see following) produce extensive keratin. A number of chemicals that induce squamous cell carcinomas in this region of the nose also induce severe epithelial damage in the early stages of the carcinogenic process.

The progression of squamous cell carcinomas from "putative preneoplastic lesions" (Morgan and Monticello 1990) is shown in Figs. 114–119. A similar progression is observed in respiratory or transitional epithelial regions. Initial formation of nonkeratinized epithelial plaques (Figs. 114, 115) precedes the appearance of heavily keratinized

▶

**Fig. 116.** (*above*) Heavily keratinized "putative preneoplastic" lesion induced by 15 ppm formaldehyde in a male F344 rat. Note prominent keratohyalin granules, surface layers of keratinized squames, and dysplastic changes in the basal layer. These lesions differ morphologically from "adaptive squamous metaplasia" (Fig. 113), from which they should be distinguished and classified separately. H&E, ×280

**Fig. 117.** (*below*) Squamous papilloma in the lateral meatus of a F344 rat exposed to 15 ppm formaldehyde. Note prominent formation of keratinized squamous debris filling much of the nasal lumen. Loss of bone around the tooth may be due to pressure atrophy and thus should be interpreted with caution when assessing the degree of malignancy of such neoplasms. H&E, ×28

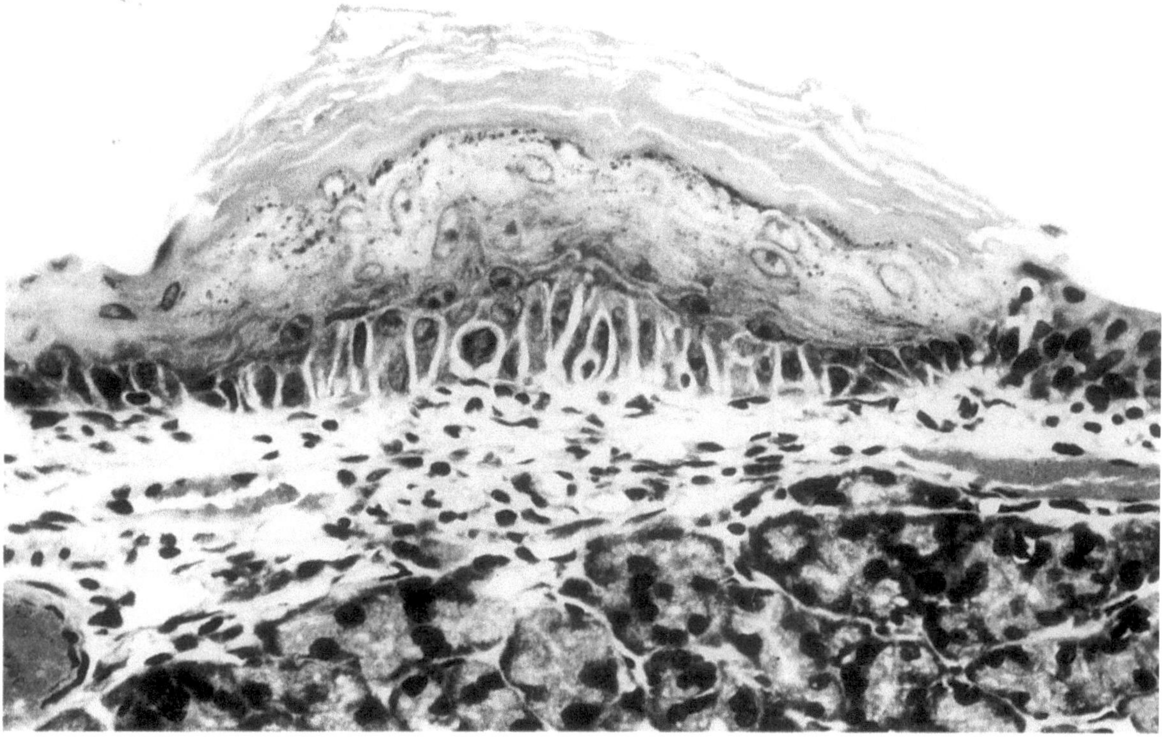

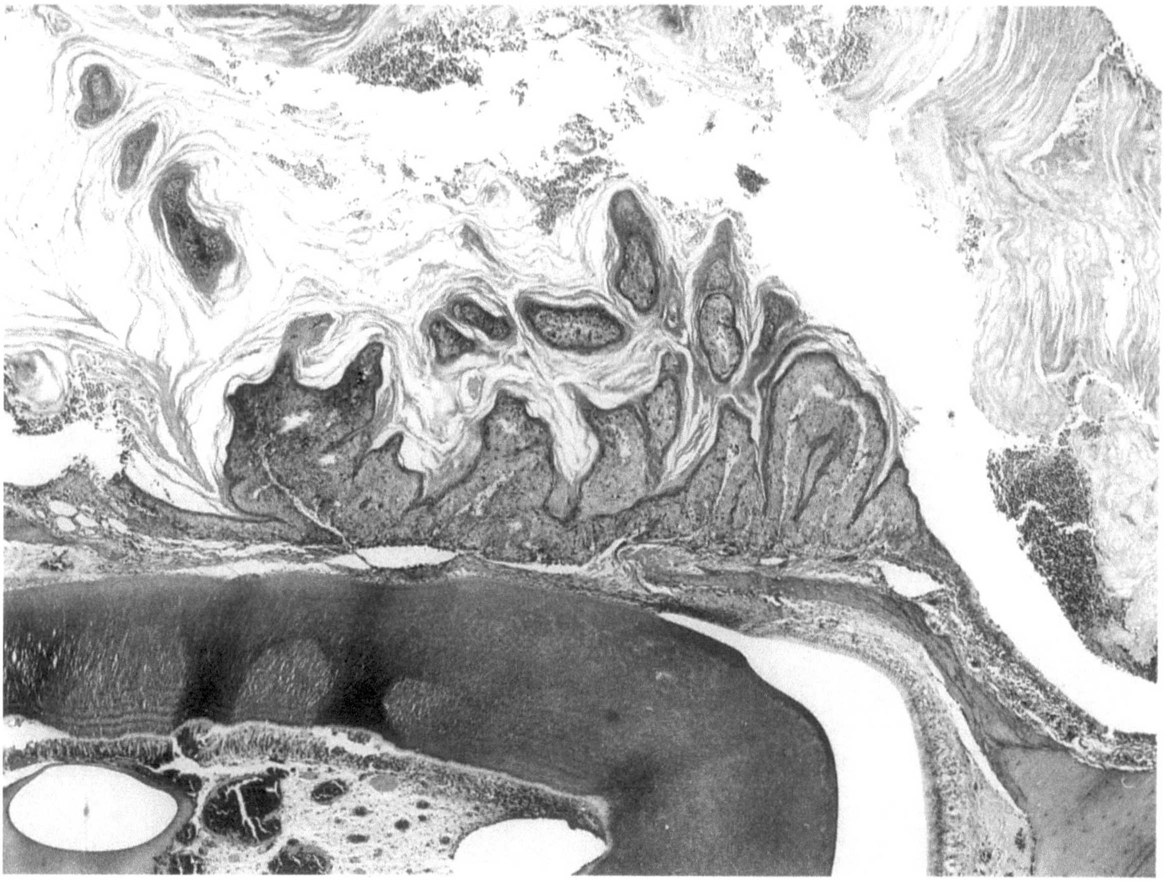

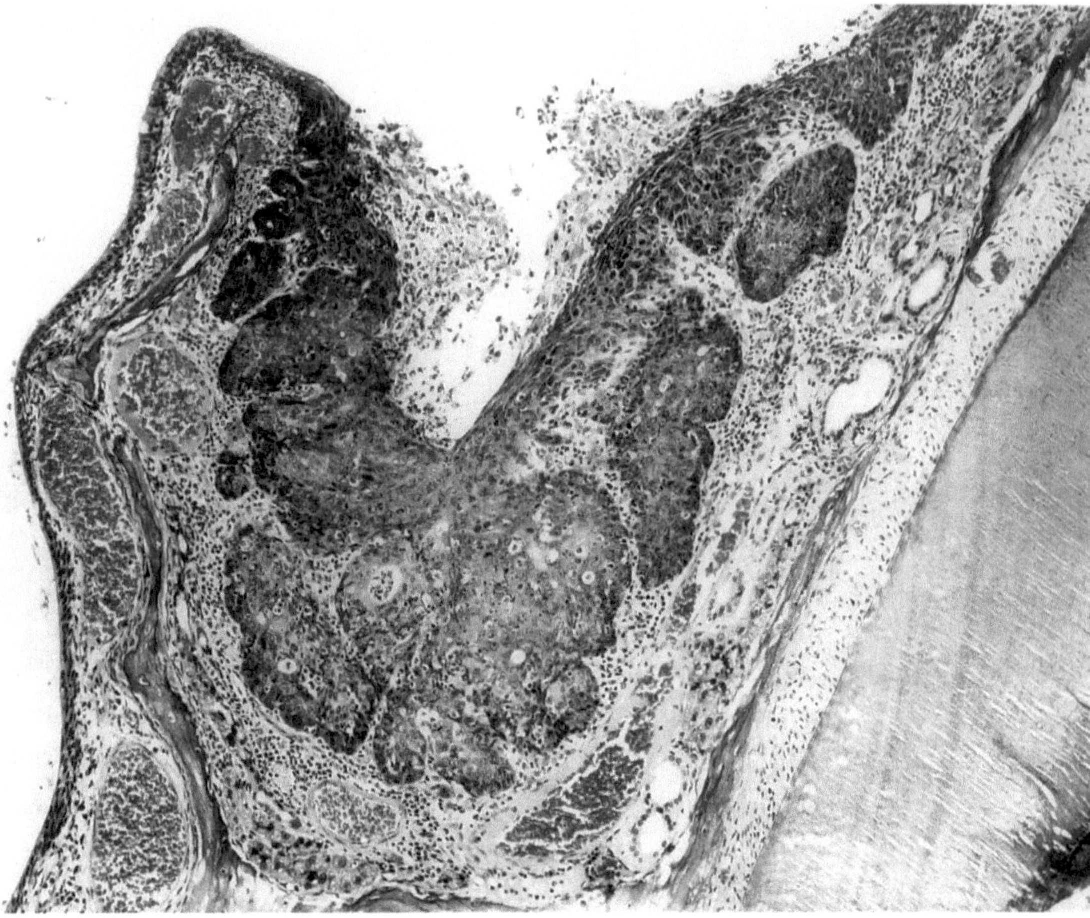

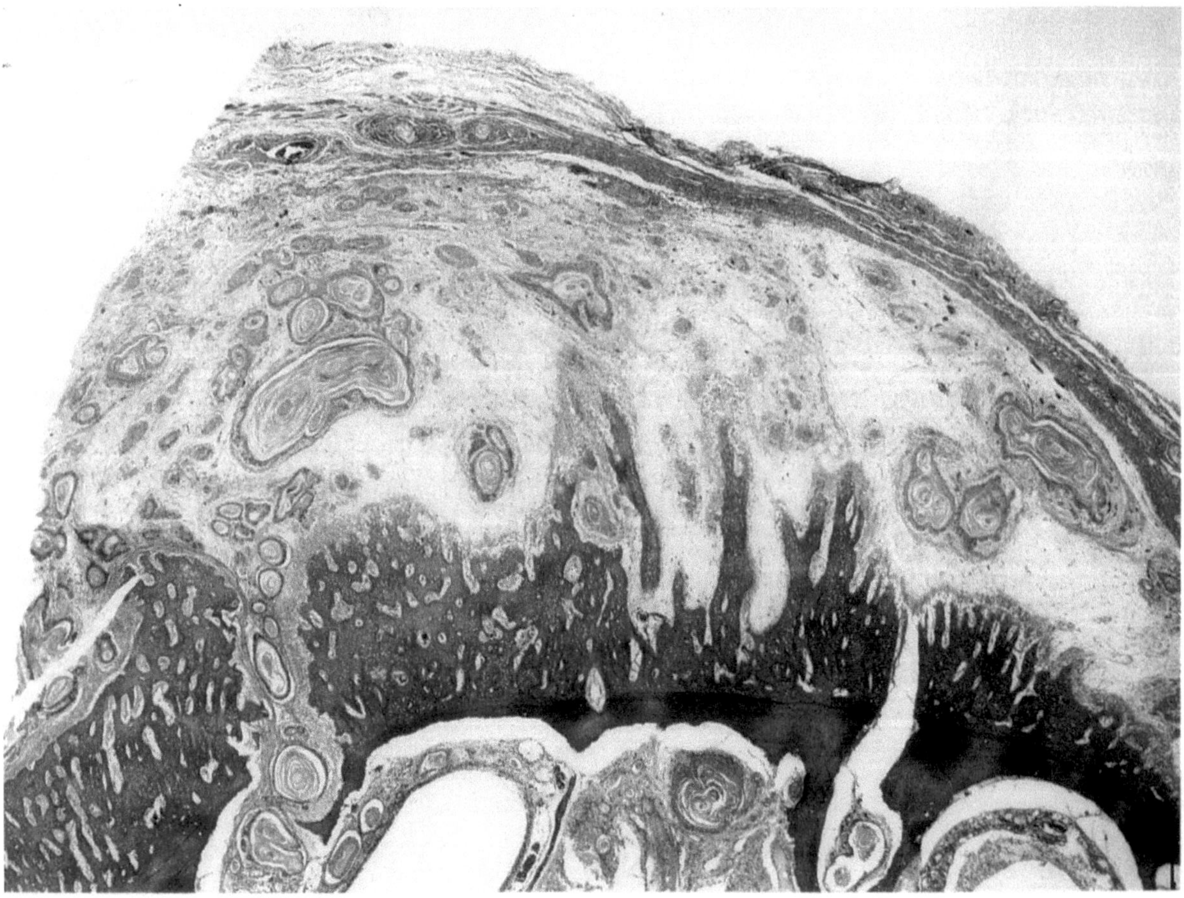

plaques with variable degrees of basal dysplasia (Fig. 116). These keratinizing lesions may produce large quantities of squames that can occlude the airways, lead to pressure atrophy of adjacent structures, and if present in a critical airway such as the nasopharyngeal meatus result in the early death of the animal. More extensive keratization may be associated with folding and formation of papillary structures (Fig. 117). However, carcinoma formation appears to result from active downgrowth of the basal layers of "preneoplastic" plaques with the induction of carcinoma in situ (Fig. 118) or frank squamous cell carcinoma (Fig. 119). Once formed, these squamous cell carcinomas are highly invasive and readily penetrate between or through the bones of the nose to form subcutaneous masses. These neoplasms rarely penetrate the nasal cartilages, but track extensively along soft tissues such as those of the vomeronasal organ. Large squamous cell carcinomas of the anterior nose may invade posteriorly to enter the cranial vault via the cribriform plate and lead to extensive compression or distortion of the olfactory bulbs and other anterior brain structures. Nasal squamous cell carcinomas vary considerably in their morphology, making diagnosis problematic in some cases. These neoplasms range from highly keratinized tumors with extensive pearl formation, through increasingly cellular or solid forms, to purely cellular nonkeratinized tumors made up of spindle cells.

## Olfactory Epithelium

Olfactory mucosal neoplasms occur in a wide range of morphological patterns, which is in part attributable to multiple potential cellular precursors. A systematic approach to classification of these neoplasms in rodents is still needed, and morphology alone may be insufficient to determine the origin of neoplastic cells. Future studies using cellular markers may clarify this issue. These neoplasms may derive from a number of olfactory epithelial elements, including basal cells and globose (immature) sensory cells, sustentacular cells, and cells lining the intraepithelial ducts of Bowman's glands. Neoplasms may also arise from elements of the lamina propria, with Bowman's glands being the most frequent target.

*Neuroepithelial Carcinoma.* Neoplasms of the olfactory epithelium frequently arise as foci of hyperplasia of basal cells, which may occur as marked basophilia and hypercellularity of the basal layer, or alternately there is formation of plaque of large cells with homogeneous eosinophilic cytoplasm (Fig. 120). Increasing proliferation of these modified basal (or at least basally located) cells leads to epithelial thickening and folding (Fig. 121) and subsequent differentiation along a number of potential morphological lines including "epidermoid" or adenosquamous, sustentacular cell (Fig. 122), neuroblastic (Fig. 123), or mixed patterns of sustentacular and sensory cells. The latter neoplasms may form variably well-organized epithelial structures. Epithelial cells in sheets may occur around cystic lumena containing cellular debris (Figs. 124, 125) and often form rosettes or pseudorosettes (Brown et al. 1991; Fig. 125 inset). Neuroendocrine cell neoplasms have also been reported as a common response to certain nasal carcinogens (Schüller 1989). Olfactory epithelial neoplasms frequently penetrate the cribriform plate to extensively involve the anterior brain (Fig. 124).

*Bowman's Gland Carcinoma.* Neoplasms may also arise in the Bowman's glands, initially appearing as foci of hyperplasia of the ductular and secretory components of these glands. Carcinoma of Bowman's glands is seen as a complex array of glandular structures with variable degrees of dedifferentiation from the normal appearance (Fig. 126). These neoplasms are highly invasive locally, and their margins may be indistinct. Neoplasms induced by a number of nitrosamines may contain complex morphological patterns due to the presence of lesions simultaneously involving other target cell populations (Fig. 126).

## Mesenchymal Tumors

Several mesenchymal neoplasms have been reported in the nose of rodents (Brown 1990;

◄

**Fig. 118.** (*above*) Carcinoma in situ in the ventral lateral meatus of a male rat exposed to 15 ppm formaldehyde. H&E, ×140

**Fig. 119.** (*below*) Squamous cell carcinoma in a rat exposed to 15 ppm formaldehyde. This neoplasm exhibits extensive squamous epithelial pearl formation and has penetrated between the bones of the skull to enter the subcutis. Such neoplasms are evident grossly as a mass on the anterior snout. The presence of exostoses, radiating as fine spicules from the nasal bones, contribute to the mass in this location. H&E, ×28

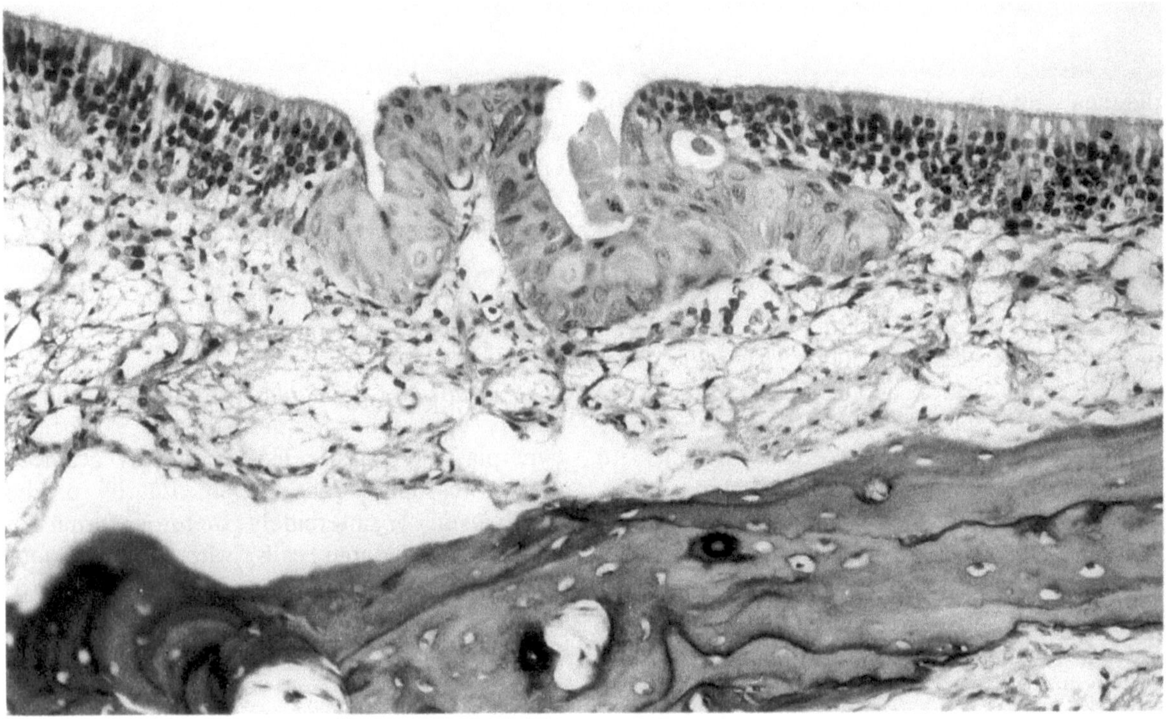

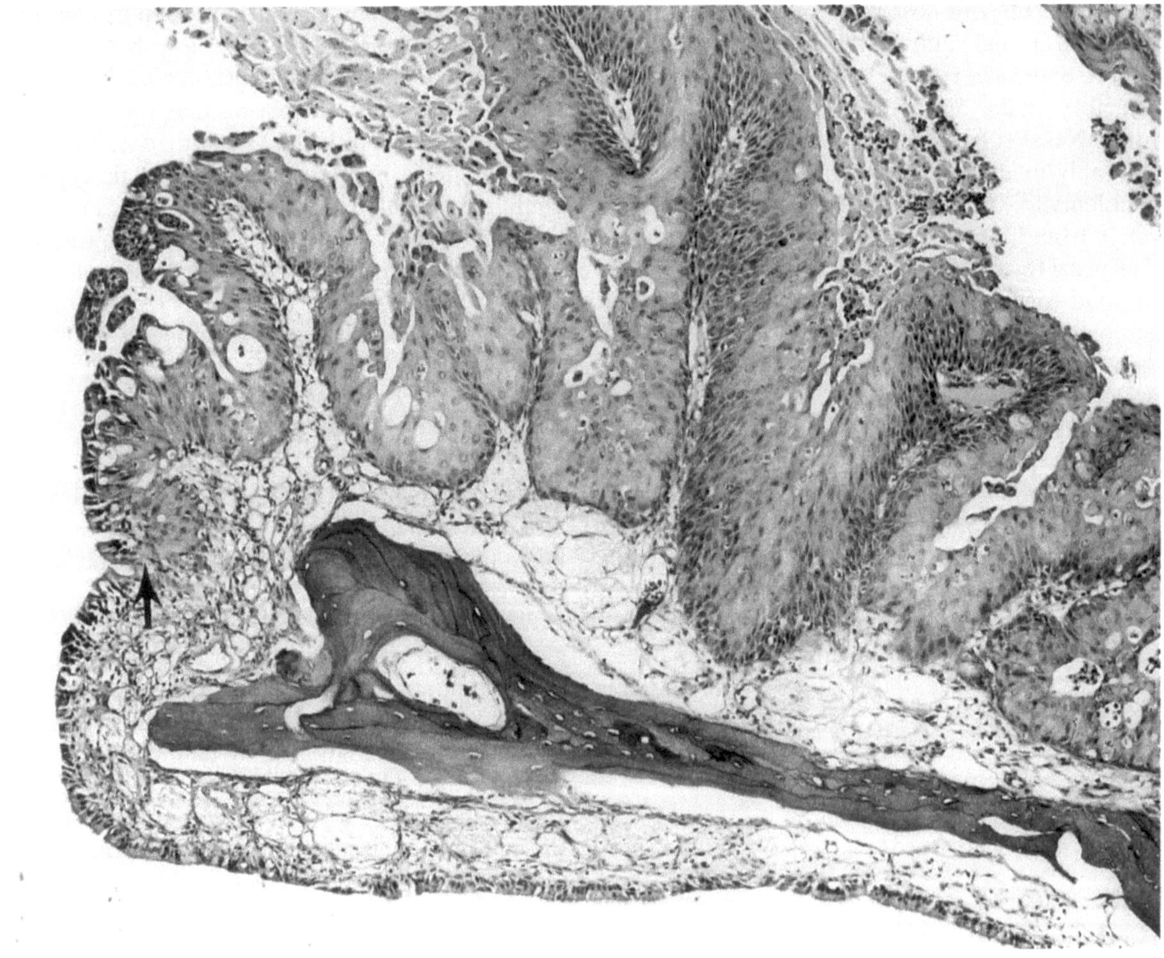

**Fig. 120.** (*above*) Focus of olfactory epithelial basal cell hyperplasia in a rat treated with 4(*N*-methyl-*N*-nitrosamino)-1-(3-pyridyl)-l-butanone (*NNK*). H&E, ×280

**Fig. 121.** (*below*) Dorsal scroll of the first endoturbinate of a rat treated with NNK exhibiting basal cell hyperplasia (*arrow*) progressing (*from left to right*) to severe epithelial folding. These lesions progress to form adenosquamous or olfactory neuroepithelial carcinomas. H&E, ×140

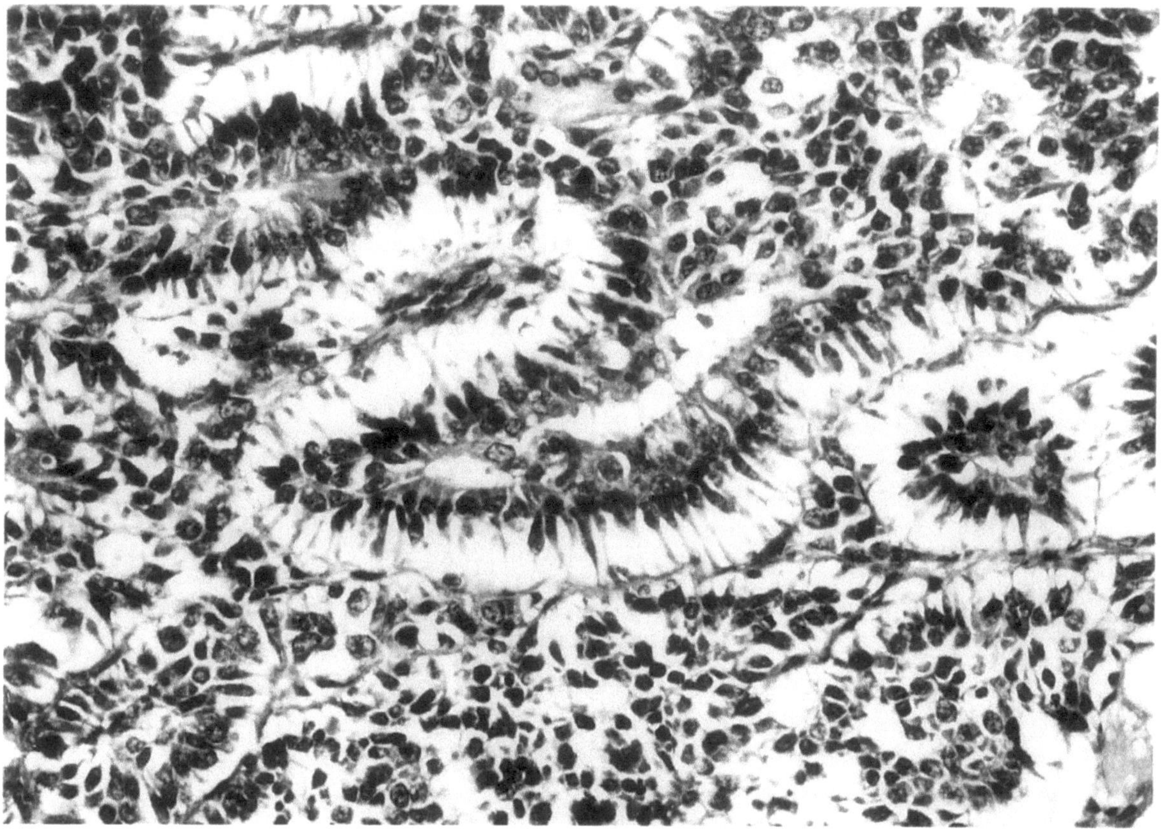

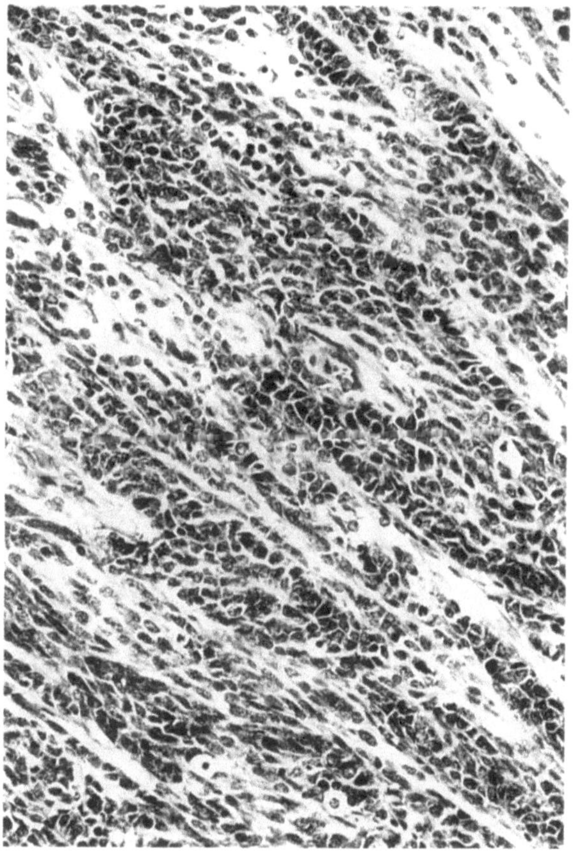

**Fig. 122.** (*above*) Olfactory neuroepithelial carcinoma exhibiting sustentacular pattern of differentiation with epithelial sheets interspersed with more solid regions. The morphological pattern seen in the sheets of presumed sustentacular cells is sometimes seen in degenerating olfactory epithelium where this cell type is more readily identified. Final identification of the cell types in these neoplasms will await studies using suitable markers. H&E, ×280

**Fig. 123.** (*below*) Poorly differentiated region of an olfactory neuroepithelial carcinoma in a rat treated with nitroso-2-hydroxypropyl-2-oxopropylamine. (Material for this figure and Figs. 124, 125, and 126 kindly provided by Dr. Torgney N. Fredrickson, Registry of Experimental Cancer, National Institutes of Health and National Cancer Institute.) H&E, ×140

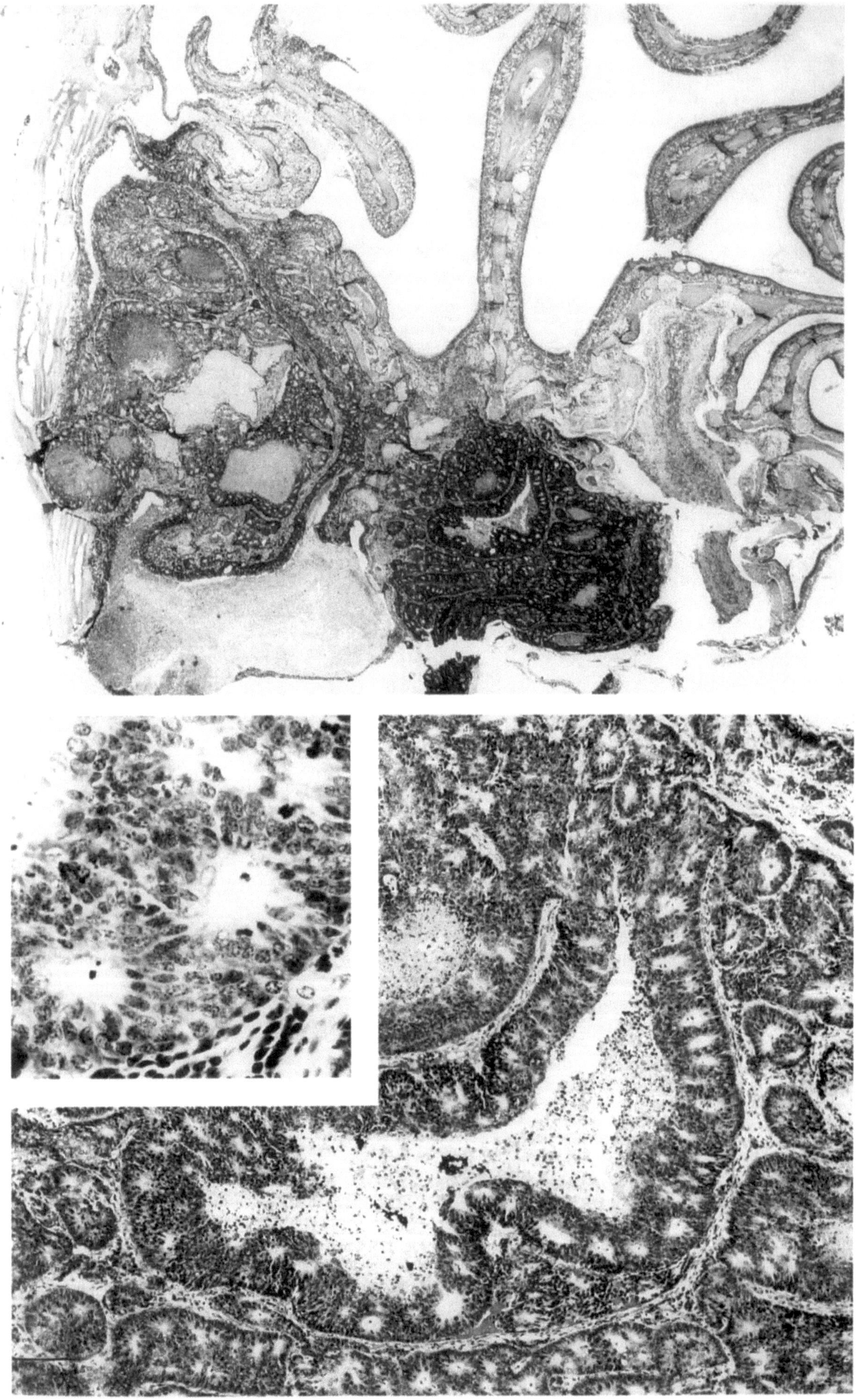

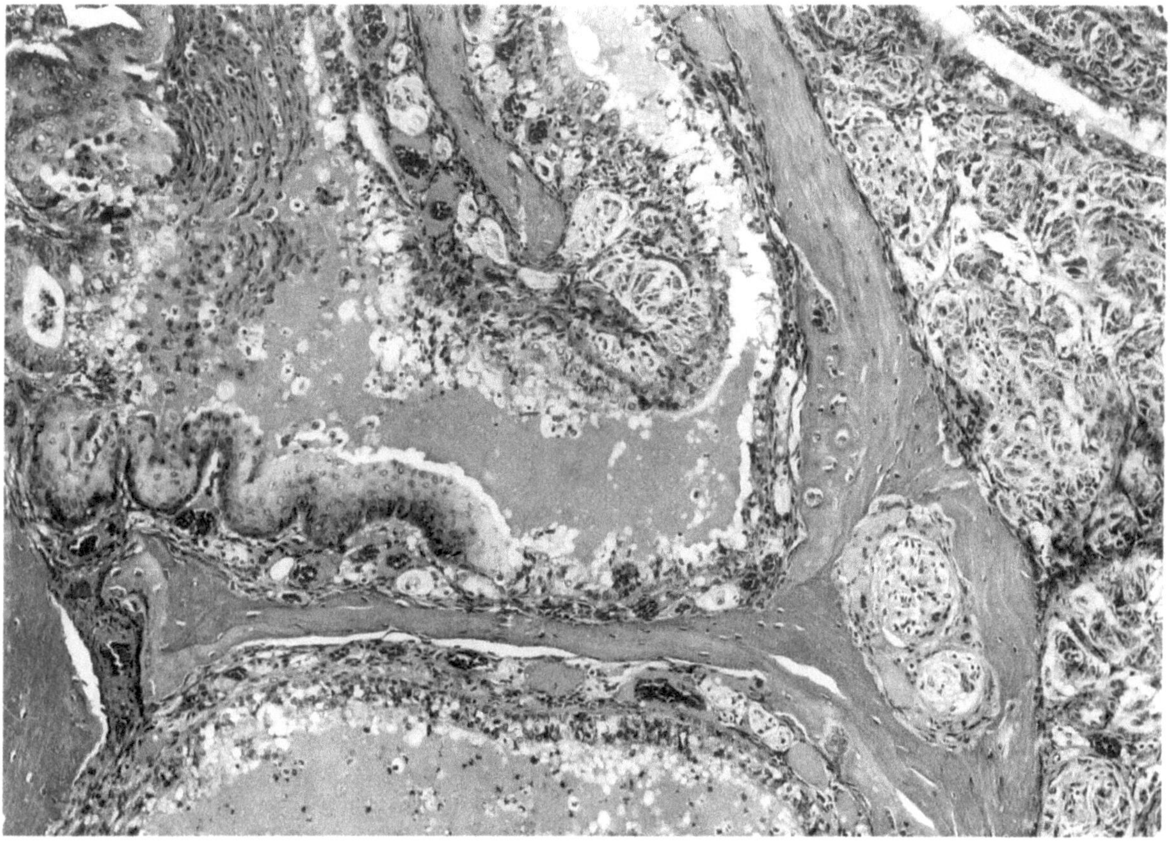

**Fig. 126.** Complex lesions associated with exposure to a nitrosamine. On the right of the figure the lamina propria of the medial aspect of the 2′-ectoturbinate is extensively infiltrated and replaced by a Bowman's gland carcinoma. *Left*, the lateral wall, in this region normally lined by respiratory epithelium, has undergone squamous metaplasia which is probably a prelude to the development of a squamous cell carcinoma at this site. H&E, ×140

Feron et al. 1986), including rhabdomyosarcoma, hemangiosarcoma, chondroma, and malignant schwannoma. Most of these neoplasms closely resemble their counterparts in other sites. An example of a rhabdomyosarcoma is shown in Figs. 127 and 128.

## Nasal Glands

Adenomas and carcinomas of the nasal septal, mural, and other glands underlying the transitional and respiratory epithelial regions of the nose are apparently rare, except in animals exposed to certain nitrosamines (Schüller 1989). Adenocarcinomas arising from these glands are distinctly different from those derived from transitional adenomas. On the nasal septum adenocarcinomas arising from the septal glands are composed of small ductular structures with secretory material in the lumina, slight stromal proliferation, and extensive destruction of the nasal septum (Brown et al. 1991). Adenocarcinomas of the maxillary sinus glands have been seen to invade the adjacent periodontal ligament of the root of an incisor tooth (Brown et al. 1991).

## Accessory Nasal Structures

Neoplasms may arise from a number of paranasal or accessory nasal structures (Sills et al. 1994). Such neoplasms include adenomas and carcinomas of the paranasal sinuses, nasolachrymal duct papilloma (Fig. 129) and squamous cell carcinoma

◄

**Fig. 124.** (*above*) Olfactory neuroepithelial carcinoma that has invaded the olfactory bulbs and lateral nasal wall. H&E, ×28

**Fig. 125.** (*below*) Portion of the neoplasm in Fig. 124 to show cyst formation and organized patterns of rosettes. H&E, ×140 (*inset* ×400)

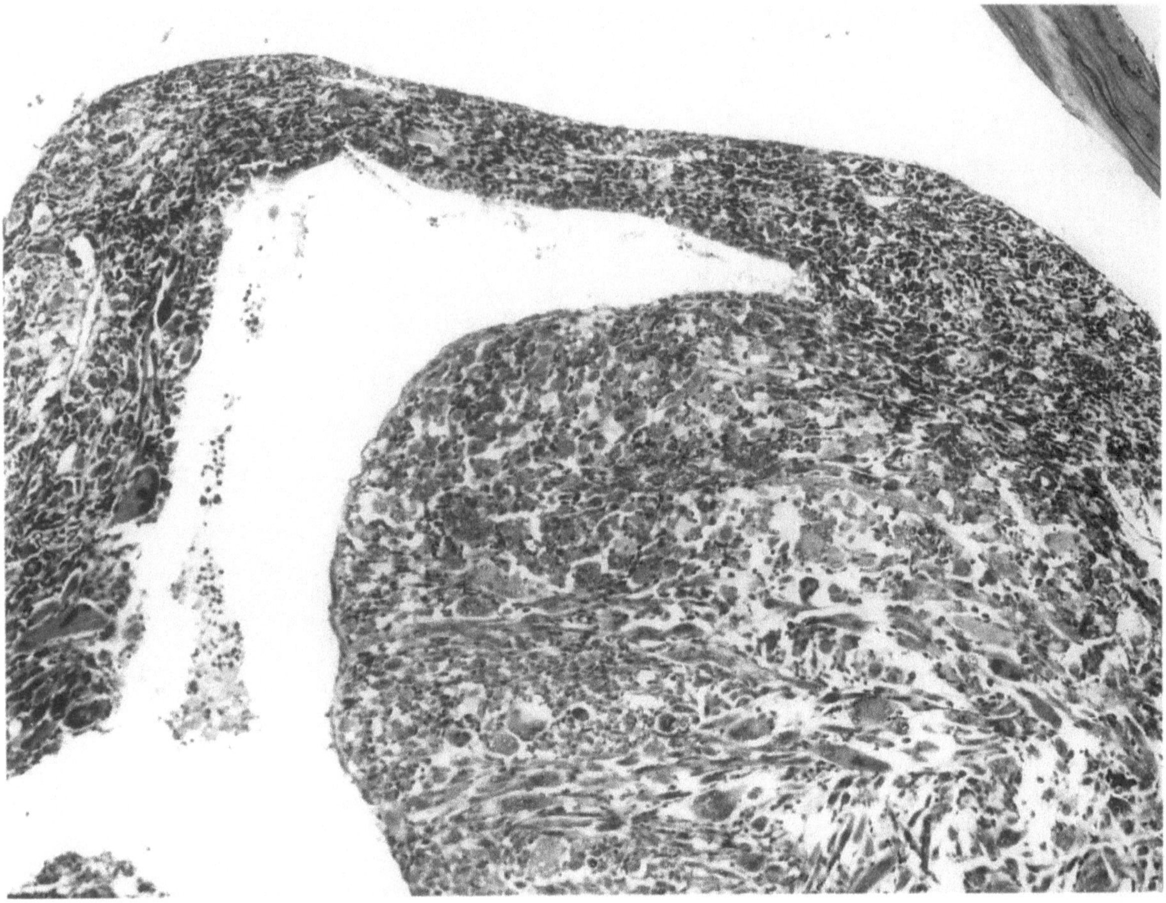

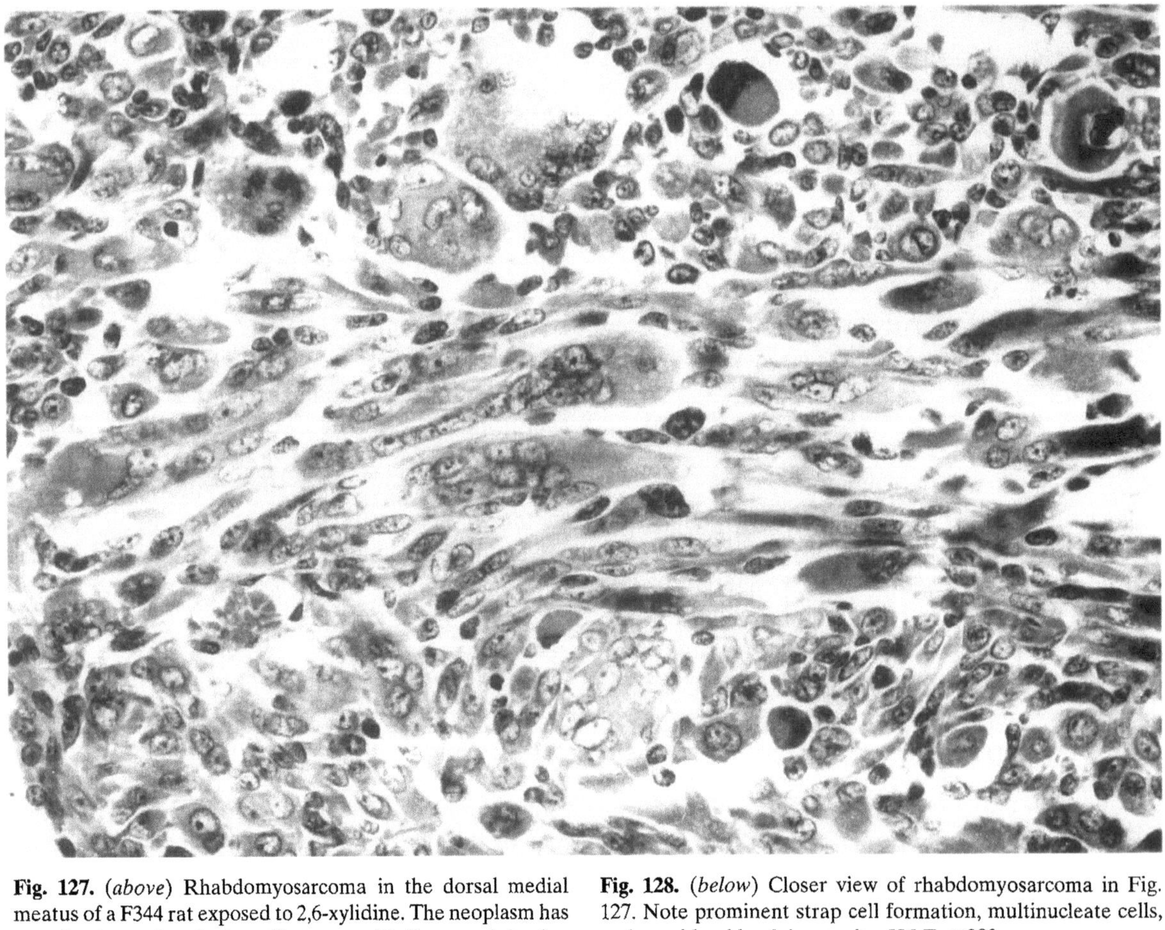

**Fig. 127.** (*above*) Rhabdomyosarcoma in the dorsal medial meatus of a F344 rat exposed to 2,6-xylidine. The neoplasm has completely replaced the olfactory epithelium and lamina propria in this site. H&E, ×56

**Fig. 128.** (*below*) Closer view of rhabdomyosarcoma in Fig. 127. Note prominent strap cell formation, multinucleate cells, and considerable pleiomorphy. H&E, ×280

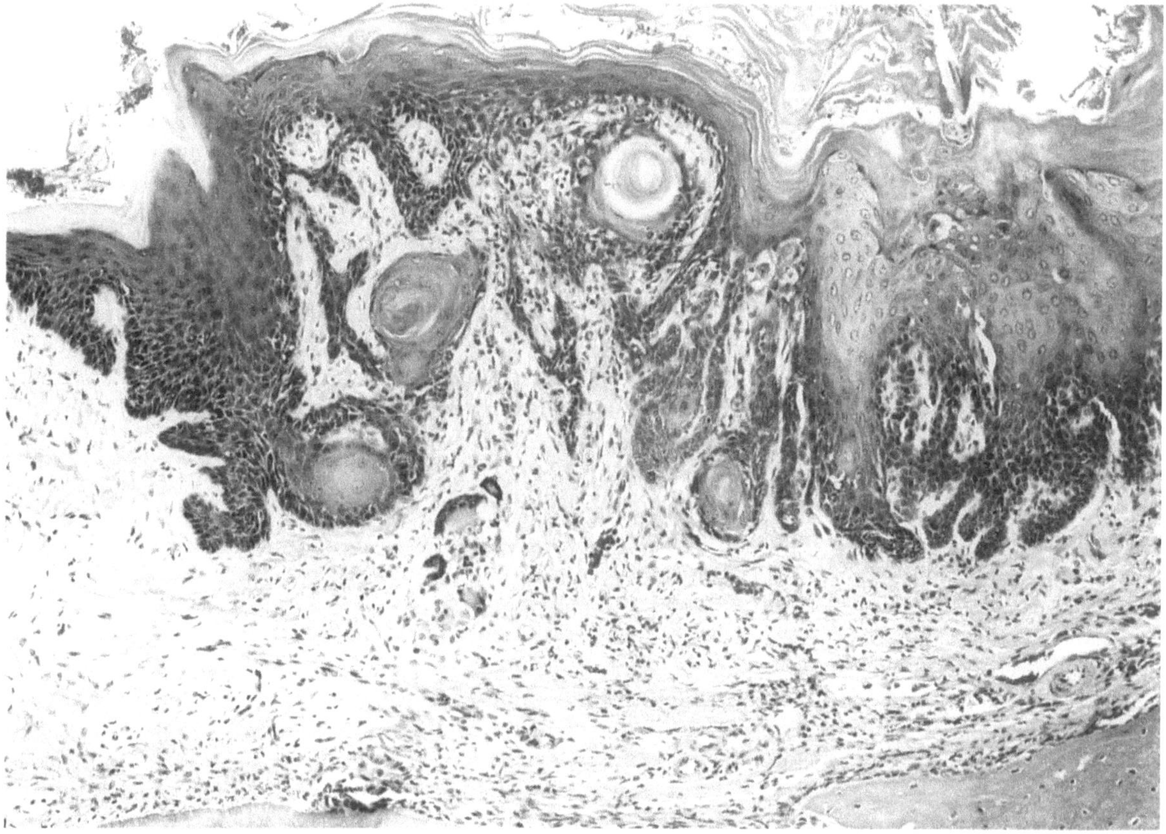

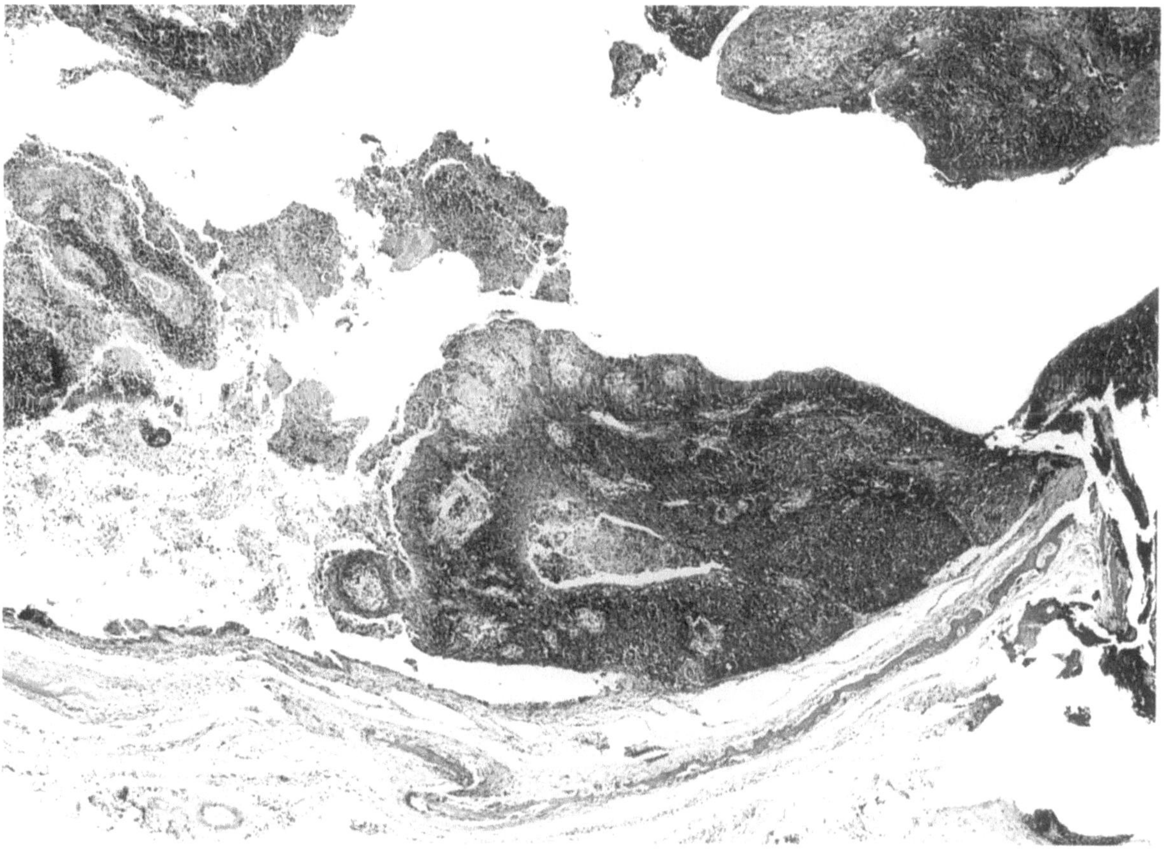

**Fig. 129.** (*above*) Periodontal squamous cell carcinoma adjacent to a molar tooth in a F344 rat. Note prominent squamous epithelial pearls. Such neoplasms readily invade the posterior nasal cavity and may be mistaken for primary nasal tumors. H&E, ×140

**Fig. 130.** (*below*) Papilloma of a nasolachrymal duct in a F344 rat. H&E, ×56

(Schoevera et al. 1994), squamous cell carcinomas of the periodontal membranes of the incisor (Feron and Woutersen 1989) and molar teeth (Fig. 130), and odontomas which generally arise from the incisor teeth and may invade and fill extensive regions of the nasal cavity.

## Cellular Markers for Studies of Tumor Progression

Light microscopic and ultrastructural studies provide essential first steps in characterization of nasal neoplasia, and these techniques may be complemented by the use of a number of enzyme histochemical and immunocytochemical markers. Extensive knowledge of the progression of squamous cell carcinomas, largely based on investigations of skin carcinogenesis, has been derived from the application of biochemical, immunocytochemical, and molecular biological techniques (Yuspa 1994). Markers suitable for such investigations include δ-glutamyl transpeptidase, a number of cytokeratins, and the products of certain oncogenes and tumor suppressor genes. Understanding of nasal squamous cell carcinomas could increase significantly from such approaches. In the case of olfactory mucosal neoplasms a number of potential markers are available for identification of cell types involved, including olfactory marker protein, sustentacular cell specific markers, and a wide range of enzymes, including multiple forms of P450 (Dahl and Hadley 1991) and other enzymes (Bogdanffy 1990). These techniques, although available, have not been widely applied to studies of nasal carcinogenesis in rodents.

## Differential Diagnosis

A number of tumors of the head of rodents may be mistaken for primary nasal neoplasms, including squamous cell carcinomas of the periodontium

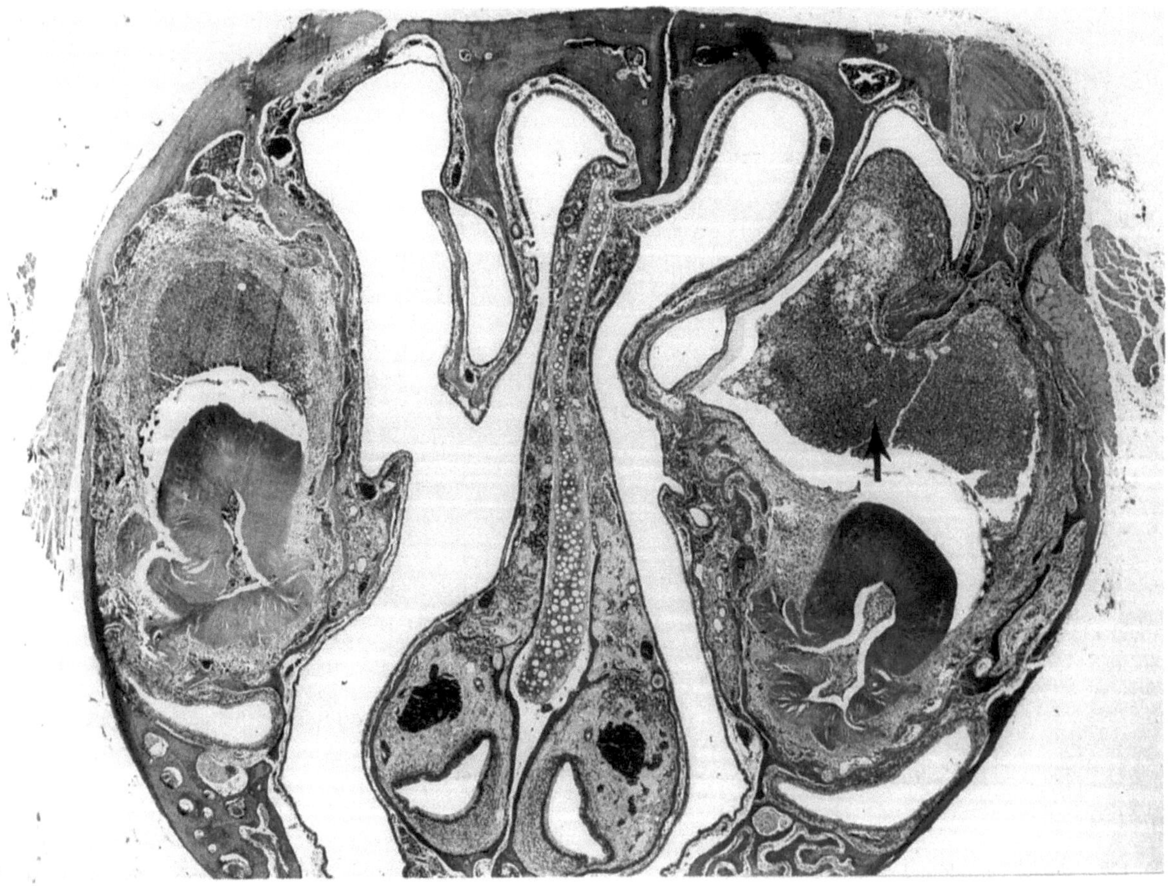

**Fig. 131.** Large granuloma fills much of the lateral meatus in this B6C3Fl mouse. Two teeth are surrounded by inflammatory exudate, indicating the association of intranasal mass (*arrow*) with the teeth. H&E, ×28

of the incisor and molar teeth and nasolachrymal ducts, and primary brain tumors invading the ethmoid region via the cribriform plate. Locally invasive harderian gland tumors may also involve the nose, while lymphomas commonly metastasize to the nasal passages. Distinction of such neoplasms from primary nasal tumors may be critical during risk assessment and determination of underlying mechanisms. Granulomas arising from periodontal inflammation may give rise to masses in the nose (Fig. 131) that may be mistaken for neoplasms if the association with odontal or periodontal inflammation is not evident in the sections.

## Biological Features

When assessing the nature of chemically induced nasal neoplasms, site of origin and the potential role of regional dosimetry are critical features. The majority of such neoplasms fall into two classes: (a) squamous cell carcinomas or polypoid adenomas in the anterior nose and (b) olfactory mucosal neoplasms in the posterior nose. Tumors may exhibit such distribution patterns whether the inducing chemical was administered by inhalation or by other routes. The location of the responses may be attributable to nasal airflow patterns, local blood flow, or metabolism, and a number of other factors (Morgan 1994). These neoplastic responses may be dramatically influenced by such factors as concurrent tissue damage, as was clearly demonstrated in the case of formaldehyde by Woutersen and colleagues (1989). In formaldehyde intoxication tissue damage and inflammation appear to play a critical role in the biology of squamous cell carcinomas induced in the nose. For many chemically-induced olfactory mucosal neoplasms, the overriding factor is likely to be local metabolism, especially that catalyzed by the mixed function oxidase system (Dahl and Hadley 1991; Reed 1993). Other factors to consider are the impact of local changes in cell replication rate and the presence of DNA adducts (Belinsky et al. 1987) or alterations of oncogenes or tumor suppressor genes (Recio et al. 1992). The majority of malignant nasal neoplasms appear to be locally invasive. Squamous cell carcinomas may metastasize to regional lymph nodes (Kerns et al. 1983) and in rare cases to the lungs (Feron et al. 1990). Both squamous cell carcinomas and olfactory neoplasms invade the anterior brain (Fig. 123).

*Etiology and Frequency.* Nasal neoplasms have been induced by a wide range of chemicals (Brown et al. 1991; Feron and Bosland 1989; Reznik and Stinson 1983; Uraih et al. 1990). In these studies the induced tumor incidence ranged from fairly low to almost 100%. In addition to chemicals, a viral etiology has been proposed for certain nasopharyngeal carcinomas in humans.

## Comparison with Other Species

*Domestic Animals.* Nasal neoplasms have been reported in a number of domestic animals, including cats, horses, cattle, pigs, and sheep (Moulton 1978). In a study of 285 sinonasal neoplasms in dogs (Patnaik 1989) epithelial neoplasms, including squamous cell carcinomas and adenocarcinomas, predominated (60%), with the second largest category (33.7%) being derived from skeletal (chondrosarcoma, osteosarcoma) and soft tissues. Almost 4% of the neoplasms in this series were of neuroendocrine origin, while olfactory neuroepithelial neoplasms (esthesioneuroblastomas) comprised less than 2% of the total. A number of melanomas (0.7%) were also reported in this study. Endemic and/or infectious outbreaks of ethmoturbinate tumors have been reported in sheep, goats, cattle, and horses (Moulton 1978).

*Humans.* Nasal neoplasms are generally rare in humans, with the exception of groups in certain occupations, such as in boot and shoe manufacture, furniture making using hard woods, and nickel refining (Brown et al. 1991). Nasopharyngeal carcinomas occur with a significant frequency in certain populations in southern China and Hong Kong, and this has been attributed to a number of potential etiological factors, including certain types of fish diet and, recently, Epstein-Barr virus. The exact etiological factors causing this human disease in these populations remain to be determined. Melanomas also have been reported in humans, and formaldehyde, among other factors, has been implicated in their etiology (Holmström and Lund 1991).

## References

Belinsky SA, Walker VE, Maronpot RR, Swenberg JA, Anderson MW (1987) Molecular dosimetry of DNA adduct formation and cell toxicity in rat nasal mucosa following

exposure to the tobacco specific nitrosamine 4-(N-methylnitrosamino)-1-(3-pyridyl)-1-butanone and their relationship to induction of neoplasia. Cancer Res 47:6058–6065
Bogdanffy MS (1990) Biotransformation enzymes in the rodent nasal mucosa: the value of a histochemical approach. Environ Health Perspect 85:177–186
Brown HR (1990) Neoplastic and potentially preneoplastic changes in the upper respiratory tract of rats and mice. Environ Health Perspect 85:291–304
Brown HG, Monticello TM, Maronpot RR, Randall HW, Hotchkiss JR, Morgan KT (1991) Proliferative and neoplastic lesions in the rodent nasal cavity. Toxicol Pathol 19:358–372
Dahl AR, Hadley WM (1991) Nasal cavity enzymes involved in xenobiotic metabolism: effects on the toxicity of inhalants. Crit Rev Toxicol 21:345–372
Feron VJ, Bosland MC (eds) (1989) Nasal carcinogenesis in rodents: relevence to human health risk. Proceedings of the TNO-CIVO/NYU Nose Symposium, Veldhoven, Netherlands, 24–28 Oct 1988: Pudoc Wageningen
Feron VJ, Woutersen RA (1989) Role of tissue damage in nasal carcinogenesis. In: Feron VJ, Bosland MC (eds) Nasal carcinogenesis in rodents: relevance to human health risk. Proceedings of the TNO-CIVO/NYU Nose Symposium, Veldhoven, Netherlands, 24–28 Oct 1988, Pudoc Wageningen, pp 76–84
Feron VJ, Woutersen RA, Spit BJ (1986) Pathology of chronic nasal toxic responses including cancer. In: Barrow CS (ed) Toxicology of the nasal passages. Hemisphere, Washington DC, pp 67–89
Feron VJ, Woutersen RA, Van Garderen-Hoetmer A, Dreef-van der Meulen HC (1990) Upper respiratory tract tumors in Cpb:WU (Wistar random) rats. Environ Health Perspect 85:305–315
Hebel R, Strombert MW (1976) Anatomy of the laboratory rat. Williams and Wilkins, Baltimore
Holmström M, Lund VJ (1991) Malignant melanomas of the nasal cavity after occupational exposure to formaldehyde. Br J Ind Med 48:9–11
Kerns WD (1985) Polypoid adenoma of the nasal cavity in the laboratory rat. In: Jones TC, Mohr U, Hunt RD (eds) Monographs on pathology of laboratory animals, respiratory system. Springer, Berlin Heidelberg New York, pp 41–47
Kerns WD, Pavkov KL, Donofrio DJ, Gralla EJ, Swenberg JA (1983) Carcinogenicity of formaldehyde in rats mice after long-term inhalation exposure. Cancer Res 43:4382–4392
Mery S, Gross EA, Joyner DR, Godo M, Morgan KT (1994) Nasal diagrams: a tool for recording the distribution of nasal lesions in rats and mice. Toxicol Pathol 22:353–372
Morgan KT (1994) Nasal dosimetry, lesion distribution, and the toxicologic pathologist: a brief review. Inhal Toxicol 6:41–57
Morgan KT, Monticello TM (1990) Formaldehyde toxicity: respiratory epithelial injury and repair. In: Thomassen DG, Nettesheim P (eds) Biology, toxicology, and carcinogenests of respiratory epithelium. Hemisphere, New York, pp 155–171
Morgan KT, Jiang XZ, Starr TB, Kerns WD (1986) More precise localization of nasal tumors associated with chronic exposure of F-344 rats to formaldehyde gas. Toxicol Appl Pharmacol 82:264–271
Morgan KT, Kimbell JS, Monticello TM, Patra AL, Fleishman A (1991) Studies of inspiratory airflow patterns in the nasal passages of the F344 rat and rhesus monkey using nasal molds: relevance to formaldehyde toxicity. Toxicol Appl Pharmacol 110:223–240
Moulton JE (1978) Tumors of the respiratory system. In: Moulton JE (ed) Tumors in domestic animals, 2nd edn. California Press, Berkeley, pp 205–239
Negus V (1958) The comparative anatomy and physiology of the nose and paranasal sinuses. Livingstone, Edinburgh
Patnaik AK (1989) Canine sinonasal neoplasms: clinicopathological study of 285 cases. J Am An Hosp Assoc 25:103–114
Recio L, Sisk S, Pluta L, Bermudez E, Gross EA, Chen Z, Morgan KT, Walker C (1992) Mutations in formaldehyde-induced nasal squamous cell carcinomas in rats. Cancer Res 52:6113–6116
Reed CJ (1993) Drug metabolism in the nasal cavity: relevance to toxicology. Drug Metab Rev 173–205
Reznik G (1983) Comparative anatomy and histomorphology of the nasal and paranasal cavities in rodents. In: Reznik G, Stinson SF (eds) Nasal tumors in animals and man, vol 1. CRC, Boca Raton, pp 35–44
Reznik G, Stinson SF (1983) (eds) Nasal tumors in animals and man. CRC, Boca Raton
Schoevers EJ, Kuijpers MH, Woutersen RA, Feron VJ (1994) Spontaneous squamous cell carcinoma of nasal and paranasal structures in the Cpb:WU (Wistar random) rat: nasolachrymal duct as major site of origin. J Environ Pathol Toxicol Oncol 13:49–57
Schüller HM (1989) Nitrosamine-induced nasal cavity carcinogenesis in rodents. In: Feron VJ, Bosland MC (eds) Nasal carcinogeneses in rodents: Relevance to human health risk. Proceedings of the TNO-CIVO/NYU nose symposium, Veldhoven, Netherlands, 24–28 Oct 1988, Pudoc Wageningen, pp 63–69
Sills RC, Morgan KT, Boorman GA (1994) Accessory nasal structures in toxicology studies. Inhal Toxicol (in press)
Sorokin SP (1983) The respiratory system. In: Weiss L (ed) Histology, cell and tissue biology, 5th edn. Elsevier Biomedical, New York, pp 788–868
Uraih LC, Morgan KT, Maronpot RR (1990) Symposium on toxicologic pathology of the upper respiratory system. Environ Health Perspect 85:161–352
Woutersen RA, Appelman LM, Van Garderen-Hoetmer A, Feron VJ (1986) Inhalation toxicity of acetaldehyde in rats. III. Carcinogenicity study. Toxicology 41:213–231
Woutersen RA, Van Garderen-Hoetmer A, Bruijntjes JP, Zwart A, Feron J (1989) Nasal tumors in rats after severe injury to the nasal mucosa and prolonged exposure to 10 ppm formaldehyde. J Appl Toxicol 9:39–46
Yuspa SH (1994) The pathogenesis of squamous cell cancer: lessons learned from studies of skin carcinogenesis-thirty-third GH. Cancer Res 54:1178–1189

# Hemangiosarcoma, Nasal Cavity, Mouse

Roger A. Renne

*Synonyms.* Hemangioendothelioma

## Gross Appearance

The lesion is not usually visible grossly because it arises in the lamina propria of the nasal mucosa. If, however, invasion occurs through the maxilla to the subcutis, a slight focal bulging of the skin results. When the skin is removed, the underlying subcutis is seen to be dark red.

## Microscopic Features

Hemangiosarcomas arise from the submucosa of the lateral walls of the nasal cavity. The normal pattern of loose connective tissue and submucosal glands is disrupted by proliferation of endothelial cells with large vesicular or hyperchromatic nuclei. Some of these cells contain mitotic figures. They form small vascular channels and sinusoids (Figs. 132, 133). These neoplastic channels are often filled with blood, giving the tumor a

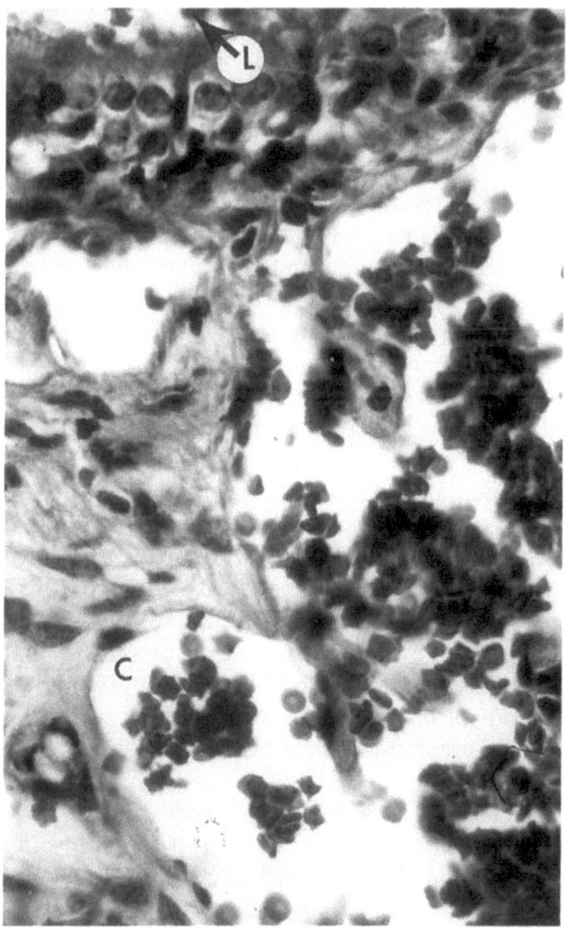


**Fig. 132.** (*left*) Hemangiosarcoma, submucosa, nasal cavity, mouse. Submucosal glands are disrupted by the proliferation of endothelial cells which form small vascular channels (*C*). Hemorrhage in nasal cavity (*L*). A mouse that chronically inhaled 400 ppm propylene oxide. H&E, ×640

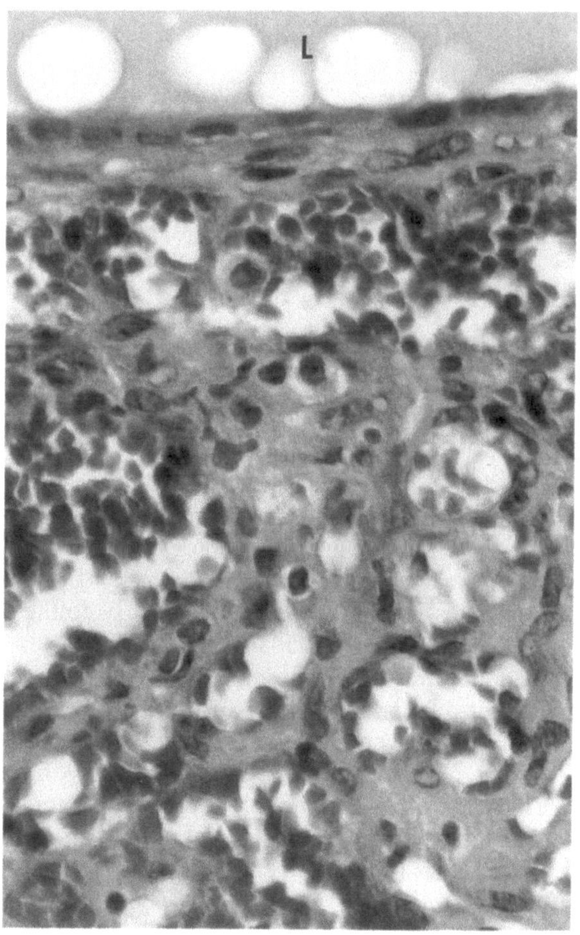


**Fig. 133.** (*right*) Hemangiosarcoma, submucosa, nasal cavity. Mouse exposed to 400 ppm propylene oxide. Note serous exudate in the lumen (*L*). H&E, ×640

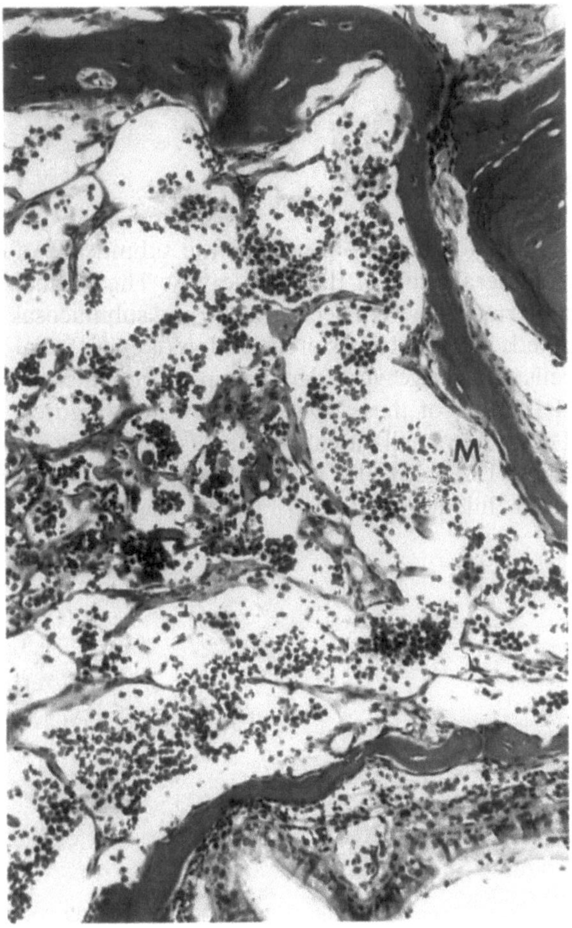


**Fig. 134.** Hemangiosarcoma, submucosa of dorsal part of nasal cavity, mouse, following long-term inhalation of 400 ppm propylene oxide. Note the invasion of the marrow (*M*) of the maxilla. H&E, ×160

hemorrhagic appearance. Occasionally areas of thrombosis, hemorrhage, and necrosis occur in the neoplasms in those portions nearer the lumen of the nasal cavity. As the neoplasms expand, erosion and loss of the overlying respiratory epithelium follow, but the principal direction of invasion is lateral toward the turbinate bones, maxillary sinus, maxilla, marrow space of the maxilla, and the subcutis overlying the maxilla (Fig. 134). These hemangiosarcomas are locally invasive, but there is no evidence of metastasis by way of blood vessels or lymphatics. Transplantation and growth of tumor cells within the respiratory tract has not been observed.

## Differential Diagnosis

Hemangiosarcomas must be distinguished from hemangiomas and from angiectasis, both of which are also induced by inhalation exposure to propylene oxide. Angiectasis can be distinguished because it is not a neoplasm. The cells are cytologically differentiated and therefore benign. New vascular channels are not formed, but preexisting ones are merely dilated. Hemangiomas are more difficult to distinguish but tend to have larger vascular channels than those in hemangiosarcomas. Mitotic figures are fewer or absent, and the endothelial cells are flattened and have a smaller nucleus to cytoplasm ratio. Hemangiomas do not invade the maxilla or maxillary space.

A complicating factor in inhalation studies is that rhinitis is often present. In the propylene oxide study described below, inflammation led to the accumulation of serous or purulent exudate in the lumen of the nasal cavity. The nasal mucosa and submucosa were often heavily infiltrated with lymphocytes, neutrophils, histiocytes, and plasma cells. Fibroplasia and congestion were ofen observed.

## Biological Features

Hemangiosarcoma of the nasal cavity as a spontaneous event is extremely rare in humans (Bomer and Arnold 1971) and animals. Only one report (Rabstein and Peters 1973) of spontaneous hemangiosarcoma in animals could be found. In this report only one of 358 BALB/Cf/Cd mice which died or were killed when moribund had a hemangiosarcoma of the ethmoid turbinates.

Experimentally induced hemangiosarcoma in the nasal cavity of mice was observed in a 2-year propylene oxide inhalation study (National Toxicology Program 1984; Renne et al. 1986). In this study (Table 3) 300 $B6C3F_1$ mice were divided into three male and three female groups of 50 each with high-dose (400 ppm), low-dose (200 ppm), and control groups for each sex. Mice were exposed by inhalation 6 h each day, 5 days per week, for 103 weeks.

Angiectasis, hemangiomas, and hemangiosarcomas were found at the end of the study in both male and female mice that received the high dose of 400 ppm propylene oxide (Table 3). All but one of the neoplasms were discovered in apparently normal mice that were killed at the end of the study. In this mouse death occurred as a result of a separate primary neoplasm in another tissue.

**Table 3.** Nasal lesions in B6C3F$_1$ mice exposed to propylene oxide and in controls[a]

| | Male mice | | | Female mice | | |
|---|---|---|---|---|---|---|
| | 0ppm | 200ppm | 400ppm | 0ppm | 200ppm | 400ppm |
| Angiectasis | 0/50 | 0/50 | 3/50 | 0/50 | 0/50 | 3/50 |
| Hemangioma | 0/50 | 0/50 | 5/50 | 0/50 | 0/50 | 3/50 |
| Hemangiosarcoma | 0/50 | 0/50 | 5/50 | 0/50 | 0/50 | 3/50 |

[a] Nasal structure of 50 animals per group was examined microscopically; e.g., 5 of 50 male high-dose mice had hemangiosarcomas and 13 mice bore lesions.

### Comparison with Other Species

In the mouse study described, hemangiosarcomas of the nasal cavity were locally invasive, extending into submucosal glands, bone, and bone marrow of the maxilla, and subcutis around the maxilla. There was no evidence of vascular or lymphatic spread to other tissues. Primary hemangiosarcomas of the nasal cavity in man, although extremely rare, tend to recur locally after excision. They also tend to metastasize via hematogenous or lymphatic channels to other tissues (Bomer and Arnold 1971).

### References


Bomer DS, Arnold GE (1971) Rare tumors of the ear, nose and throat. Acta Otolaryngol [Suppl] (Stockh) 289:1–25

National Toxicology Program (1984) Inhalation bioassay of propylene oxide for possible carcinogenicity. Terminal report. US Department of Health and Human Services, National Institutes of Health, National Technical Information Service, Springfield, VA

Rabstein LS, Peters RL (1973) Tumors of the kidneys, synovia, exocrine pancreas and nasal cavity in BALB/cf/Cd mice. JNCI 51:999–1006

Renne RA, Giddens WE Jr, Boorman GA, Kovatch R, Haseman JE, Clarke WJ (1986) Nasal cavity neoplasia in F344/N rats and (C57BL/6 × C3H) F1 mice inhaling propylene oxide for up to two years. JNCI 77:573–582


# Neuroendocrine Hyperplasias and Tumors, Larynx and Trachea, Syrian Hamster

Heinrich Ernst, Martin Heinrichs, Gerhard Bargsten, Birgit Kittel, Susanne Rittinghausen, Donald L. Dungworth, and Ulrich Mohr

*Synonyms.* Carcinoid, carcinoid tumor, tumorlet, clear cell carcinoma, neuroendocrine carcinoma

### Gross Appearance

The range of lesions described here was observed in hamsters of the strain Han:AURA from a chronic toxicity/carcinogenicity study involving inhaled particles. Since there was no difference in the frequency of the neuroendocrine proliferations between the exposure and control groups, all lesions were considered to be of spontaneous origin.

Large neuroendocrine tumors may be detected with the naked eye when they cause narrowing of the laryngeal or tracheal lumen (Fig. 135). If the larynx and trachea are split into two halves, smaller lesions may also be visible grossly as pale to pink focal protrusions of the mucosa or as glistening nodules which project from the lining of larynx or trachea.

### Microscopic Features

Neuroendocrine proliferations typically consisted of solid sheets and bands of uniform polygonal

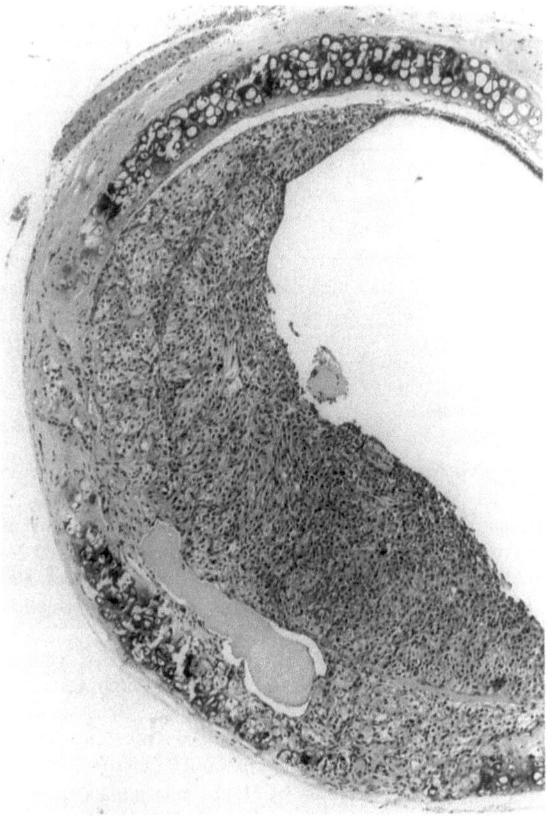

**Fig. 135.** Neuroendocrine tumor occupying nearly half of the laryngeal lumen of a hamster. Note destruction of cartilage by invading tumor cells. H&E, ×50

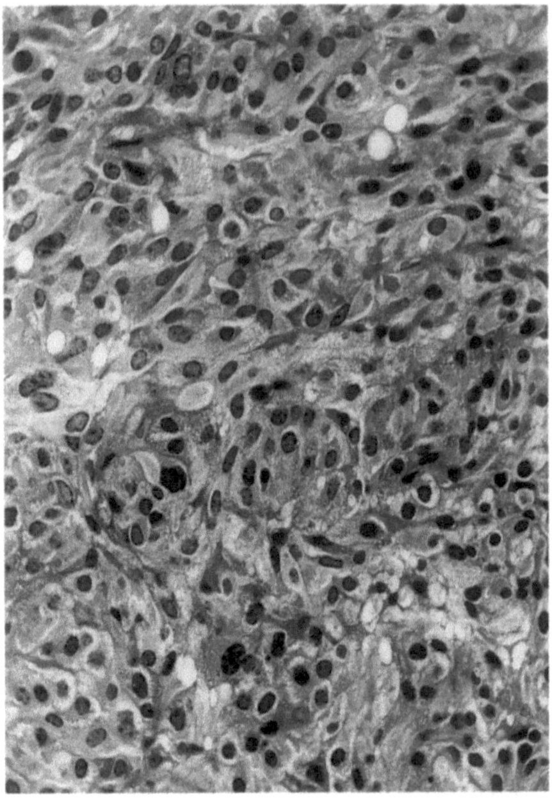

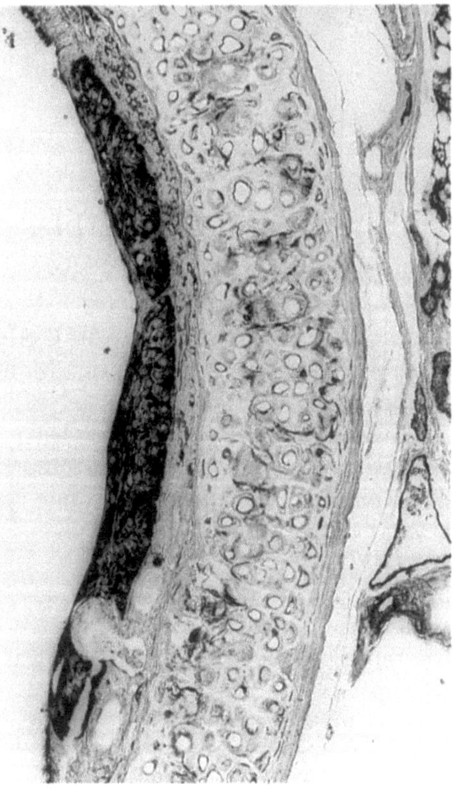

cells with abundant pale or weakly eosinophilic cytoplasm and distinct cell borders (Fig. 136). The large nuclei were centrally located, round to ovoid, and contained finely distributed chromatin and large eccentric nucleoli. Mitotic figures were rare, even in invasive tumors. The cells were negative on PAS and Alcian blue staining but displayed prominent cytoplasmic argyrophilia using the Grimelius silver impregnation method (Fig. 137).

There was a morphological continuum from minute intraepithelial hyperplasia to large exophytic and invasive tumors. Differentiation between hyperplasia and neoplasia was somewhat arbitrary since there was no significant cytological

▶

**Fig. 136.** (*above*) Higher magnification of tumor in Fig. 135. Note lack of stromal tissue and slight nuclear pleomorphism. H&E, ×300

**Fig. 137.** (*below*) Neuroendocrine hyperplasia of larynx, hamster. The cells are strongly argyrophilic. Grimelius silver, ×120

difference between the two types of proliferation. Thus the diagnosis had to rely on criteria such as size of the lesion and local invasion.

The lesions appeared to arise within the basal cell layer of the respiratory epithelium with subsequent progression to intraepithelial plaques (hyperplasias) and elevation of the overlying respiratory epithelial cells (Fig. 138). The proliferating neuroendocrine cells often extended into the underlying glands to form nodular clusters in the submucosa (Fig. 139), and sometimes these proliferating cells appeared to originate within the laryngeal submucosal glands. When proliferations involved the submucosa, there was a definite endocrine type packeting which was not imposed on the cells by preexisting structures, such as is seen in thyroid C cell tumors. This pattern was also present, but less evident, in lesions with a predominantly intraluminal growth.

About one-third of these tumors grew as intraluminal exophytic growths with little invasion into the submucosal tissue (Fig. 140). The intraluminal portion of some of these tumors was so large that the laryngeal or tracheal lumen was almost completely obstructed. Dilated submucosal glands filled with an eosinophilic homogeneous material were frequently entrapped within the larger tumors (Fig. 141). Rupture of the glands allowed this material to be present among the neuroendocrine cells. In addition, large tumors often had areas of necrosis and hemorrhage. With the exception of a few large tumors with distinct vascularized fibrous stalks, intercellular connective tissue was always inconspicuous.

Some tumors, even very small ones, obviously invaded into submucosal tissue, around submucosal glands or between cartilage rings (Fig. 141). Infiltration and destruction of cartilage was rarely observed (Fig. 135). A few tumors grew around the whole inner circumference of the larynx or trachea as demonstrated by the presence of tumor tissue on both sides of the longitudinally sectioned organs.

Distant metastases were not found in this series of lesions, but they have been reported in the lung ▶

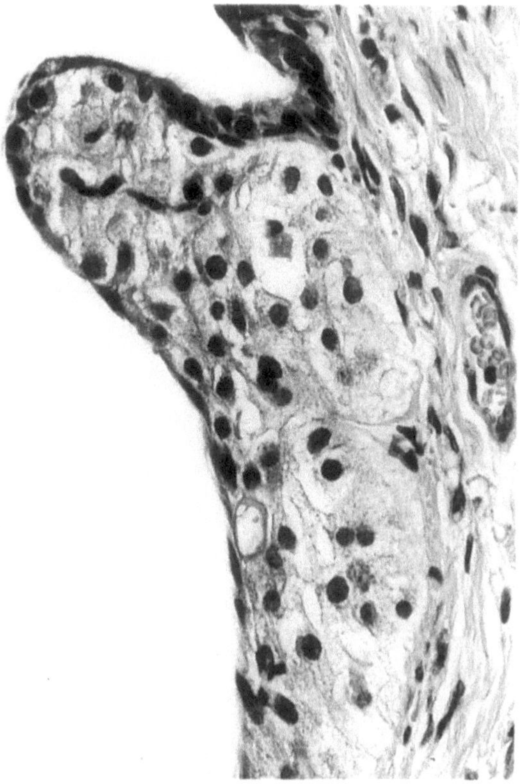

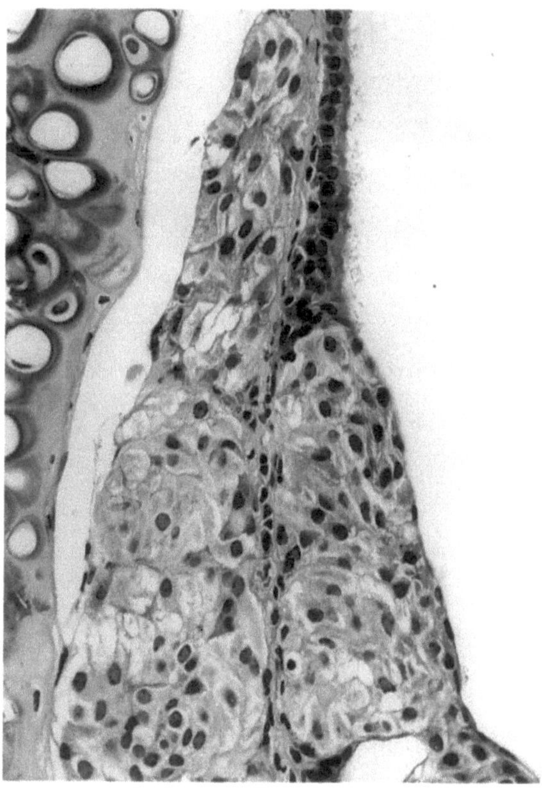

**Fig. 138.** (*above*) Neuroendocrine hyperplasia of trachea, hamster. Note elevation of the respiratory epithelium by proliferating NE cells. H&E, ×360

**Fig. 139.** (*below*) Higher magnification of tumor in Fig. 135. Peripheral expansion of tumor by combined intraepithelial and submucosal growth. H&E, ×300

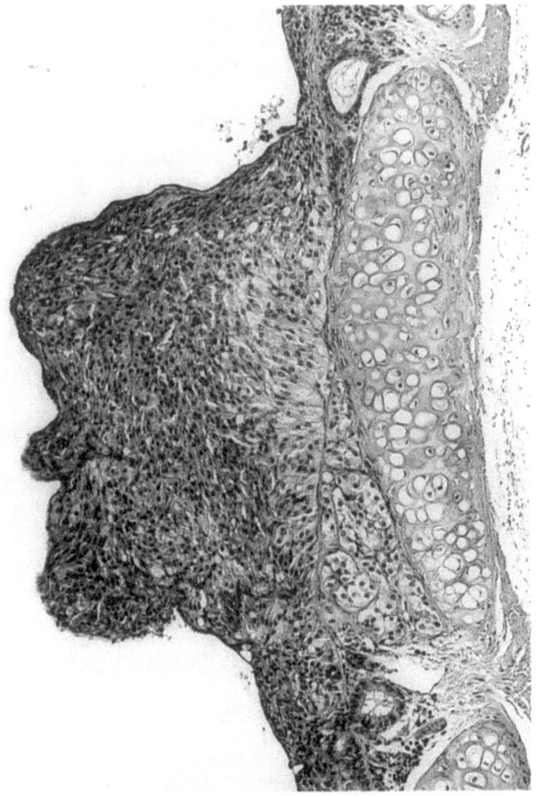

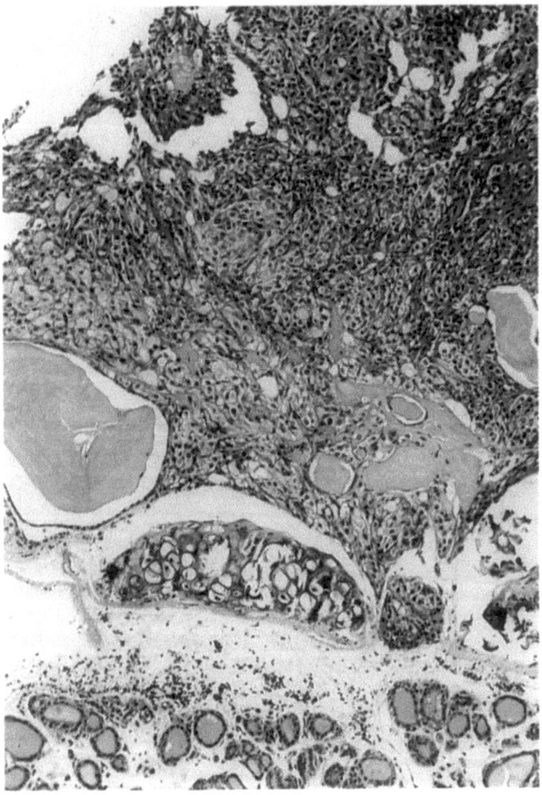

**Fig. 140.** (*above*) Neuroendocrine tumor of trachea, hamster. Note a predominant exophytic growth. Small nests of tumor cells are separated by thin fibrous septa within submucosa. H&E, ×90

**Fig. 141.** (*below*) Neuroendocrine tumor of trachea of hamster, with infiltration between cartilage rings adjacent to thyroid gland. Note homogeneous secretory product within dilated submucosal glands and between tumor cells. H&E, ×80 ◄

(Pour 1985). Tumor cell emboli entrapped within paratracheal vessels were found, however, in two tumors of our series.

*Immunohistochemistry.* For a further characterization of the neuroendocrine cells immunohistochemical investigations were performed on plastic- (semithin-) and paraffin-embedded sections of 15 representative lesions using the ABC immunoperoxidase technique (Hsu et al. 1981). The sources of reagents and results are summarized in Table 4.

No difference was found in the immunoreactivity between hyperplastic and neoplastic lesions. A strong immunoreactivity was observed in all specimens for calcitonin, calcitonin gene-related peptide (CGRP) and serotonin (Figs. 142–144). The detection of more general neuroendocrine markers such as neuron-specific enolase and synaptophysin was possible only in paraffin-embedded sections. The reaction was much weaker in paraffin-embedded material even with higher concentrated antisera. With all positive markers the staining pattern was diffuse to finely granular and confined to the cytoplasm. The lesions did not stain for ACTH, pan-cytokeratin (lu-5), chromogranin A, or somatostatin.

Neuroendocrine cells which were positive for calcitonin were also immunoreactive for CGRP. A comparable coexpression of the two peptides

►

**Fig. 142.** (*upper left*) Neuroendocrine hyperplasia of trachea of hamster. Note intense immunoreactivity for calcitonin. ABC immunohistochemistry, plastic-embedded sample, no counterstain, ×210

**Fig. 143.** (*below*) Neuroendocrine tumor of larynx of hamster, strongly reactive for CGRP. ABC immunohistochemistry, plastic-embedded sample, no counterstain, ×80

**Fig. 144.** (*upper right*) Neuroendocrine tumor of trachea. Numerous tumor cells stain positive for serotonin. ABC immunohistochemistry, plastic-embedded sample, no counterstain, ×190

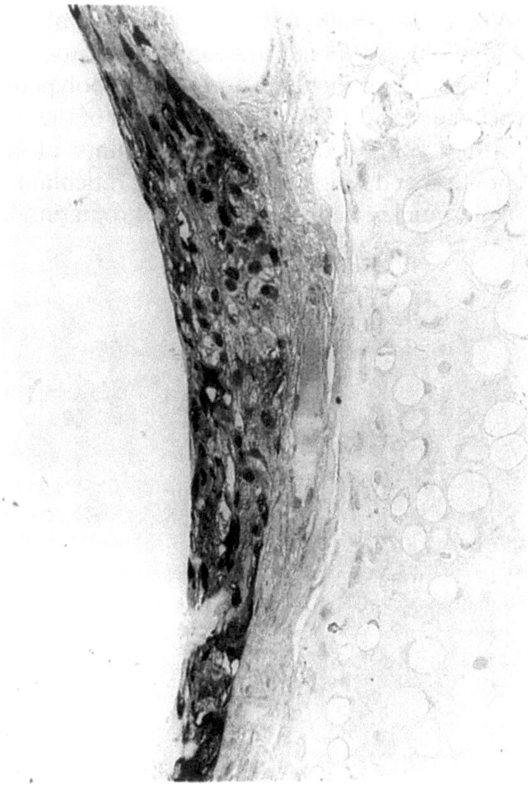

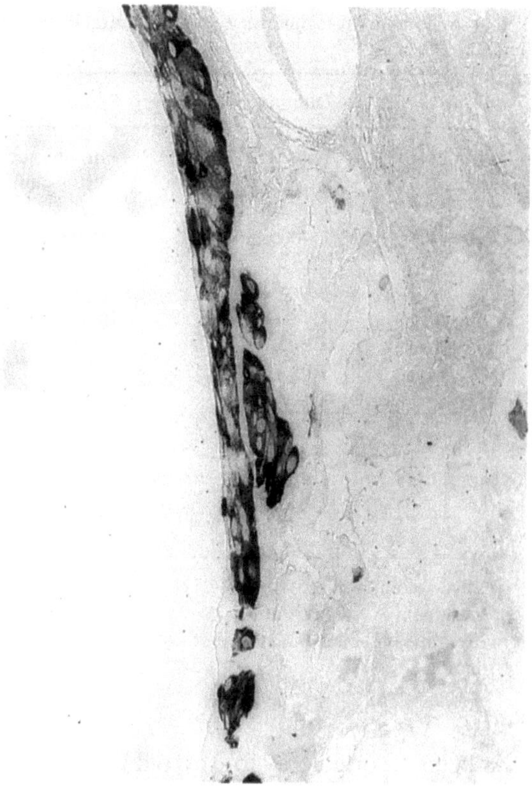

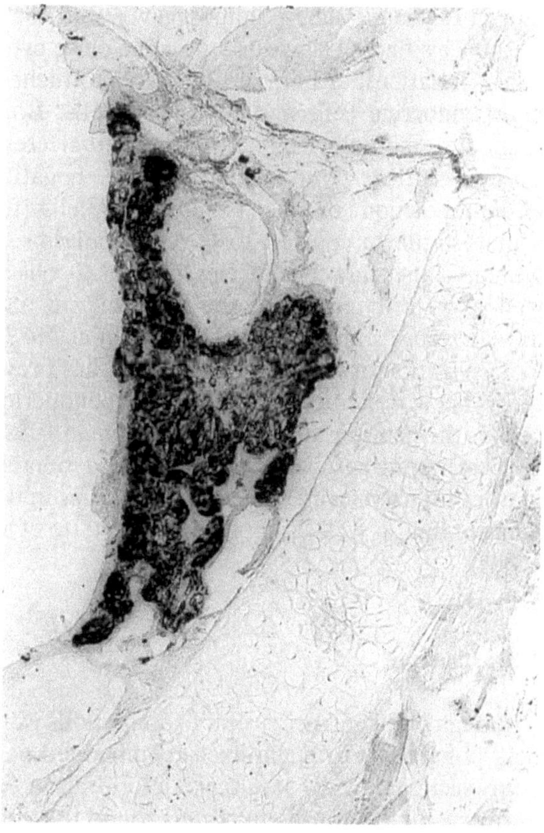

**Table 4.** Immunohistochemistry of laryngotracheal neuroendocrine lesions

| Antisera | Dilution | Reactivity | Source |
|---|---|---|---|
| Calcitonin (p) | 1:4000 | +++ | Immunonuclear; Stillwater, USA |
| CGRP (p) | 1:4000 | +++ | Peninsula; Heidelberg, Germany |
| Serotonin (p) | 1:10000 | ++ | Immunonuclear; Stillwater, USA |
| NSE (p) | 1:1000 | + | Dakopatts, Hamburg, Germany |
| Synaptophysin (m) | 1:40 | + | Progen; Heidelberg, Germany |

Negative immunoreactivity: ACTH, cytokeratin (lu-5), chromogranin A, somatostatin.
p, Polyclonal; m, monoclonal antibodies; + to +++, intensity of staining.

has been reported only for thyroid C cells and for some neuroendocrine cells of the human and rat lung (Tsutsumi 1989; Shimosegawa and Said 1991). This finding suggests a possible close cytological relationship between the laryngotracheal neuroendocrine cells and thyroid C cells. Both originate embryologically from the neural crest. This is further emphasized by the negative immunoreaction of the proliferated cells for somatostatin. In contrast to C cell neoplasms of humans, rats, and other species, normal C cells as well as C cell tumors of the hamster are also unreactive for somatostatin (DeLellis et al. 1987). Colocalization of CGRP and serotonin has previously been described for some neuroendocrine cells in the hamster lung (Keith and Ekman 1988), and calcitonin has been shown to be a reliable marker for chemically induced hyperplasias in the hamster lung as well (Linnoila et al. 1984; Ito et al. 1988).

## Ultrastructure

Although electron microscopic examinations were only possible on formalin-fixed reembedded paraffin sections, with resulting deterioration of ultrastructural features, numerous round to ovoid cytoplasmic dense core granules measuring 100–200 nm in diameter were identifiable (Figs. 145, 146). These granules are the hallmark of neuroendocrine cells and are considered to be the storage site of biogenic amines and polypeptides (Scheuermann 1987). The cytoplasm of these cells further contained moderate amounts of mitochondria and rough endoplasmatic reticulum. The ovoid nuclei had marginated chromatin, large

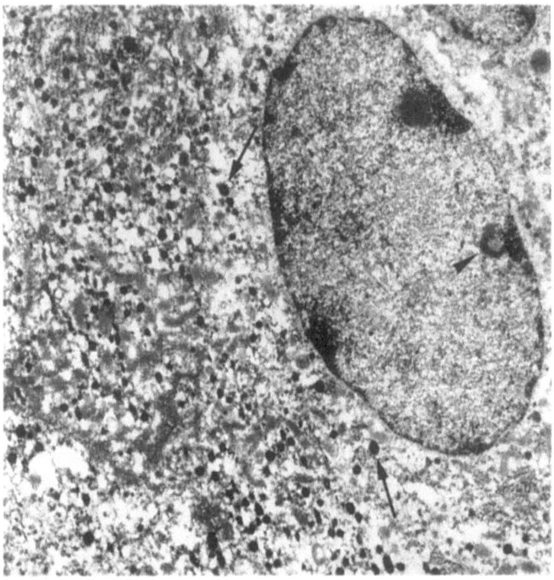

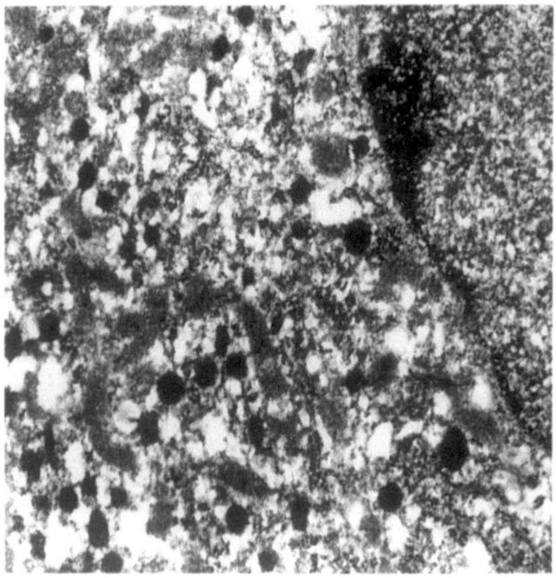

**Fig. 145.** (*above*) Neuroendocrine cell containing numerous dense core granules (*DCG*; *arrows*). Note nuclear inclusion body (*arrowhead*). Reprocessed formalin-fixed paraffin section, TEM, ×6300

**Fig. 146.** (*below*) Higher magnification of cell in Fig. 145. Note DCG and remnants of mitochondria and rough endoplasmic reticulum. Reprocessed formalin-fixed paraffin section, TEM, ×12600

nucleoli and occasional spherical, electron-dense inclusion bodies (Fig. 146).

### Differential Diagnosis

Papillomas composed of either squamous cells or of a mixed squamous and respiratory epithelial cell population may occur spontaneously in the larynx or trachea of hamsters, but at very low frequencies (Pour et al. 1979; Strandberg 1987). These tumors can be easily distinguished from neuroendocrine neoplasms by their characteristic histological and cytological appearance.

### Biological Features

*Natural History*. Hyperplasias and tumors of neuroendocrine cells are believed to arise from solitary cells or from innervated clusters called neuroepithelial bodies which are normally found in the respiratory epithelium of many vertebrates, including man (Scheuermann 1987; Sorokin and Hoyt 1989). Neuroendocrine cells were first described as *helle Zellen* (clear cells) by Fröhlich (1949) and were later regarded as components of the "diffuse endocrine epithelial system" (Feyrter 1954). These cells are all argyrophilic and are members of the bodywide amine precursor uptake and decarboxylation system (Pearse 1969). They therefore have the potential to produce amines and a wide variety of regulatory peptides such as serotonin, calcitonin, and CGRP. Although their exact physiological role is still largely unknown, they have been associated with chemoreceptor, endocrine, or neurohormonal paracrine functions (Sorokin and Hoyt 1989).

Solitary and clusters of neuroendocrine cells are found at all levels of the extrapulmonary and intrapulmonary conducting airways and in bronchial and laryngeal glands. Preferentially they occur at the laryngotracheal junction, at bronchial bifurcations, and at bronchioloalveolar junctions (Edmondson and Lewis 1980; Sorokin et al. 1983). In the Syrian hamster ten clusters of neuroendocrine cells and six solitary cells have been reported to be present per millimeter along the long axis of intrapulmonary bronchi (Sorokin et al. 1983).

*Etiopathogenesis*. The etiology of the laryngo-tracheal neuroendocrine proliferations in the hamster is unknown. In the present series lifetime inhalation of particles such as crystalline silica did not increase the frequency of these lesions in comparison to untreated hamsters, although there was extensive pulmonary damage. Furthermore, in none of the affected animals was there detected a concomitant proliferation of neuroendocrine cells in the distal trachea, bronchi, or lung parenchyma. There was also no obvious relationship between laryngotracheal neuroendocrine proliferation and other pathological changes in various organs.

According to Pour (1985), the rate of these laryngeal and tracheal tumors and their precursor lesions is not influenced by exposure to certain carcinogens. In contrast, proliferative lesions involving pulmonary neuroendocrine cells can be induced in hamsters by various chemical carcinogens (Reznik-Schüller 1976; Tateishi and Ishikawa 1985; Ito et al. 1988), cigarette smoke (Tabassian et al. 1989), and hyperoxia (Schüller et al. 1988). In human lungs hyperplasia and dysplasia of neuroendocrine cells has been reported to be associated frequently with various forms of chronic injury such as bronchiectasis, scarring and the proximity of other neoplasms (Gould et al. 1988). It has been speculated that some neuroendocrine carcinomas of the larynx in humans may represent ectopic thyroid C cell carcinomas because they elaborate calcitonin (Smets et al. 1990). These tumors are assumed to originate from embryonic rests of C cells which failed to migrate to the thyroid (Sweeney et al. 1981). The site of origin at the laryngotracheal junction, the morphological features, and the immunocytochemical findings of the present neuroendocrine tumors of the hamster appear to support such a hypothesis. The frequency of C cell tumors of the thyroid was also unexpectedly high in these Han:AURA hamsters (4.8%). This markedly exceeded the frequency in other hamster strains, which has been reported to be in the range of about 1% (Schmidt et al. 1983). However, none of the individual hamsters with neuroendocrine proliferation had a concomitant C cell tumor of the thyroid.

A characteristic feature of these laryngotracheal proliferations is the absence of pronounced cytological pleomorphism and atypia, irrespective of the size or behavior of the lesions. This imposes a major diagnostic problem in differentiating between neoplasia and the hyperplastic precursor lesion. Even those tumors which invade into blood vessels have an apparently benign histological appearance. They retain their organoid (endocrine

**Table 5.** Occurrence of spontaneous laryngotracheal neuroendocrine hyperplasias and tumors in aged Han:AURA hamsters

| Lesion | Sex | Larynx | Trachea | Both organs |
|---|---|---|---|---|
| Neuroendocrine hyperplasia | M | 9/399 (2.2%) | 15/399 (3.8%) | 24/399 (6.0%) |
| | F | 3/399 (0.8%) | 14/399 (3.5%) | 17/399 (4.3%) |
| Neuroendocrine tumor | M | 4/399 (1.0%) | 7/399 (1.8%) | 11/399 (2.8%) |
| | F | – | 10/399 (2.5%) | 10/399 (2.5%) |
| Both lesions | M + F | 16/798 (2.0%) | 46/798 (5.8%) | 62/798 (7.8%) |

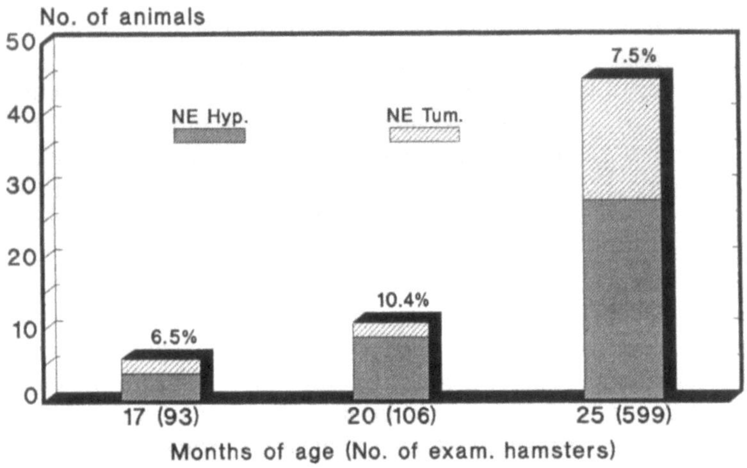


**Fig. 147.** Age distribution of laryngo-tracheal neuroendocrine proliferations in Han:AURA hamsters

organlike) architecture and express the same spectrum of immunological markers as the hyperplastic stages of the lesion.

The pathological criteria of these observed tumors correspond very well to the "carcinoid" or "carcinoid tumor" in the human respiratory system. In the classification system of Gould et al. (1983, 1988) carcinoids are low-grade neuroendocrine neoplasms which show a classical organoid histological pattern, are locally invasive, metastasize very late, and stain positively for a variety of specific markers. They comprise the beginning of a tumor spectrum which additionally includes well-differentiated intermediate cell and small cell carcinomas. "Linear neuroendocrine cell hyperplasias" (Gould et al. 1983) and "tumorlets" which correspond to nodular neuroendocrine hyperplasias (Torikata 1991) are defined as nonneoplastic precursor lesions.

*Frequency*. Hyperplasias and tumors of neuroendocrine origin were observed in the larynx of 16 (2%) and in the trachea of 46 (5.8%) of 798 Han:AURA hamsters from which these organs were histologically examined (Table 5). When numbers of laryngeal and tracheal proliferations are combined, males were affected to a slightly higher degree than females (35/399 = 8.8% versus 27/399 = 6.8%). Further examination, however, reveals that there was a striking preponderance of laryngeal proliferations in males (13/399 = 3.3% versus 3/399 = 0.8%) in females. In contrast, the frequency of tracheal proliferations was similar in males and females (5.5% versus 6.0%). The predominance of laryngeal tumors in males is consistent with the data of Pour (1985) who found the ratio of laryngeal clear cell carcinomas between males and females was 3:1.

The ratio of involvement of proximal trachea to larynx was 2.9:1 (Table 5). Some of the larger tumors involved both larynx and trachea. These cases were allocated to the organ which contained the bulk of tumor tissue.

The frequency of laryngotracheal proliferations increased with age (Fig. 147). This agrees with a previous report in which laryngeal clear cell carcinomas were described as a disease of aged hamsters, although they can be observed in hamsters as young as 30 weeks of age (Pour 1985). In the present investigation no proliferations were detected in 93 hamsters killed at 11 months of age.

The lesions were first observed in 6/93 (6.5%) hamsters aged 17 months. The frequency in 20-month-old hamsters increased to 11/106 (10.4%) and then declined to 45/599 (7.5%) in the 25-month age group, which corresponded to the terminal killing and contained the bulk of the animals examined (Fig. 147).

## Comparison with Other Species

Neuroendocrine tumors of the larynx have been reported as rare events in human beings and consist of well to poorly differentiated carcinomas (El-Naggar et al. 1991; Gnepp 1991; Smets et al. 1990; Wenig and Gnepp 1989).

A spontaneous clear cell carcinoma of the trachea has been described as occurring in a 696-day-old male Sprague-Dawley rat (Chandra et al. 1991). This tumor infiltrated the cranial trachea and consisted of lobules and cords of polygonal cells with numerous argyrophilic neurosecretory granules. We are not aware of any reports of such tumors in the larynx or trachea of other animal species.

## References


Chandra M, Riley MGI, Johnson DE (1991) Clear-cell carcinoma in the trachea of a rat. Lab Anim Sci 41:262–263

DeLellis RA, Wolfe HJ, Mohr U (1987) Medullary thyroid carcinoma in the Syrian hamster: an immunohistochemical study. Exp Pathol 31:11–16

Edmondson NA, Lewis DJ (1980) Distribution and ultrastructural characteristics of Feyrter cells in the rat and hamster airway epithelium. Thorax 35:371–374

El-Naggar AK, Batsakis JG, Vassilopoulou-Sellin R, Ordonez NG, Luna MA (1991) Medullary (thyroid) carcinoma-like carcinoids of the larynx. J Laryngol Otol 105:683–686

Feyrter F (1954) Zur Pathologie des argyrophilen Helle-Zelle-Organes im Bronchialbaum des Menschen. Virchows Arch Pathol Anat 325:723–732

Fröhlich F (1949) Die "Helle Zelle" der Bronchialschleimhaut und ihre Beziehungen zum Problem der Chemorezeptoren. Frank Z Pathol 60:517–559

Gnepp DR (1991) Small cell neuroendocrine carcinoma of the larynx: a critical review of the literature. ORL 53:210–219

Gould VE, Linnoila RI, Memoli VA, Warren WH (1983) Neuroendocrine components of the bronchopulmonary tract: hyperplasias, dysplasias, and neoplasms. Lab Invest 49:519–537

Gould VE, Lee I, Warren WH (1988) Immunohistochemical evaluation of neuroendocrine cells and neoplasms of the lung. Pathol Res Pract 183:200–213

Hsu SM, Raine L, Fanger H (1981) Use of avidin-biotin-peroxidase complex (ABC) in immunoperoxidase techniques: a comparison between ABC and unlabeled antibody (PAP) procedures. J Histochem Cytochem 29:577–580

Ito T, Kitamura H, Inayama Y, Kanisawa M (1988) Pulmonary adenoma and endocrine cell hyperplasia in Syrian golden hamster treated with 4-nitroquinoline 1-oxide. Acta Pathol Jpn 38:1097–1104

Keith IM, Ekman R (1988) Calcitonin gene-related peptide in hamster lung and its coexistence with serotonin: a chemical and immunocytochemical study. Regul Pept 22:315–323

Linnoila RI, Becker KL, Silva OL, Snider RH, Moore CF (1984) Calcitonin as a marker for diethylnitrosamine-induced pulmonary endocrine cell hyperplasia in hamsters. Lab Invest 51:39–45

Pearse AG (1969) The cytochemistry and ultrastructure of polypeptide hormone-producing cells of the APUD series and the embryologic, physiologic, and pathologic implications of the concept. J Histochem Cytochem 17:303–313

Pour PM (1985) Clear cell carcinoma, larynx, Syrian hamster. In: Jones TC, Mohr U, Hunt RD (eds) Monographs on pathology of laboratory animals: respiratory system. Springer, Berlin Heidelberg New York, pp 75–77

Pour PM, Althoff J, Salmasi SZ, Stepan K (1979) Spontaneous tumors and common diseases in three types of hamsters. J Natl Cancer Inst 63:797–811

Reznik-Schüller H (1976) Proliferation of endocrine (APUD-type) cells during early N-diethylnitrosamine-induced lung carcinogenesis in hamsters. Cancer Lett 1:255–258

Scheuermann DW (1987) Morphology and cytochemistry of the endocrine epithelial system in the lung. Int Rev Cytol 106:35–88

Schmidt RE, Eason RL, Hubbard GB, Young JT, Eisenbrandt DL (1983) Pathology of aging Syrian hamsters. CRC, Boca Raton, pp 141–174

Schüller HM, Becker KL, Witschi HP (1988) An animal model for neuroendocrine lung cancer. Carcinogenesis 9: 293–296

Shimosegawa T, Said SI (1991) Co-occurrence of immunoreactive calcitonin and calcitonin gene-related peptide in neuroendocrine cells of rat lungs. Cell Tissue Res 264:555–561

Smets G, Warson F, Dehou MF, Storme G, Sacre R, Van Belle S, Somers G, Gepts W, Klöppel G (1990) Metastasizing neuroendocrine carcinoma of the larynx with calcitonin and somatostatin secretion and CEA production, resembling medullary thyroid carcinoma. Virchows Arch [A] Pathol Anat Histopathol 416:539–543

Sorokin SP, Hoyt RF Jr (1989) Neuroepithelial bodies and solitary small-granule cells. In: Massaro D (ed) Lung cell biology. Dekker, New York, Basel pp 191–344

Sorokin SP, Hoyt RF Jr, Pearsall AD (1983) Comparative biology of small granule cells and neuroepithelial bodies in the respiratory system: short review. Am Rev Respir Dis 128:526–531

Strandberg JD (1987) Neoplastic diseases. In: Van Hoosier GL Jr, McPherson CW (eds) Laboratory hamsters. Academic, Orlando, pp 157–168

Sweeney EC, McDonnell L, O'Brien C (1981) Medullary carcinoma of the thyroid presenting as tumours of the pharynx and larynx. Histopathology 5:263–275

Tabassian AR, Nylen ES, Linnoila RI, Snider RH, Cassidy MM, Becker KL (1989) Stimulation of hamster pulmonary neuroendocrine cells and associated peptides by repeated exposure to cigarette smoke. Am Rev Respir Dis 140:436–440

Tateishi R, Ishikawa O (1985) The effect of N-nitrosobis(hydroxypropyl)amine on pulmonary neuro-epithelial cells in Syrian golden hamsters. Am J Pathol 119:326–335

Torikata C (1991) Intriguing case: tumorlets of the lung – an ultrastructural study. Ultrastructural Pathol 15:189–195

Tsutsumi Y (1989) Immunohistochemical analysis of calcitonin and calcitonin gene-related peptide in human lung. Hum Pathol 20:896–902

Wenig BM, Gnepp DR (1989) The spectrum of neuro-endocrine carcinomas of the larynx. Semin Diagn Pathol 6:329–350

# Murine Respiratory Mycoplasmosis, Rat and Mouse

Trenton R. Schoeb, Jerry K. Davis, and J. Russell Lindsey

*Synonyms.* Murine chronic respiratory disease, infectious catarrh, chronic murine pneumonia, enzootic bronchiectasis

## Gross Appearance

Gross lesions in the upper respiratory tract are not evident in most cases. Some affected rats have red-tinged fluid or red-brown crusty material around the eyes and external nares, which is porphyrin-containing secretion from the harderian glands, not serosanguinous exudate. Less commonly there is mucopurulent nasal discharge, and purulent exudate can sometimes be found in the nasal passages, tympanic bullae, and trachea.

The causative organism *Mycoplasma pulmonis* preferentially affects the nasal passages and middle ears, and the incidence of lesions decreases from the nasal passages distally. The lungs are externally normal in the majority of infected rats and mice, gross lesions being poorly correlated with clinical signs and microscopic changes. The bronchi are the most commonly affected parts of the lungs, and purple, depressed areas of atelectasis may occur in lungs in which exudate obstructs airways. Rats and mice with advanced disease may have gray- or yellow-purple consolidated areas of pneumonia in some cases. Yellow, slightly elevated foci representing bronchioles dilated with purulent exudate can affect entire lobes, imparting a cobblestone appearance (Figs. 148, 149). Frank abscesses are rare. The bronchial and paratracheal lymph nodes may be enlarged to three or four times normal size.

## Microscopic Features

The principal lesions of murine respiratory mycoplasmosis in the upper respiratory tract are, in decreasing order of frequency, rhinitis, otitis media, laryngitis, and tracheitis. All are characterized by: (a) epithelial changes, including hypertrophy, hyperplasia, metaplasia to nonkeratinizing squamous or stratified squamous epithelium, and goblet cell hyperplasia, (b) neutrophilic exudation, and (c) accumulation of lymphocytes and plasma cells.

*Rhinitis.* Normal rat nasal mucosa (Fig. 150) contains few lymphocytes except small numbers around and just anterior to the nasopharynx. In affected animals lymphoid cells accumulate diffusely in the subepithelial stroma. Loss of cilia, pseudoglandular epithelial hyperplasia, and goblet cell hyperplasia can be extensive and severe (Fig. 151).

*Otitis Media.* The middle ears are nearly as frequently affected as the nasal passages. The tympanic cavity may be completely filled with neutrophils (Fig. 152). The lining epithelium, normally simple squamous or low cuboidal, becomes hyperplastic. Goblet cells are often numerous. Commonly the lumen becomes filled with immature collagenous connective tissue, leaving only a few glandular spaces containing neutrophils at the boundary representing the original lining. The cavity may eventually clear, but the lining membrane remains thickened by connective tissue (Fig. 153).

*Laryngitis and Tracheitis.* The laryngeal submucosal glands are commonly dilated with mucopurulent exudate. Epithelial changes are as in other tissues, and the tracheal mucosa can become extremely thickened by epithelial hypertrophy and hyperplasia, with formation of glandlike crypts and severe accumulation of lymphoid cells (Figs. 154, 155).

*Bronchi and Lungs.* Pathogen-free and even germ-free laboratory rats have small amounts of

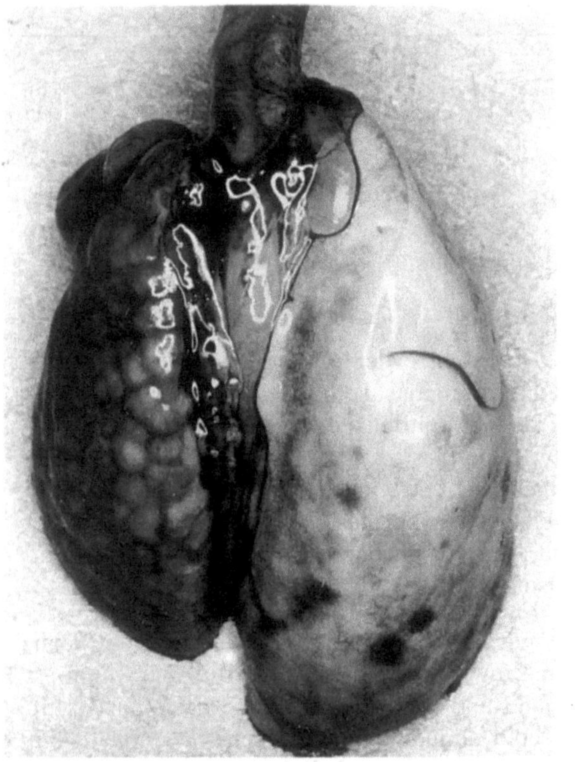

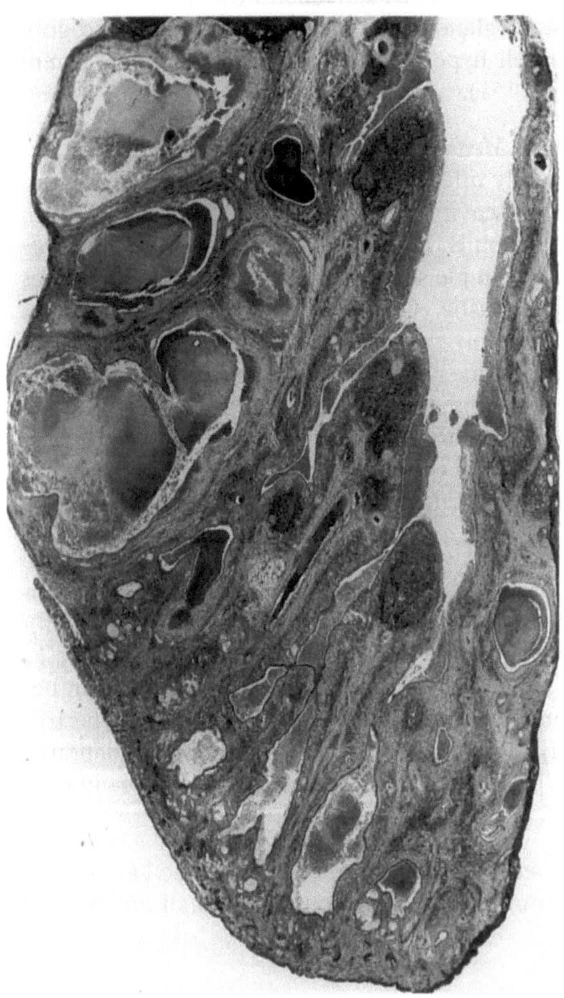

bronchus-associated lymphoid tissue, especially at the acute angles of bronchial bifurcations. Similar lymphoid aggregates occur between the bronchi and adjacent blood vessels (Figs. 156, 157). The trachea, bronchi, and bronchioles are lined by cuboidal to low columnar, rather than columnar and pseudostratified, epithelium. Lesions in the lung occur mainly in the major airways and are characterized by neutrophilic exudate, epithelial hyperplasia and hypertrophy, and increased peribronchial lymphoid tissue (Figs. 158–160). The distribution and severity of these changes within the lungs, and even within an individual lobe, are quite variable. Bronchiectasis and bronchiolectasis can result as airways become distended with purulent exudate. The epithelium of these distended airways becomes flattened and can become stratified, nonkeratinizing squamous. Rarely, the epithelium is destroyed completely, and is lost in the resulting abscess. The epithelium of alveoli around these severely affected airways may become cuboidal, imparting a glandular appearance (Fig. 160). Variably distributed alveolar exudation of neutrophils and macrophages can occur in advanced disease.

Microscopic lesions of respiratory mycoplasmosis in mice are similar to those in rats, with a few minor differences. Syncytia in the epithelium of the nasal passages occur in mice with the disease, but not in rats, and middle ear fibrosis such as that seen in rats does not occur in mice. Unlike rats, normal mice have minimal bronchial lymphoid tissue, making slight increases readily evident. Lymphoid accumulations in mice contain a greater proportion of plasma cells than those in rats, as do the regional lymph nodes.

## Ultrastructure

*M. pulmonis* parasitizes the surface of ciliated and nonciliated respiratory epithelial cells. In mild disease the organisms are sparsely distributed and can be extremely difficult to find, whereas in

◄

**Fig. 148.** (*above*) Murine respiratory mycoplasmosis, rat. Severe diffuse bronchiolectasis, atelectasis, and pneumonia in the left lung. ×2

**Fig. 149.** (*below*) Murine respiratory mycoplasmosis, rat. Severely affected left lung with bronchiectasis, bronchiolectasis, atelectasis, pneumonia, and greatly increased bronchial lymphoid tissue. ×8

severe disease they often are extremely numerous (Fig. 161). Ultrastructural changes in affected epithelium closely parallel those evident by light microscopy. Mildly affected epithelial cells may be increased in height but otherwise normal. In more severely affected epithelium degenerative changes are evident, including cytoplasmic vacuolation, loss of cilia, necrosis of scattered individual cells, and increased proportions of Clara and goblet cells.

## Differential Diagnosis

In naturally occurring *M. pulmonis* infection in rats and mice other agents are almost always present, such as Sendai virus, sialodacryoadenitis or rat coronavirus, pneumonia virus of mice, *Streptococcus pneumoniae*, *Corynebacterium kutscheri*, *Bordetella bronchiseptica*, *Pasteurella pneumotropica*, *Streptobacillus moniliformis*, *Pseudomonas aeruginosa*, *Klebsiella pneumoniae*, and cilia-associated respiratory (CAR) bacillus. CAR bacillus infection (pp. 325, this volume) is the major differential diagnostic problem. Lesions associated with CAR bacillus infection include chronic rhinitis, otitis media, laryngitis, tracheitis, and bronchitis that are indistinguishable morphologically from those of murine respiratory mycoplasmosis. CAR bacillus infection can be detected by silver impregnation staining of affected tissues, serological testing, culture, and DNA sequence amplification. Inasmuch as concurrent *M. pulmonis* infection is common in rats with natural CAR bacillus infections, identification of both agents should always be sought.

In rats *S. pneumoniae* causes fibrinopurulent bronchopneumonia, pleuritis, and pericarditis, and *C. kutscheri* induces multifocal suppurative pneumonia (Lindsey et al. 1991). In each case the diagnosis can be established by cultural identification and by demonstration of the organisms in sections stained with tissue gram stains, but because affected rats usually have concurrent *M. pulmonis* infection, cultural, morphological, and

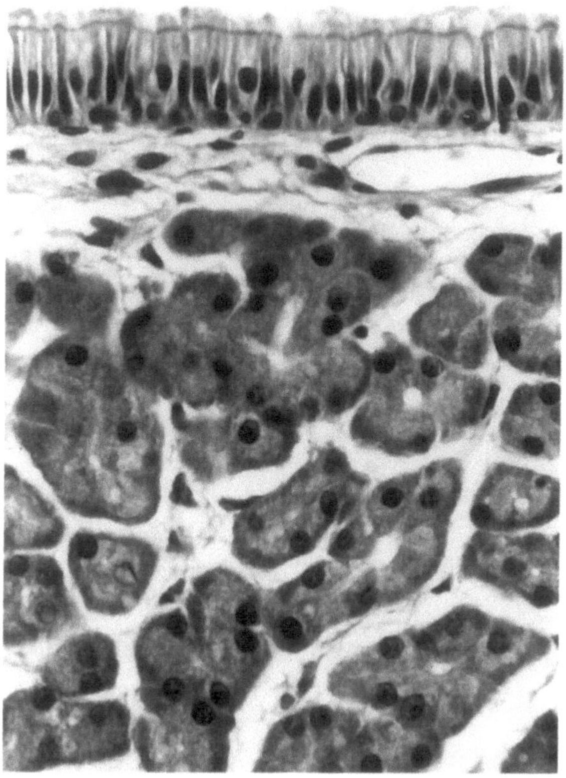

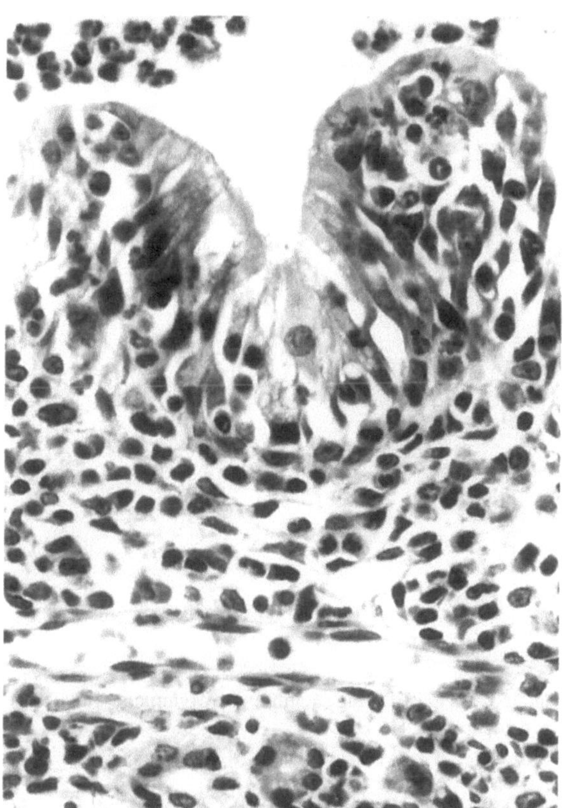

◄

**Fig. 150.** (*above*) Normal nasal septal mucosa. H&E, ×500

**Fig. 151.** (*below*) Nasal septal mucosa in severe murine respiratory mycoplasmosis, with neutrophilic exudate, loss of cilia, goblet cell hyperplasia with formation of glandular epithelial infoldings, and diffuse accumulation of lymphocytes and plasma cells. H&E, ×500

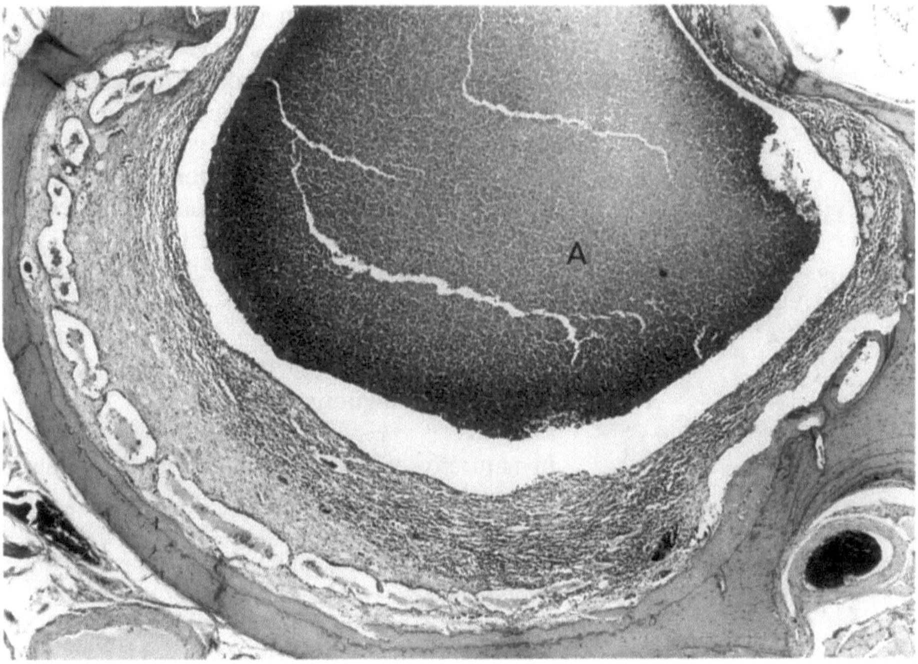


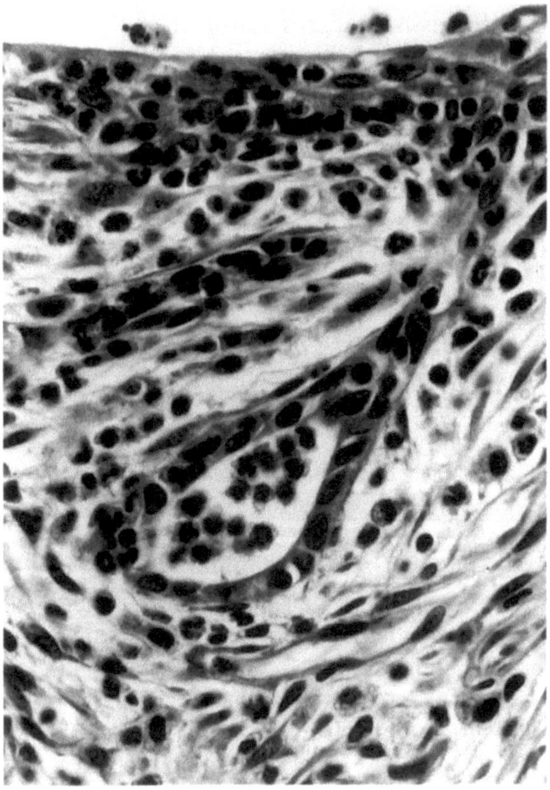

**Fig. 152.** (*above*) Tympanic bulla with purulent exudate in the lumen (*A*) and fibrosis of the lining membrane. H&E, ×35

**Fig. 153.** (*below*) Lining membrane of tympanic bulla thickened by fibrosis. H&E, ×500

serological evidence of respiratory mycoplasmosis should still be sought. The other bacteria listed probably are only opportunistic pathogens. Sendai virus infection in mice and rats and sialodacryoadenitis virus infection in rats cause focally necrotizing rhinotracheitis with accumulation of lymphoid cells, sometimes with pneumonitis. These lesions are transient, and, if found, are easily differentiated from those of respiratory mycoplasmosis. Serological test results indicate that infection with pneumonia virus of mice is common in conventional mice and rats, but no natural disease is known in either species.

At present there is no single diagnostic test for *M. pulmonis* infection that is satisfactory in all situations (Davidson et al. 1994). Cultural recovery is definitive, but failure to isolate the organism does not rule out subclinical infection, inasmuch as the organism can be difficult to isolate from rats with minimal or mild disease. Enzyme-linked immunosorbent assay for serum antibodies to *M. pulmonis* is commercially available but also can fail to detect subclinical infections and can be confounded by infection with other species of mycoplasmas. Immunoblotting is useful in such cases but is impractical for routine use. The probability of detecting *M. pulmonis* infection is increased by use of serological tests in combination with culture of multiple sites.

Methods for diagnosis of *M. pulmonis* infection based on the polymerase chain reaction (PCR) are reported to be able to detect 0.5–1 pg *M. pulmonis* DNA and identify *M. pulmonis* in rat respiratory tract specimens from which the organism could not be cultured (Goto et al. 1994; Harasawa et al. 1990; Kunita et al. 1990; Sanchez et al. 1994; van Kuppeveld et al. 1992). Use of reverse transcriptase PCR to amplify ribosomal RNA sequences increases sensitivity up to 1000-fold, and efficiently detected *M. pulmonis* in throat swabs from rats for up to 248 days after inoculation (van Kuppeveld et al. 1992, 1993). As with other diagnostic methods, PCR-based techniques require the use of adequate controls. A detection limit of 0.5–1 pg *M. pulmonis* DNA, for example, is the

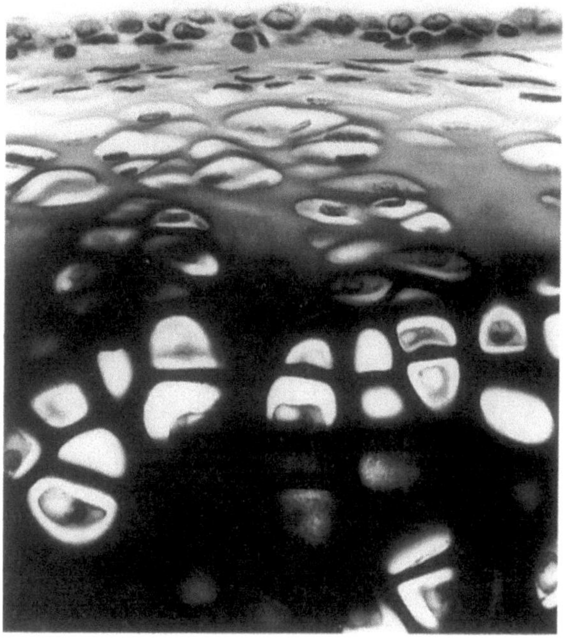

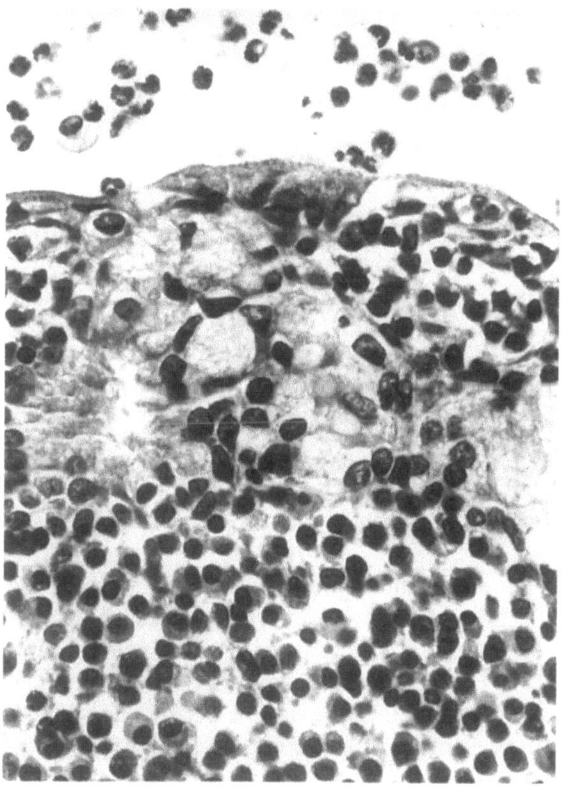

◄

**Fig. 154.** (*above*) Normal rat tracheal mucosa. H&E, ×500

**Fig. 155.** (*below*) Tracheal mucosa in severe chronic murine respiratory mycoplasmosis, with neutrophilic exudate, epithelial hyperplasia with glandlike infoldings, loss of cilia, and accumulation of lymphocytes and plasma cells. H&E, ×500

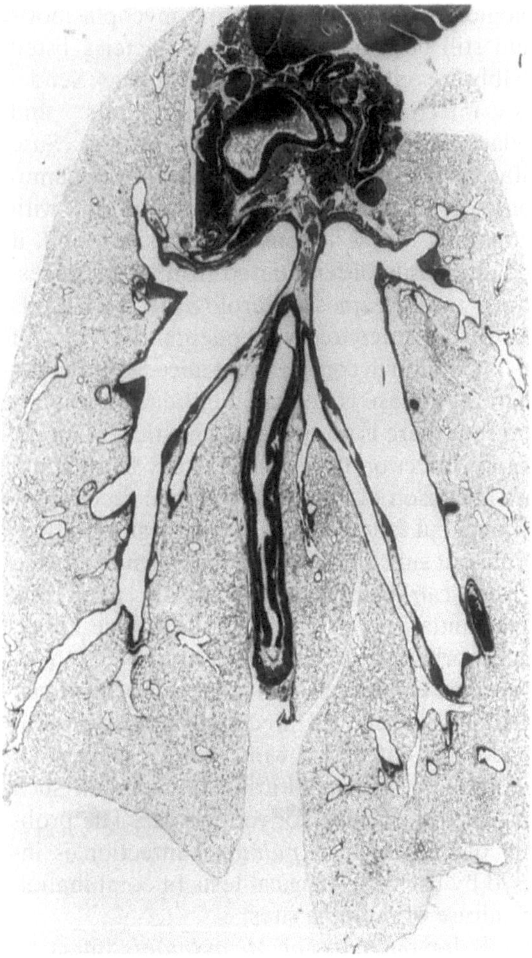

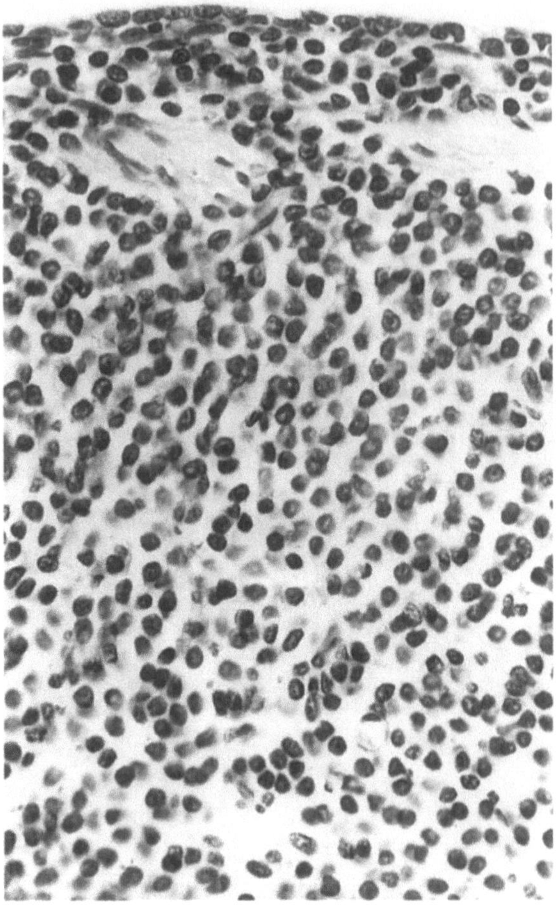

**Fig. 156.** (*left*) Normal lungs of a rat, with small amounts of lymphoid tissue predominantly at major bronchial bifurcations. ×4

**Fig. 157.** (*right*) Normal bronchial lymphoid tissue of rat, with flat epithelium and mostly small lymphocytes. H&E, ×500

equivalent of about 500–1000 mycoplasma cells, little better than the limit of sensitivity of carefully optimized culture methods. In addition, efficiency of amplification can vary due to the type of sample, the sample preparation method, and various impurities, not all of which are necessarily removed even by chloroform-phenol extraction. Thus a sample that is only moderately inhibitory could contain a considerable number of mycoplasmas but fail to yield enough amplicon to be detected without blotting and probing. Use of an internal control in each sample tested shows that with some types of samples amplification is inhibited in one-third or more of the reactions (Ursi et al. 1992; Schoeb et al. 1993a). Therefore internal controls are necessary to ensure accurate results, and additional or modified procedures such as reverse transcriptase or nested PCR, dot or Southern blotting and probing of the reaction product, or both, may be necessary to ensure detection of very small numbers of mycoplasmas or to compensate for inhibitory samples.

## Biological Features

*M. pulmonis* infection once was common among rats and mice from commercial sources, but it has been essentially eliminated from specific pathogen-free rats and mice from modern commercial vendors. Nonetheless, only a decade ago it was still present in some commercial barrier-maintained colonies (Cassell et al. 1986), and this probably is still the case. *M. pulmonis* still is prevalent among conventional rats and to a lesser extent mice.

The major *mode of transmission* of *M. pulmonis* is

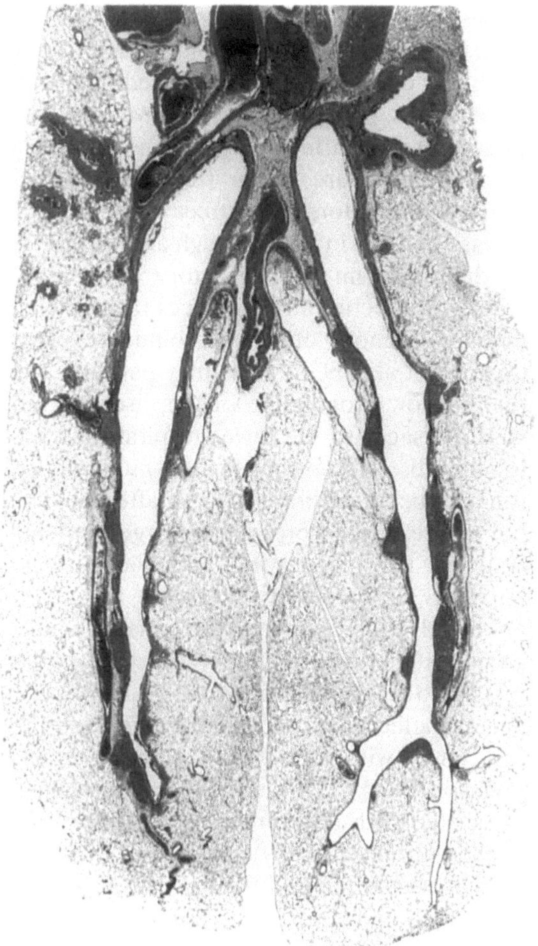

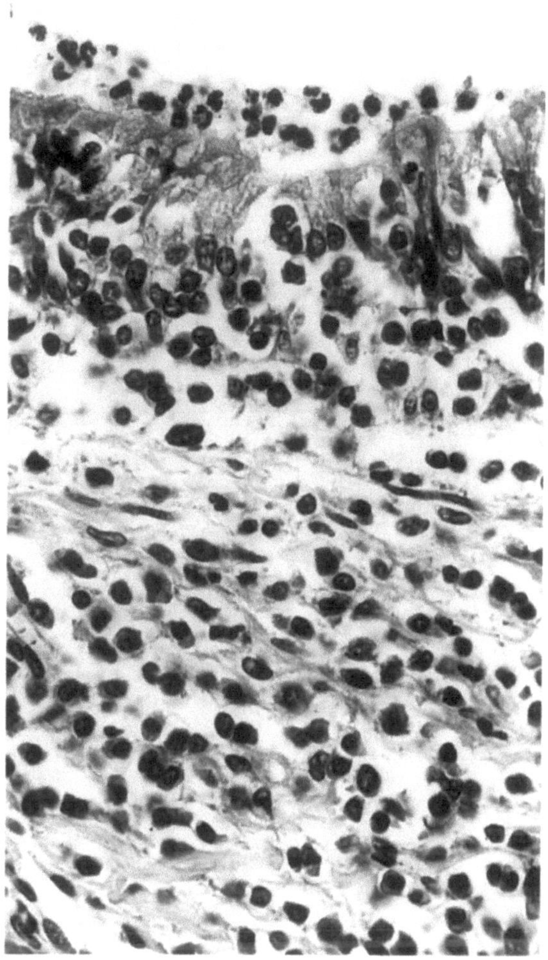

**Fig. 158.** Mildly affected lungs of a rat with mild to moderate increase in bronchial lymphoid tissue and early bronchiolitis in the right cranial lobe and cranial part of the left lung. ×4

**Fig. 159.** Bronchus in murine respiratory mycoplasmosis, with neutrophilic exudate, respiratory epithelial hyperplasia, intraepithelial lymphocytes, and large lymphocytes and plasmacytoid cells in the lamina propria. H&E, ×500

probably via aerosol or direct contact from mothers to neonates. *M. pulmonis* also infects the genital tract in both rats and mice, causing purulent endometritis, salpingitis, and perioophoritis (Banerjee et al. 1985; Lindsey et al. 1986). *M. pulmonis* infection has been identified in cesarean-derived rats housed in isolators (Ganaway et al. 1973; Cox et al. 1988), and in utero transmission in rats has been experimentally documented (Steiner et al. 1993). Infection of the respiratory tract probably persists throughout the animal's life, although the severity of lesions may wane with age. Infected rats can transmit the infection to others, but horizontal transmission is slow, even within a cage, and is considerably reduced by increasing the space between cages. Transmission of *M. pulmonis* via food, water, bedding, and other materials has been suggested but not proved. Inasmuch as *M. pulmonis* has been isolated from wild rats, cotton rats, rabbits, Syrian hamsters, and guinea pigs, these animals could be potential sources of infection.

The nasal passages and middle ears, the most commonly infected sites, appear to be the source of infection for the distal respiratory tract. Disease is minimal or mild under conditions favorable to the host, extending to the distal airways and lungs under the influence of complex interactions among host, organism, and environment. Factors known to affect disease expression include differences in susceptibility among rats and mice of different inbred strains (Davis and Cassell 1982; Davis et al. 1985a; Lai et al. 1993), virulence of *M. pulmonis* strains (Davidson et al. 1988b; Schoeb et al. 1993b), exposure to ammonia (Broderson et al.

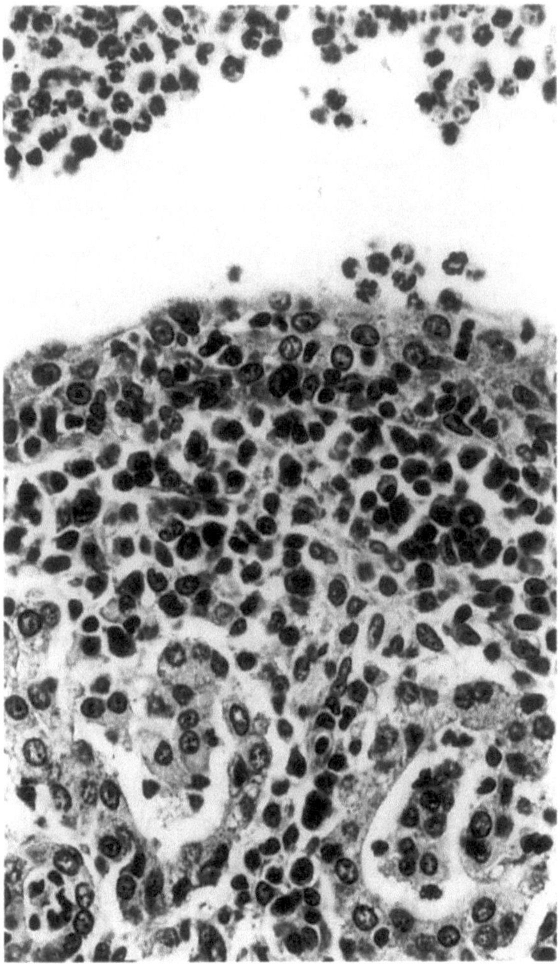

**Fig. 160.** Bronchiole in severe murine respiratory mycoplasmosis, with neutrophilic exudate, severe epithelial distortion and ciliary loss, lymphoid accumulation, and peribronchiolar glandular structures. ×500

1976), concurrent infection with Sendai virus (Howard et al. 1978; Schoeb et al. 1985) or sialodacryoadenitis virus (Schoeb and Lindsey 1987), and advancing age (Cassell et al. 1979). Expression of the disease also can be influenced by experimental manipulations.

The *pathogenesis* is not fully understood. The close relationship of *M. pulmonis* with the surface of respiratory epithelium undoubtedly is fundamental to establishing and maintaining infection and may help the organism escape elimination by the mucociliary system, cellular and noncellular inflammatory processes, and specific immune effector mechanisms. Adherence of *M. pulmonis* to rat respiratory epithelium is at least partially mediated by a trypsin-resistant 46-kDa protein of the organism's membrane (Beyers et al. 1994), but the corresponding receptor on epithelial cells has not been identified. Adherence of the organism to rat tracheal epithelium is increased in sialodacryoadenitis virus infection and vitamin A deficiency but is not affected by Sendai virus infection, ammonia exposure, or age (Schoeb et al. 1993b). Thus, some factors that affect expression of the disease may act in part through altered adherence of the organism to respiratory epithelium. *M. pulmonis* infection itself induces rat tracheal epithelium to more effectively bind the organism (Schoeb et al. 1993b). This may partially account for the slow progression of the disease from the nasal passages to the lower respiratory tract and for the observation that few *M. pulmonis* organisms can be found in rats shortly after inoculation, but as the disease progresses, large numbers appear on the respiratory epithelial surface. *M. pulmonis* strains vary in ability to adhere to epithelial cells. Among the small number of strains studied to date, adherence appears to be related to virulence (Schoeb et al. 1993b). Differences in adherence among *M. pulmonis* strains are associated with variations in the V-1 antigen (Watson et al. 1988), and V-1 heterogeneity is associated with differences in virulence for mice (Talkington et al. 1989). *M. pulmonis* has a high rate of recombination, which can be associated with phenotypic variation (Bhugra and Dybvig 1992). These phenomena may be related to defensive mechanisms of the organism. In mice variation in virulence of *M. pulmonis* strains is related to their ability to resist mucociliary clearance and intrapulmonary killing by alveolar macrophages (Davidson et al. 1988a), but the basis for these properties is not known.

LEW rats develop more severe disease in response to *M. pulmonis* inoculation than F344 rats, and lung lesions are characterized by more severe and more prolonged accumulation of both B and T lymphocytes (Davis et al. 1982). This may be due, at least in part, to the stronger nonspecific mitogenic responses to *M. pulmonis* of lymphocytes of LEW rats than those of F344 rats, which probably results from larger numbers of T helper cells in LEW rats (Davis et al. 1985b; Williamson et al. 1986). Surface membrane proteins of *M. pulmonis* have chemoattractant activity, mediated largely by the V-1 antigen, for both B lymphocytes and macrophages (Ross et al. 1992), and *M. pulmonis* induces expression of class II major histocompatibility antigens on both B lymphocytes and macrophages (Stuart et al.

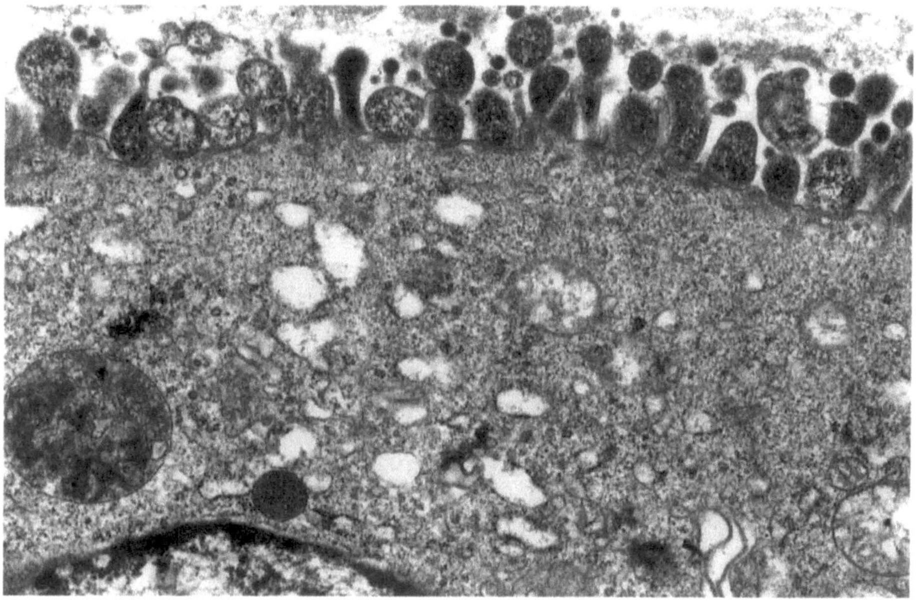

**Fig. 161.** Tracheal epithelial cell with *M. pulmonis* organisms on its surface. TEM, ×12000

1989), which may increase interactions of these cells with T helper cells.

Rats and mice produce serum and secretory immunoglobulin (Ig) M, IgG, and IgA antibodies in response to *M. pulmonis* infection (Simecka et al. 1991, 1992, 1993). The lymph nodes of the upper respiratory tract are the initial site of antibody production in rats and remain the major site as the disease progresses. LEW rats produce equal or greater amounts of the major classes of serum antibody to *M. pulmonis* than F344 rats, although LEW and F344 rats have similar numbers of antibody forming cells of all major immunoglobulin classes in their lymphoid tissues. However, the subclass distribution of IgG antibodies differs among rat strains. The IgG antibodies of LEW rats are largely of the $IgG_1$ and $IgG_{2a}$ subclasses, whereas those of F344 rats are primarily $IgG_{2b}$ and those of Sprague-Dawley rats are predominantly $IgG_{2a}$ (Brown and Reyes 1991). The roles of these responses in resistance to *M. pulmonis* are unclear. High concentrations of specific antibody are associated with severe disease with large numbers of the organisms in the respiratory tract rather than elimination of the organisms and resolution of lesions. Transfer of immune cells, but not serum, confers resistance in rats, whereas the reverse is the case in mice (Lai et al. 1991; Taylor and Taylor-Robinson 1976).

*Nonspecific responses* to *M. pulmonis* (those not requiring recognition by receptors of B or T lymphocytes) are best studied in mice. The greater susceptibility of C3H/HeN mice relative to C57BL/6N mice is related to impaired pulmonary mycoplasmacidal activity (Parker et al. 1987). Genetically determined differences in susceptibility to murine respiratory mycoplasmosis and to exacerbation by nitrogen dioxide are mediated at least in part by effects on alveolar macrophages (Davis et al. 1992; Lai et al. 1993). Interactions of *M. pulmonis* with natural killer (NK) cells are unclear. *M. pulmonis* infection is reported to increase activity of splenic and lung NK cells (Kamiyama et al. 1991; Lai et al. 1990), and NK cells appear to be able to aid clearance of *M. pulmonis* from the lungs by an interferon-γ dependent process, possibly macrophage activation (Lai et al. 1990). Others have found that virulence of *M. pulmonis* strains, susceptibility of mouse strains, and stimulation of NK were not related, and that *M. pulmonis* stimulated significant NK cell activity only in susceptible C3H/HeN mice (Swing et al. 1995). Nonetheless, interferon-γ and other cytokines probably have prominent roles in pathogenesis. Messenger RNAs of tumor necrosis factor-α, interferon-γ, interleukin-1, and interleukin-6 appear in the lungs of mice shortly after inoculation, and susceptible C3H/HeN mice have increased interleukin-6 in serum and higher and more persistent concentrations of tumor necrosis factor-α and interleukin-6 in bronchoalveolar lavage fluid than resistant C57BL/6N mice

(Faulkner et al. 1995b; Nishimoto et al. 1994). *M. pulmonis* infection also potentiates neurogenic inflammation of the respiratory mucosa, probably by inducing increases in the number and responsiveness of mediator-sensitive postcapillary venules (McDonald et al. 1991). Exposure to ammonia further increases the severity of the response.

The *mechanisms of host cell injury* by *M. pulmonis* are not known but may include deprivation of nutrients, alteration of host cell components and metabolism, and production of toxic substances. *M. pulmonis* has membrane-associated nuclease and hemolysin activities that could be involved in such processes (Minion and Jarvill-Taylor 1993, 1994). The inflammatory and immune responses that accompany infection probably contribute to host injury. Mice with acute *M. pulmonis* pneumonia develop severe lung lesions associated with coagulopathy (Faulkner et al. 1995a), which may be related to tumor necrosis factor-α production. Specific responses also appear to be injurious as well as beneficial, inasmuch as both rats and mice with T cell deficiency develop less severe lung disease due to *M. pulmonis* infection than immunocompetent animals (Simecka et al. 1992).

## Comparison with Other Species

Several features are common among most mycoplasmal respiratory diseases, including parasitism of the epithelial surface; chronic, predominantly lymphocytic, inflammation; and rare fatality. An exception is contagious pleuropneumonia, caused by *M. mycoides*, of cattle and goats, which is characterized by fibrinous pleuropneumonia and is frequently fatal. As in murine respiratory mycoplasmosis, host and environmental factors strongly affect disease progression and lesion severity in enzootic pneumonia of swine and the genital and respiratory diseases caused by mycoplasmas in poultry. Avirulent strains of *M. pulmonis* and most other animal mycoplasmas occur naturally, and at least some animals carry the organisms with no signs of disease.

Lesions of *M. gallisepticum* infection in chickens include chronic suppurative rhinitis, sinusitis, tracheitis, and bronchitis, with epithelial hypertrophy and hyperplasia, increased mucus production, and lymphoid cell accumulation with follicle formation in the lamina propria. The lesions are thus similar to those of murine respiratory mycoplasmosis. *M. gallisepticum* alone usually causes a rather mild upper respiratory disease, but infection frequently is complicated by wild or vaccine Newcastle disease virus, infectious bronchitis virus, avian adenovirus, or *Escherichia coli*, resulting in more severe disease with extension to the lungs and air sacs.

In turkeys *M. gallisepticum* produces a disease similar to that in chickens but with even more of a tendency for upper respiratory tract lesions, especially sinusitis, to predominate. Thus, the disease is usually called infectious sinusitis. *M. meleagridis* causes a spontaneously resolving air sacculitis also characterized by chronic suppurative inflammation, lymphoid infiltration, and epithelial hyperplasia.

Swine with porcine enzootic pneumonia, caused by *M. hyopneumoniae*, develop lesions similar to those of murine respiratory mycoplasmosis, although bronchiectasis does not occur. Alveolitis with macrophage and neutrophil accumulation is more prominent than in the rodent disease. The gross lesions, discrete gray-red firm areas predominantly in the dependent parts of the lungs, are characteristic. The natural disease is frequently complicated by other agents such as *Pasteurella multocida*, *M. hyorhinis*, and swine adenovirus.

Lesions of human disease caused by *M. pneumoniae* are not well known because the disease is rarely fatal. However, available descriptions indicate that lesions include peribronchial and perivascular lymphoid infiltrates, acute bronchitis and bronchiolitis, transformation of alveolar epithelium to cuboidal type, and an alveolar exudate made up chiefly of macrophages. These changes are similar to those of other respiratory mycoplasmoses.

## References

Banerjee AK, Angulo AF, Polak-Vogelzang AA, Kershof AM (1985) Naturally occurring genital mycoplasmosis in mice. Lab Anim 19:275–276

Beyers TM, Lai WC, Read RW, Pakes SP (1994) Mycoplasma pulmonis 46-kDa trypsin-resistant protein adheres to rat tracheal epithelial cells. Lab Anim Sci 44:573–578

Bhugra B, Dybvig K (1992) High-frequency rearrangements in the chromosome of Mycoplasma pulmonis correlate with phenotypic switching. Mol Microbiol 6:1149–1154

Broderson JR, Lindsey JR, Crawford JE (1976) The role of environmental ammonia in respiratory mycoplasmosis of rats. Am J Pathol 85:115–130

Brown MB, Reyes L (1991) Immunoglobulin class- and subclass-specific responses to Mycoplasma pulmonis in sera and secretions of naturally infected Sprague-Dawley female rats. Infect Immun 59:2181–2185

Cassell GH, Lindsey JR, Baker HJ, Davis JK (1979) Mycoplasmal and rickettsial diseases. In: Baker HJ, Lindsey JR, Weisbroth SH (eds) The laboratory rat, vol 1: biology and diseases. Academic, New York, chap 10

Cassell GH, Cox NR, Davis JK, Brown MB, Minion FC, Lindsey JR (1986) State-of-the-art detection methods for rodent mycoplasmas. In: Hamm TE Jr (ed) Complications of viral and mycoplasmal infections in rodents to toxicology research and testing. Hemisphere, Washington DC, chap 7

Cox NR, Davidson MK, Davis JK, Lindsey JR, Cassell GH (1988) Natural mycoplasmal infections in isolator-maintained LEW/Tru rats. Lab Anim Sci 38:381–388

Davidson MK, Davis JK, Lindsey JR, Cassell GH (1988a) Clearance of different strains of Mycoplasma pulmonis from the respiratory tract of C3H/HeN mice. Infect Immun 56:2163–2168

Davidson MK, Lindsey JR, Parker RF, Tully JG, Cassell GH (1988b) Differences in virulence for mice among strains of Mycoplasma pulmonis. Infect Immun 56:2156–2162

Davidson MK, Davis JK, Gambill GP, Cassell GH, Lindsey JR (1994) Mycoplasmas of laboratory rodents. In: Whitford HW, Rosenbusch RF, Lauerman LH (eds) Mycoplasmosis in animals: laboratory diagnosis. Iowa State University Press, Ames, IA, pp 97–133

Davis JK, Cassell GH (1982) Murine respiratory mycoplasmosis in LEW and F344 rats: strain differences in lesion severity. Vet Pathol 19:280–293

Davis JK, Thorp RB, Maddox PA, Brown MB, Cassell GH (1982) Murine respiratory mycoplasmosis in F344 and LEW rats: evolution of lesions and lung lymphoid cell populations. Infect Immun 36:720–729

Davis JK, Parker RF, White H, Dziedzic D, Taylor G, Davidson MK, Cox NR, Cassell GH (1985a) Strain differences in susceptibility to murine respiratory mycoplasmosis in C57BL/6 and C3H/HeN mice. Infect Immun 50:647–654

Davis JK, Simecka JW, Williamson JS, Ross SE, Juliana MM, Thorp RB, Cassell GH (1985b) Nonspecific lymphocyte responses in F344 and LEW rats: susceptibility to murine respiratory mycoplasmosis and examination of cellular basis for strain differences. Infect Immun 49:152–158

Davis JK, Davidson MK, Schoeb TR, Lindsey JR (1992) Decreased intrapulmonary killing of Mycoplasma pulmonis after short-term exposure to NO2 is associated with damaged alveolar macrophages. Am Rev Respir Dis 145:406–411

Faulkner CB, Davidson MK, Davis JK, Schoeb TR, Simecka JW, Lindsey JR (1995a) Acute Mycoplasma pulmonis infection is associated with coagulopathy in C3H/HeN mice. Lab Anim Sci (in press)

Faulkner CB, Simecka JW, Davidson MK, Davis JK, Schoeb TR, Lindsey JR, Everson MP (1995b) Gene expression and production of TNF-α, IL-1, IL-6, and IFN-γ in C3H/HeN and C57BL/6N mice in acute Mycoplasma pulmonis disease. Infect Immun (in press)

Ganaway JR, Allen AM, Moore TD, Bohner HJ (1973) Natural infection of germfree rats with Mycoplasma pulmonis. J Infect Dis 127:529–537

Goto K, Kunita S, Terada E, Itoh T (1994) Comparison of polymerase chain reaction and culture methods for detection of Mycoplasma pulmonis from nasal, tracheal and oral swab samples of rats. Jikken Dobutsu 43:413–415

Harasawa R, Koshimizu K, Uemori T, Takeda O, Asada K, Kato I (1990) The polymerase chain reaction for Mycoplasma pulmonis. Microbiol Immunol 34:393–395

Howard CJ, Stott EJ, Taylor G (1978) The effect of pneumonia induced in mice with Mycoplasma pulmonis on resistance to subsequent bacterial infection and the effect of a respiratory infection with Sendai virus on the resistance of mice to Mycoplasma pulmonis. J Gen Microbiol 109:79–87

Kamiyama T, Saito M, Nakagawa M (1991) Effects of Mycoplasma pulmonis infection and exposure to nitrogen dioxide on activities of natural killer cells and macrophages of the mouse. Jikken Dobutsu 40:255–257

Kunita S, Terada E, Goto K, Kagiyama N (1990) Sensitive detection of Mycoplasma pulmonis by using the polymerase chain reaction. Jikken Dobutsu 39:103–107

Lai WC, Bennett M, Pakes SP, Kumar V, Steutermann D, Owusu I, Mikhael A (1990) Resistance to Mycoplasma pulmonis mediated by activated natural killer cells. J Infect Dis 161:1269–1275

Lai WC, Bennett M, Lu YS, Pakes SP (1991) Vaccination of Lewis rats with temperature-sensitive mutants of Mycoplasma pulmonis: adoptive transfer of immunity by spleen cells but not by sera. Infect Immun 59:346–350

Lai WC, Linton G, Bennett M, Pakes SP (1993) Genetic control of resistance to Mycoplasma pulmonis infection in mice. Infect Immun 61:4615–4621

Lindsey JR, Davidson MK, Schoeb TR, Cassell GH (1986) Murine mycoplasmal infections, diseases, and research complications. A critique of current knowledge. In: Hamm TE Jr (ed) Complications of viral and mycoplasmal infections in rodents to toxicology research and testing. Hemisphere, Washington DC, chap 5

Lindsey JR, Boorman GA, Collins MJ Jr, Hsu CK, Van Hoosier GL Jr, Wagner JE (1991) Infectious diseases of mice and rats. National Academy Press, Washingtion DC

McDonald DM, Schoeb TR, Lindsey JR (1991) Mycoplasma pulmonis infections cause long-lasting potentiation of neurogenic inflammation in the respiratory tract of the rat. J Clin Invest 87:787–799

Minion FC, Jarvill-Taylor KJ (1993) Membrane-associated nuclease activities in mycoplasmas. J Bacteriol 175:7842–7847

Minion FC, Jarvill-Taylor K (1994) Membrane-associated hemolysin activities in mycoplasmas. FEMS Microbiol Lett 116:101–106

Nishimoto M, Akashi A, Kuwano K, Tseng CC, Ohizumi K, Arai S (1994) Gene expression of tumor necrosis factor alpha and interferon gamma in the lungs of Mycoplasma pulmonis-infected mice. Microbiol Immunol 38:345–352

Parker RF, Davis JK, Blalock DK, Thorp RB, Simecka JW, Cassell GH (1987) Pulmonary clearance of Mycoplasma pulmonis in C57BL/6N and C3H/HeN mice. Infect Immun 55:2631–2635

Ross SE, Simecka JW, Gambill GP, Davis JK, Cassell GH (1992) Mycoplasma pulmonis possesses a novel chemoattractant for B lymphocytes. Infect Immun 60:669–674

Sanchez S, Tyler K, Rozengurt N, Lida J (1994) Comparison of a PCR-based diagnostic assay for Mycoplasma pulmonis with traditional detection techniques. Lab Anim 28:249–256

Schoeb TR, Lindsey JR (1987) Exacerbation of murine respiratory mycoplasmosis by sialodacryoadenitis virus infection in gnotobiotic F344 rats. Vet Pathol 24:392–399

Schoeb TR, Kervin KC, Lindsey JR (1985) Exacerbation of murine respiratory mycoplasmosis in gnotobiotic F344/N rats by Sendai virus infection. Vet Pathol 22:272–282

Schoeb TR, Dybvig K, Davidson MK, Davis JK (1993a) Cultivation of cilia-associated respiratory bacillus in artificial medium and determination of the 16S rRNA gene sequence. J Clin Microbiol 31:2751–2757

Schoeb TR, Juliana MM, Nichols PW, Davis JK, Lindsey JR (1993b) Effects of viral and mycoplasmal infections, ammonia exposure, vitamin A deficiency, host age, and organism strain on adherence of Mycoplasma pulmonis in cultured rat tracheas. Lab Anim Sci 43:417–424

Simecka JW, Patel P, Davis JK, Ross SE, Otwell P, Cassell, GH (1991) Specific and nonspecific antibody responses in different segments of the respiratory tract in rats infected with Mycoplasma pulmonis. Infect Immun 59:3715–3721

Simecka JW, Davis JK, Davidson MK, Ross SE, Stadtlander CTK, Cassell GH (1992) Mycoplasma diseases of animals. In: Maniloff J, McElhaney RN, Finch LE, Baseman JB (eds) Mycoplasmas: molecular biology and pathogenesis. American Society for Microbiology, Washington DC, chap 24

Simecka JW, Ross SE, Cassell GH, Davis JK (1993) Interactions of mycoplasmas with B cells: antibody production and nonspecific effects. Clin Infect Dis 17 [Suppl 1]:S176–S182

Steiner DA, Uhl EW, Brown MB (1993) In utero transmission of Mycoplasma pulmonis in experimentally infected Sprague-Dawley rats. Infect Immun 61:2985–2990

Stuart PM, Cassell GH, Woodward JG (1989) Induction of class II MHC antigen expression in macrophages by Mycoplasma species. J Immunol 142:3392–3399

Swing SP, Davis JK, Egan ML (1995) In vitro effects of Mycoplasma pulmonis on murine natural killer cell activity. Lab Anim Sci (in press)

Talkington DF, Fallon MT, Watson HL, Thorp RK, Cassell GH (1989) Mycoplasma pulmonis V-1 surface protein variation: occurrence in vivo and association with lung lesions. Microb Pathog 7:429–436

Taylor G, Taylor-Robinson D (1976) Effects of active and passive immunization on Mycoplasma pulmonis-induced pneumonia in mice. Immunology 30:611–618

Ursi JP, Ursi D, Ieven M, Pattyn SR (1992) Utility of an internal control for the polymerase chain reaction. Application to detection of Mycoplasma pneumoniae in clinical specimens. APMIS 100:635–639

van Kuppeveld FJ, van der Logt JT, Angulo AF, van Zoest MJ, Quint WG, Niesters HG, Galama JM, Melchers WJ (1992) Genus- and species-specific identification of mycoplasmas by 16S rRNA amplification. Appl Environ Microbiol 58:2606–2615 (published erratum appears in Appl Environ Microbiol 59: 655, 1993)

van Kuppeveld FJ, Melchers WJ, Willemse HF, Kissing J, Galama JM, van der Logt JT (1993) Detection of Mycoplasma pulmonis in experimentally infected laboratory rats by 16S rRNA amplification. J Clin Microbiol 31:524–527

Watson HL, McDaniel LS, Blalock DK, Fallon MT, Cassell GH (1988) Heterogeneity among strains and a high rate of variation within strains of a major surface antigen of Mycoplasma pulmonis. Infect Immun 56:1358–1363

Williamson JS, Davis JK, Cassell GH (1986) Polyclonal activation of rat splenic lymphocytes after in vivo administration of Mycoplasma pulmonis and its relation to in vitro response. Infect Immun 52:594–599

# Rat Coronavirus Infection, Upper Respiratory Tract, Rat

David G. Brownstein

*Synonyms.* Rat submaxillary gland virus infection, sialodacryoadenitis virus, Parker's rat coronavirus

## Gross Appearance

Gross lesions are usually extrarespiratory and limited to mixed or serous salivary glands, exorbital glands, harderian glands, periglandular connective tissue, cervical lymph nodes, and thymus. The submaxillary and parotid salivary glands are enlarged, pale, and edematous. Intermandibular and cervical connective tissue is gelatinous due to periglandular edema. This edema restricts the venous return in the neck, resulting in distention of the great veins entering the thoracic inlet. Exorbital glands are occasionally enlarged. Harderian glands are swollen and flecked with yellow-gray spots. These foci must be distinguished from normal brown-red mottling of the harderian gland imparted by its normal content of porphyrin pigment. The cervical lymph nodes are enlarged, and the thymus is atrophic. In these cases ocular lesions may include corneral opacity, corneal ulcers, pannus, hypopyon, hyphema, and megalogobus (Innes and Stanton 1961; Jacoby et al. 1975, 1979).

## Microscopic Features

Respiratory lesions are restricted primarily to the upper respiratory tract. They precede inflammatory changes in the exocrine tissues of the head. Over the course of approximately 5 days, beginning on the 2nd day of infection, there is spreading necrosis of respiratory epithelium in the nasal cavity accompanied by congestion, edema, and mixed inflammatory infiltrate of the lamina propria (Figs. 162, 163). The epithelial lining of the turbinates is most severely affected; olfactory epithelium is usually spared. Some meatuses are covered by exudate composed of necrotic epithelium, neutrophils, and mucus. Despite a tropism of these viruses for serous or mixed salivary glands the serous mucosal glands of the nasopharynx sustain relatively mild injury. Necrotic ducts and acini within mucosal glands do occur, however, and afford some specificity to the lesion. There is qualitatively similar inflammation in the trachea, but changes are milder and less uniform than in the nasopharynx. Upper respiratory lesions are resolved by the end of the 2nd week of infection. Lung changes are confined to mild hyperplasia within peribronchial lymphoid nodules (Jacoby et al. 1975, 1979).

Severe inflammatory changes occur within mixed or serous salivary glands, exorbital glands, and harderian glands. Description of these changes is beyond the scope of this volume. The reader is referred to several excellent studies of sequential changes in these tissues (Innes and Stanton 1961; Jacoby et al. 1975, 1979).

## Ultrastructure

We have found no report of the ultrastructural features of respiratory tract lesions caused by rat coronavirus, but these features have been studied in infected submaxillary gland epithelium (Jonas

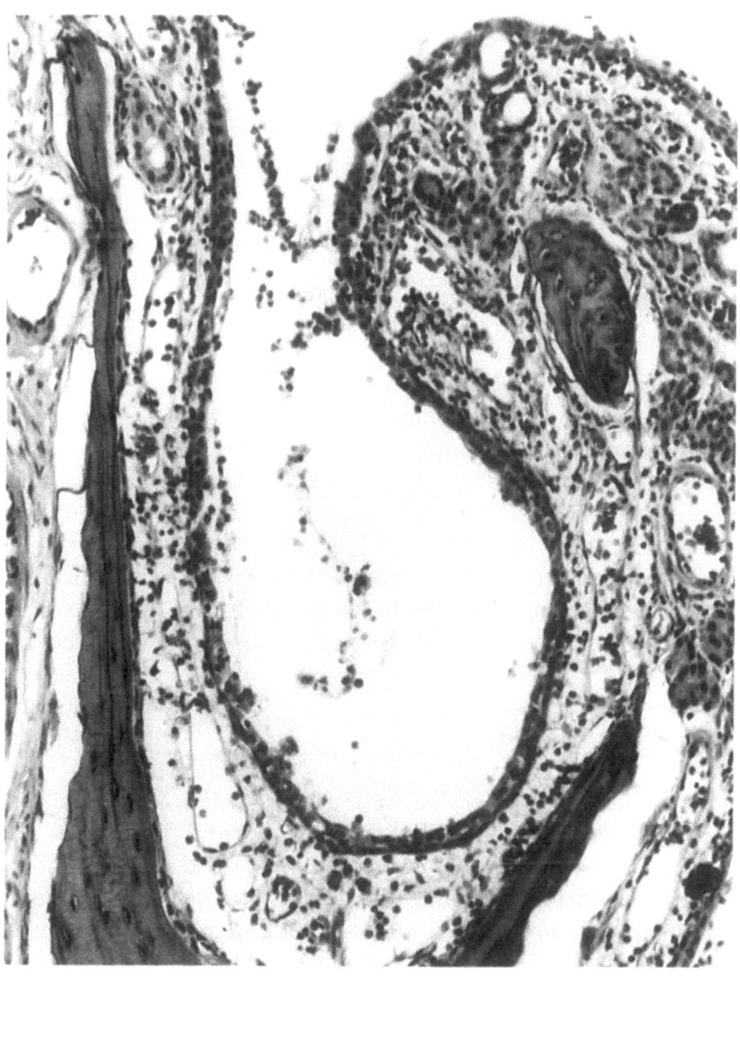

**Fig. 162.** Ventral turbinate and lateral wall of nasal cavity in rat experimentally infected with rat coronavirus. Note exudative inflammation of the mucosa with gaps in epithelial integrity. H&E, ×240

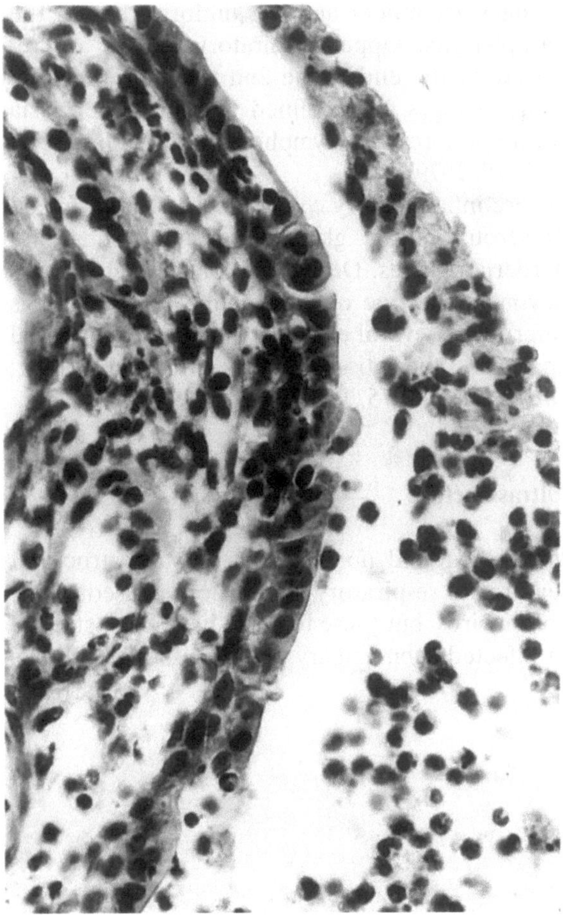

**Fig. 163.** Ventral turbinate of a rat experimentally infected with rat coronavirus. Much of the epithelium is necrotic and desquamated. Some leukocytes are present in the lumen. H&E, ×740

et al. 1969). Infected epithelial cells have focally dilated cisternae of endoplasmic reticulum and cytoplasmic vesicles which contain spherical dense or hollow cores 60–70 nm in diameter surrounded by an envelope 80–120 nm in diameter. The characteristic corona, seen in negatively stained preparations, is not observed by transmission ultramicroscopy.

## Differential Diagnosis

Upper respiratory tract lesions must be distinguished from those caused by Sendai virus, pneumonia virus, *Mycoplasma pulmonis*, and pathogenic bacteria. Pneumonic changes, which frequently accompany rhinitis caused by Parker's rat coronavirus, Sendai virus, and pneumonia virus, have not been reported in rat coronavirus infection. A careful histopathological examination of the exocrine tissues of the head is usually sufficient to enable one provisionally to diagnose rat coronavirus infection, but rhinotracheitis can precede changes in these tissues.

## Biological Features

*Natural History*. Rat coronavirus causes acute limited infections; there is no evidence for a carrier state. The virus is highly contagious and is transmitted by aerosol, direct contact, and fomites. There are two patterns of infection. Enzootic infections occur primarily in breeding colonies, where sucklings are passively immune, adults are actively immune, and weanlings are a continuous source of susceptible individuals due to waning passive immunity. It is therefore weanlings that generally exhibit clinical signs. Explosive epizootics occur in nonimmune colonies with the highest morbidity in weanlings. Signs are usually transient and consist of intermandibular and cervical edema, swelling of submaxillary glands, sneezing, and nasal and ocular discharges which are often red-tinged due to a high content of porphyrin, photophobia, and keratoconjunctivitis and its sequelae. Some complications of keratoconjunctivitis, such as glaucoma and phthisis, cause permanent disfigurement (Jacoby et al. 1979). Subclinical infections are common. Extensive host range studies have not been carried out but rat coronavirus can experimentally infect mice by the respiratory route (Bhatt et al. 1977).

*Pathogenesis*. Rat coronavirus is epitheliotropic with replication limited to the respiratory tract and certain exocrine tissues of the head and neck. It replicates at all levels of the respiratory tract but produces disease primarily in the upper respiratory tract, where the highest titers are achieved. Virus is excreted for 7 days, after which it is cleared, and neutralizing and complement-fixing antibodies appear in the serum (Jacoby et al. 1975, 1979).

*Etiology*. Rat coronavirus (Coronaviridae) is a pleomorphic, enveloped RNA virus with plump pedunculated surface projections (corona). It is approximately 114 nm in diameter. The virus replicates intracytoplasmically and virions are formed in cytoplasmic vesicles and endoplasmic reticulum (Jacoby et al. 1979). The virus is closely related antigenically to sialodacryoadenitis virus (Bhatt et al. 1972).

*Frequency*. Coronavirus infections are common in commercial and institutional rat colonies (Jacoby et al. 1979; Parker et al. 1970). Because of the close antigenic relationship of Parker's rat coronavirus to SDAV seroconversion to both viruses occurs in coronavirus-infected rats. It is therefore difficult to confirm coronavirus infection by serology alone (Bhatt et al. 1972; Jacoby et al. 1979).

## Comparison with Other Species

Coronaviruses are ubiquitous in humans, animals, and birds (Bohl 1981). Although coronaviruses cause respiratory infections in chickens, humans, and rats, SDAV (and to a limited degree Parker's rat coronavirus) is the only coronarvirus that replicates and produces disease in salivary, exorbital, and harderian glands.

## References

Bhatt PN, Percy DH, Jonas AM (1972) Characterization of the virus of sialodacryoadenitis of rats: a member of the coronavirus group. J Infect Dis 126:123–130

Bhatt PN, Jacoby RO, Jonas AM (1977) Respiratory infection in mice with sialodacryoadenitis virus, a coronavirus of rats. Infect Immun 18:823–827

Bohl EH (1981) Coronaviruses: diagnosis of infections. In: Kurstak E, Kurstak C (eds) Comparative diagnosis of viral diseases, vol 4. Academic, New York, chap 7

Innes JRM, Stanton MF (1961) Acute diseases of the submaxillary and harderian glands (sialodacryoadenitis) of rats with cytomegaly and no inclusion bodies. Am J Pathol 38:455–468

Jacoby RO, Bhatt PN, Jonas AM (1975) Pathogenesis of sialodacryoadenitis in gnotobiotic rats. Vet Pathol 12:196–209

Jacoby RO, Bhatt PN, Jonas AM (1979) Viral diseases. In: Baker HJ, Lindsey JR, Weisbroth SH (eds) The laboratory rat, vol 1. Academic, New York, chap 11

Jonas AM, Craft J, Black CL, Bhatt PN, Hilding D (1969) Sialodacryoadenitis in the rat. A light and electron microscopic study. Arch Pathol 88:613–622

Parker JC, Cross SS, Rowe WP (1970) Rat coronavirus (RCV): a prevalent, naturally occurring pneumotropic virus of rats. Arch Virusforsch 31:293–302

# The Lung (Bronchi, Bronchioles, Alveolar Ducts, Alveoli, Pleura)

# Structure and Function of the Lung

Charles G. Plopper

## Introduction

The respiratory system is one of the primary interfaces between the organism and the environment. As a result of air passage through the respiratory system it is the target for toxic gases, airborne particulates, and microbial infectious agents. Because the entire output of the right heart also passes through the vascular bed of the lung, it is also a target for bloodborne toxicants and pathogens. The respiratory system, especially the conducting airways and gas exchange area of the lungs, is organized in a highly polarized fashion. As a consequence most of the pathological responses within the lung tend to be highly focal and generally target one or more small subpopulations of the over 40 different cell types found in the lung. Further, the cellular composition and architectural organization of airway and gas exchange tissue have major impacts on the pathological responses within the system. Recent work has documented the great heterogeneity in cellular composition and architectural organization of the distal parts of the respiratory system in various mammalian species. This chapter deals with differences in cellular composition, architectural organization, and size differences as they are reflected in species commonly used in laboratory studies: mouse, hamster, rat, guinea pig, rabbit, and macaque monkey.

## Compartmental Organization of the Lungs

Most of the thoracic cavity is occupied by the right and left lungs. In laboratory mammals, the right lung is divided into four lobes (Table 6). This is true for all the commonly used species ranging from macaque monkeys to mice. Division of the left lung, however, is not uniform between species (Table 6). For some species, such as rabbits and macaques, the left lung is divided into two lobes, while in others, for example, the rat and mouse, it is a single lobe.

The air passages of the lungs are organized into intrapulmonary conducting airways and parenchyma as diagrammed in Fig. 164. The intrapulmonary airways (*bronchi and bronchioles*) compose between 6% and 10% of lung volume. The *parenchyma*, or gas exchange area, consisting of alveolar sacs and alveoli, comprises approximately 85% of lung volume. A *transitional zone* joins small distal bronchioles with the gas exchange tissue. The lung is encapsulated by a layer of connective tissue and mesothelial cells, the visceral pleura. Along with the pleura, the intrapulmonary nervous and vascular tissue (pulmonary arteries, pulmonary veins, and bronchiole arteries) comprise the remaining 9%–10% of the lung. In mammals commonly used for laboratory studies the functional units of gas exchange, acini or lobules, are not separated by intralobular septal bands of connective tissue as they are in humans and some larger mammals (horses and cattle).

**Table 6.** Comparison of lung lobation and teminology

| | Species |
|---|---|
| Left lung | |
| Undivided | Gerbil, hamster, rat, mouse |
| Divided | Macaque monkey, rabbit, guinea pig |
| Cranial | |
| Cranial part | |
| Caudal part | |
| Caudal | |
| Right lung | Macaque monkey, rabbit, guinea pig, gerbil, hamster, rat, mouse |
| Cranial | |
| Middle | |
| Caudal | |
| Accessory | |

See Tyler et al. (1991) for more details.

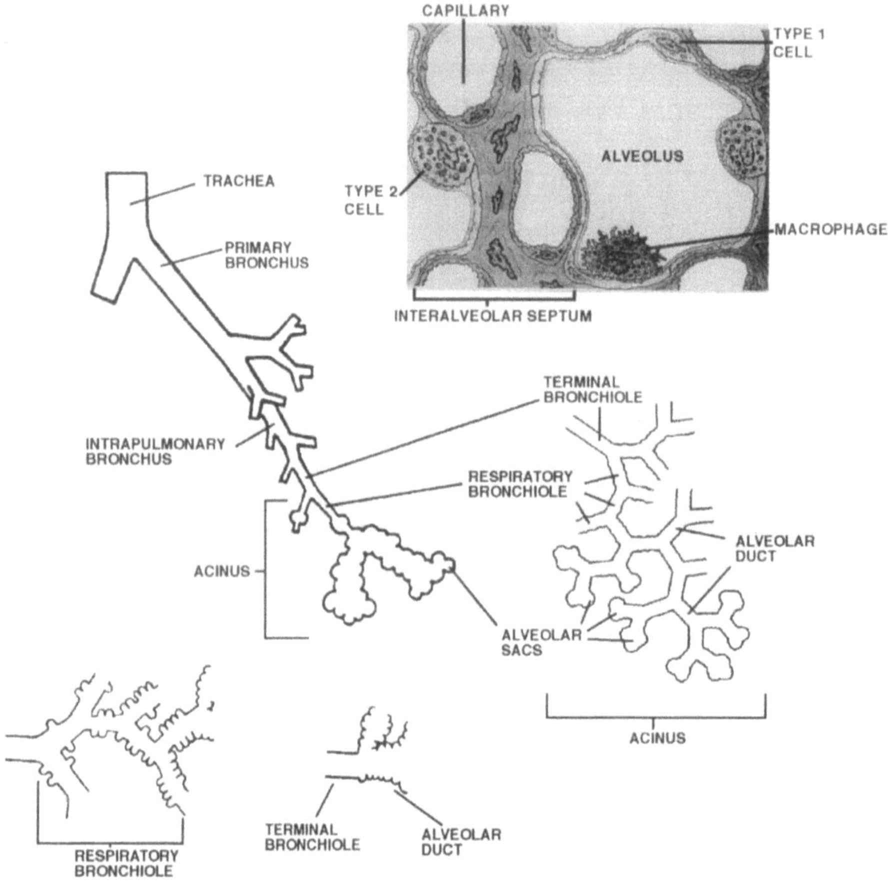


**Fig. 164.** Diagrammatic representation of the organization of the distal respiratory system. The intrapulmonary conducting airways (intrapulmonary bronchi, terminal bronchioles and respiratory bronchioles) join the gas exchange area at the central portion of the acinus. The transition zone may be abrupt, having a direct junction between the terminal bronchiole and the alveolar ducts, or much more gradual, being characterized by alveolarization in the walls of bronchioles forming respiratory bronchioles. The gas exchange area is organized into acini, which are composed of alveoli organized into alveolar ducts and alveolar sacs. The alveolar airspace is bounded by interalveolar septa composed of a capillary bed, alveolar type I and type II epithelial cells and interstitial connective tissue

## Bronchi

The bronchial tree for each half of the lung is formed by a primary bronchus and the various orders of airways that it supplies with air. The largest segments of the intrapulmonary conducting airways are the *lobar bronchi*, each of which is a branch of a primary bronchus and enters a lobe of the lung at its hilum (Fig. 164). Each of the lobar bronchi divides into two smaller branches, each of which divides again. These branches also divide, and this process continues until the gas exchange area is reached. For most laboratory mammals this system of division is called pseudodichotomous, because one daughter branch is larger in cross-sectional area than the other, and because each of these branches exits the parent branch at a different angle. The smaller of the two daughter branches exits at a greater angle from the parent. The number of times the bronchial tree branches before the gas exchange area is reached varies from species to species, from lobe to lobe in the same species, and by position within any particular lobe (McBride 1992). The number of generations of branching between the trachea and the parenchymal airspace can vary in the same lobe from as few as 6 for gas exchange areas closest to the hilum to as many as 28–30 for gas exchange areas located in the most distal portion of a lobe. Each of the first two or three generations of branching from a lobar bronchus supplies portions of the lung lobe identified as bronchopulmonary segments in some species. Each succeeding generation of branching is composed a greater number of airways and has a larger total cross-sectional area than the generation before it.

The organization of the wall of a bronchus is generally similar to that of the trachea except that the various layers are less abundant. In macaques, rabbits, and guinea pigs, the proximal bronchi are lined by a pseudostratified columnar epithelium (Fig. 165). The following seven epithelial cell types have been identified in the lining epithelium of the tracheobronchial airways: basal cells, goblet (or mucous) cells, ciliated cells, brush cells, serous cells, Clara cells, and neuroendocrine cells. *Basal cells* are oriented with long axes parallel to and in contact with the basal lamina. The cytoplasm, containing many filaments and few organelles, is usually small in relation to the size of the nucleus. This cell is thought to be the progenitor cell for the other epithelial cell types. *Goblet, ciliated, and brush cells* of the trachea are similar to those of the upper respiratory system. *Serous cells* have basal, lobated nuclei and apical microvilli; they contain abundant rough endoplasmic reticulum (rER) and apical electron-dense secretory granules. The structure of *Clara cells* is described under *Bronchioles*. *Neuroendocrine cells*, also known as amine precursor uptake decarboxylation cells, are typically pyramid shaped with their bases containing osmiophilic granules, abundant ER, Golgi complex, ribosomes, and many filaments. These cells are most abundant in young animals and are sometimes associated with nerve endings. Other *unidentifiable cells* represent a small proportion of the epithelial cell population and are characterized by a generalized cell structure with none of the individual specific characteristics of the seven cell types described. A variety of *migratory cells* are also observed in the epithelium. These include lymphocytes, globule leukocytes, and mast cells. *Globule leukocytes are* mononuclear cells containing acidophilic, metachromatic granules. Although their function is unknown in the respiratory system, similar cells occur in urinary and digestive epithelia. Interspecies variation is great in the composition of the tracheobronchial epithelium. Goblet cells are the predominant secretory cell type in domestic mammals and macaques, whereas Clara or serous cells are the major secretory cell of other species. Other variations between species include the relative abundance of brush cells, neurosecretory cells, and basal cells.

The composition of the epithelium changes by airway generation in a proximal to distal direction in a single species. A complete summary of species differences in tracheobronchial epithelium is included in Mariassy (1992). Figure 166 compares the relative abundance of the major epithelial cell types in the airways of rhesus monkeys and rabbits. Fewer total cells and proportionally fewer secretory cells line the proximal bronchi than line the trachea. In rabbits and rats, proximal bronchi have more epithelial cells and more basal cells per unit surface area than do more distal bronchi. In many species in which mucous cells are the predominant surface secretory cell type, the percentage of the population composed of mucous cells decreases and that for Clara cells increases in more distal airways. This is not true, however, for the macaque monkeys, where mucous goblet cells are found in abundance even in distal bronchioles. The epithelial height and the thickness of the lamina propria progressively decrease proximally to distally. The differences in the abundance of all epithelial cells and in ciliated, nonciliated, and basal cells lining the lobar bronchus between three laboratory species is compared in Fig. 167.

Submucosal glands are fewer and smaller in proximal bronchi than those in the trachea; in species in which glands are sparse or nonexistent in the distal trachea submucosal glands do not occur in intrapulmonary bronchi. In those species which have them they are tubuloacinar seromucous glands that remain connected to the surface by a series of ducts, some of which are lined by a ciliated epithelium. The primary cell types of the ducts include ciliated cells, mucus-secreting cells with granules in their apical portion and various intermediate cells. Most of the secretory portions of these glands are located within the submucosal region. The proximal portions are composed of tubules and are lined by mucus-secreting cells, and the distal portions are composed of acini and lined primarily by serous secretory cells. The differences in content of submucosal glands is summarized by St. George and Wang (1992). The mucus-secreting cells lining the tubules and acini generally secrete sulfated acid glycoproteins. In hamsters the secretory mucins are acidic but unsulfated, while in rats and mice they are mixed acidic and/or sulfated, and exclusively sulfated in rhesus monkeys and rabbits. In most species se-

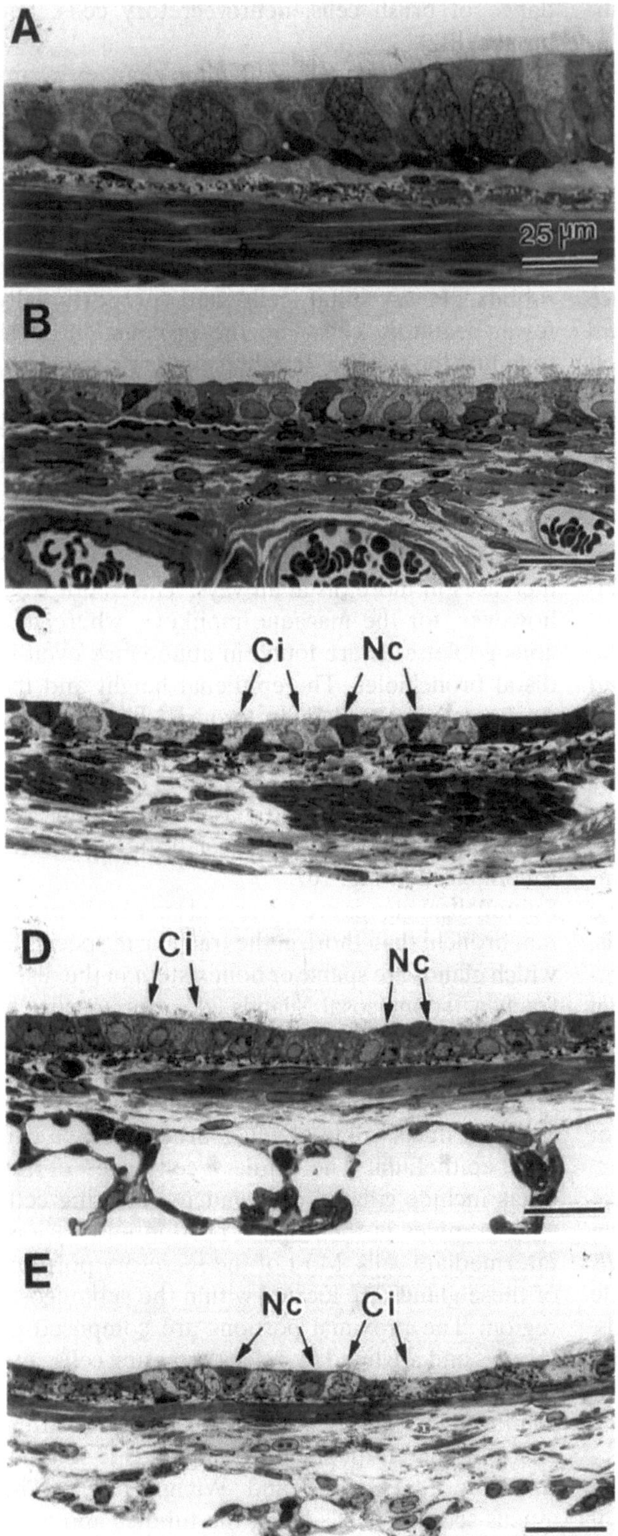


**Fig. 165.** Histological comparison of the organization of the wall of the lobar bronchus in five species; *A*, rhesus monkey; *B*, rabbit; *C*, rat; *D*, hamster; *E*, mouse. *Ci*, Ciliated cells; *Nc*, nonciliated (Clara) cells

Fig. 166. Graphic representation of the relative proportions of epithelial cell types throughout the airway tree in rabbit (A) and rhesus monkey (B). In the rabbit, the maximum number of generations of branching between the trachea (generation 0) and the terminal bronchiole (generation 22) is much greater than it is for the same pathway in the rhesus monkey, which includes down to the respiratory bronchiole (generation 14). In the rabbit the majority of the intrapulmonary airways are lined by two cell types, ciliated and nonciliated bronchiolar (or Clara) cells. In the rhesus monkey basal cells are found lining the walls of respiratory bronchioles. The other principal cell types are ciliated cells and mucous goblet cells

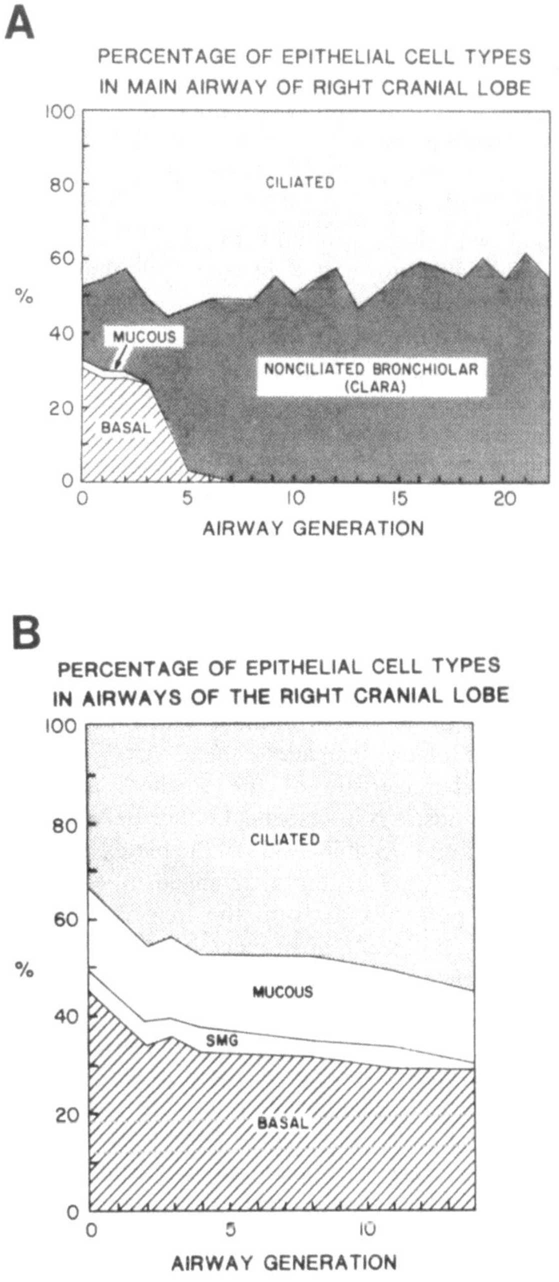


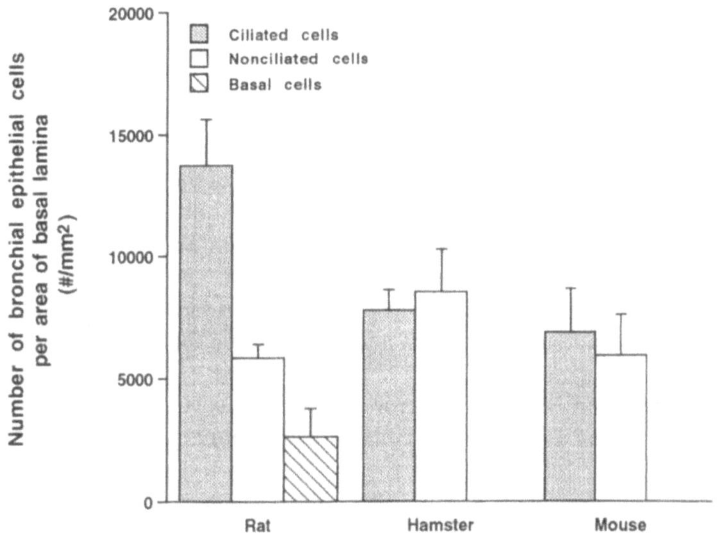


Fig. 167. A quantitative comparison of epithelial cell abundance in the lobar bronchus of three species: rat, hamster, and mouse. The absolute number of cells per unit surface area varies from species to species, as does the relative abundance of different cell types and the extent of basal cells in intrapulmonary airways

rous cells are the major secretory cells of the glands. Their secretory product is a neutral glycoprotein that is sometimes sulfated. The serous cells that produce this protein have small, dense, discrete granules and a cytoplasm filled with large amounts of rER. Acini and tubules are surrounded by myoepithelial cells. Nonmyelinated nerve fibers and nerve endings are generally adjacent to the secretory portions of submucosal glands. Migratory cells in the vicinity of the glands include lymphocytes, plasma cells, globular leukocytes, and mast cells. Submucosal glands are thought to provide most of the secretory material that lines the ciliary surface in the tracheobronchial airways. Intrapulmonary bronchi contain glands in macaques and rabbits, but glands are not found distal to the trachea in rats, mice, or hamsters.

Other components of the bronchial walls also vary by airway generation and species. The hyaline cartilage of the proximal bronchi is in the form of irregular plates, instead of the C- or U-shaped pieces characteristic of the trachea, and the smooth muscle is interspersed either between the plates or on the luminal side of the plates. Smooth muscle cells are generally arranged in a circular fashion perpendicularly to the long axis of the airway. The extent of bronchial cartilage within the tracheobronchial tree varies greatly from species to species. In the rabbit the amount of cartilage decreases in more distal bronchial generations and disappears at about airway generation number 7, whereas the relative abundance of smooth muscle increases to completely replace cartilage from generation number 7 distally. In the rhesus monkey cartilage plates are found even as far distally as respiratory bronchioles (Tyler and Plopper 1985). Cartilage has not been identified in the walls of intrapulmonary airways of rats, hamsters, or mice. The connective tissue external to bronchial cartilage in the adjoining adventitia is primarily loose, with many collagen fibers and variable numbers of elastic fibers. Many of the fibers are oriented longitudinally, whereas others are oriented perpendicularly to the long axis of the airway. Small groups of myelinated and nonmyelinated nerves and parasympathetic ganglia are in the adventitia and submucosa of the bronchi. Nerve endings have been identified within the surface epithelium and surrounding the glands.

Based primarily on the lack of submucosal cartilage and glands in the proximal intrapulmonary airways of rats, mice, and hamsters, it is not unreasonable to consider these airways as bronchioles instead of bronchi. The difficulty with this approach is that it masks the very real cellular and metabolic differences in the epithelial and interstitial compartments which exist between proximal and distal intrapulmonary airways in these species. All of which have been shown to have an impact on their pathobiology. When the position of a particular segment is defined, it becomes apparent that proximal airways vary from distal airways in the following ways: (a) composition of the epithelium (Plopper et al. 1992b; Plopper 1993); (b) antioxidant enzyme activity (Duan et al. 1993); (c) reduced glutathione content (Buckpitt et al. 1995); (d) ability to activate potentially toxic compounds via the cytochrome P450 mono-oxygenase system (Buckpitt et al. 1995); (e) pathological response to inhaled toxic fibers and gases (Plopper et al. 1994; Pinkerton et al. 1986); (f) pathological response to bioactivated toxic compounds (Plopper et al. 1992a,b); and (g) the ability to detoxify reactive cellular injurants (Buckpitt et al. 1995). Whether all the conducting airways within the lungs of these three species are considered bronchi or bronchioles seems of less importance than ensuring that evaluations of pathological responses in intrapulmonary airways account for the position within the airway tree of airway profiles under evaluation. This should help to ensure that all intrapulmonary airways in these three species are not considered equal, which they definitely are not.

## Bronchioles

The most distal intrapulmonary air passages have been termed bronchioles (Fig. 164). The bronchioles, whose cross-sectional profiles are roughly circular, may be distinguished from bronchi histologically. In general, walls of bronchioles are composed of epithelium, smooth muscle, and small amounts of connective tissue without glands or cartilage. Virtually all the intrapulmonary conducting airways in rats, hamsters, and mice meet this description. Bronchioles without alveoli opening directly through their walls are said to be nonalveolarized. Several generations of nonalveolarized bronchioles are present in most species; generally only one or two generations of nonalveolarized bronchioles are present in the lungs of macaque monkeys. The most distal branches of the conducting airway which are free of alveoli are termed the terminal bronchioles. Its lining epithelium is a simple columnar or cuboidal epithelium composed of ciliated cells and Clara cells (Fig. 168). The abundance of each cell type varies by species (Table 7; Fig. 169). The *Clara cells* (bronchiolar exocrine cells) have characteristics of both secretory cells and cells capable of metabolizing xenobiotic compounds. The secretory granules are discrete membrane-bounded, electron-dense structures that contain either neutral glycoprotein or low molecular weight proteins.

The identity and functions of these proteins is still being characterized (Singh and Katyal 1992). The most characteristic protein is a uteroglobinlike protein of around 10-kDa apparent molecular weight, which appears to have inhibitory properties for a number of inflammatory events. Also identified in Clara cells is a leucoprotease inhibitor and some of the surfactant-associated proteins including surfactant-associated proteins A and C. Species variability in expression of Clara cell proteins is not completely understood, but it is apparently not uniform. Metabolism of xenobiotic compounds in Clara cells via the cytochrome P-450 (CYP) and flavin-containing (FMO) mono-

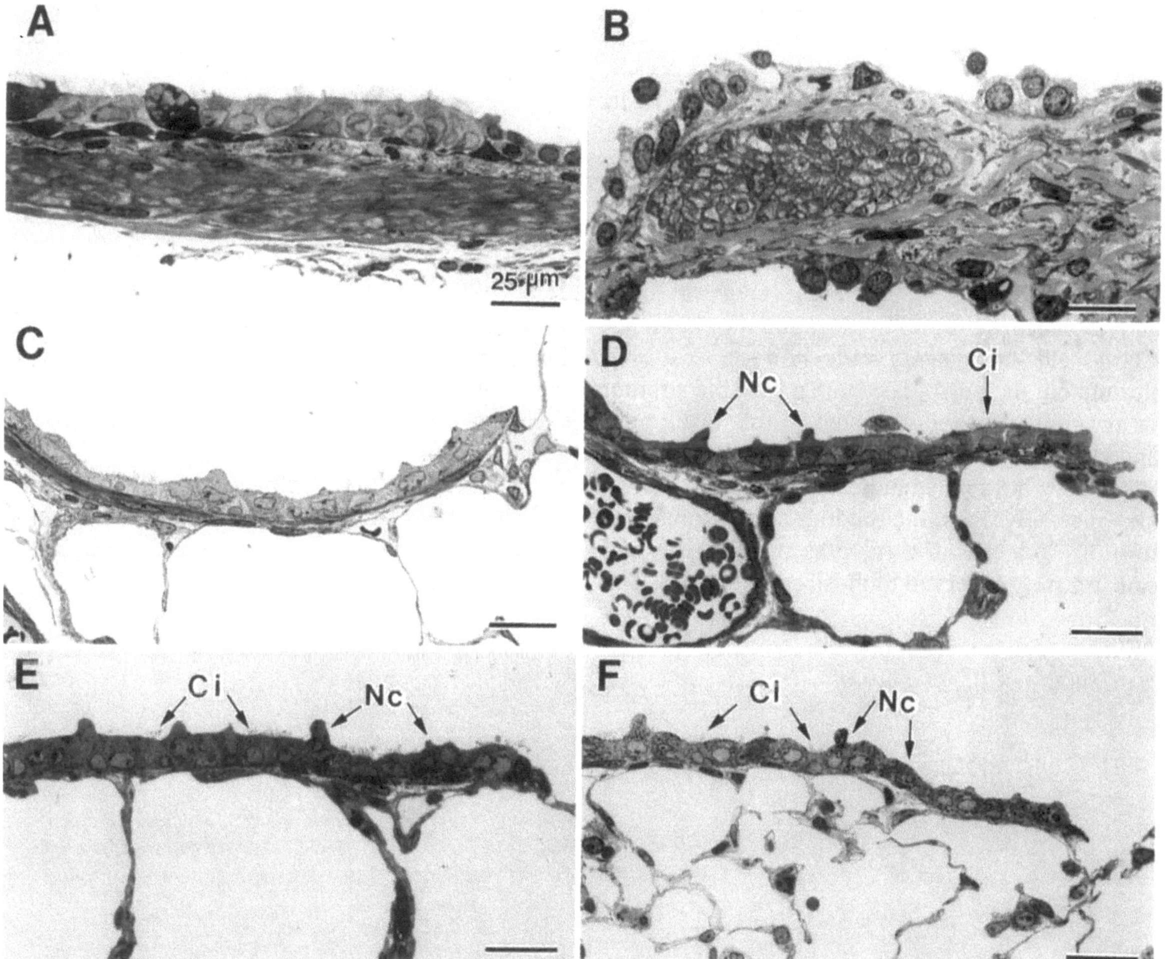


**Fig. 168.** Histological comparison of the wall of the terminal bronchiole in five species: *A*, *B*, rhesus monkey; *C*, rabbit; *D*, rat; *E*, hamster; *F*, mouse. Terminal bronchiolar epithelium contains ciliated and nonciliated cells in rabbit, rat, hamster, and mouse. In the rhesus monkey the terminal bronchiole and the blood vessel side of the respiratory bronchiole are lined by a pseudostratified epithelium in which basal cells, ciliated cells, and mucous goblet cells are the primary cell types. The respiratory bronchiole (*B*) in the rhesus monkey contains a mixture of epithelium characteristic of alveolar gas exchange areas and simple cuboidal epithelium which forms a border between the gas exchange areas and the pseudostratified epithelium. *Ci*, Ciliated cells; *Nc*, nonciliated

**Table 7.** Comparison of nonciliated bronchiolar epithelial (Clara) cell distribution and organization of the transitional zone

| Species | Transitional or respiratory bronchiole | | Nonciliated bronchiolar cells in lobar bronchi |
|---|---|---|---|
| | Extensive | Minimal | |
| Mouse | | + | >60% |
| Hamster | | + | >15% |
| Rat | | + | 0 |
| Guinea pig | | + | 0 |
| Rabbit | | + | >25% |
| Macaque monkey | + | | 0 |

oxygenases is species specific (Devereux et al. 1989). Clara cells of most laboratory species express P-450 isozymes CYP2B and CYP4B, which are phenobarbital inducible in the liver. The benzopyrene-metabolizing forms, such as CYP1A1, have been identified in, or are inducible in, Clara cells of rabbits and rats, but are absent in mice. Flavin mono-oxygenases have been found in rabbits, but not thoroughly evaluated in other species (Overby et al. 1992). Little CYP or FMO activity has been found in macaque monkeys.

Clara cells have many mitochondria scattered throughout their cytoplasm and a variable amount of agranular ER and glycogen (Table 8; Plopper and Hyde 1992). Agranular ER is abundant within Clara cells in rabbits, guinea pigs, rats, hamsters, and mice. Glycogen, the predominant cellular feature of Clara cells in carnivores such as dogs and cats, is rarely observed in most other species. The predominant organellular feature of nonciliated bronchiolar cells in macaques is rER. The presence of cytoplasmic extensions on the lateral surfaces of bronchiolar epithelium suggests a role in regulation of fluid balance in distal airways. The Clara cell is the predominant nonciliated cell in all generations of intrapulmonary airways in laboratory mammals (Table 7). The exception is the macaque, in which only the epithelium of the most distal (alveolarized) bronchioles contain Clara cells, with few ciliated cells present.

The thickness of the lamina propria and submucosa of bronchioles is less than that of the lamina propria and submucosa of bronchi (Sannes 1992). Smooth muscle is in separate fascicles that branch and anastomose such that the fibers course both circularly and obliquely. The surrounding connective tissue includes collagen fibers oriented in all directions and elastic fibers oriented circularly or obliquely. Numerous nerve fibers occur in the area immediately below the epithelium and interspersed between muscle fascicles.

## Transition Zone

*The transition zone*, the area where small air passages of the tracheobronchial tree join the gas exchange area, is the focus of many lung disorders. This transition occurs by the formation of outpocketings of gas exchange tissue in the walls of bronchioles. Bronchioles that are alveolarized are termed *respiratory bronchioles*. Their histological appearance is similar to that of terminal

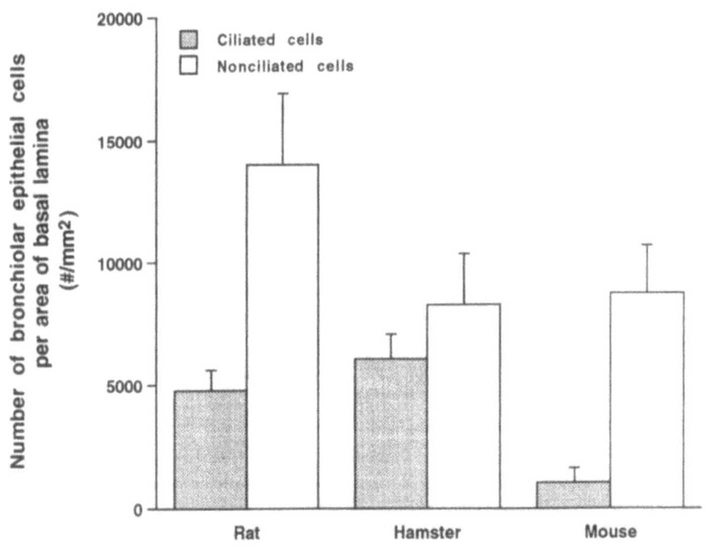


**Fig. 169.** A quantitative comparison of epithelial abundance in the terminal bronchioles of rat, hamster, and mouse. The absolute number, as well as the relative proportions of the two dominant cell types, ciliated and nonciliated (or Clara) bronchiolar epithelial cells, vary among species

**Table 8.** Comparison of relative proportions (percentages) of cellular components in Clara cells (percentage of cytoplasmic volume; from Plopper and Hyde 1992)

| Species | Nucleus | Agranular endoplasmic reticulum | Secretory granules | Cytoplasmic glycogen | Mitochondria | Large mitochondria | Lateral cytoplasmic extension |
|---|---|---|---|---|---|---|---|
| Mouse | 21.8 ± 6.5 | 54.8 ± 7.5 | + | 0 | 34.7 ± 6.4 | + | + |
| Hamster | 25.2 ± 6.1 | 79.3 ± 7.6 | + | 0 | 10.7 ± 4.4 | − | + |
| Rat | 28.5 ± 10.4 | 66.2 ± 9.4 | + | 0.1 ± 0.4 | 16.3 ± 6.0 | + | + |
| Guinea pig | 28.6 ± 8.9 | 58.3 ± 9.0 | + | 0 | 25.1 ± 8.5 | + | + |
| Rabbit | 23.8 ± 8.8 | 61.6 ± 5.4 | + | 7.0 ± 5.4 | 19.1 ± 7.6 | + | + |
| Macaque monkey | 28.6 ± 4.4 | 5.2 ± 3.3 | + | 0 | 14.1 ± 2.8 | − | + |

+, Present; −, not present.

bronchioles, with the exception that the epithelium is interrupted by alveoli (Fig. 164). The smooth muscle is arranged in fascicles that underlie the simple cuboidal or columnar epithelium. The alveoli open between these muscle bundles.

The organization of the transitional zone is highly variable among species, with two extremes being present. In one condition the transition is abrupt (Fig. 170) with a short or absent respiratory bronchiole, such as occurs in laboratory rodents as well as rabbit and guinea pig (Table 7). The other condition is characterized by extensive alveolarization of the distal bronchioles (Fig. 171), with alveolar outpocketings per generation of branching generally fewer in number proximally and greater in number distally. This organization is typical of macaque monkeys. In this species three populations of epithelial cells occupy respiratory bronchioles: pseudostratified columnar with mucous goblet cells, nonciliated cuboidal and alveolar with type I and type II cells (Fig. 168).

## Respiratory Area

The respiratory area, or *parenchyma*, consists of alveolar ducts, alveolar sacs, alveoli, and the airspaces contained within these structures (Fig. 164). A detailed comparison of the differences in parenchymal organization is included in Mercer and Crapo (1992) and Pinkerton et al. (1992). In the inflated lung of laboratory species the pa-

A 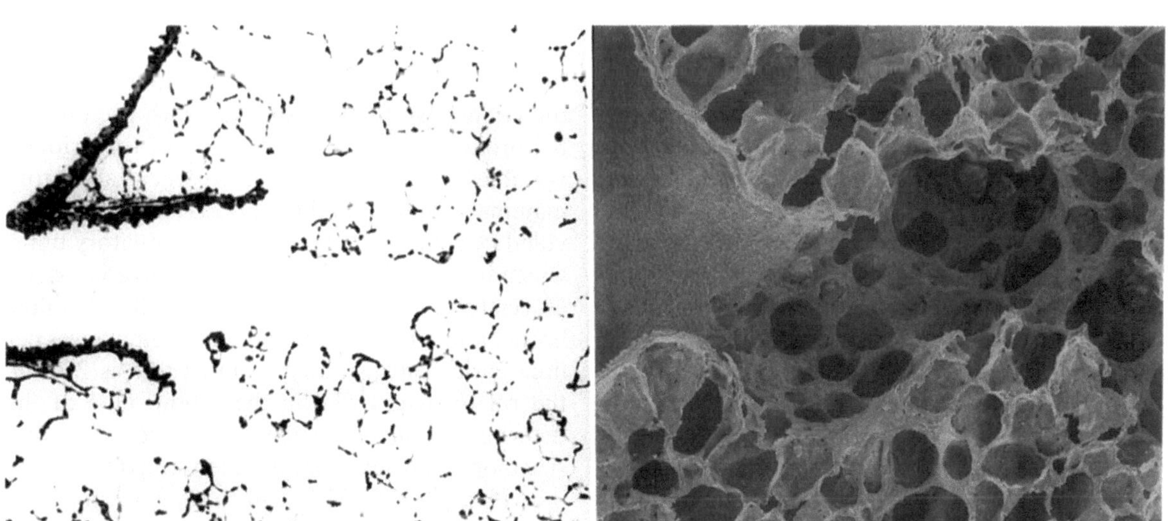 B

**Fig. 170A,B.** Comparison of the transition zone in species with short or undetectable respiratory bronchioles. **A** Light microscope. **B** Scanning electron microscope

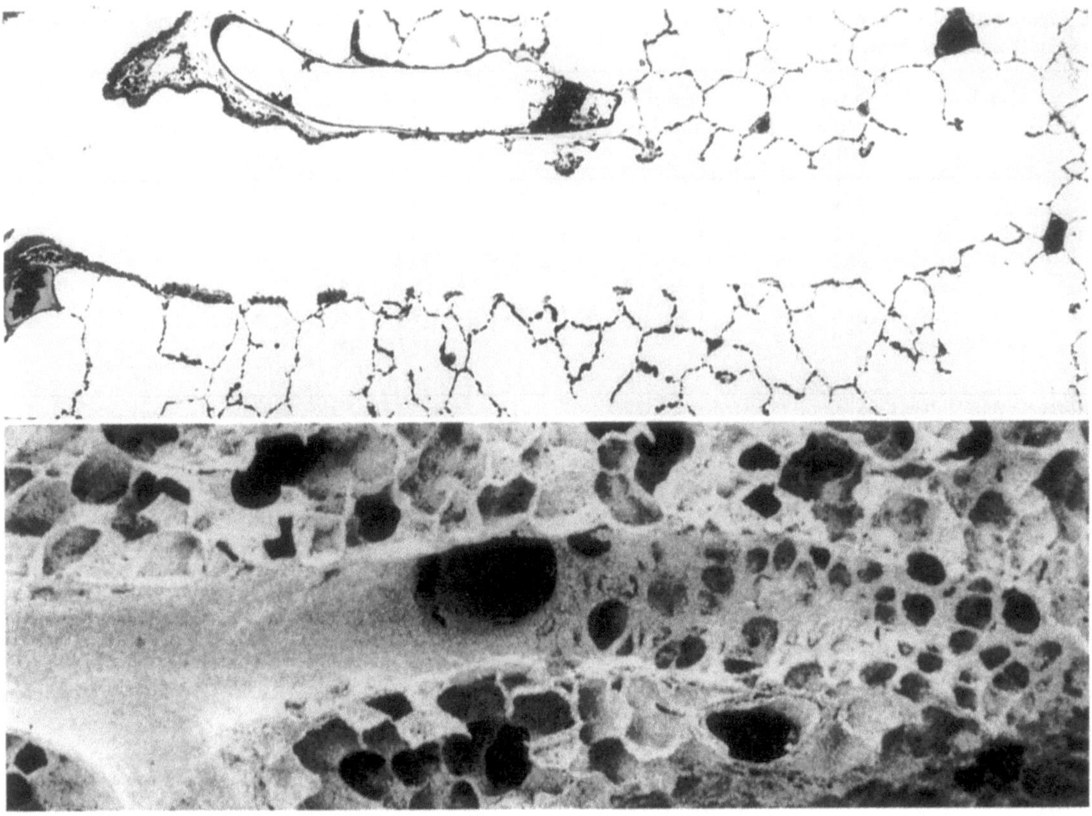

**Fig. 171A,B.** Comparison of the transition zone in species with extensive respiratory bronchioles. **A** Light microscope. **B** Scanning electron microscope

renchyma, which is between 80% and 90% of lung volume, consists of around 70% airspace and 30% gas exchange tissue which surrounds the airspace. This tissue includes epithelium, some connective tissue, arterioles and venules, and the pulmonary capillary bed (Fig. 164). The gas exchange membrane, or *blood-air barrier* (Fig. 164) has a large surface with capillary bed on one side and air on the other. The surface area on the air side of this membrane ranges from less than $0.07\,m^2$ in the mouse (average body weight: 0.023kg) to $13.3\,m^2$ in the macaque monkey (average body weight: 3.7kg; Fig. 172). The surface area of the capillary side of this membrane is only slightly less than that of the air side. This large surface, which is manyfold the surface area of the skin, is packed into a small total lung volume (0.8ml in the mouse, 180ml in the macaque; Fig. 172). All of these characteristics, as well as capillary blood volume (Fig. 172), have a close allometric relationship to body mass when body mass is plotted logarithmically (Pinkerton et al. 1992).

The air passages of the parenchymal tissue are organized into functional units, the *acini or terminal respiratory units* (Fig. 164). The acini are generally defined as all the airspaces distal to one terminal bronchiole, which includes all the respiratory bronchioles branching from one terminal bronchiole and all alveolar ducts, alveolar sacs, and alveoli joined to these respiratory bronchioles. Unoxygenated blood is supplied to this unit by a *pulmonary arteriole* which courses in the connective tissue associated with each terminal bronchiole. Acinar size is one of the primary variables in the parenchyma between laboratory mammals (Mercer and Crapo 1992). Acini are divided by some investigators into ventilatory units, which include all of the alveoli and alveolar ducts associated with one branch off the terminal bronchiole. The total number of terminal units per lung varies substantially, from as few as 2500 in the rat to over 18000 in the rabbit. One of the determining factors which appears to affect unit size more than any other feature is the diameter of individual alveoli. Although these have not been evaluated for all laboratory species, there appears to be a close correlation between alveolar diameter (approximately 50 μm in the mouse, 100 μm in

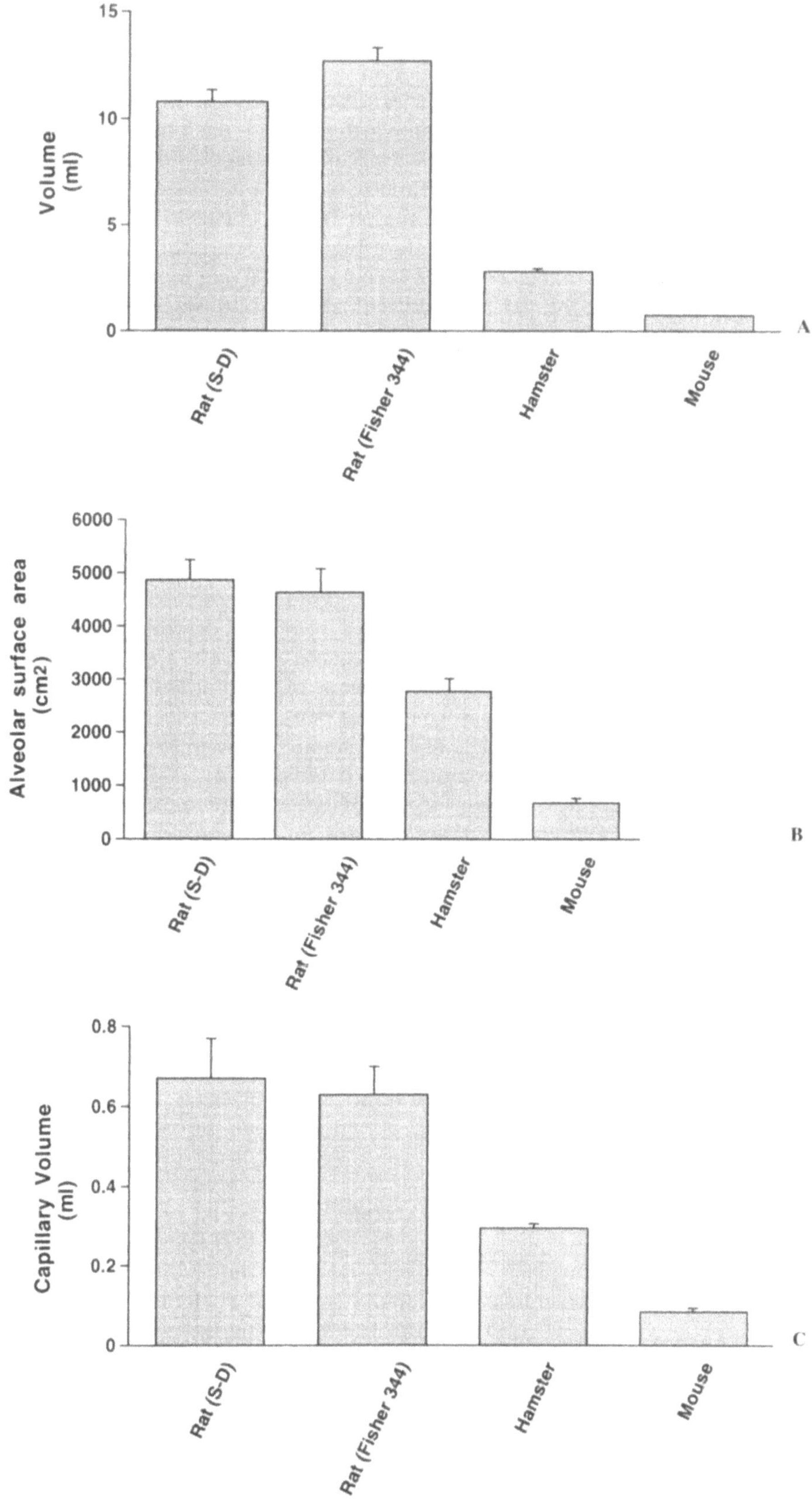


**Fig. 172.** Comparison of the differences in absolute values for total lung volume (**A**), pulmonary alveolar surface area (**B**), and capillary blood volume (**C**) in the three species: rat, hamster, and mouse. (From Gehr 1981)

the rat, and almost 200 μm in the macaque) and overall ventilatory unit diameter (mouse: 1 mm; rat: 1.5 mm; monkey: 2.5 mm). Variation in size of ventilatory units within the same species has only been characterized in the rat. The findings to date indicate that there is considerable variability within a single species, varying by as much as 15-fold between ventilatory units receiving air from the same bronchus. An even more interesting aspect of this finding is that alveolar size is comparable between alveoli located in large ventilatory units and those located in small units. This is also true for the alveolar surface to volume ratio. One of the major functional effects of variation in ventilatory unit size when combined with the dead space associated with the more proximal airways is the tremendous variation in the fraction of new inspired air which is received in each ventilatory unit. A primary result is that units located a fewer number of generations of branching from the trachea receive a larger percentage of new inspired gas than a ventilatory unit which is separated from the trachea by a much larger number of generations of branching. Obviously, ventilatory units of larger size also receive more gas which then penetrates further into the unit. The primary impact of these changes on the pathobiology of parenchyma is to produce a wide range of variability in the inflammatory and cellular injury patterns for toxicants and pathogens whose targets are the central portion of the pulmonary acinus. An additional factor which may affect pathology in the lung parenchyma from bloodborne pathogens and toxicants is the transient time for unoxygenated gas through a ventilatory unit. It appears that larger units have longer transient times, in other words, the distance between arterioles and venules within an acinus is greater in larger units than in smaller units.

## Alveolar Ducts, Alveolar Sacs, and Alveoli

Most of the parenchyma is organized as either tubular or saclike structures. The tubular structures, or *alveolar ducts*, are comparable to hallways lined by rooms on all sides (Figs. 170, 171). Each of these rooms is a single pocket or alveolus. From 6 to 12 generations of alveolar ducts are supplied by a single terminal or respiratory bronchiole. The variation in number is greatest between acini of a single species and not between acini in different species. The walls of an alveolar duct are composed of the open sides of alveolar spaces and the terminations of the interalveolar septa that separate these alveoli. Spiraling bands of smooth muscle and elastic fibers, perpendicular to the long axis of the alveolar ducts, occupy space deep to the epithelium at the terminations of the interalveolar septa. The alveolar ducts terminate in clusters of alveoli, the *alveolar sacs*.

The interalveolar septa, the sheets of connective tissue containing a capillary plexus and covered on both sides by a layer of epithelium, separate individual alveolar airspaces (Fig. 173A,B). Differences in the cellular composition of the septa are summarized by Pinkerton et al. (1992). Two epithelial cell types line the interalveolar septa, forming the air side of the blood-air barrier. The *squamous, or type I, alveolar epithelial cell* is a squamated cell with a centrally placed nucleus (Fig. 173A), and has a large cytoplasmic volume with few organelles. Mitochondria, minimal amounts of rER, and a moderate number of endocytotic vesicles are present. This cell type covers approximately 96% of the interalveolar septal surface in all the species studied thus far, yet forms only 45% of the cells lining the alveolus. The average surface area of a type I cell ranges from 5000 to 7000 μm$^2$. The tissue side of this vast sheet of cells is lined by a continuous basal lamina (Sannes 1992).

The second type of epithelial cell (Fig. 173B) is the *granular, or type II, alveolar epithelial cell.* It is a cuboidal cell with a central nucleus. This cell type covers the remainder of the interalveolar septal surface area (approximately 3%). The alveolar type II cell constitutes approximately 12% of the cells composing the interalveolar septum. Its average cell surface ranges from 100 to 280 μm$^2$ per cell. This cell is filled with many organelles, including mitochondria (5%–9% of cell volume), rER, microvesicles, and a Golgi complex. The alveolar surface bears microvilli. Its characteristic feature is the presence of many osmiophilic, laminated vesicles called lamellar bodies (12% of cell volume in the rat and 21% in the rabbit). The lamellar bodies are thought to contain primarily phospholipid and to be the source of the phospholipids that compose the *pulmonary surfactant* that lines the airspaces. The type II alveolar cell is now recognized to be the source of a variety of other surfactant related materials (Singh and Katyal 1992). The most important of these are the surfactant associated proteins whose cellular distribution appears to be relatively spe-

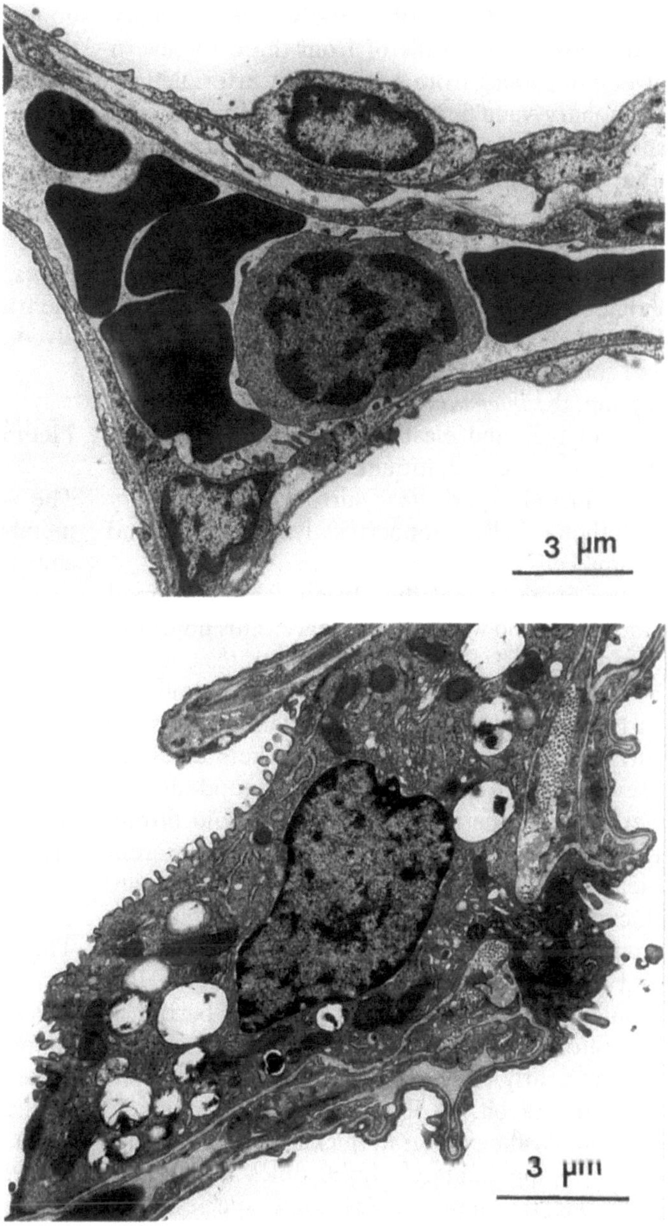


A

B

**Fig. 173A,B.** Cellular organization of the interalveolar septum in the rat. **A** The blood-air barrier is composed of the squamous epithelial cells lining the airspace and the capillary epithelial cells within the interalveolar septum. TEM, ×5000. **B** The histological characteristics of the alveolar type II cell are relatively similar among species. TEM, ×5500

cies specific both in terms of molecular weight and cellular distribution. At present four associated proteins have been identified (A, B, C, D). Another major secretory protein of type II cells is lysozyme, a naturally occurring antibacterial agent. Lysozyme is present in the rat, but may not be present in humans. Alveolar type II cells have also been shown to be the source of several complement proteins in humans and rats. The type II alveolar cell is thought to function as the progenitor cell for both type I and type II cells (Singh and Katyal 1992).

The capillary bed of the interalveolar septa is an intermeshed network of short, branching vessels. Alveolar capillary blood volume in mammals ranges from 0.08 ml in the mouse to 15.5 ml in the macaque monkey (Fig. 172C; Pinkerton et al. 1992). Capillary *endothelial cells* resemble endothelial cells in other organs (Fig. 173A). They are characterized by few organelles and relatively large amounts of endocytotic vesicles. The average surface area of an endothelial cell is approximately 1000 $\mu m^2$. Endothelial cells are attached to a continuous basal lamina. The intercellular junctions tend to be loose or leaky; the tight junctions have few parallel arrays of contact. The surface area of the gas exchange capillary bed is between 66% and 75% of the surface area of the air side of the interalveolar septa. Individual capillary beds traverse the walls of from three to severn alveoli in passing from a pulmonary arteriole to a pulmonary venule. Most of the endothelial cells surrounding the capillaries have one side with a thin extension of cytoplasm which faces the epithelial cells lining the air portion of the blood-air barrier (Fig. 173A,B). The endothelium of the opposite side of the capillary is separated from the lining epithelial cells by a band of elastic and collagen fibers. The space between alveolar epithelial and endothelial cells within the interalveolar septum, the *interstitium*, contains a variety of cells and collagen and elastic fibers. The majority of the cells in the interstitium are fibroblasts. Other cells include pericytes surrounding capillary endothelial cells, monocytes, lymphocytes, and plasma cells.

In the living animal the alveoli contain a small amount of fluid within the airspace. This fluid consists of a biphasic layer of plasma filtrates overlaid by a thin layer of phospholipids called pulmonary surfactant. The pulmonary surfactant reduces the surface tension in these small pockets of air to prevent them from collapsing. The blood-air barrier prevents the massive release of fluid filtrate from capillaries into the airspace. Two different measurements are currently used to evaluate thickness of the barrier. Harmonic mean thickness emphasizes the thinnest portions of the barrier and estimates potential for gas diffusion. Harmonic mean thickness of the blood-air barrier in laboratory mammals can vary among various species by nearly twofold: mouse, 0.32 μm; hamster, 0.42 μm; rabbit, 0.50 μm; macaque monkey, 0.50 μm. Arithmetic mean thickness of the barrier averages approximately three times larger than harmonic thickness for the same species. This measurement averages all the thick as well as thin segments equally. It is not useful for estimating gas diffusing capacity but is very effective in detecting subtle changes in the cellular and acellular compartments of the interalveolar septa, such as: alveolar type H cell hyperplasia, capillary endothelial cell necrosis or loss, and interstitial fibrosis or edema. At its thinnest the blood-air barrier consists of the surface-lining layer of pulmonary surfactant and fluid, the thin cytoplasm of an alveolar type I cell, fused basal laminae of the alveolar epithelial cell and the underlying capillary endothelial cell, the capillary endothelial cell, and the plasmalemma of a red blood cell (Fig. 173A). At the thickest this barrier consists of the above-mentioned layers and interstitial connective tissue and cells between the basal laminae of epithelial and endothelial cells. Openings in the interalveolar septa interconnect adjacent alveoli. These openings, *alveolar pores*, are lined by epithelial cells and permit air and alveolar macrophages to pass from one alveolus to another. All the laboratory species have alveolar pores, but the impact that their presence has on the transfer of pathogens and toxic gases between alveoli and acini is not understood.

## Pleura

The *visceral, or pulmonary pleura*, is the serous membrane that completely covers both lungs except at the hilum and pulmonary ligament, consists of squamous to cuboidal mesothelial cells overlaying varying amounts of elastic fibers and dense irregular connective tissue. Pleural mesothelial cells contain large amounts of rER and mitochondria; their free surfaces are covered by microvilli. At its thickest in humans and large domestic mammals the connective-tissue elements of the pleura consist of two or more layers of elastic laminae, many dense irregular bundles of collagen fibers, pulmonary capillaries, and two additional sets of vessels (Tyler and Julian 1992). These two sets of vessels include capillaries and small arterioles from the bronchial circulatory system and lymph vessels. The pulmonary capillaries supply the superficial portion of the gas exchange area. The connective tissue of the pulmonary pleura is continuous with that of the interalveolar septa. The thickness of the pulmonary pleura varies from species to species and within different regions of the same species. The pleura is thinnest in laboratory mammals. In these species the subpleural connective tissue is minimal, and the only blood supply derives from the pulmonary artery via pulmonary capillaries also involved in gas exchange with subpleural alveoli.

## Pulmonary Circulatory System

Blood is supplied to the lungs through two different circulatory systems, *pulmonary* and *bronchial* (Kay 1992). Most of the blood flow to the lungs moves through the pulmonary arteries which carry the entire output of the right ventricle as unoxygenated blood. Variation in the pulmonary vascular system is summarized by Kay (1992). The pulmonary circulatory system is a low-pressure system, with the walls of the large, medium, and small arteries being considerably thinner than walls of vessels of comparable volume in the systemic circulatory system. Pulmonary arteries have fewer elastic and collagen fibers and fewer smooth muscle cells. There are interspecies variations in the organization of the pulmonary arterial wall. In guinea pigs the wall averages 4.3% of vessel diameter, the elastin is arranged as fragmented, discontinuous lamellae, and the smooth muscle is in discontinuous segments. In the rat the wall averages 2.6%–26% of the diameter (20–350 μm), the elastin is in long parallel lamellae, and the smooth muscle is arranged in oblique sheets. The amount of pulmonary artery smooth muscle found in each species in the steady state has a major impact on that species hypertensive response to chronic hypoxia. The pulmonary arterial circulatory system shares its connective tissue adventitia with that of the tracheobronchial tree. The integrity of this connection varies considerably by species. In the mouse the artery is closely applied throughout the airway tree and is nearly impossible to separate from it. In the rabbit and macaque monkey the arterial supply separates easily from the tree.

The bronchial arteries are under high pressure, as a part of the systemic arterial circulatory system. The blood vessels in this system have the same wall structure as that of other systemic arteries of the same size. It is a low-flow system, with less than 1% of the left ventricular output. In all laboratory species the bronchial artery supplies blood to the walls of the large bronchi, the major pulmonary vessels, and the pulmonary lymph nodes. Except in the rat and mouse the bronchial artery also supplies blood to the walls of bronchioles as far distal as the terminal bronchioles. In species with a thick pleura (human, horse, cattle, sheep, and pig) the bronchial artery also supplies blood to the pleural connective tissue and interlobular septa. In humans the bronchial artery also supplies capillaries in the interalveolar septa. Anastomoses between bronchial and pulmonary arterial circulatory systems have been identified in the walls of medium-sized bronchi and bronchioles of the rabbit, rat, and guinea pig but not macaque monkeys. All blood from the lungs is carried back to the heart by the *pulmonary veins*, a low-pressure system. The tunica interna is composed of endothelium and an internal elastic membrane. In most species the tunica media is composed of irregularly arranged smooth muscle and elastic and collagen fibers. The demarcation between the media and the externa is not clear. However, in mouse and rat the pulmonary veins contain a thick medial coat of cardiac muscle which continues into the atrium. In larger veins it is arranged into two layers: outer longitudinal and inner circular. In most species the pulmonary vein is located at the periphery of lobules and courses to the hilum in parenchymal gas exchange tissue or interlobular septa. In the mouse and rat the pulmonary veins accompany the bronchial tree on the side opposite the pulmonary arteries. The pulmonary veins have thin fibrous walls with little smooth muscle in all the laboratory species.

*Acknowledgements.* Portions of work reported here were supported by NIEHS grants ES00628, ES04311, and ES06700. The author appreciates the assistance of Susan Nishio and Alison Weir in preparing the figures and Pam Wallace in preparing the manuscript.

## References

Buckpitt A, Chang A, Weir A, Van Winkle L, Duan X, Philpot R, Plopper GC (1995) Relationship of cytochrome P450 activity to Clara cell cytotoxicity. IV. Metabolism of naphthalene and naphthalone oxide in microdissected airways from the mouse, rat, and hamster. Mol Pharmacol 47:74–81

Devereux TR, Domin BA, Philpot RM (1989) Xenobiotic metabolism by isolated pulmonary cells. Pharmacol Ther 41:243–256

Duan X, Buckpitt AR, Plopper CG (1993) Variation in antioxidant enzyme activities in anatomic subcompartments within rat and rhesus monkey lung. Toxicol Appl Pharmacol 123:73–82

Kay JM (1992) Blood vessels of the lung. In: Parent RA (ed) Comparative biology of the normal lung. CRC, Boca Raton, pp 163–171

Mariassy AT (1992) Epithelial cells of trachea and bronchi. In: Parent RA (ed) Comparative biology of the normal lung. CRC, Boca Raton, pp 63–76

Mcbride JT (1992) Architecture of the tracheobronchial tree. In: Parent RA (ed) Comparative biology of the normal lung. CRC, Boca Raton, pp 49–61

Mercer RR, Crapo JD (1992) Architecture of the acinus. In: Parent RA (ed) Comparative biology of the normal lung. CRC, Boca Raton, pp 109–119

Overby L, Nishio S, Lawton M, Plopper CG, Philpot R (1992) Cellular localization of flavin-containing monooxygenase in rabbit lung. Exp Lung Res 18:131–144

Pinkerton KE, Plopper CG, Mercer RR, Roggli VL, Patra AL, Brody AR, Crapo JD (1986) Airway branching patterns influence asbestos fiber location and the extent of tissue injury in the pulmonary parenchyma. Lab Invest 55:688–695

Pinkerton KE, Gehr P, Crapo JD (1992) Architecture and cellular composition of the air-blood barrier. In: Parent RA (ed) Comparative biology of the normal lung. CRC, Boca Raton, pp 121–128

Plopper CG (1993) Pulmonary bronchiolar epithelial cytotoxicity: Microanatomical considerations. In: Gram TE (ed) Metabolic activation and toxicity of chemical agents to lung tissue and cells. Pergamon, New York, pp 1–24

Plopper CG, Hyde DM (1992) Epithelial cells of bronchioles. In: Parent RA (ed) Comparative biology of the normal lung. CRC, Boca Raton, pp 85–92

Plopper CG, Suverkropp C, Morin D, Nishio S, Buckpitt A (1992a) Relationship of cytochrome P-450 activity to Clara cell cytotoxicity. I. Histopathologic comparison of the respiratory tract of mice, rats and hamsters after parenteral administration of naphthalene. J Pharmacol Exp Ther 261:353–363

Plopper CG, Macklin J, Nishio SJ, Hyde DM, Buckpitt AR (1992b) Relationship of cytochrome P450 activity to Clara cell cytotoxicity. III. Morphometric comparison of changes in the epithelial populations of terminal bronchioles and lobar bronchi in mice, hamsters, and rats after parenteral administration of naphthalene. Lab Invest 6:553–565

Plopper CG, Chu FP, Haselton CJ, Peake J, Wu J, Pinkerton KE (1994) Dose-dependent tolerance to ozone. I. Tracheobronchial epithelial reorganization in rats after 20 months exposure. Am J Pathol 144:404–420

Sannes PL (1992) Basement membrane and extracellular matrix. In: Parent RA (ed) Comparative biology of the normal lung. CRC, Boca Raton, pp 129–144

Singh G, Katyal SK (1992) Secretory proteins of Clara cells and type II cells. In: Parent RA (ed) Comparative biology of the normal lung. CRC, Boca Raton, pp 93–108

St George JA, Wang S (1992) Secretory glycoconjugates of trachea and bronchi. In: Parent RA (ed) Comparative biology of the normal lung. CRC, Boca Raton, pp 77–83

Tyler NK, Plopper CG (1985) Morphology of the distal conducting airways in rhesus monkey lungs. Anat Rec 211:295–303

Tyler WS, Julian MD (1992) Gross and subgross anatomy of lungs, pleura, connective tissue septa, distal airways, and structural units. In: Parent RA (ed) Comparative biology of the normal lung. CRC, Boca Raton, pp 37–48

# In Vitro Differentiation of an Epithelial Stem Cell Line Derived from the Fetal Syrian Hamster Lung

Makito Emura

## Introduction

Investigation of the development of an organ from the embryonic to the perinatal stage can be of considerable help in understanding its pathobiology. In the lung the developmental process includes various cellular and molecular events which are relevant to the regeneration of mature respiratory epithelium. Epithelial regeneration involves cellular differentiation, which has been proposed to recapitulate, at least phenotypically, the ontogenic process during fetal development (McDowell 1987; McDowell et al. 1990). This differentiation may start from a small pool of immature pluripotent precursor cells within the mature epithelium or may originate by dedifferentiation of differentiated secretory cells (Evans and Shami 1989). Although progenitor cells can arise by dedifferentiation of phenotypically mature cells, by as yet unknown mechanisms, the likelihood is high that in the adult respiratory epithelial tissue there is a population of undifferentiated pluripotent stem cells (McDowell and Trump 1983; Liu et al. 1994).

This chapter deals with recent findings from in vitro studies using a cloned stem cell line derived from Syrian hamster fetuses. The findings provide several lines of evidence that a single stem cell type can be a precursor of different cell types such as Clara cells, alveolar type II pneumocytes and pulmonary neuroendocrine cells depending on the specialized culture conditions.

## Characteristics of the Fetal Stem Cell Line Under Conventional Culture Conditions

The initial cell culture was started as a mixed population of cells obtained from the lung of Syrian golden hamster fetuses on day 15 of gestation. The extrapulmonary airways were removed before preparing a cell suspension from the lung tissue by trypsinization (Emura et al. 1979). The first cloning was performed at the 10th passage and was followed by three further sequential clonings (Emura et al. 1982). The cultures were then incubated with 200 μg/ml *cis*-4-hydroxy-L-proline for two sequential passages to eliminate collagen-synthesizing fibroblasts.

Several clones derived from a single epithelial cell were isolated from the 18th passage cultures. One of these epithelial cell lines, M3E3/C3, was characterized in more detail (Emura et al. 1982) for later use in various experiments. The cell line possesses a female, pseudodiploid karyotype. The stock cell line is not neoplastically transformed although it is immortalized. Spontaneous transformation (for anchorage independency) first occurred after 150 passages (Peiser et al. 1993). Under conventional in vitro conditions (RPMI 1640 medium containing pyruvate and fetal bovine serum and a solid plastic surface as a substrate) the cells of this line grow rapidly. In a monolayer they usually form intermediate junctions rather than desmosomes at cell-to-cell contact sites. Immunohistochemical reaction with anticytokeratin antibodies (raised against cytokeratin of various molecular sizes) is usually negative under conventional conditions, although antivimentin antibodies react positively. This is consistent with the observation that vimentin can develop rapidly in epithelial cells cultivated in vitro (Dairkee et al. 1985). When the cells are transplanted subcutaneously in the newborn Syrian hamsters after neoplastic transformation in vitro by benzo(a)pyrene (BaP), poorly differentiated carcinomas develop containing foci of cells reacting with a monoclonal anticytokeratin antibody raised against cytokeratin extracted from a human hepatoma (Emura et al. 1986; Fig. 174). From this it appears that cytokeratins are not required for cells growing in a monolayer (two-dimensional fashion). They are probably needed when the cells first adopt a three-dimensional architecture usually seen in an intact epithelium.

After spontaneous transformation around 150 passages (Peiser et al. 1993) the cells formed colonies in soft agar through anchorage-independent growth. In many such colonies cells developed cross-linking protein envelopes (Fig. 175) easily detectable morphologically in semisolid suspension culture (Green 1977). This envelope formation corresponds to epithelial cell cornification in vivo.

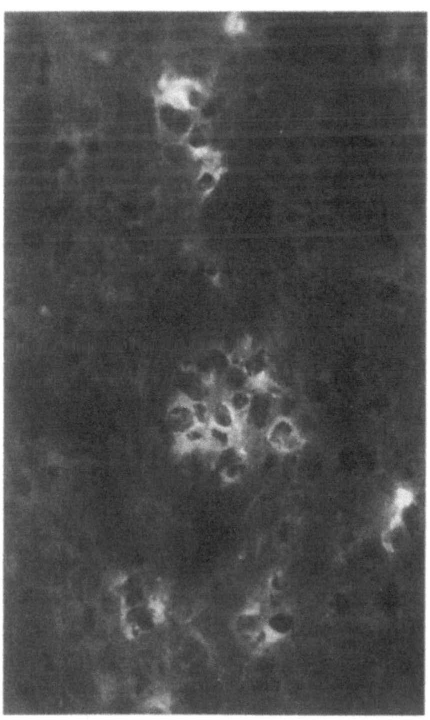

**Fig. 174.** Positive cytokeratin immunofluorescence in a tumor developed by the cells of M3E3/C3 line that were neoplastically transformed in vitro by BaP and implanted subcutaneously in a newborn Syrian hamster (Emura et al. 1987). Besides these cytokeratin-positive foci, vimentin was also expressed more widely (data not shown). ×150

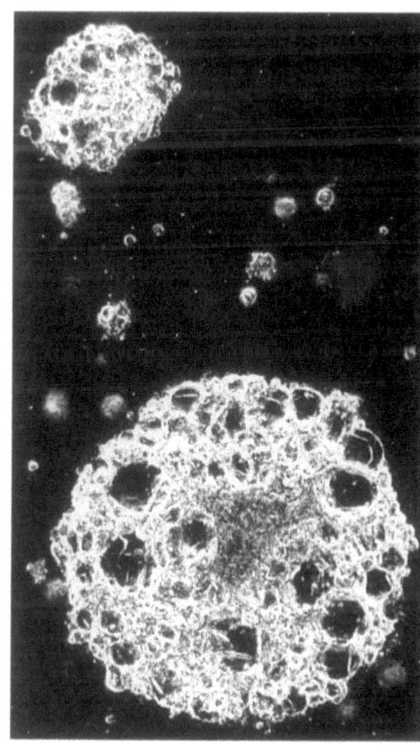

**Fig. 175.** Dark-field picture of two colonies formed in soft agar by the cells of M3E3/C3 line transformed spontaneously around 150 passages. Dark round to ovoid spaces of various sizes inside the colonies indicate the cross-linking envelopes which are transparent to a large extent under a light microscope. ×120

Under these conventional culture conditions vitamin A (10–25 μg/ml) is inhibitory for cell proliferation (Emura et al. 1982) and fails to stimulate cellular differentiation. The overall ultrastructural features of the cells growing under conventional conditions resemble those of intermediate cells described by McDowell and Trump (1983) and those of undifferentiated nonciliated bronchiolar epithelial (Clara) cells described by Plopper et al. (1992). They do not possess features of basal cells (Inayama et al. 1989). The cytoplasm lacks secretory granules, basal bodies, cilia (except occasional solitary cilia), or any other organelles to indicate specialized functions, including tonofilaments. The cytoplasm contains scattered glycogen granules, a small amount of both smooth (s) and rough (r) endoplasmic reticulum (ER) and a poorly developed Golgi apparatus. There are sparse single or polyribosomes, and the smooth-contoured nuclei contain an inconspicuous amount of heterochromatin (Emura et al. 1987). A polycyclic aromatic hydrocarbon, benz(a)anthracene is only slightly metabolized by the cells at this undifferentiated stage (Emura et al. 1987).

### Development of Clara Cell Features

The differentiation process toward a Clara cell type can be experimentally divided into two consecutive stages (Emura et al. 1988). The initial stage is inducible when the cells are cultivated on a collagen gel in a hormone-supplemented medium (Emura et al. 1987). It can be characterized functionally by the capacity of the cells metabolically to activate certain polycyclic aromatic hydrocarbons (Jacob et al. 1987, 1993). Morphologically, the first stage is characterized by development of a large amount of rER and a prominent Golgi apparatus. Occasionally present are small periodic acid–Schiff (PAS) positive granules. This first stage may be regarded as a predifferentiation stage, at which many of the ultrastructural features resemble those of the small mucus granule cells observed in a regenerating human and hamster airway epithelium (McDowell and Trump 1983). Unless additional factors are added to the culture, this predifferentiated state persists in the cells. When vitamin A is added at any time during cultivation, however, the differentiation process proceeds into the second stage during which PAS-positive granules are developed in large amounts. These granules contain glycoconjugates bound with a small amount of sialic acid which gives a faint blue-green tinge in sections stained with PAS–Alcian blue. Ultrastructurally, the contents of the granules are moderately to highly electron-dense and rather homogeneous in contrast to the secretory granules of goblet cells. In addition to these granules, only a small amount of vesicular sER is observed. Although the secretory granules bear little resemblance to those of goblet cells, we first considered that the cells differentiated under the influence of vitamin A (and on colagen gel) might be an in vitro cell type corresponding to a native goblet cell because of the occasional slight acidity of the granule contents and the paucity of sER. In the meantime, however, we detected antigenicity of Clara cell specific 10 kDa protein within these cells using a polyclonal antibody (Singh et al. 1988) raised against this protein (Fig. 176). Whereas only a small fraction of the undifferentiated cells showed this protein antigenicity, about 30% of the predifferentiated cells demonstrated it. Vitamin A appears to enhance the development of this antigen in a dose-dependent manner, with more than 70% of the differentiated cells positive for this antigen at 24 μg/ml.

Since 30% of the cells growing on collagen gel in hormone-supplemented medium and in the absence of vitamin A already possess antigenicity to the Clara cell specific 10-kDa protein, it seems that under these conditions vitamin A is not an essential factor for the development of the antigen, but an enhancer.

A substrate such as collagen seems to play a more decisive role, as does hormone supplementation. Nevertheless, the fact that the intracytoplasmic formation of secretory granules containing mainly neutral glycoconjugates requires vitamin A as a factor (Emura et al. 1988) provides an attractive link between the evident role of vitamin A in the differentiation and the maturation of lung epithelium in vivo (Chytil 1992) and the in vitro development of certain biological feataures of native Clara cells. In addition, our unpublished data (manuscript in preparation) show that the 10-kDa protein, when enhanced by vitamin A, is released from the cells into the culture medium in a cyclic manner. The first peak is on day 6 of culture followed by the second peak on day 12. Meanwhile, the level of the antigenicity within the cells remains almost constant, with a barely recogniz-

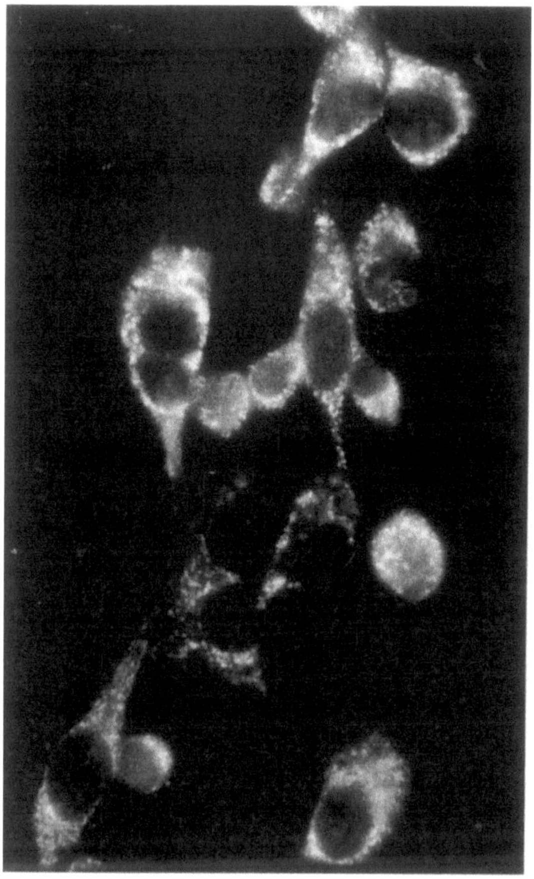

**Fig. 176.** Positive immunofluorescence for 10-kDa hamster Clara cell specific protein in the cytoplasm of the cells grown for 7 days under differentiation-inducing conditions (vitamin A and collagen gel). ×480

able peak on day 8. Chromatographic data further suggest that the protein is released in larger molecular sizes (>15 kDa) and can be digested by protease into various smaller sizes without much loss of antigenicity. The glycoconjugates labeled with [$^3$H]glucosamine behave completely differently on fractionation through a Bio-Gel A-15m. Further information on the Clara cell specific proteins is provided by Singh et al. (1985, 1988); Patton et al. (1986); Massaro (1989); Plopper et al. (1991); Hackett et al. (1992); Cardoso et al. (1993).

The sER is one of the most important features of Clara cells in the mature Syrian hamster lung (Plopper et al. 1991) but has not been observed in these in vitro differentiated cells on such a large scale. Although a close association has been observed between the lysis of previously accumulated glycogen and the genesis of sER in perinatally developing rabbit Clara cells, exact mechanisms of sER differentiation are not known (Massaro 1989; Plopper et al. 1991). In our in vitro system one or more crucial factors are presumably lacking. Nevertheless, the cells differentiated in vivo demonstrate the capacity to metabolize BaP.

Since the presence of vitamin A in the incubation medium disturbs the activation of BaP (Hill and Shih 1974; Shah et al. 1992), cells were grown on plastic for a day without vitamin A after detachment from the collagen gel and thorough rinsing in trypsin solution. Then they were incubated with BaP (10 μg/flask) for 2 days in the absence of vitamin A. The measured BaP turnover rate was 670 pmol/μg DNA/2 days. When the BaP turnover was similarly measured 15 days after the end of exposure to vitamin A, it was reduced to about 40%. These observations indicate that the cells possess a high capacity to metabolize BaP immediately after in vitro differentiation has been induced, but they lose it quickly when no longer under inducing conditions.

## Development of Features Belonging to Alveolar Type II Pneumocytes

The cells of the cell line M3E3/C3 can also undergo in vitro differentiation into a cell type possessing some features of alveolar type II pneumocytes under different culture conditions. Studies to date indicate that this direction of differentiation occurs best when there is use of hormone-supplemented medium and an agar overlay containing 10 μg/ml insulin and 6.5 μg/ml hydrocortisone (Germann et al. 1993). Morphological characteristics observed so far include the positive immunocytochemical reaction of intracytoplasmic inclusion bodies (Fig. 177) with a rabbit polyclonal antibody raised against the Syrian hamster lung surfactant (Katyal et al. 1977; Emura et al. 1989), positive reaction of these inclusion bodies with Phosphin 3R, detection of alkaline phosphatase activity, and positive Papanicolaou staining. Utrastructurally, the inclusions have lamellar structure (Germann et al. 1993). The role of the agar overlay is apparently to trap certain components secreted by the differentiating cells and make them readily available in autocrine fashion as further differentiation-stimulating factors.

High performance liquid chromatography analysis has revealed that the differentiated cells contained

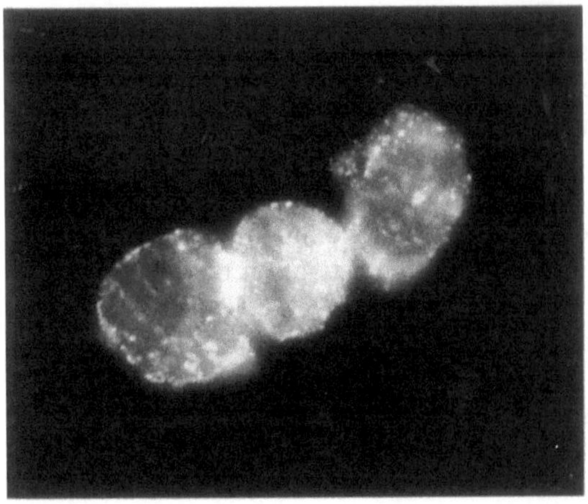

**Fig. 177.** Positive immunofluorescence for surfactant complex in the cytoplasm of the cells grown under an agar overlay for 7 days (Emura et al. 1989). ×1500

more surfactant-specific phosphatidylcholine (more than 64% of the total phospholipids) than the undifferentiated cells (phosphatidylcholine less than 50% of the total phospholipids) growing under conventional conditions (Germann et al. 1993).

In spite of evidence that in some pathological alterations (e.g., development of pulmonary adenocarcinomas) Clara cells and alveolar type II pneumocytes can have a common precursor (McDowell 1987; Marchevsky 1990), there is still a lack of direct evidence to demonstrate this relationship between the two cell types (Broers et al. 1992).

Although our findings need to be confirmed and extended, the data presented indicate the close relationship between Clara cells and type II pneumocytes and support the hypothesis that transdifferentiation from one to the other can occur in pathological situations.

## Development of Neuroendocrine Cell Phenotype

The third phenotypic expression that can be induced in vitro in this cell line is that of pulmonary neuroendocrine cells (PNEC; Emura et al. 1992). The culture condition specific for the induction of this phenotype is a reduction of oxygen pressure in the air to 5% (approximately 87 mmHg in the medium). A higher carbon dioxide pressure in the culture flask (probably corresponding to hypercapnia in vivo) also appears to stimulate the induction of PNEC phenotype. The substrate on which the cells grow can be plastic, but a collagen gel appears to be more effective. The same hormone-supplemented medium as used for the induction of Clara cell phenotype seems to be adequate. Using immunohistochemistry, functional features so far found inducible after 6 days of exposure to hypoxia have been the production of bombesin (gastrin-releasing peptide), serotonin (Fig. 178), and chromogranin (Fig. 179). Histochemically, Grimelius staining is also positive. A small fraction of cells also tend to be positive for calcitonin reactivity. Electron microscopy reveals dense-cored granules as large as 100–400 nm in diameter.

The amount of serotonin in the spent medium of the culture under hypoxia is about 14 n*M*, compared to 2 n*M* in the culture under normal oxygen pressure. The cell homogenates from the hypoxic cultures contain 560 ng per gram of cells, in contrast to 190 ng per gram of undifferentiated cells (Emura et al. 1994). The serotonin is released into the culture medium in a cyclic manner with the first peak on day 2, followed by the second peak on day 8 (unpublished results). Since the cells replicate very slowly or even scarcely at all under the hypoxic condition, many of the cells with PNEC phenotype are assumed to have developed directly from the undifferentiated stage (Emura et al. 1994).

Thus the above observations support the hypothesis (DiAugustine et al. 1984) that PNEC hyperplasia observed in infants with hyaline membrane disease can be derived from a pluripotent precursor of pulmonary epithelium. The observations also support the view that not all PNEC cells originate from cells which migrate from the neural crest during embryogenesis. The pulmonary neuroendocrine cells are considered to be an important chemoreceptor (especially for hypoxia and hypercapnia) in the adult lung and to play a significant role in the developing lung of infants (Sorokin and Hoyt 1989; Johnson 1991; Springall and Polak 1993; Hoyt et al. 1993). From this point of view it is conceivable that in an epithelial cell line obtained from the fetal lung the response in vitro to a low concentration of oxygen or high concentration of carbon dioxide (Linnoila et al. 1993) is towards induction of a neuroendocrine phenotype.

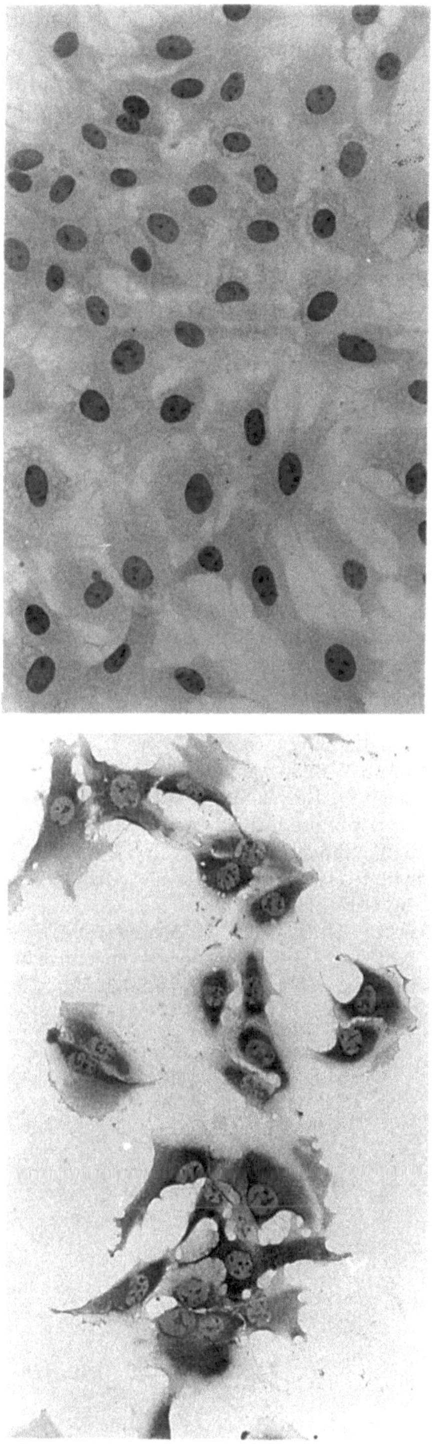

**Fig. 178a,b.** Positive immunofluorescence for serotonin. The cells were fixed with paraformaldehyde in phosphate buffer, and reacted with an antiserotonin antiserum, then with diaminobenzidine. **a** Control cells grown under normoxia. **b** Serotonin-positive cells under hypoxia. Note different growth patterns between the two conditions. ×200

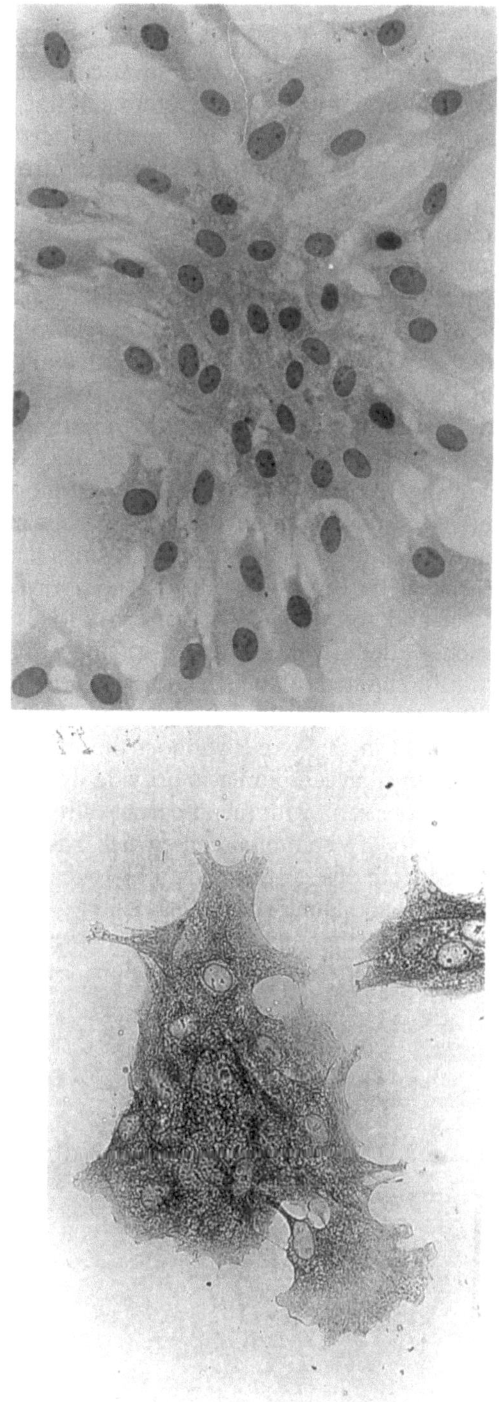

**Fig. 179a,b.** Positive immunofluorescence for chromogranin A. The cells were fixed in paraformaldehyde, reacted with a monoclonal antichromogranin A antibody, then with diaminobenzidine. **a** Control cells grown under normoxia. **b** Chromogranin-positive cells under hypoxia. ×200

## Conclusion

This chapter presents information concerning in vitro culture of an epithelial stem cell line of the fetal lung under various culture conditions. Interpretations relevant to the currently controversial question as to what is the progenitor cell of the tracheobronchial and bronchioloalveolar epithelium are summarized in Fig. 180.

Until fairly recently the most widely accepted viewpoint has been that progenitor (stem) cells of the various specialized types of epithelial cells of the lung are different (Jetten 1991). Since McDowell (1987) proposed the existence of a common stem cell; however, there has been increasing recognition that ciliated, secretory, and metaplastic cells can have precursor cells in common. Recent evidence along these lines has been provided by Liu et al. (1994) who showed that basal and secretory cells grafted onto denuded trachea dedifferentiate into a single type of undifferentiated cell which later gives rise to fully differentiated mucociliary epithelium. The studies described in this paper support the existence of common stem cells and also provide dynamic evidence consistent with the apparent differentiation of pulmonary epithelial cells which has been inferred from observations of pathological material (Plopper and Dungworth 1987).

From both a theoretical and experimental point of view, an in vitro system utilizing pluripotent respiratory epithelial cells provides an attractive opportunity for further investigation. A challenging question is whether the hamster stem cell fine develops basal cells and ciliated cells under the appropriate conditions.

*Acknowledgements.* We wish to thank Dr. M. Osborn, Max Planck Institute, Göttingen, who supplied us with a monoclonal antibody against cytokeratin extracted from human hepatoma cells. Dr. G. Singh, Department of Veterans Affairs, University of Pittsburgh, PA, USA, kindly supplied us with an antiserum against Clara cell specific 10-kDa protein.

## References

Broers JLV, Jensen SM, Travis WD, Pass H, Whitsett JA, Singh G, Katyal SL, Gazdar AF, Mina JD, Linnoila RI (1992) Expression of surfactant associated protein-A and Clara cell 10 kilodalton mRNA in neoplastic and non-neoplastic human lung tissue as detected by in situ hybridization. Lab Invest 66:337–346

Cardoso WV, Stewart LG, Pinkerton KE, Ji C, Hook GER, Singh G, Katyal SL, Thurlbeck WK, Plopper CG (1993) Secretory product expression during Clara cell differentiation in the rabbit and rat. Am J Physiol 264:L543–L552

Chytil F (1992) The lungs and vitamin A. Am J Physiol 262:L517–L527

Dairkee SH, Blayney CM, Asarnow DM, Smith HS, Hackett AJ (1985) Early expression of vimentin in human mammary cultures. In Vitro Cell Dev Biol 21:321–327

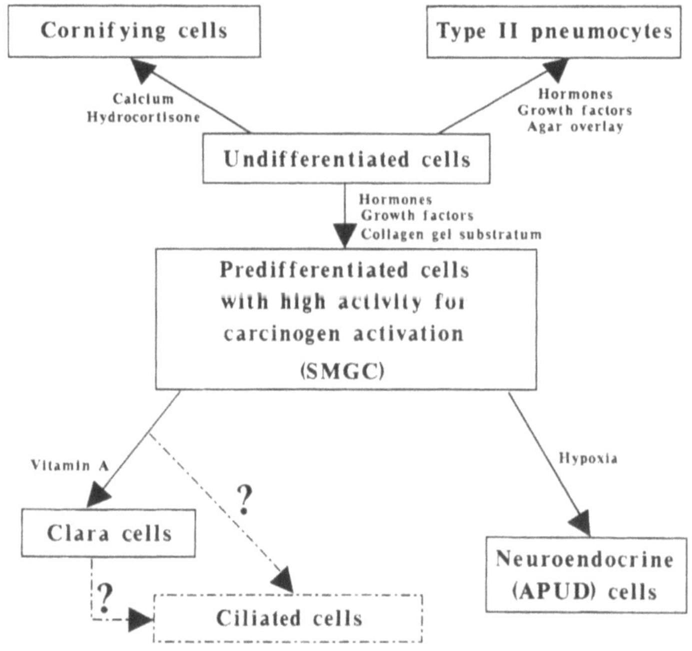


**Fig. 180.** Diagram illustrating the observed pluripotency of M3E3/C3 line. The expression of specialized phenotypes requires correspondingly specific culture conditions. Ciliated cells have not yet been observed

DiAugustine RP, Jahnke GD, Talley F (1984) Endocrine cells of the guinea pig upper airways. Morphology, distribution, and disposition after xenotransplantation in the nude mouse. In: Becker KL, Gazdar AF (eds) The endocrine lung in health and disease. Saunders, Philadelphia, pp 232–248

Emura M, Richter-Reichhelm H-B, Matthei S, Mohr U (1979) Effects of serum concentrations on the clonal growth of Syrian golden hamster fetal lung cells. Exp Pathol 17:340–346

Emura M, Richter-Reichhelm H-B, Böning W, Eichinger R, Schoch C, Althoff J, Mohr U (1982) A fetal respiratory epithelial cell line for studying some problems of transplacental carcinogenesis in Syrian golden hamsters. J Cancer Res Clin Oncol 104:133–144

Emura M, Riebe M, Aufderheide M, Mohr U (1986) A fetal Syrian hamster lung epithelial cell line as an in vitro model for respiratory carcinogenesis. Exp Pathol 29:211–216

Emura M, Mohr U, Riebe M, Aufderheide M, Dungworth DL (1987) Predisposition of cloned fetal hamster lung epithelial cells to transformation by a precarcinogen, benzo(a)pyrene, using growth hormone supplementation and collagen gel substratum. Cancer Res 47:1155–1160

Emura M, Mohr U, Riebe M, Aufderheide M, Dungworth DL (1988) Regulation of growth and differentiation by vitamin A in a cloned fetal lung epithelial cell line cultured on collagen gel in hormone-supplemented medium. In Vitro Cell Dev Biol 24:639–648

Emura M, Riebe M, Germann P, Brockmeyer C, Aufderheide M, Mohr U (1989) Functional culture of hamster and human airway epithelial cells and its application to pulmonary toxicology. Exp Pathol 37:224–227

Emura M, Ochiai A, Riebe-Imre M, Panning B, Paulini I, Mohr U, Dungworth DL (1992) In vitro differentiation of hamster pulmonary neuroendocrine cells. In Vitro Cell Dev Biol 28:133A

Emura M, Ochiai A, Gobert-Bohlen A, Panning B, Dungworth DL (1994) Neuroendocrine phenotype differentiation in a hamster lung epithelial cell line under low oxygen pressure or after transformation by diethylnitrosamine. Toxicol Lett 72:59–64

Evans MJ, Shami SG (1989) Lung cell kinetics. In: Massaro D (ed) Lung cell biology. Dekker, New York, pp 1–36

Germann P-G, Ueberschär S, Gerull A, Emura M (1993) In vitro induction of type II pneumocyte-related differentiation in a clonal fetal bronchioloalveolar epithelial cell line (M3E3/C3). Exp Toxicol Pathol 45:315–324

Green H (1977) Terminal differentiation of cultured human epidermal cells. Cell 11:405–416

Hackett BP, Shimizu N, Gitlin JD (1992) Clara cell secretory protein gene expression in bronchiolar epithelium. Am J Physiol 262:L399–L404

Hill DL, Shih TW (1974) Vitamin A compounds and analogs as inhibitors of mixed function oxidases as carcinogenic polycyclic hydrocarbons and other compounds. Cancer Res 34:564–570

Hoyt RF Jr, Sorokin SP, McDowell EM, McNally NA (1993) Neuroepithelial bodies and growth of the airway epithelium in developing hamster lung. Anat Rec 236:15–22

Inayama Y, Hook GE, Brody AR, Jetten AM, Gray T, Mahler J, Netteshein P (1989) In vitro and in vivo growth and differentiation of clones of tracheal basal cells. Am J Pathol 134:539–549

Jacob J, Grimmer G, Raab G, Emura M, Riebe M, Mohr U (1987) Comparison of chrysene metabolism in epithelial human bronchial and Syrian hamster lung cells. Cancer Lett 38:171–180

Jacob J, Grimmer G, Mohr U, Emura M, Riebe-Imre M, Raab G, Knebel J (1993) Metabolic activation of chrysene and benzo(a)pyrene in hamster, rat and human in vitro lung cell cultures. In: Proceedings of the 13th International Symposiums on Polynuclear Aromatic Hydrocarbons. Gordon and Breach Science, Langhorne, pp 1175–1182

Jetten AM (1991) Growth and differentiation factors in tracheobronchial epithelium. Am J Physiol 260:L361–L373

Johnson DE (1991) Pulmonary neuroendocrine cells. In: Farmer SG, Hay DWP (eds) The airway epithelium: physiology, pathophysiology, and pharmacology. Dekker, New York, pp 335–397

Katyal SL, Estes LW, Lombardi B (1977) Method for the isolation of surfactant from homogenates and lavages of lung of adult, newborn, and fetal rats. Lab Invest 36:585–592

Linnoila RI, Gazdar AF, Funa K, Becker KL (1993) Long-term selective culture of hamster pulmonary endocrine cells. Anat Rec 236:231–240

Liu JY, Nettesheim P, Randel SH (1994) Growth and differentiation of tracheal epithelial progenitor cells. Am J Physiol 266:L296–L307

Marchevsky A (1990) Pathogenesis and experimental models of lung cancer. In: Marchevsky AM (ed) Surgical pathology of lung neoplasms. Dekker, New York, pp 7–27

Massaro GDC (1989) Nonciliated bronchiolar epithelial (Clara) cells. In: Massaro D (ed) Lung cell biology. Dekker, New York, pp 81–114

McDowell EM (1987) Bronchogenic carcinomas. In: McDowell EM (ed) Lung carcinomas. Churchill Livingstone, Edinburgh, pp 255–285

McDowell EM, Trump BF (1983) Histogenesis of preneoplastic and neoplastic lesions in tracheobronchial epithelium. Surv Synth Pathol Res 2:235–279

McDowell EM, Ben T, Newkirk C, Chang S, De Luca LM (1987) Differentiation of tracheal mucociliary epithelium in primary cell culture recapitulates normal fetal development and regeneration following injury in hamsters. Am J Pathol 129:511–522

McDowell EM, Zhang XM, Philpot RM, De Santi AM, Strum JM (1990) Immunohistochemical demonstration of cytochrome P-450 monooxygenase in regenerating tracheal epithelium: a recapitulation of fetal development. Virchows Arch [B] 59:243–249

Patton SE, Gilmore LB, Jetten AM, Nettesheim P, Hook GER (1986) Biosynthesis and release of proteins by isolated pulmonary Clara cells. Exp Lung Res 11:277–294

Peiser C, Riebe-Imre M, Emura M, Mohr U (1993) Influence of culture passages on growth kinetics, xenobiotic metabolism, chromosomal stability and transformation in a clonal fetal hamster lung epithelial cell line. Mutat Res 28:281–290

Plopper CG, Dungworth DL (1987) Structure, function, cell injury and cell renewal of bronchiolar and alveolar epithelium. In: McDowell EM (ed) Lung carcinomas. Churchill Livingstone, Edinburgh, pp 94–128

Plopper CG, Hyde DM, Buckpitt AR (1991) Clara cells. In: Crystal RG, West JB, Barnes PJ, Cherniak NS, Weibel ER (eds) The lung: scientific foundations. Raven, New York, pp 215–228

Plopper CG, Nishio SJ, Alley JL, Kass P, Hyde DM (1992) The role of the nonciliated bronchiolar epithelial (Clara) cell as the progenitor cell during bronchiolar epithelial differentia-

tion in the perinatal rabbit lung. Am J Respir Cell Mol Biol 7:606–613
Shah GM, Goswami UC, Bhattacharya RK (1992) Action of some retinol derivatives and their provitamins on microsome-catalyzed formation of benzo[a]pyrene-DNA adduct. J Biochem Toxicol 7:177–181
Singh G, Katyal SL, Gottron GA (1985) Antigenic, molecular and functional heterogeneity of Clara cell secretory proteins in the rat. Biochem Biophys Acta 829:156–163
Singh G, Singh J, Katyal SL, Brown WE, Kramps JA, Paradis IL, Dauber JH, Macpherson TA, Squeglia N (1988) Identification, cellular localization, isolation, and characterization of human Clara cell-specific 10 KD protein. J Histochem Cytochem 36:73–80
Sorokin SP, Hoyt RF Jr (1989) Neuroepithelial bodies and solitary small-granule cells. In: Massaro D (ed) Lung cell biology. Dekker, New York, pp 191–344
Springall DR, Polak JM (1993) Calcitonin gene-related peptide and pulmonary hypertension in experimental hypoxia. Anat Rec 236:96–104

# Comparative Aspects of Pulmonary Carcinogenesis

Sabine Rehm

## Introduction

Tumor classification systems are generally established to give the physician, scientist, toxicologist, or regulatory agency a means of relating to findings in a given patient, experiment, or toxicological study. Classification systems reflect the occurrence of lesions and the knowledge of a process regarding morphology and biological behavior (Table 9). A classification system based solely on histogenesis (McDowell et al. 1978; Becci et al. 1978) may be impossible to achieve, but several instances could allow for classifications according to cell types involved in both animals and humans.

There is much controversy over possible cells of origin of lung tumors: undifferentiated cells, as suggested by Sell and Pierce (1994), are not present in adults of all species and are not involved in metabolic activation, a prerequisite for some carcinogens (Boyd and Reznik-Schüller 1984; Alworth et al. 1993; Bartsch et al. 1992). Cells with the capacity to divide have commonly been considered as probable cells of origin for epithelial lung tumors: alveolar type II, bronchiolar Clara, mucous and mucous gland, neuroendocrine, and basal cells (Kennedy et al. 1977; McDowell and Trump 1983; McDowell et al. 1985; Evans et al. 1975, 1978; Evans and Moller 1991; Plopper and Dungworth 1987; Plopper et al. 1991; Nettesheim et al. 1990; Linnoila 1991; Baldwin 1994).

Specific markers are employed for the confirmation of cell lineage (Table 10; Mulshine et al. 1992; Linnoila 1991; Linnoila et al. 1992; Wiedenmann and Huttner 1989; Singh and Katyal 1991). However, properties once considered specific for a single epithelial cell type have been found to be associated with both alveolar and bronchiolar epithelium, making a histogenetic classification system difficult (Auten et al. 1990; Strum et al. 1992; Ten Have-Opbroek and De Vries 1993; Wang et al. 1993; Broers et al. 1992). Furthermore, genes in carcinogen-exposed or neoplastic cells may be derepressed, allowing dual marker expression or the development of amphicrine tumors (Reznik-Schüller and Reznik 1979; Chejfec et al. 1985; McDowell et al. 1985; Ito 1985; Ten Have-Opbroek et al. 1993; Thiedemann et al. 1989). It may therefore be more appropriate to use markers as indication for the degree of tumor differentiation or dedifferentiation rather than as a

**Table 9.** Comparative lung tumor classifications

| Rat[a] | Human[b] |
|---|---|
| Bronchioloalveolar | Adenocarcinoma |
| Adenoma | Acinar |
| Carcinoma | Papillary |
| | Lepidic bronchioloalveolar |
| | Solid |
| Adenocarcinoma, not otherwise specified | |
| Adenosquamous carcinoma | Adenosquamous carcinoma |
| Squamous cell carcinoma | Squamous cell carcinoma |
| | Large cell carcinoma |
| | Small cell carcinoma |
| | Carcinoid |

[a] Schwartz et al. 1991; Rittinghausen et al. 1992.
[b] WHO 1981.

**Table 10.** Epithelial lung cell markers

| Alveolar Type II | Cell type | | | |
|---|---|---|---|---|
| | Clara | Mucous | Ciliated | Neuroendocrine |
| Specific cell organelles | | | | |
| Lamellar/multivesicular bodies | Smooth endoplasmic reticulum<br>Secretory granules | Secretory granules | Cilia | Dense core granules |
| Specific cell products/function | | | | |
| Surfactant apoprotein | Clara cell protein<br>P450 metabolic capacity | Mucins | NA | Neuropeptides |

NA, Not applicable.

measure from which cell type the neoplasm originated.

Carcinogeic agents are etiological factors shared by most cases of human and experimental lung tumors. Studying tumor development in humans is difficult since biopsies are not readily obtained, and tumors are usually detected in later stages. In experimental animals, however, timed killing allows examination of origin and cellular changes ranging from atypia and hyperplasia to adenoma and carcinoma. The present review analyzes cellular features (alveolar, bronchiolar, or mixed) and growth patterns of chemically induced mouse and hamster lung tumors and explores the extent to which these models contribute to the understanding of biological and morphological features of both human and rodent lung tumors.

## Proliferative Lesions with Alveolar Cell Features

Proliferative peripheral lesions of lung composed of cells with alveolar cell features have been examined in detail in the mouse and in the rat (Toth and Shimizu 1974; Kauffman and Sato 1985a; Ward et al. 1985; Rehm et al. 1991a; Foley et al. 1991; Dixon and Maronpot 1991; Belinsky et al. 1990, 1992; Maase 1980; Ohshima et al. 1985; Herbert et al. 1994) but have also been documented in other animal species and man (Straks and Feron 1973; Cutlip and Young 1982; Rosadio et al. 1988; Hoch-Ligeti et al. 1982; Mollo et al. 1973; Fantone et al. 1982; Singh et al. 1984; Kurotaki et al. 1993). Hyperplastic and neoplastic alveolar cells may produce surfactant apoproteins and are characterized ultrastructurally by lamellar and multivesicular cytoplasmic bodies (Dairaku et al. 1983). In humans intranuclear tubular structures are also considered a hallmark for alveolar type II cell tumors.

Alveolar neoplasms are frequently preceded by focal hypertrophy and hyperplasia of alveolar type II cells. This phenomenon is well known in animals but has only recently been identified in humans (Nakayama et al. 1990; Weng et al. 1992; Mori et al. 1993). In mice alveolar tumors have been shown to progress from well-differentiated tumors composed of round cells with alveolar or solid pattern to less well-differentiated papillary structures lined by cuboidal to columnar cells. An example of a papillary lung tumor with cells exhibiting alveolar cell features is shown in Figs. 181–184. Mixed solid/papillary tumors represent intermediate stages. Therefore solid lesions are frequently diagnosed as adenomas whereas papillary growth is considered carcinomatous (Heath et al. 1982; Kimura 1971; Foley et al. 1991; Belinksy et al. 1992). Papillary tumors may also develop de novo from alveolar walls without passing through a stage of solid growth, and less common pleomorphic alveolar microcarcinomas have also been observed (Rehm et al. 1991a; Belinsky et al. 1992). Papillary growth patterns are also found typically in tumors with alveolar cell features of other animal species and humans. Alveolar tumors of sheep, mice, and humans do not undergo squamous or mucous differentiation which may be associated with neoplasms of airway cell origin.

Some investigators believe that papillary lung tumors in the mouse originate in Clara cells (Kauffman and Sato 1985b; Thaete and Malkinson 1991; Gunning et al. 1991). Other investigators, with a contrary view, have described experimental systems in which tumors arise from alveolar walls, lack specific markers for Clara cells (secretory granules, abundant smooth endo-

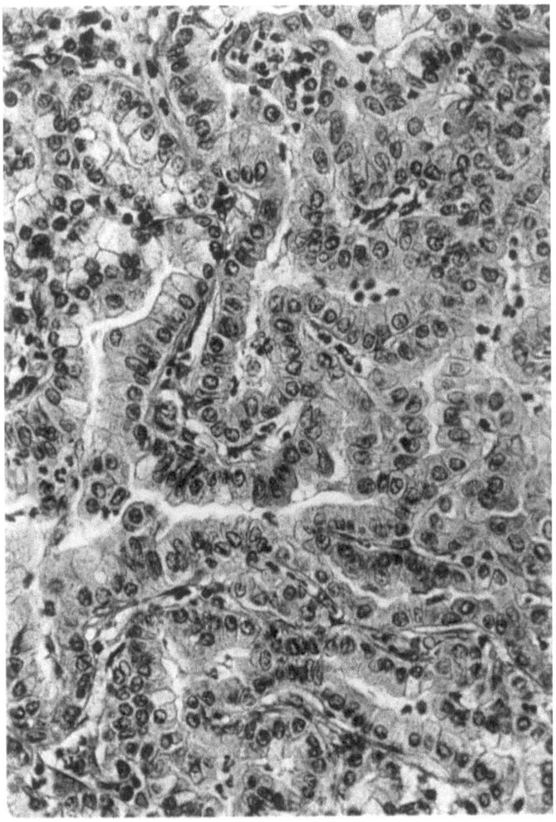

**Fig. 181.** Papillary pulmonary adenocarcinoma, hamster, induced by *N*-nitrosomethyl-*n*-heptylamine (Rehm et al. 1993). Papillary fronds lined by cuboidal to columnar cells, some with vacuolated, pale cytoplasm. Ultrastructure is shown in Figs. 182–184. H&E, ×250

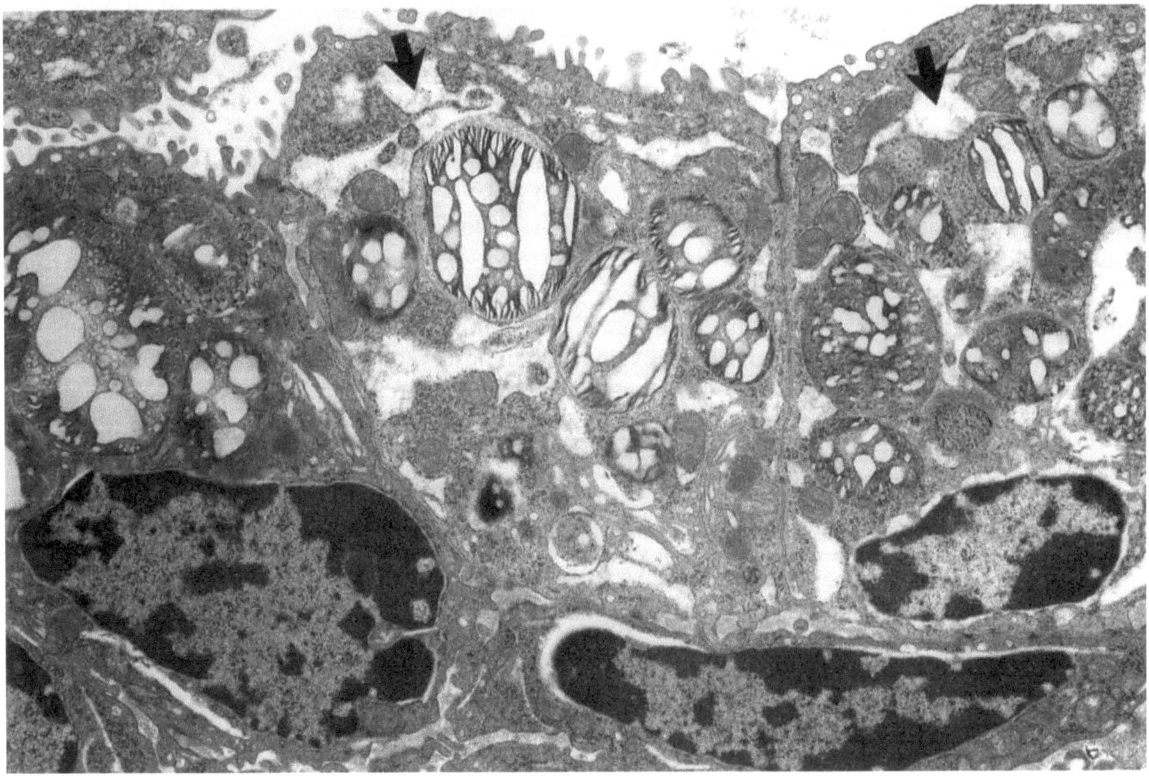

**Fig. 182.** Alveolar cell tumor, hamster, same tumor as in Fig. 181, characterized by variably sized, atypically vacuolated lamellar bodies and dilated rough endoplastic reticulum (*arrows*). Uranyl acetate/lead citrate, TEM, ×1000

**Fig. 183.** (*above*) Alveolar cell tumor, hamster, same tumor as in Fig. 182 at higher magnification showing multivesicular bodies (*large arrow*), dense body (*arrowhead*), and rough endoplasmic reticulum (*small arrow*). *L*, Lamellar body. Uranyl acetate/lead citrate, TEM, ×14000

**Fig. 184.** (*below*) Alveolar cell tumor, hamster, same tumor as in Fig. 182. Numerous dense bodies (*arrowheads*) are present besides lamellar bodies (*L*) and slightly dilated rough endoplasmic reticulum (*arrow*). Uranyl acetate/lead citrate, TEM, ×12000

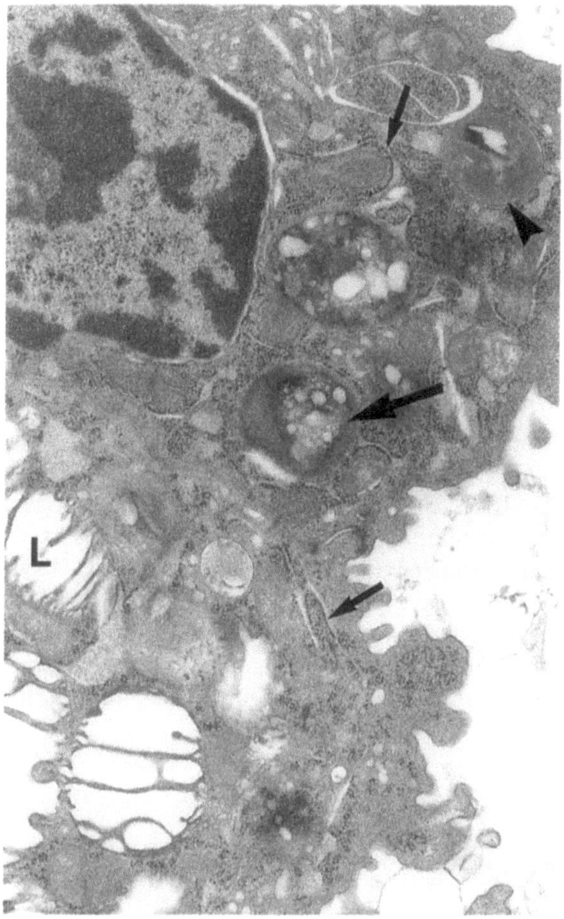

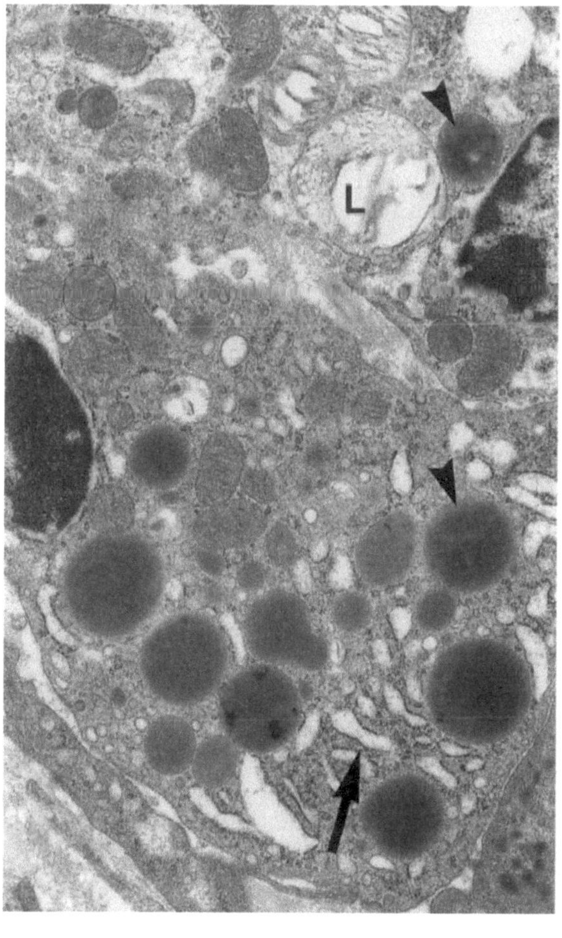

plasmic reticulum, Clara cell protein), and tumor cells are unable to metabolize xenobiotics as is normally done by Clara cells (Ward et al. 1985; Rehm et al. 1991a; Forkert et al. 1992; Rehm and Devor 1993).

The basis for light microscopic and ultrastructural changes, as is commonly seen with malignant progression, is most likely based on changes in the genome. Tumor cell dedifferentiation (or retrodifferentiation; Mulshine et al. 1992) may easily lead to misinterpretation and misdiagnosis. Lamellated structures may be reduced in size and number, or they are no longer detectable (Figs. 185, 186). However, the presence of heterogeneous osmiophilic dense bodies and a dispersed dilated rough endoplasmic reticulum (Fig. 185) are reminiscent of alveolar features as shown in Fig. 184. Irregular nuclei with multiple indentations signal increased malignancy. Some criteria used for Clara cell derivation of lung tumors in humans and the mouse are the presence of peg-shaped or columnar cells and dense bodies (Kauffman and Sato 1985b; Gunning et al. 1991; Mori et al. 1993; Broers et al. 1992). As a consequence the presence of dense bodies together with lamellar bodies in columnar cells is interpreted as dual expression of alveolar and Clara cell features (Kurotaki et al. 1993; Fantone et al. 1982). Such a conclusion, without further evidence, is not justified. Dense bodies are present not only in neoplastic but also in normal alveolar type II cells as precursors of lamellar bodies, in intermediate alveolar type II/I cells, and in fetal alveolar cells (Mollo et al. 1973; Evans et al. 1975; Ten Havė-Opbroek et al. 1990; Rehm and Lijinsky 1994).

Features of malignant alveolar tumors are tissue invasion, necrosis and fibrosis, formation of spindle cells, aerogenous intrapulmonary spread, deposits on pleural surfaces, and metastases to mediastinal lymph nodes and other organs. The

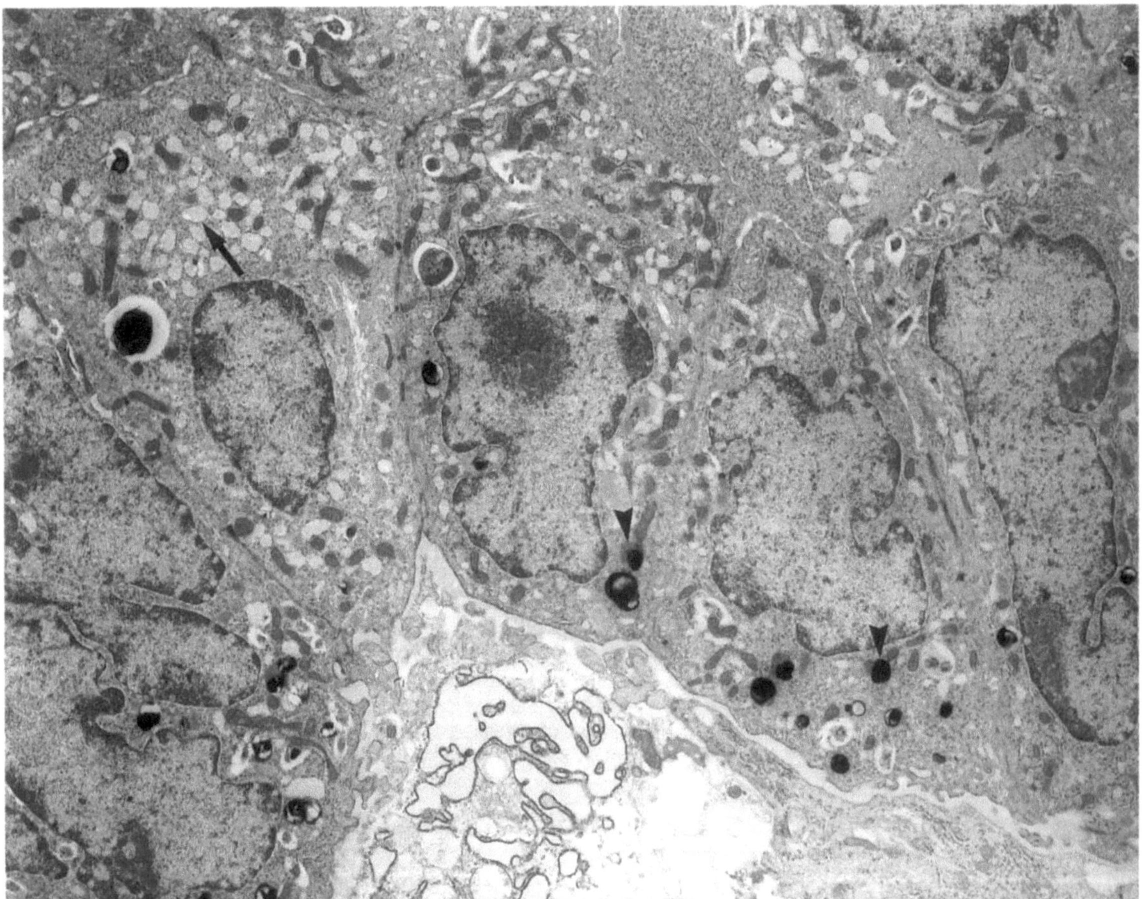

**Fig. 185.** Alveolar cell tumor, hamster, less well differentiated, induced by *N*-nitrosomethyl-*n*-heptylamine. Cells show indented nuclei, few dense bodies (*arrowheads*), and dilated rough endoplasmic reticulum (*arrow*). On H&E this neoplasm was classified as papillary pulmonary adenocarcinoma. Uranyl acetate/lead citrate, TEM, ×6300

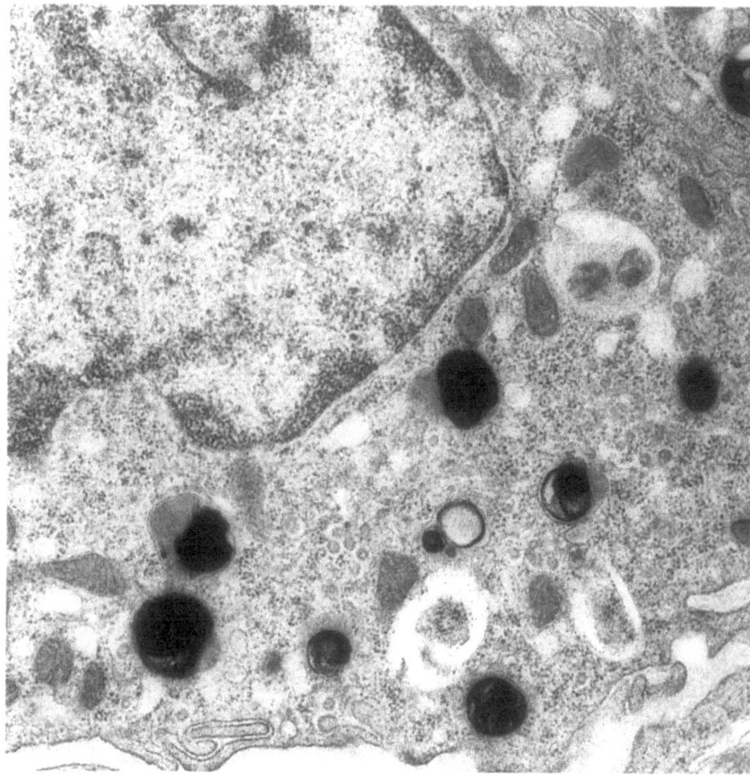

**Fig. 186.** Alveolar cell tumor, hamster, same tumor as in Fig. 185. Higher magnification of area showing variable morphology of osmiophilic dense bodies. Uranyl acetate/lead citrate, TEM, ×20000

ability of alveolar cells to produce extracellular matrix components (Mason and Williams 1991) may be responsible, directly or indirectly, for the fibrotic thickening of alveolar walls, scar formation, and scirrhous responses. Increased connective tissue in alveolar lesions led to the erroneous diagnosis of "sclerosing hemangiomas" in humans (Table 9; Satoh et al. 1989). There is no separate category in the human classification system for alveolar lesions. In man this type of tumor is grouped as subcategory of nonmucinous (Clara or alveolar) bronchioloalveolar hyperplasia or neoplasia (Espinoza et al. 1984; Clayton 1986). Proliferative alveolar lesions of humans, as in experimental animals, may be multifocal, and it may be difficult to distinguish between various proliferative stages such as hyperplasia, adenoma, or carcinoma (Nakayama et al. 1990; Mori et al. 1993; Barsky et al. 1994).

The etiology of naturally occurring alveolar lung tumors varies depending on the species. In sheep alveolar carcinomas are associated with a retrovirus whereas genetic predisposing factors are responsible in mouse strains with high incidences of lung tumors, such as in strain A (Devereux et al. 1994; Fijneman et al. 1995; Hegi et al. 1994). Little is known about etiological factors of alveolar tumors in man. Only limited information is available in rodents on oncogene or tumor-suppressor gene expression in lung tumors depending on the cell type, and it is not clear to what extent the cell of origin plays a role in carcinogenic mutational events. In rats as well as mice alveolar tumors have been associated most commonly with K-*ras* oncogene mutations (You et al. 1991; Belinsky et al. 1992; Nickell-Brady et al. 1994). The lack of mutations reported in some studies, however, indicates other yet unknown carcinogen-related genetic events (Nickell-Brady et al. 1994). Endogenous mutations of the p53 tumor suppressor gene are rarely observed in rodent papillary lung tumors (Fig. 187) whereas they constitute the most frequent genetic alteration in human lung cancer (Greenwell et al. 1994; Goodrow et al. 1992; Li et al. 1994). A high incidence of lung tumors has, however, been observed in various transgenic mice (Lavigueur et al. 1989; Wikenheiser et al. 1992).

## Proliferative Lesions with Bronchial/Bronchiolar Cell Features

Proliferative lesions exhibiting features of airway cells are uncommon spontaneous lesions in animals but represent the majority of pulmonary le-

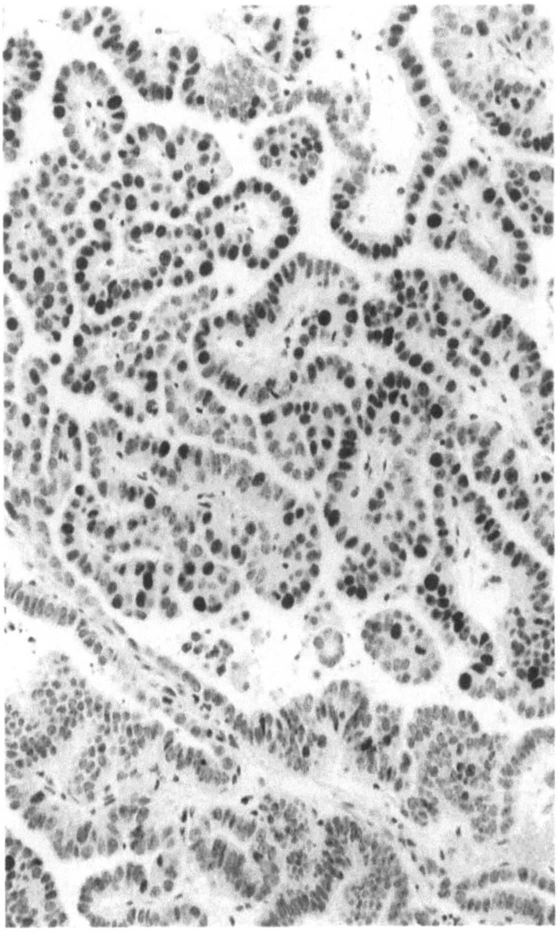

**Fig. 187.** Papillary lung tumor of mouse exposed to 1,3 butadiene (Greenwell et al. 1994). Nuclear expression of p53 mutations. ABC immunohistochemistry, hematoxylin counter stain, ×200. (Courtesy of A. Greenwell)

sions in man. Generally these lesions may be subdivided into those occurring in bronchi or in more peripheral regions.

In humans most bronchial neoplasms are squamous cell carcinomas and are thought to be of basal cell origin (Baldwin 1994). However, mucin production and the presence of mucous granules also imply secretory cells as cell of origin (McDowell and Trump 1983; McDowell et al. 1985). Human bronchial squamous cell carcinomas are often preceded by squamous metaplasia, dysplasia, and carcinoma in situ (Nagamoto et al. 1987; Leube and Rustad 1991; Trump et al. 1978; Müller and Müller 1983). There is also evidence that squamous cell cancers can develop without going through the above sequence (Matthews and Linnoila 1988; Nagamoto et al. 1987). Experimental systems have been developed to mimic the human situation by intratracheal carcinogen instillation or by placing the carcinogen at a localized area of the trachea or mainstem bronchi (Yoshimoto et al. 1980; Henry et al. 1981; Becci et al. 1978, 1980; Hammond and Benfield 1993; Benfield and Hammond 1992; Keenan et al. 1989). Most commonly, squamous cell carcinomas and/or adenosquamous carcinomas are the type of tumors found at these sites. The morphology and biological behavior of experimental bronchial carcinomas are comparable to those of humans, i.e., they are invasive and metastasize.

The incidence of adenocarcinoma in the United States has recently become greater than that of squamous cell carcinoma (Auerbach and Garfinkel 1991; Barsky et al. 1994). Most adenocarcinomas in the human develop distal to the large airways and obvious histological transitions, i.e., precursor lesions, have not clearly been established (Li et al. 1994; Solomon et al. 1990). The majority of human adenocarcinomas are thought to be of Clara cell origin due to the presence of dense or mucous granules (Matthews and Linnoila 1988; Broers et al. 1992; Espinoza et al. 1984; Clayton 1986; Linnoila et al. 1992). However, about only 10% of these neoplasms express Clara cell proteins and mRNA (Singh et al. 1988). A histogenetic tumor classification may seem academic, particularly with the generally poor prognosis of most human lung cancer cases. However, it does become important when specifically targeting Clara cell derived neoplasms for treatment since tumors with alveolar cell differentiation should then be excluded (Christian et al. 1989; Rehm and Devor 1993; Rowinsky et al. 1993).

A variety of cells may be considered as progenitors for airway cell tumors. It has been established that Clara and mucous cells serve as progenitors for themselves and ciliated cells (Plopper et al. 1991; Christensen et al. 1987); basal cells (not present in mouse and hamster) may be the progenitor for any cell type, and observations in humans indicate secretory cells as progenitors for neuroendocrine cells (Plopper and Dungworth 1987; McDowell et al. 1985). Squamous differentiation may occur in secretory, neuroendocrine, or basal cells (Becci et al. 1978; Trump et al. 1978; Leube and Rustad 1991; Rehm and Lijinsky 1994). Therefore individual neoplastic airway cells can be expected to show a variety of features singly or in various combinations.

In experimental animals hyperplasia of airway cells may occur within airway lumens or within the alveolar parenchyma (Figs. 188, 189; Yoshimoto et al. 1980; Rehm et al. 1991b, 1993). Both types of hyperplasia are usually considered a preneoplastic condition when associated with cellular atypia and dysplasia. Cells types involved include: Clara, mucous, ciliated, squamous, and undifferentiated neuroendocrine cells. The proportion of different cell types may vary between individual animals, species, and types of experiments. Cavitary neoplasms have been observed mainly in a transgenic mouse model (Maronpot et al. 1991). Many chemically induced lung tumors with airway cell features in rodents are derived from bronchiolar cells lining alveolar walls (Kotin and Wiseley 1963; Little and O'Toole 1974; Reznik-Schüller and Gregg 1981; Maase 1980; Chang et al. 1992; Rehm et al. 1991b, 1993). This condition is frequently referred to as alveolar bronchiolization (Fig. 189; Nettesheim and Szakal 1972), is associated with airway cell toxicity, and is localized mainly in the bronchioloalveolar region. This localization is observed irrespective of the applied test substance, i.e., aerogenous or systemic (gavage, subcutaneous, dermal). Alveolar type II cells may also proliferate, and the condition therefore is also referred to as bronchioloalveolar hyperplasia. Controversy exists on the yet unresolved pathogenesis of alveolar bronchiolization mainly about the relative importance of bronchiolar cell migration and alveolar type II metaplasia. Some investigators consider "metaplasia of alveolar type II" cells as source for parenchymal bronchiolar cells (Adamson and Bowden 1979; Nolte et al. 1993; Pinkerton et al. 1993). Others perceive bronchiolar cells to have populated alveolar walls by migration from open terminal bronchioles and through pores, or by invasion of the basement membrane of the proximal alveolar

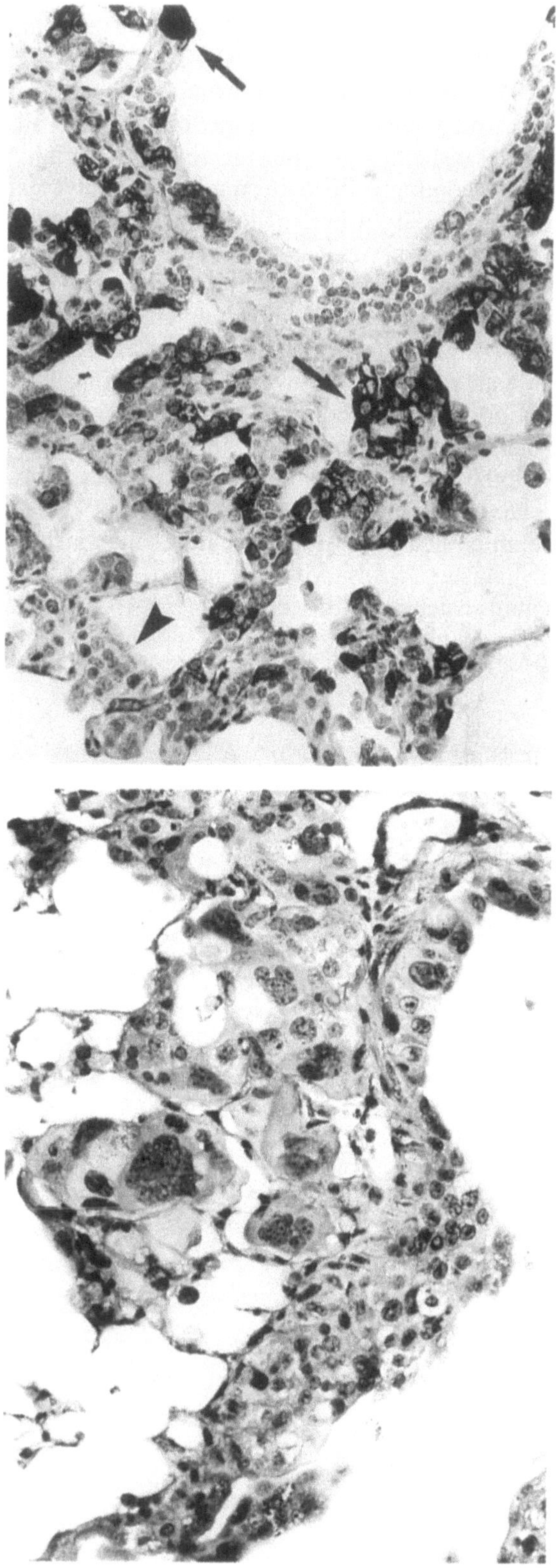

▶

**Fig. 188.** (*above*) Mouse, parenchymal bronchiolar cell hyperplasia adjacent to bronchiole with atypical cellular lining, induced by *N*-nitrosomethyl-*n*-heptylamine (Rehm et al. 1991b). Localization of Clara cell protein (*arrows*), and focal area of squamous differentiation (*arrowhead*). Most bronchiolar lining Clara cells are replaced by ciliated or squamous cells. ABC immunohistochemistry, H&E, ×250

**Fig. 189.** (*below*) Hyperplasia and cellular atypia (dysplasia) of bronchiolar lining cells of mouse induced by *N*-nitrosomethyl-*n*-heptylamine. Adjacent anaplastic multinucleated giant cells belong to invasive squamous cell carcinoma, nonkeratinizing. H&E, ×250

duct (Fig. 189; Nettesheim and Szakal 1972; Rehm et al. 1993; Plopper et al. 1991).

Initially bronchiolar cells growing in the parenchyma may blend into the frame of alveolar walls without distorting or replacing airspaces, forming a honeycomb growth pattern mimicking alveolar hyperplasia. According to the human classification system, this pattern is referred to as lepidic bronchioloalveolar (BAC pattern; Table 9). These lesions may progress by crowding alveolar spaces and giving rise to acinar/glandular structures with nodular, expansile, or invasive growth (Fig. 190). Tumor cells may produce Clara cell protein and/or mucus, possess secretory granules, abundant smooth endoplasmic reticulum, cilia, or show squamous differentiation (Table 10; Figs. 190–192; Rehm et al. 1993). Atypical features may include in hamsters, cells with elongated membrane-bound structures with secretions (Fig. 192), and in mice deeply eosinophilic cells associated with crystals (Rehm et al. 1991b). Carcinomas may also exhibit larger areas composed of primarily a single cell type such as Clara, mucous, or ciliated cells. Neoplasms with features of bronchiolar cells may, as mentioned above for alveolar neoplasms, be likewise deficient in marker expression making a histogenetic classification difficult (Figs. 193, 194). Cilia are lost, secretory granules are reduced in size and number, smooth endoplasmic reticulum is replaced by rough endoplasmic reticulum and ribosomes, and nuclei attain cleaved, irregular shapes. Neoplasms may also show squamous differentiation, forming adenosquamous, solid or cystic squamous cell carcinomas (Fig. 190; Kittel et al. 1993). Benign tumors composed of bronchiolar cells are uncommon following experimental induction. Local invasion usually occurs early during tumor development, with growth beyond the pleural surface with formation of metastases. Selective induction of bronchiolar-cell derived neoplasms may be achieved in mice depending on compound or strain (Yoshimoto et al. 1980; Rehm et al. 1991b).

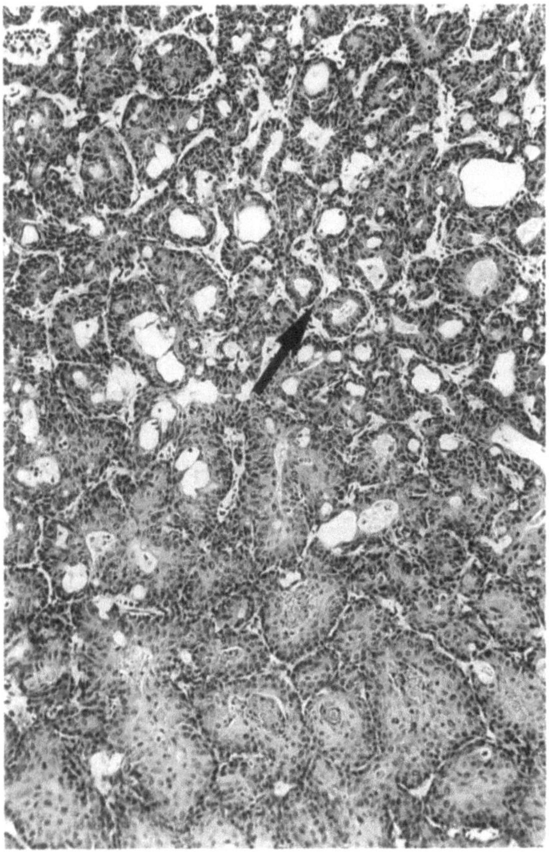

**Fig. 190.** Adenosquamous cell carcinoma of mouse treated with 3-methylcholanthrene (Rehm et al. 1991b). Glandular portion showing acinar structures (*arrow*) and adjacent area (*lower left*) with squamous differentiation with overt keratinization. H&E, ×100

Bronchial carcinomas with neuroendocrine cell features (small cell lung cancer and carcinoids) represent 20%–25% of all human lung cancers and rarely occur in the absence of a smoking history (Matthews and Linnoila 1988; Addis 1988). Neuroendocrine lung tumors, however, are uncommon spontaneous lesions in animals (Harkema et al. 1992) and are not readily induced experimentally. Hyperplasia of neuroendocrine cells, however, is readily induced by nitrosamines in rodents and rabbits maintained at ambient air or exposed to hyperoxia (Figs. 195, 196; Huntrakoon et al. 1989; Linnoila et al. 1981; Sunday et al. 1994). Likewise, in humans neuroendocrine cell hyperplasia has been observed in lung tissue surrounding resected lung tumors, possibly indicating exposure to carcinogens (Linnoila 1991). Neuroendocrine differentiation has also been observed in adenocarcinomas and in large cell and squamous cell carcinomas of humans but not of animals, and neuroendocrine cancers develop after chemotherapy or radiotherapy of other lung tumors. If such variability of neuroendocrine features is due to the multipotentiality of bronchial basal cells (Matthews and Linnoila 1988), species differences in tumor formation may be related to differences in cellular ontogeny. Basal cells for the most part are not present in the rodent lung, and no mucous cells with dense core granules have been found in these species.

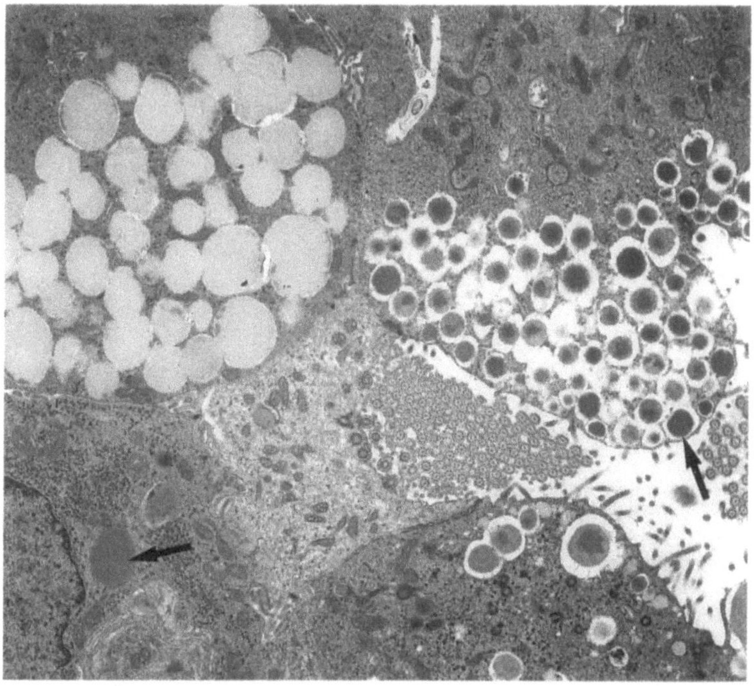

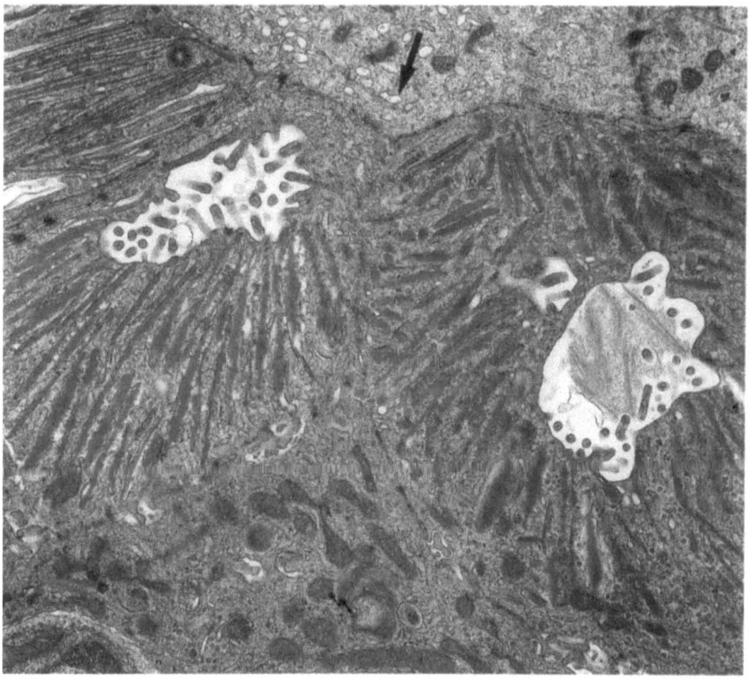

**Fig. 191.** (*above*) Lepidic well differentiated bronchioloalveolar carcinoma of hamster treated with *N*-nitrosomethyl-*n*-heptylamine. Clara cells with dense secretion granules (*arrows*), some with artifactual empty spaces, next to mucous cell with pale granules (*upper left*) and ciliated cell. Uranyl acetate/lead citrate, TEM, ×6000

**Fig. 192.** (*below*) Lepidic well differentiated bronchioloalveolar carcinoma of hamster treated with *N*-nitrosomethyl-*n*-heptylamine. Atypical Clara cells with elongated structures derived from Golgi system or smooth endoplasmic reticulum. Structures contain secretory product and are arranged perpendicularly to intracytoplasmic lumens with microvillous border. Note abundant smooth endoplasmic reticulum (*arrow*) in all cells. Uranyl acetate/lead citrate, TEM, ×9000

## Proliferative Lesions with Both Alveolar and Bronchiolar Cell Features

As outlined above, it is to be expected that tumors derived from the bronchiolar epithelium show variable marker expression typical for the cell lineage. However, the formation of alveolar cells from airway cells or vice versa is not generally accepted and has not been documented adequately. The potential for bidirectional differentiation may be supported by in vitro studies (Emura et al. 1989) showing human and hamster cell lines that may differentiate into Clara cells or alveolar cells depending on the composition of the matrix.

Recent work has demonstrated the expression of alveolar type II cell markers (m-RNAs for surfactant apoprotein A and Clara cell protein) in

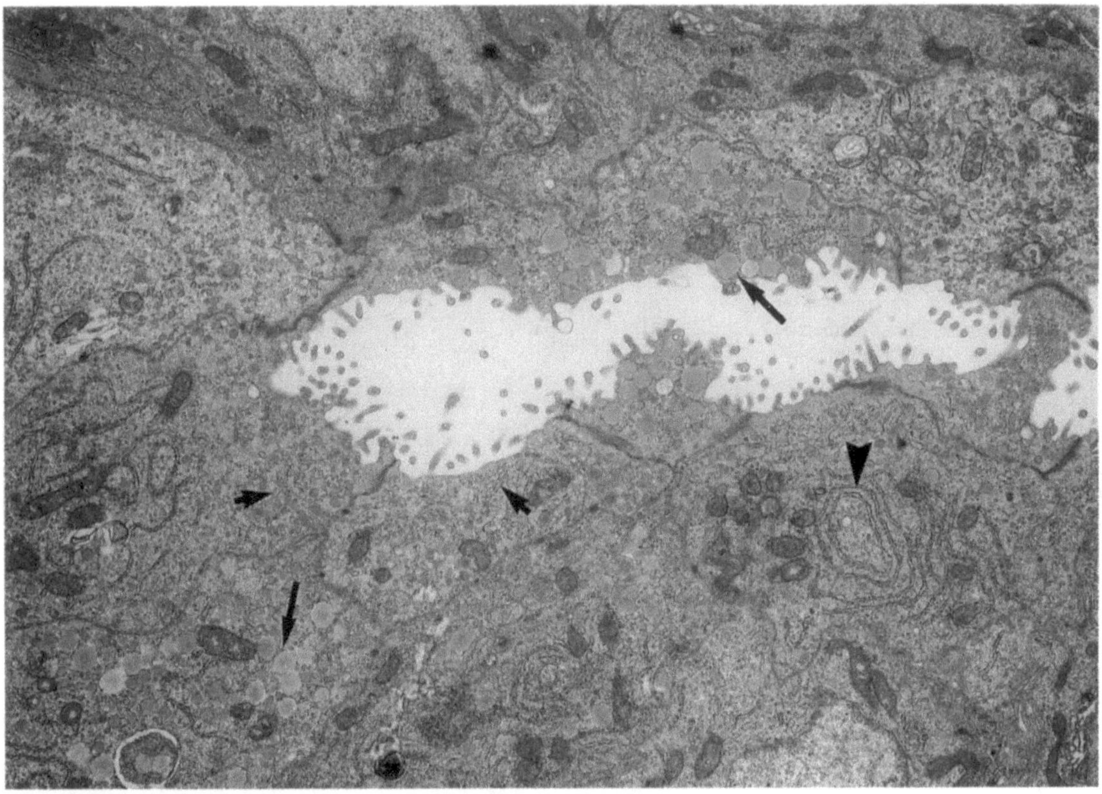

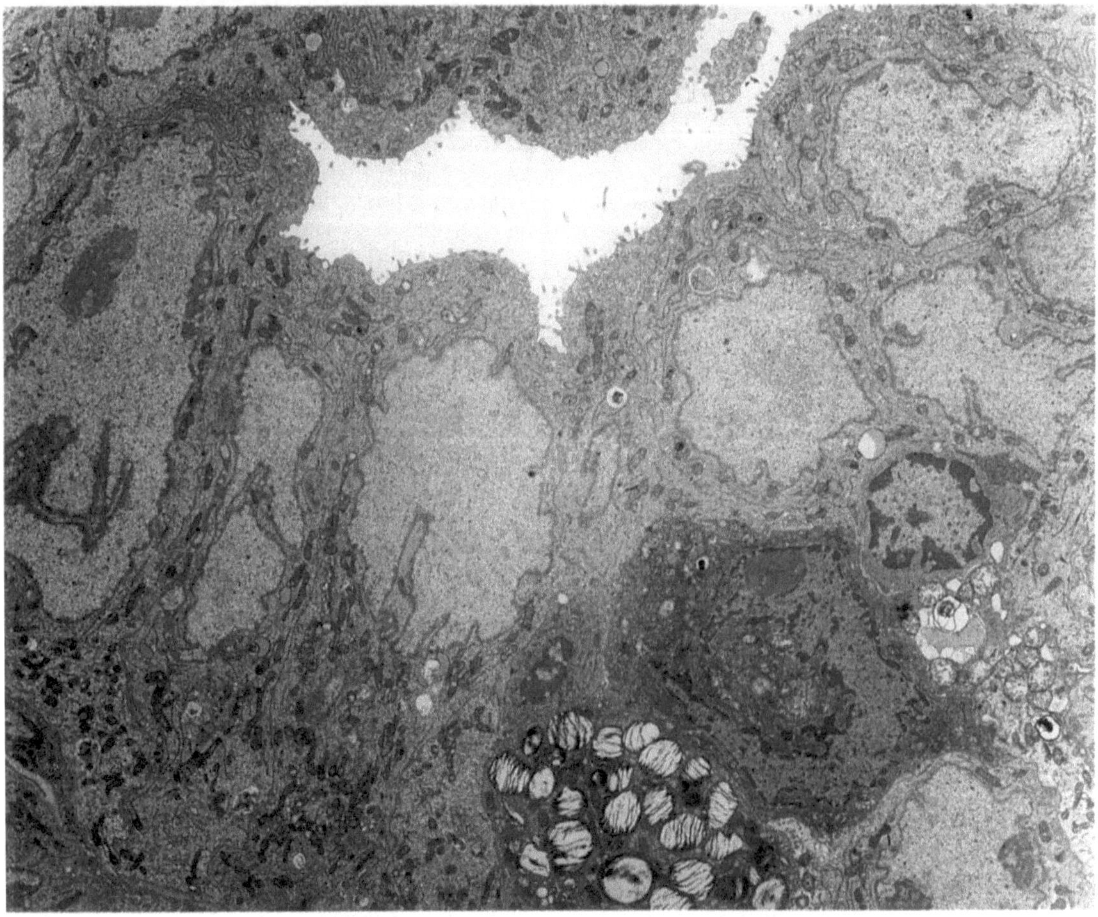

bronchiolar epithelium during fetal development and in mature epithelium of various species (Auten et al. 1990; Strum et al. 1992; Broers et al. 1992; Wikenheiser et al. 1992). Less commonly it has been possible to demonstrate the actual proteins and the issue of surfactant apoprotein A production by airway epithelium remains controversial (Ten Have-Opbroek and De Vries 1993). Lung tumors from humans and rats have been identified as expressing mRNAs for surfactant and Clara cell protein as well the corresponding proteins (Broers et al. 1992; Linnoila et al. 1992; Ohshima et al. 1985; Herbert et al. 1994). Tumors from bronchial explants in dogs have been shown to produce surfactants and lamellar bodies (Ten Have-Opbroek et al. 1993), and carcinogen-treated hamsters have lamellar bodies in Clara cells and develop Clara cell tumors with lamellar bodies (Reznik-Schüller and Reznik 1979; Ito 1985; Thiedeman et al. 1989).

Studies on bidirectional differentiation require particular scrutiny. Lamellar bodies are lysosomally derived structures that can form in any cell, where they usually are referred to as myelin figures and are inducible by drugs. Therefore lamellated structures by themselves do not make an alveolar type II cell (Plopper and Dungworth 1987; Ten Have-Opbroek et al. 1993). Similarly, the presence of dense bodies or granules do not make a Clara or a neuroendocrine cell (Mollo et al. 1973; Mooi et al. 1990; Rehm et al. 1991a; Rehm and Lijinsky 1994). One of the best ways to identify these organelles is probably by immunoelectron microscopy. Erroneous interpretation of ultrastructural granules may, for example, be responsible for the unexpectedly low frequency of human adenocarcinomas expressing Clara cell protein or mRNA. In the future it may be anticipated that new analytical methods and improved in vivo as well as in vitro models will improve the understanding of epithelial differentiation in both the lung and other organs.

◀

**Fig. 193.** (*above*) Acinar carcinoma of hamster treated with *N*-nitrosomethyl-*n*-heptylamine. Acinus lined by less well-differentiated cells with small secretory granules (*large arrows*) that may be labeled for Clara cell protein by immunoelectron microscopy (Rehm and Lijinsky 1994). Note finely dispersed smooth endoplasmic reticulum (*small arrows*) and strands of rough endoplasmic reticulum (*arrowhead*). Uranyl acetate/lead citrate, TEM, ×7200

**Fig. 194.** (*below*) Poorly differentiated acinar carcinoma of hamster treated with *N*-nitrosomethyl-*n*-heptylamine. Acinus lined by columnar cells with highly irregular nuclei, and devoid of specific organelles. Note trapped parenchymal alveolar type II cell (*center*, *bottom*) with numerous lamellar bodies. Uranyl acetate/lead citrate, TEM, ×3600

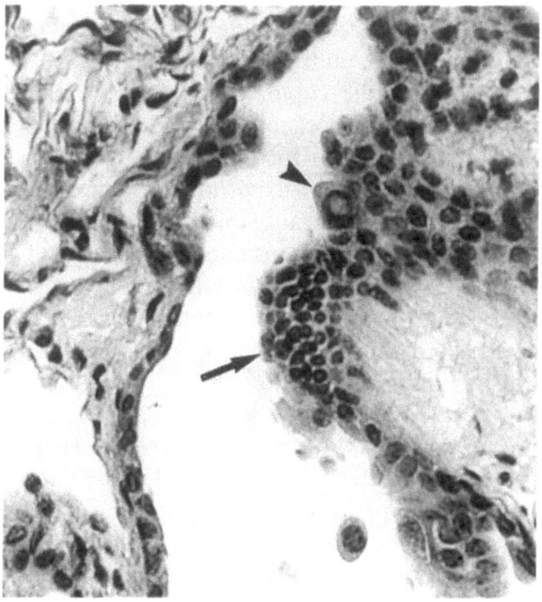

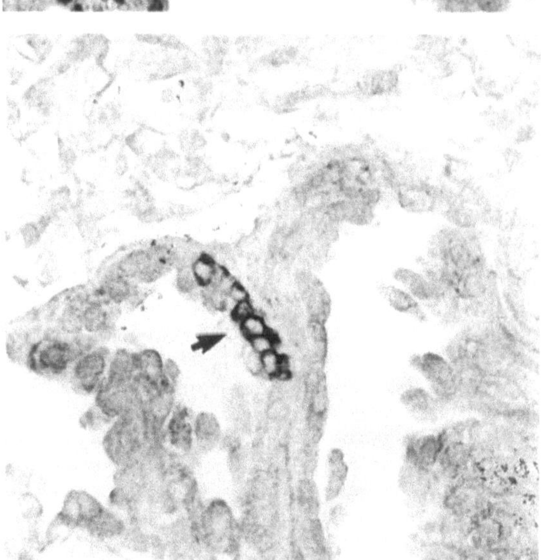

**Fig. 195.** (*above*) Mouse, focal bronchiolar neuroendocrine cell hyperplasia (*arrow*). Tangential section through base of focus. Crowded nuclei are small and round with stippled chromatin. *Arrowhead*, carcinogen-induced cellular atypia of Clara cell. H&E, ×340

**Fig. 196.** (*below*) Mouse, focal bronchiolar neuroendocrine cell hyperplasia (*arrow*). Atypical cell perpendicular section through focus immunoreactive for chromogranin. ABC immunohistochemistry, no counterstain. ×400

## Conclusions

Despite existing species differences such as the rare occurrence of neuroendocrine small cell lung cancer in animals it has been possible in man and animals to identify lung tumors that clearly are composed of cells expressing markers of only alveolar cells or only bronchial/bronchiolar cells. More work is needed to determine the extent to which tumors or individuals cells (neoplastic or normal) have the capacity to express markers characteristic for both airway and parenchymal cell types. The successful application of new techniques to well-known experimental systems and the development of transgenic mice or new models may bring greater insights into processes of pulmonary carcinogenesis. Ultimately research may lead to classification systems, incorporating location, growth patterns, cell types, marker expression, and species differences.

*Acknowledgements.* Most figures are from experimental studies that were performed at the Laboratory of Comparative Carcinogenesis, National Cancer Institute, National Institutes of Health, Frederick, Maryland, USA. The excellent technical assistance of Dawn M. Zimmerman and Thomas J. Covatta, SmithKline Beecham, King of Prussia, Pennsylvania, is gratefully acknowledged. The author would further like to thank Drs. H.A. Solleveld and S. Eustis for critical reading of the manuscript.

## References

Adamson IYR, Bowden DH (1979) Bleomycin-induced injury and metaplasia of alveolar type II cells. Relationship of cellular responses to drug presence in the lung. Am J Pathol 96:531–544

Addis (1988) Pathology of lung cancer. In: Hoogstraten B, Addis BJ, Hansen HH, Martini N, Spiro SG (eds) Lung tumors. Lung, mediastinum, pleura, and chest wall. Springer, Berlin Heidelberg New York, pp 17 36

Alworth WL, Young-Sciame R, Hecht SS (1993) Inhibition of 4-(methylnitrosamino)-I-(3-pyridyl)-1-butanone mouse lung tumorigenesis by arylalkynes, mechanism-based inactivators of cytochrome P450. Carcinogenesis 14:1711–1713

Auerbach O, Garfinkel L (1991) The changing pattern of lung carcinoma. Cancer 68:1973–1977

Auten RL, Watkins RH, Shapiro DL, Horowitz S (1990) Surfactant apoprotein A (SP-A) is synthesized in airway cells. Am J Respir Cell Mol Biol 3:491–496

Baldwin F (1994) Basal cells in human bronchial epithelium. Anat Rec 238:360–367

Barsky SH, Cameron R, Osann KE, Tomita D, Holmes EC (1994) Rising incidence of bronchioloalveolar lung carcinoma and its unique clinicopathologic features. Cancer 73:1163–1170

Bartsch H, Petruzzelli S, De Flora S, Hietanen E, Camus A-M, Castegnaro M, Alexandrow K, Rojas M, Saracci R, Giuntini C (1992) Carcinogen metabolism in human lung tissues and the effect of tobacco smoking: results from a case-control multicenter study on lung cancer patients. Environ Health Persp 98:119–124

Becci PJ, McDowell EM, Trump BF (1978) The respiratory epithelium. VI. Histogenesis of lung tumors induced by benzo[a]pyrene-ferric oxide in the hamster. J Natl Cancer Inst 61:607–618

Becci PJ, Thompson HJ, Grubbs CJ, Moon RC (1980) Histogenesis and dose dependence of N-methyl-N-nitrosourea-induced carcinoma in a localized area of the hamster trachea. J Natl Cancer Inst 64:1135–1140

Belinsky SA, Foley JF, White CM, Anderson MW, Maronpot RR (1990) Dose-response relationship beween $O^6$-methylguanine formation in Clara cells and induction of pulmonary neoplasia in the rat by 4-(methylnitrosarnino)-l-(3-pyridyl)-l-butanone. Cancer Res 50:3772–3780

Belinky SA, Devereux TR, Foley JF, Maronpot RR, Anderson MW (1992) Role of the alveolar type II cell in the development and progression of pulmonary tumors induced by 4(methylnitrosamino)-1-(3-pyridyl)-l-butanone in the A/J mouse. Cancer Res 52:3164–3173

Benfield JR, Hammond WG (1992) Bronchial and pulmonary carcinogenesis at focal sites in dogs and hamsters. Cancer Res [Suppl] 52:2687s-2693s

Boyd MR, Reznik-Schüller HM (1984) Metabolic basis for the pulmonary Clara cell as a target for pulmonary carcinogenesis. Toxicol Pathol 12:56–61

Broers JLV, Jensen SM, Travis WD, Pass H, Whitsett JA, Singh G, Katyal SL, Gazdar AF, Minna JD, Linnoila RI (1992) Expression of surfactant associated protein-A and Clara cell 10 kilodalton mRNA in neoplastic and non-neoplastic human lung tissue as detected by in situ hybridization. Lab Invest 66:337–346

Chang F, Wang L, Zhao Q, Zhu Q, Wu Y, Chen C, Syrjänen S, Syrjänen K (1992) Investigation on the carcinogenic effects of coal tar pitch in rat respiratory tract by intratracheal instillations. Carcinogenesis 13:233–239

Chejfec G, Capella C, Solcia E, Jao W, Gould VE (1985) Amphicrine cells, dysplasias and neoplasias. Cancer 56:2683–2690

Christensen TG, Breuer R, Homstra LJ, Lucey EC, Stone PJ, Snider GL (1987) An ultrastructural study of the response of hamster bronchial epithelium to human neutrophil elastase. Exp Lung Res 13:279–297

Christian MC, Wittes RE, Leyland-Jones B, McLemore TL, Smith AC, Grieshaber CK, Chabner BA, Boyd MR (1989) 4-Ipomeanol: a novel investigational new drug for lung cancer. J Natl Cancer Inst 81:1133–1143

Clayton F (1986) Bronchioloalveolar carcinomas. Cell types, patterns of growth, and prognostic correlates. Cancer 57:1555–1564

Cutlip RC, Young S (1982) Sheep pulmonary adenomatosis (jaagsiekte) in the United States. Am J Vet Res 43:2108–2113

Dairaku M, Sueishi K, Tanaka K, Horie A (1983) Immunohistological analysis of surfactantapoprotein in the bronchiole-alveolar carcinoma. Virchows Arch A Pathol Anat Histopathol 400:223–234

Devereux TR, Wiseman RW, Kaplan N, Garren S, Foley JF, White CM, Anna C, Watson MA, Patel A, Jarchow S, Maronpot RR, Anderson MW (1994) Assignment of a locus for mouse lung tumor susceptibility to proximal chromosome 19. Mam Genome 5:749–755

Dixon D, Maronpot RR (1991) Histomorphologic features of spontaneous and chemically-induced pulmonary neoplasms in B6C3F1 mice and Fischer 344 rats. Toxicol Pathol 19:540–556

Emura M, Riebe M, Germann P, Brockmeyer C, Aufderheide M, Mohr U (1989) Functional culture of hamster and human airway epithelial cells and its application to pulmonary toxicology. Exp Pathol 37:224–227

Espinoza CG, Balis JU, Saba SR, Paciga JE, Shelley SA (1984) Ultrastructural and immunohistochemical studies of bronchiole-alveolar carcinoma. Cancer 54:2182–2189

Evans MJ, Moller PC (1991) Biology of airway basal cells. Exp Lung Res 17:513–531

Evans MJ, Cabral U, Stephens RJ, Freeman G (1975) Transformation of alveolar type II cells to type I cells following exposure to $NO_2$. Exp Mol Pathol 22:142–150

Evans MJ, Cabral-Anderson LJ, Freeman G (1978) Role of the Clara cell in renewal of the bronchiolar epithelium. Lab Invest 38:648–653

Fantone JC, Geisinger KR, Appelman HD (1982) Papillary adenoma of the lung with lamellar and electron dense granules. An ultrastructural study. Cancer 50:2839–2844

Fijneman RJA, Oomen LCJM, Snoek M, Demant P (1995) A susceptibility gene for alveolar lung tumors in the mouse maps between Hsp 70.3 and G7 in the H2 complex. Immunogenetics 41:106–109

Foley JF, Anderson MW, Stoner GD, Gaul BW, Hardisty JF, Maronpot RR (1991) Proliferative lesions of the mouse lung: progression studies in strain A mice. Exp Lung Res 17:157–168

Forkert PG, Parkinson A, Thaete LG, Malkinson AM (1992) Resistance of murine lung tumors to xenobiotics-induced cytotoxicity. Cancer Res 52:6997–6803

Goodrow TL, Storer RD, Leander KR, Prahalada SR, van Zwieten M, Bradley MO (1992) Murine p53 intron sequences 5–8 and their use in polymerase chain reaction/direct sequencing analysis of p53 mutations in CD-1 mouse liver and lung tumors. Mol Carcinog 5:9–15

Greenwell A, Sills R, Söderkvist P, Wiseman R (1994) Characterization of p53 mutations by immunohistochemistry, single strand conformation analysis and DNA sequencing in B6C3F1 mice exposed to 1,3-butadiene. Toxicologist 14:147

Gunning WT, Castonguay A, Goldblatt PJ, Stoner GD (1991) Strain A/J mouse lung adenoma growth patterns vary when induced by different carcinogens. Toxicol Pathol 19:168–175

Hammond WG, Benfield JR (1993) Hamster bronchial carcinogenesis induced by carcinogen containing sustained release implants placed endobronchially: a clinically relevant model. J Cell Biochem [Suppl] 17F:104–117

Harkema JR, Jones SE, Naydan DK, Wilson DW (1992) An atypical neuroendocrine tumor in the lung of a beagle dog. Vet Pathol 29:175–179

Heath JE, Frith CH, Wang PM (1982) A morphologic classification and incidence of alveolarbronchiolar neoplasms in BALB/c female mice. Lab Anim Sci 32:638–647

Hegi ME, Devereux TR, Dietrich WF, Cochran CJ, Lander ES, Foley JF, Maronpot RR, Anderson MW, Wiseman RW (1994) Allelotype analysis of mouse lung carcinomas reveals frequent allelic losses on chromosome 4 and an association between allelic imbalances on chromosome 6 and K-ras activation. Cancer Res 54:6257–6264

Henry CJ, Billups LH, Avery MD, Rude TH, Dansie DR, Lopez A, Sass B, Whitmire CE, Kouri RE (1981) Lung cancer model system using 3-methylcholanthrene in inbred strains of mice. Cancer Res 41:5027–5032

Herbert RA, Stegelmeier BS, Gillett NA, Rebar AH, Carlton WW, Singh G, Hahn FF (1994) Plutonium-induced proliferative lesions and pulmonary epithelial neoplasms in the rat: immunohistochemical and ultrastructural evidence for their origin from type II pneumocytes. Vet Pathol 31:366–374

Hoch-Ligeti C, Congdon CC, Deringer MK, Strandberg JD, Sass B, Stewart HL (1982) Primary tumors and adenomatosis of the lung in untreated and in irradiated guinea pigs. Toxicol Pathol 10:1–11

Huntrakoon M, Menon CD, Hung KS (1989) Diethylnitrosamine-induced pulmonary endocrine cell hyperplasia and its association with adenomatosis and adenocarcinoma in rabbits. Am J Pathol 135:1119–1128

Ito T (1985) An ultrastructural study of the acute effects of 4-nitroquinoline I-oxide on the hamster lung. Exp Mol Pathol 42:220–233

Kauffman SL, Sato T (1985a) Alveolar type II cell adenoma, lung, mouse. In: Jones TC, Mohr U, Hunt RD (eds) Respiratory system. Monographs on pathology of laboratory animals. Springer, Berlin Heidelberg New York, pp 102–107

Kauffman SL, Sato T (1985b) Bronchiolar adenoma, lung, mouse. In: Jones TC, Mohr U, Hunt RD (eds) Respiratory system. Monographs on pathology of laboratory animals. Springer, Berlin Heidelberg New York, pp 107–111

Keenan KP, Saffiotti U, Stinson SF, Riggs CW, McDowell EM (1989) Multifactorial hamster respiratory carcinogenesis with interdependent effects of cannula-induced mucosal wounding, saline, ferric oxide, benzo[a]pyrene and N-methyl-N-nitrosourea. Cancer Res 49:1528–1540

Kennedy AR, McGandy RB, Little JB (1977) Histochemical, light and electron microscopic study of polonium-210 induced peripheral tumors in hamster lungs: evidence implicating the Clara cell as the cell of origin. Eur J Cancer 13:1325–1340

Kimura I (1971) Progression of pulmonary tumor in mice. I. Histological studies of primary and transplanted pulmonary tumors. Acta Pathol Jap 21:13–56

Kittel B, Ernst H, Dungworth DL, Rittinghausen S, Nolte T, Kamino K, Stuart B, Lake SG, Cardesa A, Morawietz G, Mohr U (1993) Morphological comparison between benign keratinizing cystic squamous cell tumours of the lung and squamous lesions of the skin in rats. Exp Toxicol Pathol 45:257–267

Kotin P, Wiseley DV (1963) Production of lung cancer in mice by inhalation exposure to influenza virus and aerosols of hydrocarbons. Prog Exp Tumor Res 3:186–215

Kurotaki H, Kamata Y, Kimura M, Nagai K (1993) Multiple papillary adenomas of type II pneumocytes found in a 13-year-old boy with von Recklinghausen's disease. Virchows Arch A Pathol Anat Histopathol 423:319–322

Lavigueur A, Maltby V, Mock D, Rossant J, Pawson T, Bernstein A (1989) High incidence of lung, bone, and lymphoid tumors in transgenic mice overexpressing mutant alleles of the p53 oncogene. Mol Cell Biol 9:3982–3991

Leube RE, Rustad TJ (1991) Squamous cell metaplasia in the human lung: molecular characteristics of epithelial stratification. Virchows Arch B Cell Pathol 61:227–253

Li ZH, Zheng J, Weiss LM, Shibata D (1994) c-K-ras and p53 mutations occur very early in adenocarcinoma of the lung. Am J Pathol 144:303–309

Linnoila RI (1991) Pathways of differentiation in human lung cancer. Proc Am Assoc Cancer Res 32:446–448

Linnoila RI, Nettesheim P, DiAugustine RP (1981) Lung endocrine-like cells in hamsters treated with diethyinitrosaffiine: alterations in vivo and in cell culture. Proc Natl Acad Sci USA 78:5170–5174

Linnoila RI, Jensen SM, Steinberg SM, Mulshine JL, Eggleston JC, Gazdar AF (1992) Peripheral airway cell marker expression in non-small cell lung carcinoma. Association with distinct clinicopathologic features (see comments). Am J Clin Pathol 97:233–243

Little JB, O'Toole WF (1974) Respiratory tract tumors in hamsters induced by benzo(a)pyrene and $^{210}$Po a-radiation. Cancer Res 34:3026–3039

Maase R (1980) Histogenesis of lung tumors induced in rats by inhalation of alpha emitters: an overview. In: Sanders A (ed) Pulmonary toxicology of respirable particles. National Technical Information Service, Springfield, Conf-791002, pp 498–521

Maronpot RR, Palmiter RD, Brinster RL, Sandgren EP (1991) Pulmonary carcinogenesis in transgenic mice. Exp Lung Res 17:305–320

Mason RJ, Williams MC (1991) Alveolar type II cells. In: Crystal RG, West JB (eds) The lung: scientific foundations. Raven, New York, pp 235–246

Matthews MJ, Linnoila RI (1988) Pathology of lung cancer-an update. In: Bitran JD, Golomb HM, Little AG, Weichselbaum RR (eds) Lung cancer a comprehensive treatise. Harcourt Brace Jovanovich, New York, pp 5–34

McDowell EM, Trump BF (1983) Histogenesis of preneoplastic and neoplastic lesions in tracheobronchial epithelium. Surv Synth Pathol Res 2:235–279

McDowell EM, McLaughlin JS, Merenyl DK, Kieffer RF, Harris CC, Trump BF (1978) The respiratory epithelium. V. Histogenesis of lung carcinomas in the human. J Natl Cancer Inst 61:587–606

McDowell EM, Keenan KP, Trump BF (1985) The pathogenesis of hormone-producing tumors of the lung. In: Havenann K, Sorenson GD, Gropp C (eds) Peptide hormones in lung cancer. Springer, Berlin Heidelberg New York, pp 94–106 (Recent results in cancer research, vol 99)

Mollo F, Canese MG, Campobasso O (1973) Human peripheral lung tumours: light and electron microscopic correlation. Br J Cancer 27:173–182

Mooi WJ, Dingemans KP, Wagenaar SS, Hart AAM, Wagenvoort CA (1990) Ultrastructural heterogeneity of lung carcinomas: representativity of samples for electron microscopy in tumor classification. Hum Pathol 21:1227–1234

Mori M, Chiba R, Takahashi T (1993) Atypical adenomatous hyperplasia of the lung and its differentiation from adenocarcinoma. Characterization of atypical cells by morphometry and multivariate cluster analysis. Cancer 72:2331–2340

Müller KM, Müller G (1983) The ultrastructure of preneoplastic changes in the bronchial mucosa. In: Müller KM (ed) Pulmonary diseases. Clinicopathological correlations. Spinger, Berlin Heidelberg New York, pp 233–263 (Current topics in pathology, vol 73)

Mulshine JL, Linnoila RI, Treston AM, Scott FM, Quinn K, Avis I, Shaw GL, Jensen SM, Brown P, Birrer MJ, Cuttitta F (1992) Candidate biomarkers for application as intermediate end points of lung carcinogenesis. J Cell Biochem [Suppl] 16G:183–186

Nagamoto N, Saito Y, Imai T, Suda H, Takahashi S, Usuda K, Kanma K, Sagawa M, Ohta S, Sato M, Nakada T, Sato H, Hashimoto K (1987) Histogenesis and characterization of minimal bronchogenic carcinoma observed in heavy smokers. Tohoku J Exp Med 153:265–284

Nakayama H, Noguchi M, Tsuchiya R, Kodama T, Shimosato Y (1990) Clonal growth of atypical adenomatous hyperplasia of the lung: cytofluorometric analysis of nuclear DNA content. Mod Pathol 3:314–320P, Szakal AK (1972) Morphogenesis of alveolar bronchiolization. Lab Invest 26:210–219

Nettesheim P, Jetten AM, Inayama Y, Brody AR, George MA, Gilmore LB, Gray T, Hook GER (1990) Pathways of differentiation of airway epithelial cells. Environ Health Perspect 85:317–329

Nickell-Brady C, Hahn FF, Finch GL, Belinsky SA (1994) Analysis of K-ras, p53 and c-raf-1 mutations in beryllium-induced rat lung tumors. Carcinogenesis 15:257–262

Nolte T, Thiedemann KU, Dungworth DL, Ernst H, Paulini I, Heirich U, Dasenbrock C, Peters L, Ueberschär S, Mohr U (1993) Morphology and histogenesis of squamous cell metaplasia of the rat lung after chronic exposure to a pyrolized pitch condensate, and/or carbon black, or to combinations of pyrolized pitch condensate, carbon black and irritant gases. Exp Toxicol Pathol 45:135–144

Ohgaki H, Furukawa F, Takahashi M, Kleihues P (1993) K-ras mutations are frequent in pulmonary squamous cell carcinomas but not in adenocarcinomas of WBN/kob rats induced by N-nitrosobis(2-oxopropyl)amine. Carcinogenesis 14:1471–1473

Ohshima M, Ward JM, Singh G, Katyal SL (1985) Immunocytochemical and morphological evidence for the origin of N-nitrosomethylurea-induced and naturally occurring primary lung tumors in F344/NCr rats. Cancer Res 45:2785–2792

Pinkerton KE, Dodge DE, Cededahl-Demmler J, Wong VJ, Peake J, Haselton CJ, Mellick PW, Singh G, Plopper CG (1993) Differentiated bronchiolar epithelium in alveolar ducts of rats exposed to ozone for 20 months. Am J Pathol 142:947–956

Plopper CG, Dungworth DL (1987) Structure, function, cell injury and cell renewal of bronchiolar and alveolar epithelium. In: McDowell EM (ed) Lung carcinomas. Churchill Livingstone, New York, pp 95–128

Plopper CG, Hyde DM, Buckpitt AR (1991) Clara cells. In: Crystal RG, West JB, Barnes PJ, Cherniak NS, Weibel ER (eds) The lung: scientific foundations. Raven, New York, pp 215–228

Rehm S, Devor DE (1993) Acute effects of 4-ipomeanol on experimental lung tumors with bronchiolar or alveolar cell features in Syrian hamsters or C3H/HeNCr mice. J Cancer Res Clin Oncol 120:41–50

Rehm S, Lijinsky W (1994) Squamous metaplasia of bronchiolar cell-derived acinar adenocarcinoma induced by N-nitrosomethyl-n-heptylamine in Syrian hamsters. Vet Pathol 31: 561–571

Rehm S, Devor DE, Henneman JR, Ward JM (199la) Origin of spontaneous and transplacentally induced mouse lung tumors from alveolar type II cells. Exp Lung Res 17:181–195

Rehm S, Lijinsky W, Singh G, Katyal SL (1991b) Mouse bronchiolar cell carcinogenesis. Histologic characterization and expression of Clara cell antigen in lesions induced by N-nitrosobis-(2-chloroethyl) ureas. Am J Pathol 139:413–422

Rehm S, Lijinsky W, Thomas BJ, Kasprzak BH (1993) Clara cell antigen in normal and migratory dysplastic Clara cells, and bronchioloalveolar carcinoma of Syrian hamsters induced by N-nitrosomethyl-n-heptylamine. Virchows Arch B Cell Pathol 64:181–190

Reznik-Schüller H, Reznik G (1979) Experimental pulmonary carcinogenesis. Int Rev Exp Pathol 20:211–281

Reznik-Schüller HM, Gregg M (1981) Pathogenesis of lung tumors induced by N-nitrosoheptamethyleneimine in F344 rats. Virchows Arch A Pathol Anat Histopathol 393:333–343

Rittinghausen S, Dungworth DL, Ernst H, Mohr U (1992) Primary pulmonary tumors. In: Mohr U, Dungworth DL, Capen CC (eds) Pathobiology of the aging rat vol 1. International Life Sciences Institute, Washington DC, pp 161–172

Rosadio RH, Sharp JM, Lairmore MD, Dahlberg JE, De Martini JC (1988) Lesions and retroviruses associated with naturally occurring ovine pulmonary carcinoma (sheep pulmonary adenomatosis). Vet Pathol 25:58–66

Rowinsky EK, Noe DA, Ettinger DS, Christian MC, Lubejko BG, Fishman EK, Sartorius SE, Boyd MR, Donehower RC (1993) Phase I and pharmacological study of the pulmonary cytotoxin 4-ipomeanol on a single dose schedule in lung cancer patients: hepatotoxicity is dose limiting in humans. Cancer Res 53:1794–1801

Satoh Y, Tsuchiya E, Weng SY, Kitagawa T, Matsubara T, Nakagawa K, Kinoshita I, Sugano H (1989) Pulmonary sclerosing hemangioma of the lung. A type II pneumocytoma by immunohistochemical and immunoelectron microscopic studies. Cancer 64:1310–1317

Schwartz LW, Hahn FF, Keenan KP, Keenan CM, Brown HR, Mann PC (1991) Proliferative lesions of the rat respiratory tract. In: Guides for toxicologic pathology. STP/ARP/AFIP, Washington DC, pp 1–12

Sell S, Pierce GB (1994) Maturation arrest of stem cell differentiation is a common pathway for the cellular origin of teratocarcinomas and epithelial cancers. Lab Invest 70:6–22

Singh G, Katyal SL (1991) Pulmonary proteins as cell-specific markers. Exp Lung Res 17:245–253

Singh G, Katyal SL, Ordonez NG, Dail DH, Negishi Y, Weedn VW, Marcus PB, Weldon-Linne CM, Axiotis CA, Alvarez-Femandez E, Smith Wl (1984) Type II pneumocytes in pulmonary tumors. Implications for histogenesis. Arch Pathol Lab Med 108:44–48

Singh G, Singh J, Katyal SL, Brown WE, Kramps JA, Paradis IL, Dauber JH, Macpherson TA, Squeglia N (1988) Identification, cellular localization, isolation, and characterization of human Clara cell-specific 10 KD protein. J Histochem Cytochem 36:73–80

Solomon MD, Greenberg SD, Spjut HJ (1990) Morphology of bronchial epithelium adjacent to adenocarcinoma of the lung. Mod Pathol 3:684–687

Straks W, Feron VJ (1973) Ultrastructure of pulmonary adenomas induced by intratracheal instillation of diethylnitrosamine in Syrian golden hamsters. Eur J Cancer 9:359–362

Strum JM, Compton RS, Katyal SL, Singh G (1992) The regulated expression of mRNA for Clara cell protein in the developing airways of the rat, as revealed by tissue in situ hybridization. Tissue Cell 24:461–471

Sunday ME, Willett CG, Patidar K, Graham SA (1994) Modulation of oncogenes and tumor suppressor gene expression in a hamster model of chronic lung injury with varying degrees of pulmonary neuroendocrine cell hyperplasia. Lab Invest 70:875–888

Ten Have-Opbroek AAW, De Vries ECP (1993) Clara cell differentiation in the mouse: ultrastructural morphology and cytochemistry for surfactant protein-A and Clara cell l0kD protein. Microsc Res Tech 26:400–411

Ten Have-Opbroek AAW, Otto-Verbern CJM, Dubbeldam JA (1990) Ultrastructural characteristics of inclusion bodies of type II cells in late embryonic mouse lung. Anat Embryol 181:317–323

Ten Have-Opbroek AAW, Hammond WG, Benfield JR, Teplitz RL, Dijkman JH (1993) Expression of alveolar type II cell markers in acinar adenocarcinomas and adenoid cystic carcinomas arising from segmental bronchi. A study in a heterotopic bronchogenic carcinoma model in dogs. Am J Pathol 142:1251–1264

Thaete LG, Malkinson AM (1991) Cells of origin of primary pulmonary neoplasms in mice: morphologic and histochemical studies. Exp Lung Res 17:219–228

Thiedemann KU, Lüthe N, Paulini I, Kreft A, Heinrich U, Glaser U (1989) Ultrastructural observations in hamsters and rat lungs after chronic inhalation of cadmium compounds. Exp Pathol 37:264–268

Toth B, Shimizu H (1974) 1-Carbamyl-2-phenylhydrazine tumorigenesis in Swiss mice. Morphology of lung adenomas. J Natl Cancer Inst 52:241–251

Trump BF, McDowell EM, Glavin F, Barrett LA, Becci PJ, Schürch W, Kaiser HE, Harris CC (1978) The respiratory epithelium. III. Histogenesis of epidermoid metaplasia and carcinoma in situ in the human. J Natl Cancer Inst 61:563–575

Wang J, Souza P, Kuliszewski M, Transwell AK, Post M (1993) Expression of surfactant proteins in embryonic rat lung. Am J Respir Cell Mol Biol 10:222–229

Ward JM, Singh G, Katyal SL, Anderson LM, Kovatch RM (1985) Immunocytochemical localization of the surfactant apoprotein and Clara cell antigen in chemically induced and naturally occurring pulmonary neoplasms of mice. Am J Pathol 118:493–499

Weng SY, Tsuchiya E, Kasuga T, Sugano H (1992) Incidence of atypical bronchioloalveolar cell hyperplasia of the lung: relation to histological subtypes of lung cancer. Virchows Arch A Pathol Anat Histopathol 420:463–471

WHO (1981) Histological typing of lung tumours, 2nd edn. World Health Organization, Geneva (International histological classification of tumours, no 1)

Wiedenmann B, Huttner WB (1989) Synaptophysin and chromogranins/secretogranins – widespread constituents of distinct types of neuroendocrine vesicles and new tools in tumor diagnosis. Virchows Arch B Cell Pathol 58:95–121

Wikenheiser KA, Clark JC, Linnoila RI, Stahlman MT, Whitsett JA (1992) Simian virus 40 large T antigen directed by transcriptional elements of the human surfactant protein C gene produces pulmonary adenocarcinomas in transgenic mice. Cancer Res 52:5342–5352

Yoshimoto T, Inoue T, Iizuka H, Nishikawa H, Sakatani M, Ogura T, Hirao F, Yamamura Y (1980) Differential induction of squamous cell carcinomas and adenocarcinomas in mouse lung by intratracheal instillation of benzo(a)pyrene and charcoal powder. Cancer Res 40:4301–4307

You M, Wang Y, Lineen A, Stoner GD, You L, Maronpot RR, Anderson MW (1991) Activation of protooncogenes in mouse lung tumors. Exp Lung Res 17:389–400

# Alveolar/Bronchiolar Hyperplasia, Adenoma and Carcinoma, Lung, Rat

Gary A. Boorman and Ronald A. Herbert

*Synonyms.* Alveolar/bronchiolar hyperplasia: alveolar hyperplasia, bronchioalveolar adenomatosis, pulmonary adenomatosis, alveolar epithelialization, bronchiolar-alveolar hyperplasia; alveolar/bronchiolar adenoma: pulmonary adenoma, alveolar adenoma, adenoma, bronchiolar-alveolar adenoma; alveolar/bronchiolar carcinoma: bronchiolar carcinoma, alveolar cell carcinoma, adenocarcinoma, carcinoma, bronchiolar-alveolar adenocarcinoma.

## Gross Appearance

Alveolar/bronchiolar hyperplasia is generally not visible on gross examination. It may appear as white pinpoint foci on the pleural surface. Spontaneous alveolar/bronchiolar adenomas are usually seen as solitary spherical gray to white smooth nodules on the pleural or cut surface of the lung. Typically the lesions are 1–5 mm in diameter, sharply demarcated from the surrounding lung parenchyma, and often slightly elevated above the pleural surface.

Alveolar/bronchiolar carcinomas are usually firm, pale, white to pink irregular nodules projecting from the pleural surface. These carcinomas may involve an entire lung lobe or several lobes in advanced cases. (Whereas carcinomas in man are most often found in the upper lung lobes.) Most carcinomas have a smooth tan to yellow surface. Areas of necrosis, however, can appear as yellow to white caseous foci within the tumor. Hemorrhage within the tumor mass results in brown to red discoloration.

## Microscopic Features

Alveolar/bronchiolar hyperplasia appears as poorly circumscribed areas of increased cellularity (Fig. 197). The increased cellularity is due to proliferation of cuboidal cells lining the alveoli; an increase in intraluminal macrophages is often present (Fig. 198). The cuboidal cells comprising the hyperplastic alveolar epithelium usually resemble normal type II pneumocytes with little atypia and few mitotic figures. Important characteristic features are the lack of compression at the margins (Fig. 197) and retention of normal alveolar architecture within the lesion (Fig. 198). At the margins the hyperplastic cuboidal epithelium extends along contiguous alveoli (Fig. 199). As the hyperplasia progresses, the lining cells may become multilayered or form papillary projections into the lumen.

Alveolar/bronchiolar adenomas appear as focal solid areas of increased cellularity obliterating the underlying alveolar architecture (Fig. 200). They are sharply demarcated from the surrounding pulmonary tissue (Fig. 201) and often compress the adjacent alveolar parenchyma. These adenomas contain scant connective tissue, few blood vessels, and inflammatory infiltrates. In contrast to hyperplasia of these cells, in which cells appear to grow along existing alveolar surfaces, cells of the adenoma form glandular, papillary, or solid patterns. In the glandular pattern the cells are cuboidal to tall columnar, enclose a central lumen (Fig. 202), and exhibit moderate cellular atypia. Mitotic figures may be common. In these adenomas with a papillary pattern the cells are often oblong and form papillary projections supported by a fibrovascular core. Neoplastic cells may grow in a solid pattern (Fig. 203). The cells in

▶

**Fig. 197.** (*upper left*) Focal bronchiolar/alveolar hyperplasia, lung, rat. The pleural surface is not raised, adjacent lung is not compressed, and the underlying alveolar pattern can be seen throughout the lesion. H&E, ×120

**Fig. 198.** (*upper right*) Bronchiolar/alveolar hyperplasia, lung, rat. Alveolar surfaces are lined by a continuous layer of plump cuboidal cells. Much of the increased cellularity is due to free intraluminal cells, which appear to be pulmonary macrophages. H&E, ×200

**Fig. 199.** (*below*) Bronchiolar/alveolar hyperplasia, lung, rat. At the margin of the lesion the hyperplastic cells extend partially into contiguous alveoli. No compression or distortion of adjacent alveoli; hyperplastic cells lining the alveoli are uniform with little cellular atypia, are more basophilic, and contain few mitotic figures. The intraluminal erythrocytes are not a usual feature, and their presence is considered to be an agonal event. H&E, ×400

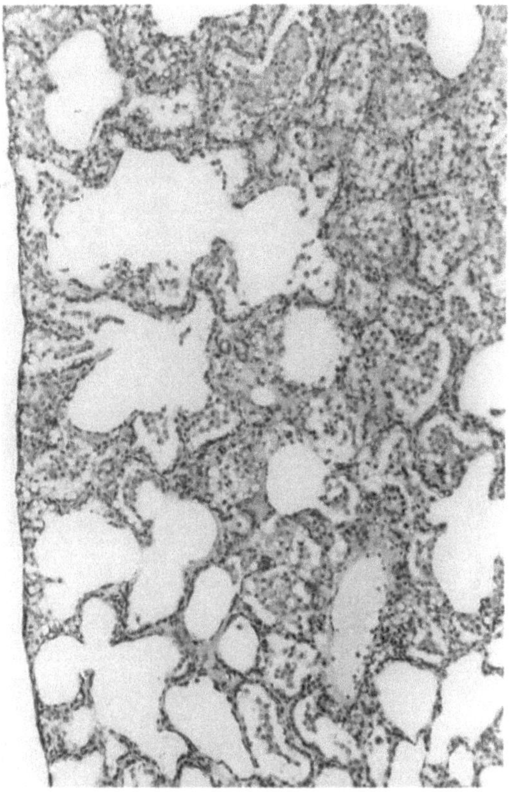

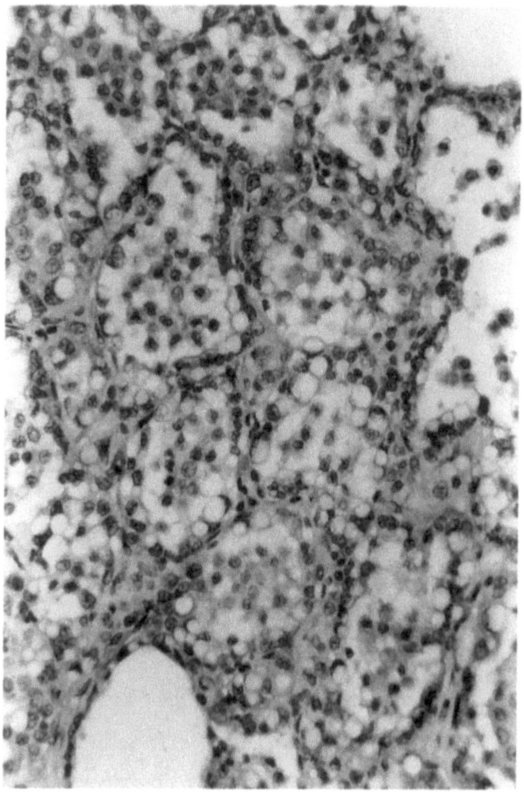

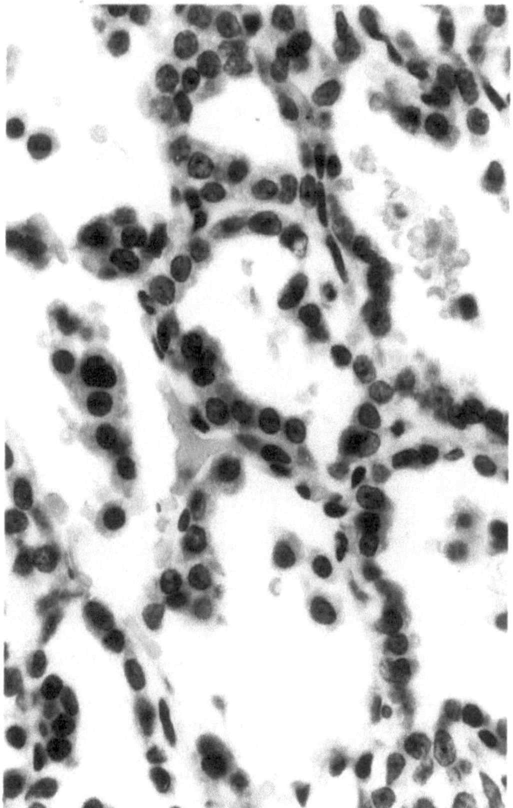

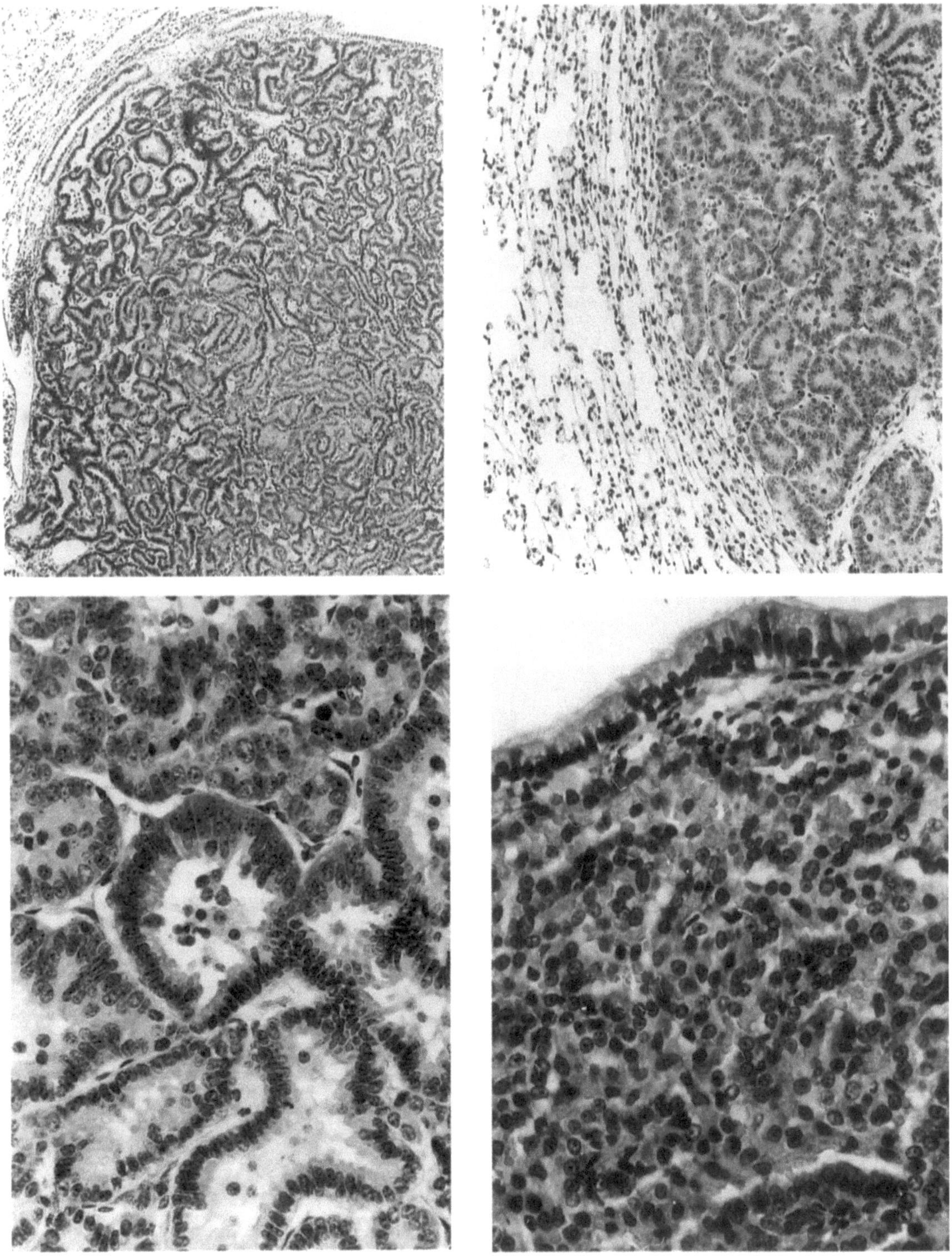

**Fig. 200.** (*upper left*) Bronchiolar/alveolar adenoma, lung, rat. A well-circumscribed lesion with a glandular pattern. H&E, ×300

**Fig. 201.** (*upper right*) Bronchiolar/alveolar adenoma with a glandular pattern. The nuclei form serpentine rows, and the cells tend to surround lumina. H&E, ×300

**Fig. 202.** (*lower left*) Bronchiolar/alveolar adenoma that is sharply demarcated from surrounding parenchyma. There is collapse and compression of the adjacent alveoli. H&E, ×100

**Fig. 203.** (*lower right*) Bronchiolar/alveolar adenoma with a solid pattern. The cells are round and have moderate cytoplasm, poorly defined cell boundaries, and few mitotic figures. The underlying alveolar architecture is not discernible. H&E, ×240

these areas are often round. Their nuclei vary in size and may exhibit mild atypia. In general cells in these adenomas are fairly uniform and have moderate amount of cytoplasm and poorly defined cell borders. In routine hematoxylin and eosin sections these tumor cells usually appear more basophilic than adjacent alveolar epithelial cells. Important features of these neoplasms are distinct borders, compression of adjacent alveolar parenchyma, and obliteration of the underlying architecture (Boorman and Eustis 1990).

Spontaneous alveolar/bronchiolar carcinomas are usually solitary masses that tend to occur in the peripheral regions of the lung (Fig. 204). The neoplasms are usually poorly circumscribed and invade the pleura, vessels, airways, or adjacent parenchyma (Fig. 205). Solid, papillary, glandular, or heterogenous patterns of growth may be observed. Well-differentiated carcinomas usually have a papillary pattern and can be difficult to distinguish from adenomas (Fig. 206). The cells of poorly differentiated neoplasms can be quite pleomorphic and may be spindle shaped. Invasion of adjacent tissue, cellular pleomorphism, and anaplasia are features of malignancy. Poorly differentiated neoplasms often incite a scirrhous response. Squamous metaplasia may be observed in some carcinomas (Fig. 207). Even when squamous metaplasia is extensive, the diagnosis of alveolar/

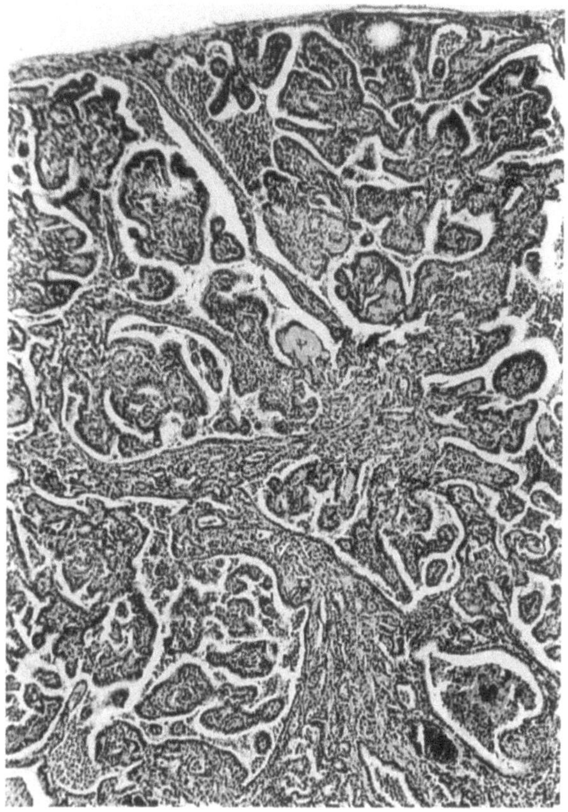

**Fig. 204.** Bronchiolar/alveolar carcinoma obliterating normal alveolar architecture. H&E, ×120

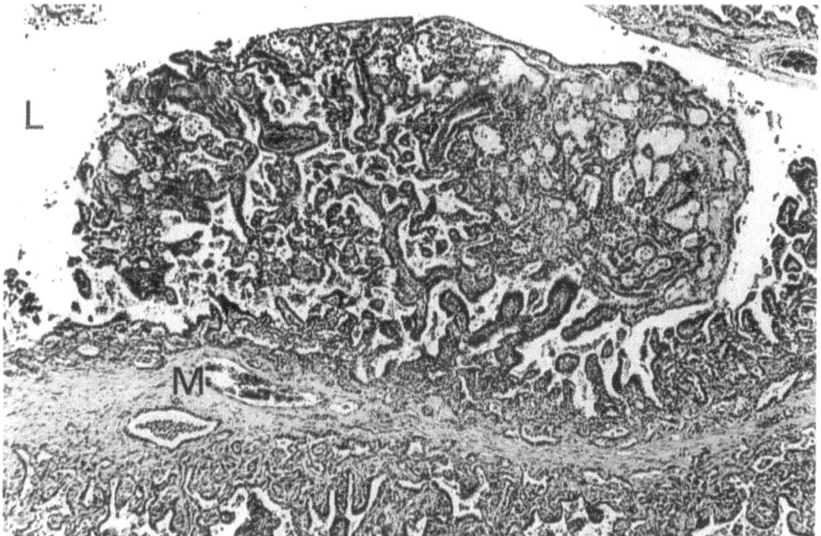


**Fig. 205.** Cells of bronchiolar/alveolar carcinoma invading wall of large bronchus. *L*, Lumen of bronchus; *M*, smooth muscle of bronchus. H&E, ×120

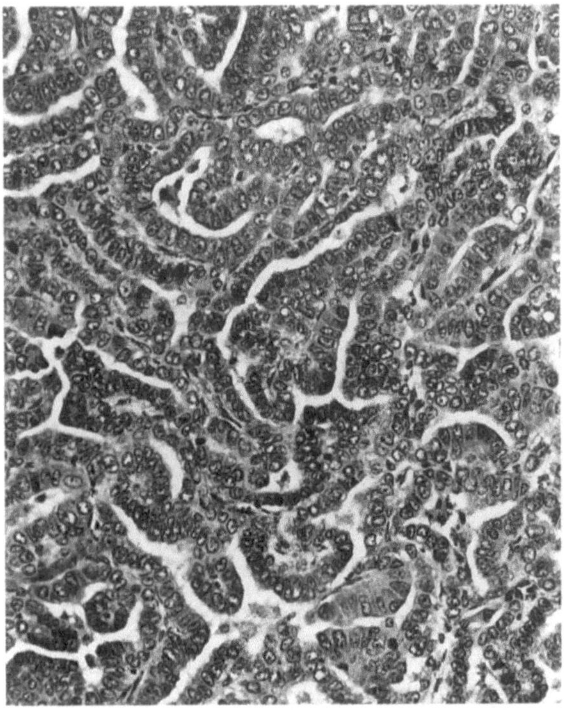

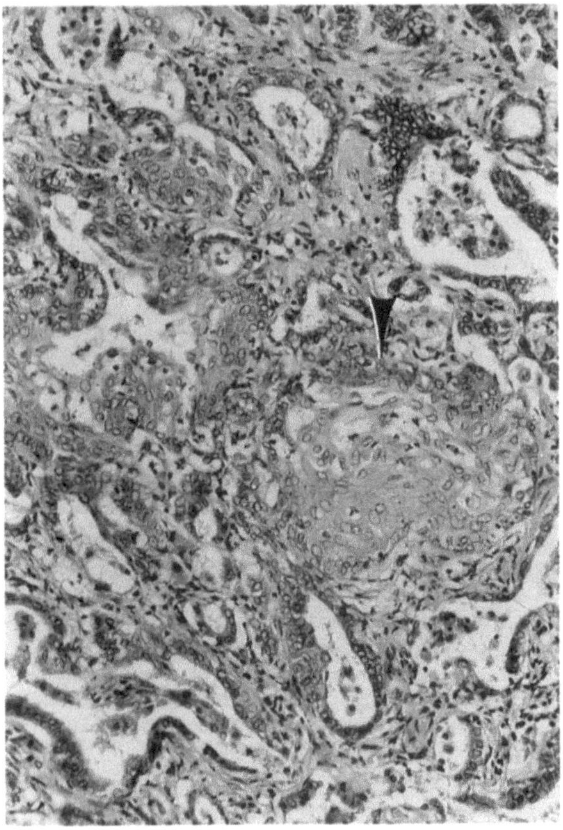

**Fig. 206.** (*above*) Alveolar/bronchiolar adenoma with a glandular pattern. The nuclei form rows and the cells tend to surround lumina. H&E, ×150

**Fig. 207.** (*below*) Bronchiolar/alveolar carcinoma with area of squamous metaplasia (*arrowhead*). H&E, ×200

bronchiolar carcinoma is appropriate if the neoplasm appears to be of alveolar/bronchiolar origin (Boorman and Eustis 1990).

## Ultrastructure

Ultrastructural examination of a limited number of spontaneous alveolar/bronchiolar adenomas and carcinomas suggests that many may originate from type II cell pneumocytes (Boorman and Eustis 1990) although occasional Clara cells may be seen within the tumors. Nitrosamine or plutonium-induced alveolar/bronchiolar adenomas and carcinomas in the F344 rat are characterized by the presence of osmiophilic cytoplasmic lamellar inclusions (Fig. 208), indicating that these tumors are also of type II cell origin (Reznik-Schüller and Gregg 1981; Reznik-Schüller and Reznik 1982; Herbert et al. 1994). Cells with ultrastructural features of Clara cells, ciliated cells, mucous cells, or cells of the amine precursor uptake and

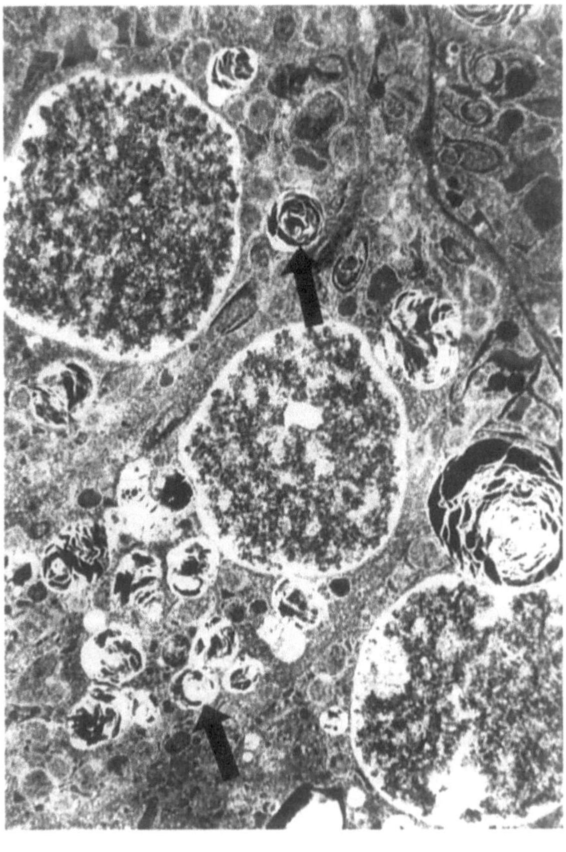

**Fig. 208.** Alveolar/bronchiolar carcinoma with cells containing lamellar bodies (*arrows*) characteristic of type II cells. TEM × approximately 10000

decarboxylation type (APUD) have not been found in these induced neoplasms.

## Differential Diagnosis

The use of standardized criteria applied in a uniform fashion is critical for comparisons of dose groups within a study, when making structure/activity inferences, evaluating different routes of exposure, and comparing relative hazards of chemicals evaluated in different studies. There is morphological evidence for progression from focal alveolar/bronchiolar cell hyperplasia to adenoma and carcinoma in rats (Boorman and Eustis 1990). Clear distinction between these categories may sometimes be difficult. Small foci of alveolar/bronchiolar hyperplasia can usually be distinguished from adenomas of similar cells. However, the distinction becomes more difficult with large foci of hyperplasia since there appears to be a gradual progression from focal hyperplasia to adenoma and finally to obvious carcinoma with local invasion, extension into the plural, or mediastinal space and metastases. Some of the diagnostic difficulty stems from the lack of significant cytological differences between hyperplastic cells and cells of these adenomas. Thus structural features and growth patterns are used to distinguish the two lesions. In hyperplasia the alveolar architecture is essentially retained. The margins of the lesion are not well defined, and the hyperplastic cells grow along the basement membrane of adjacent alveolar septa (Fig. 197). In contrast to focal hyperplasia, adenomas have more complex and/or solid patterns of growth in which the original alveolar architecture of the lung is lost (Boorman and Eustis 1990). The margin of adenomas is more discrete, and compression of the adjacent alveolar parenchyma may be seen (Fig. 201). Intraluminal macrophages and perivascular accumulations of lymphocytes are more commonly associated with areas of hyperplasia.

Alveolar/bronchiolar adenomas may also be difficult to distinguish from carcinomas involving similar cells. However, separating benign and malignant lesions is useful in characterizing the response to a chemical exposure and allows a more reasoned judgment of the potential hazard of the chemical. Size is important for distinguishing carcinomas since many neoplasms greater than 1 cm in diameter have areas of local invasion. Often at the margin of the lesion neoplastic cells can be found invading the airways, pleura, or blood vessels (Boorman and Eustis 1990). These carcinomas can often be distinguished by the scirrhous response that they incite. The occurrence of individual neoplastic cells separated by collagen fibers at the margins of the lesion is an important diagnostic criterion. Some chemically induced carcinomas may be quite anaplastic.

Alveolar/bronchiolar carcinomas must also be differentiated from squamous cell carcinomas which may arise in the lung. In man carcinomas showing features of both squamous cell carcinoma and adenocarcinoma behave as adenocarcinomas (WHO 1982). Neoplasms with features of alveolar/bronchiolar carcinoma should be diagnosed as such and the diagnosis of squamous cell carcinoma reserved only for neoplasms that appear to be comprised entirely of squamous cells.

## Biological Features

Spontaneous alveolar/bronchiolar hyperplasia is not an uncommon finding in toxicology studies (Table 11). Several cell types contribute to the development of focal alveolar/bronchiolar hyperplasia. The normal alveolar epithelium is comprised of two cell types, type I and type II pneumocytes. Type I pneumocytes are very thin, flattened cells which cover about 90% of the alveolar surface (Pinkerton et al. 1982). The remaining lining cells are type II pneumocytes, which are normally located at the junction of alveolar septa. Type II pneumocytes are cuboidal and contain cytoplasmic osmiophilic lamellar inclusions which are the source of lung surfactant (Kauffman 1980). Injury to the alveolar epithelium resulting in necrosis of type I pneumocytes stimulates the proliferation of type II pneumocytes to replace the

**Table 11.** Bronchiolar/alveolar hyperplasia in F344 rats

| Study type[a] | Males | Females |
|---|---|---|
| Gavage | 7/249 (2.8%) | 4/248 (1.6%) |
| Other | 4/198 (2.0%) | 3/200 (1.5%) |
| Total | 11/447 (2.5%) | 7/448 (1.6%) |

[a] Incidence rates from control groups. Animals in gavage studies received corn oil 5 ml/kg, five times/week for 104 weeks. Includes data from nine NTP technical reports issued through 1983.

damaged epithelium (Evans et al. 1975; Mason et al. 1977; Bocking et al. 1981). Hyperplasia is a normal response to lung injury and contributes to repair of the epithelial surface.

Cells of the terminal bronchiole may also proliferate and migrate into centriacinar alveoli in response to lung injury (Aso et al. 1976; Boorman et al. 1994). Cells of the intrapulmonary airways that have regenerative capability and possibly contribute to foci of hyperplasia include nonciliated bronchiolar (Clara) cells, Kulchitsky (APUD) cells, and ciliated cells (Jeffery and Reid 1975). This process is known as bronchiolization and is different from the focal hyperplasia that occurs spontaneously. Exposure to bleomycin results in the appearance of ciliated cells in alveoli (Kauffman 1980; Bowden 1985; p. 252, this volume), exposure to ozone causes hyperplasia of nonciliated cells (Boorman et al. 1980, 1994), and exposure to nitrosamine results in increases of Clara and APUD cells in the alveoli (Kauffman et al. 1979). Thus a variety of cell types in the lung have the potential to proliferate and may be found in areas of hyperplasia. However, type II pneumocytes have a higher mitotic potential (Dormans 1983) and are the major cell type in most areas of hyperplasia. It needs to be emphasized however, that with specific chemical exposures, for example, bleomycin (Kauffman 1980; see Bowden, p. 265, this volume), other cell types may play a more important role.

As in hyperplasia, spontaneous and chemically induced adenomas in the rat are likely to be of type II cell origin (Reznik-Schüller and Gregg 1981). Alveolar/bronchiolar adenomas are uncommon as spontaneous lesions in Fischer 344 rats. In 2-year toxicology studies 1.3% of untreated males (2.3% incidence in corn oil gavage controls) and only 0.8% in female F344 rats (either gavage or untreated controls) have alveolar/bronchiolar adenomas (Haseman et al. 1990). The incidence of neoplasms of the lung is also low in other rat strains (Table 12). In the National Toxicology Program (NTP) 2-year toxicity and carcinogenicity studies only 14 chemicals have been carcinogenic based on the occurrence of lung neoplasms (Table 13). Chemical carcinogenic studies positive for lung neoplasms have not shown a clear sex difference (there have been three studies in male rats, five in female rats, and six in which both male and female rats were positive for lung neoplasms). There is clearly a greater probability of inhalation studies being positive for lung neoplasms; of 450 long-term studies (30 of

**Table 12.** Naturally occurring bronchiolar/alveolar tumors in rats

| Strain | Sex | *n* | Age | Tumors[a] | | Reference |
|---|---|---|---|---|---|---|
| | | | | Adenomas | Carcinomas | |
| ACI/N | M | 55 | Life span | 0 | 0 | Maekawa and Odashima (1975) |
| ACI/N | F | 209 | Life span | 0 | 0 | Maekawa and Odashima (1975) |
| F344 | M | 2305 | 24 mo | 35 (1.5) | 18 (0.8) | Haseman et al. (1984) |
| F344 | F | 2354 | 24 mo | 20 (0.9) | 9 (0.4) | Haseman et al. (1984) |
| F344 | M | 3877 | 24 mo | 70 (1.8) | 45 (1.2) | Haseman, Eustis & Arnold (1990) |
| F344 | F | 3919 | 24 mo | 32 (0.8) | 13 (0.3) | Haseman, Eustis & Arnold (1990) |
| F344 | M | 160 | Life span | 0 | 0 | Sass et al. (1975) |
| F344 | F | 192 | Life span | 0 | 0 | Sass et al. (1975) |
| Holtzman-SD | M/F | 268 | 24 mo | 0 | 0 | MacKenzie and Garner (1973) |
| Oregon | M/F | 673 | 24 mo | 0 | 1 (0.1) | MacKenzie and Garner (1973) |
| Osborne-Mendel | M | 975 | 24 mo | 4 (0.4) | 5 (0.5) | Goodman et al. (1980) |
| Osborne-Mendel | F | 970 | 24 mo | 2 (0.2) | 3 (0.3) | Goodman et al. (1980) |
| Sherman | M | 60 | 24 mo | 0 | 0 | Kociba et al. (1974) |
| Sherman | F | 60 | 24 mo | 0 | 0 | Kociba et al. (1974) |
| Sprague-Dawley | M | 85 | 24 mo | 1 (1.2) | 1 (1.2) | Kociba et al. (1978) |
| Sprague-Dawley | F | 86 | 24 mo | 0 | 0 | Kociba et al. (1978) |
| Sprague-Dawley | M | 655 | Life span | 2 (0.3)[b] | 2 (0.3)[b] | Ross and Bras (1965) |
| Wistar | M | 472 | 30 mo | 0 | 1 (0.2) | Kroes et al. (1981) |
| Wistar | F | 457 | 30 mo | 0 | 0 | Kroes et al. (1981) |
| Wistar | F | 290 | Life span | 0 | 0 | Boorman and Hollander (1973) |

[a] Total tumors found (%).

[b] All tumors found in the 210 animals receiving high-protein diet.

**Table 13.** Chemicals inducing lung neoplasms in F344/N rats

| NTP TR[a] | Chemical | Sal[a] | Route | Male | Female | Other sites[b] |
|---|---|---|---|---|---|---|
| 452 | 2,2-Bis(bromomethyl)-1,3-propanediol | + | Feed | P | N | Yes |
| 405 | C. 1. acid red 114 | + | Water | N | P | Yes |
| 210 | 1,2-Dibromoethane | + | Inhal. | N | P | Yes |
| 390 | 3,3'-Dimethylbenzidine dihydrochloride | + | Water | P | P | Yes |
| 287 | Dimethyl hydrogen phosphite | +/? | Gavage | P | N | Yes |
| 329 | 1,2-Epoxybutane | + | Inhal. | P | N | Yes |
| 271 | HC blue 1 | + | Feed | N | P | Yes |
| 448 | Isobutyl nitrite | + | Inhal. | P | P | Yes |
| 451 | Nickel oxide | NT | Inhal. | P | P | Yes |
| 453 | Nickel subsulfide | ? | Inhal. | P | P | Yes |
| 118 | 5-Nitroacenaphthene | + | Feed | P | P | Yes |
| 421 | Talc | NT | Inhal. | N | P | Yes |
| 386 | Tetranitromethane | + | Inhal. | P | P | No |
| 160 | 2,4,5-Trimethylaniline | + | Feed | N | P | Yes |

NTP TR, National Toxicology Program Technical Report number; +, positive result with or without induction; ?, uncertain finding; NT, chemical not tested; P, positive for carcinogenicity in the lung; N, negative for carcinogenicity in the lung.
[a] Results of Salmonella assay for mutagenicity.
[b] Positive for carcinogenicity at sites other than the lung.

which were by inhalation) 7/14 studies in which the chemical was administered by inhalation were carcinogenic for lung neoplasms. The most dramatic positive chemical was tetranitromethane, which caused a nearly 100% incidence of lung neoplasms in both male and female rats (a similarly high percentage was found in both sexes of mice; Bucher et al. 1991). It is interesting to note that nearly all chemicals which induced lung neoplasms in rats were mutagenic in *Salmonella* and with the exception of tetronitromethane, also induced neoplasms at sites other than the lung.

Morphologically, alveolar/bronchiolar carcinomas appear to represent a progression of the alveolar/bronchiolar adenomas. The exact biological behavior has not been established. Whether some lesions are malignant from inception or undergo malignant changes over time is also not known. Using direct sequencing, mutations at codon 12, 13, or 61 of the K-*ras* proto-oncogene were not detected in 24 adenocarcinomas induced by beryllium metal in the rat (Nickell-Brady et al. 1994). A more sensitive assay detected codon 12 mutations in only 2 of 12 tumors, suggesting that activation of the K-*ras* proto-oncogene is both a rare and late event in these neoplasms in the rat (Nickell-Brady et al. 1994). Mutant p53 nuclear immunoreactivity has not been observed in any beryllium-induced neoplasms, indicating that the mechanisms underlying the development of beryllium-induced lung neoplasia in rats do not involve the gene dysfunction commonly associated with human non-small-cell lung cancer (Nickell-Brady et al. 1994).

Alveolar/bronchiolar carcinomas arise in rats exposed to inert particulate compounds such as talc (NTP 1993) and titanium dioxide (Lee et al. 1985). The mechanism of this effect is not known, but rats appear to be more prone to develop lung neoplasms induced by inert dusts than other species since mice exposed to the same concentrations do not have an increased incidence of pulmonary neoplasms (NTP 1993).

Almost all neoplasms of the lung of rats appear to be of the alveolar/bronchiolar type. One rat was reported to have a mucinous bronchiolar carcinoma characterized by tall columnar cells and mucus production analogous to the human acinar adenocarcinoma (Yang and Grice 1965). In rats spontaneous neoplasms rarely arise in the bronchi. When these neoplasms become large, they can be difficult to distinguish from alveolar/bronchiolar carcinomas which have a low tendency to metastasize (Boorman and Eustis 1990). Only one metastasis was reported in 21 carcinomas of the lung found in 3099 female and female F344 rats (Goodman et al. 1980).

## Comparison with Other Species

In man alveolar/bronchiolar carcinoma is one of the least common of the primary lung neoplasms, accounting for only 5% of the total cases (Greenberg 1982). Although the cell of origin has been controversial, it appears that both the Clara cell and the type II pneumocytes can give rise to this neoplasm (Lieber et al. 1976; Singh et al. 1981; Dermer 1982; Greenberg 1982). In the mouse alveolar/bronchiolar adenomas and carcinomas are quite common but vary with the strain (Maronpot et al. 1986; Belinsky et al. 1993). These arise from both Clara cells and type II pneumocytes (Kauffman 1981; Rehm et al. 1988, 1994). The incidence of spontaneous neoplasms of the lung in Syrian golden hamsters is less than 0.5% (Mohr 1982). Chemically induced neoplasms in the hamster are usually either alveolar cell adenocarcinoma or squamous cell carcinomas which are believed to arise from the bronchi and alveolar cells (Mohr 1982). In both the dog and the cat neoplasms of the lung are quite uncommon. Approximately 75% of the lung neoplasms are classified as adenocarcinoma. Many may arise in bronchi and bronchioles. In one report only 26/171 neoplasms of the lung in the dog and 5/47 in the cat were considered to be of alveologenic origin (Moulton et al. 1981).

## References


Aso Y, Yoneda K, Kikkawa Y (1976) Morphologic and biochemical study of pulmonary changes induced by bleomycin in mice. Lab Invest 35:558–568

Bowden DH (1985) Bleomycin-induced injury, mouse: a model for pulmonary fibrosis. In: Jones TC, Mohr U, Hunt RD (eds) Monograph on pathology of laboratory animals, respiratory system. Springer, Heidelberg, New York, Berlin pp 160–166

Belinsky SA, Stefanski SA, Anderson MW (1993) The A/J mouse lung as a model for developing new chemointervention strategies. Cancer Res 53:410–416

Bocking A, Mittermayer C, von Deimling O (1981) Urethane-induced lung hyperplasia: carboxylesterase isozymes as markers in lung pathology. Lab Invest 44:138–143

Boorman GA, Eustis SL (1990) Lung. In: Boorman, GA, Eustis SL, Elwell MR, Montgomery CA, MacKenzie WF (eds) Pathology of the Fischer rat, chap 21. Academic, San Diego, pp 339–367

Boorman GA, Hollander CF (1973) Spontaneous lesions in the female WAG/Rij (Wistar) rat. J Gerontol 28:152–159

Boorman GA, Schwartz LW, Dungworth DL (1980) Pulmonary effects of prolonged ozone insult in rats. Morphometric evaluation of the central acinus. Lab Invest 43:108–115

Boorman GA, Hailey R, Grumbein S, Chou BJ, Herbert RA, Goehl T, Mellick PW, Roycroft JH, Haseman JK, Sills R (1994) Toxicology and carcinogenesis studies of ozone and ozone/4-(N-nitrosomethylamino)-l-(3-pyridyl)-l-butanone in Fischer-344/N rats. Toxicol Pathol 22:545–554

Bucher JR, Huff JE, Jokinen MP, Haseman JK, Stedham M, Cholakis JM (1991) Inhalation of tetranitromethane causes nasal passage irritation and pulmonary carcinogenesis in rodents. Cancer Lett 57:95–101

Dermer GB (1982) Origin of bronchioloalveolar carcinoma and peripheral bronchial adenocarcinoma. Cancer 49:881–887

Dormans JA (1983) The ultrastructure of various cell types in the lung of the rat: a survey. Exp Pathol 24:15–33

Evans MJ, Cabral LJ, Stephens RJ, Freeman G (1975) Transformation of alveolar type II cells to type I cells following exposure to NO2. Exp Mol Pathol 22:142–150

Goodman DG, Ward JM, Squire RA, Paxton MB, Reichardt WD, Chu KC, Linhart MS (1980) Neoplastic and nonneoplastic lesions in aging Osborne-Mendel rats. Toxicol Appl Pharmacol 55:433–447

Greenberg SD (1982) Histology and ultrastraucture of bronchioloalveolar carcinoma. In: Shimosato Y, Melamed MR, Nettesheim P (eds) Morphogenesis of lung cancer. CRC, Boca Raton, pp 121–145

Haseman JK, Huff JE, Boorman GA (1984) Use of historical control data in carcinogenicity studies in rodents. Toxicol Pathol 12:126–135

Haseman JK, Eustis SL, Arnold J (1990) Tumor incidences in Fischer 344 rats: NTP historical data. In: Boorman GA, Eustis SL, Elwell MR, Montgomery CA, MacKenzie WF (eds) Pathology of the Fischer rat, chap 35. Academic, San Diego, pp 339–367

Herbert RA, Stegelmeier BS, Gillett NA, Rebar AH, Carlton WW, Singh G, Hahn FF (1994) Plutonium-induced proliferative lesions and pulmonary epithelial neoplasms in the rat: immunohistochemical and ultrastructural evidence for their origin from type II pneumocytes. Vet Pathol 31:366–374

Jeffery PK, Reid L (1975) New observations of rat airway epithelium: a quantitative and electron microscopic study. J Anat 120:295–320

Kauffman SL (1980) Cell proliferation in the mammalian lung. Int Rev Exp Pathol 22:131–191

Kauffman SL (1981) Histogenesis of the papillary Clara cell adenoma. Am J Pathol 103:174–180

Kauffman SL, Alexander L, Sass L (1979) Histologic and ultrastructural features of the Clara cell adenoma of the mouse lung. Lab Invest 40:708–716

Kociba RJ, McCollister SB, Park C, Torkelson TR, Gehring PJ (1974) 14-Dioxane I results of a 2-year ingestion study in rats. Toxicol Appl Pharmacol 30:275–286

Kociba RJ, Keys DG, Beyer JE, Carreon RM, Wade CE, Dittenber DA, Kalnins RP, Frauson LE, Park CN (1978) Results of a two-year chronic toxicity and oncogenicity study of 2,3,7,8-tetrachlorodibenzo-p-dioxin in rats. Toxicol Appl Pharmacol 46:279–303

Kroes RJM, Garbis-Berkvens JM, de Vries T, van Nesselrooy HJ (1981) Histopathological profile of a Wistar rat stock including a survey of the literature. J Gerontol 36:259–279

Lee KP, Trochimowicz HJ, Reinhardt DF (1985) Pulmonary response of rats exposed to titanium dioxide (Ti02) by inhalation for two years. Toxicol Appl Pharmacol 79:179–192

Lieber M, Smith B, Szakal A, Nelson-Rees W, Todaro G (1976) A continuous tumor-cell line from a human lung carcinoma with properties of type II alveolar epithelial cells. Int J Cancer 17:62–70

MacKenzie WF, Garner FM (1973) Comparison of neoplasms in six sources of rats. J Natl Cancer Inst 50:1243–1257

Maekawa A, Odashima S (1975) Spontaneous tumors in ACI/N rats. J Natl Cancer Inst 55:1437–1445
Maronpot RR, Shimkin M, Witschi HP, Smith LH, Cline JM (1986) Strain A mouse pulmonary tumor test results for chemicals previously tested in the National Cancer Institute carcinogenicity tests. J Natl Cancer Inst 76:1101–1112
Mason RJ, Dobbs LG, Greenleaf RD, Williams MC (1977) Alveolar type II cells. Fed Proc 36:2697–2702
Mohr U (1982) Tumours of the respiratory tract. In: Turusov V, Mohr U (eds) Pathology of tumours in laboratory animals: tumours of the hamster, 1st edn. IARC Scientific, Lyon, pp 115–146
Moulton JE, von Tscharner C, Schneider R (1981) Classification of lung carcinomas in the dog and cat. Vet Pathol 18: 513–528
National Toxicology Program (NTP) (1993) Toxicology and carcinogenesis studies of talc (CAS NO 14807-96-6) in F344/N rats and B6C3Fl mice (inhalation studies). Research Triangle Park, NC, United States Department of Health and Human Services Public Health Service National Institutes of Health (NTP technical report, no 421)
Nickell-Brady C, Hahn FF, Finch GL, Belinsky SA (1994) Analysis of K-ras p53 and c-raf-1 mutations in beryllium-induced rat lung tumors. Carcinogenesis 15:257–262
Pinkerton KE, Barry BE, O'Neil JJ, Raub JA, Pratt PC, Crapo JD (1982) Morphologic changes in the lung during the lifespan of Fischer 344 rats. Am J Anat 164:155–174
Rehm S, Ward JM, ten Have-Opbroek AAW, Anderson LM, Singh G, Katyal SL, Rice JM (1988) Mouse papillary lung tumors transplancentally induced by N-nitrosoethylurea: evidence for alveolar type II cell origin by comparative light microscopic, ultrastructural, and immunohistochemical studies. Cancer Res 48:148–160
Rehm S, Ward JM, Sass B (1994) Tumours of the lungs. In: Turusov V, Mohr U (eds) Pathology of tumours in laboratory animals: tumours of the mouse, 1st edn. IARC Scientific Publications, Lyon, pp 325–355
Reznik-Schüller HM, Gregg M (1981) Pathogenesis of lung tumors induced by n-nitrosoheptamehtyleneimine in F344 rats. Virchows Arch A Pathol Anat Histopathol 393:333–343
Reznik-Schüller HM, Reznik G (1982) Morphology of spontaneous and induced tumors in the bronchioloalveolar region of F344 rats. Anticancer Res 2:53–57
Ross M, Bras HG (1965) Tumor incidence patterns and nutrition in the rat. J Nutr 87:245–260
Sass B, Rabstein LS, Madison R, Nims RM, Peters RL, Kelloff GJ (1975) Incidence of spontaneous neoplasms in F344 rats through out the natural life span. J Natl Cancer Inst 54:1449–1456
Singh G, Katyal SL, Torikata C (1981) Carcinoma of type II pneumonocytes. Am J Pathol 102:195–208
World Health Organization (WHO) (1982) Histological typing of lung tumors neoplasma. 29:111–123
Yang YH, Grice HC (1965) Mucinous bronchiolar carcinoma of the rat lung: a case report. Can J Comp Med 29:15–17

# Naturally Occurring Pulmonary Tumors in Rodents

S. Rittinghausen, Donald L. Dungworth, Heinrich Ernst, and Ulrich Mohr

## Introduction

The development of naturally occurring lung tumors is related to aging. In rats, mice, and hamsters younger than 12 months naturally occurring pulmonary tumors are exceedingly rare. The majority of them are found in animals older than 20 months. Even then the prevalence in rats and Syrian hamsters is very low whereas in certain strains of mice pulmonary tumors occur quite frequently. The interpretation of long-term animal studies resulting in primary neoplasms of the respiratory tract requires classification of tumors. Because most long-term studies are carried out in rats, the recent literature contains more reports on classification and description of lung tumors for this species.

In rats and Syrian hamsters little is known about the pathobiology of naturally occurring lung tumors, in part because of their infrequent occurrence. In mice more research on naturally occurring lung neoplasms has been carried out, particularly on bronchioloalveolar tumors, and immunohistochemical methods for the identification of cells of alveolar type II or Clara cell origin have been established (Rehm et al. 1991a, 1994). Nevertheless, most descriptions of lung tumors are based on studies of induced neoplasms.

## Classification

A standardized World Health Organization classification for pulmonary tumors of the rat was published in 1992 for international use under the auspices of the International Agency for Research on Cancer (Dungworth et al. 1992). For mice a modified classification is being developed and will be published in the near future (Dungworth et al., in preparation). For Syrian hamsters descriptions have been recently published (Mohr et al. 1995).

The various types of primary pulmonary neoplasms and their occurrence in the various laboratory rodent species are listed in Table 14. In the lung of laboratory rodents bronchioloalveolar tumors, adenosquamous carcinomas, and squamous cell carcinomas are the most frequently observed naturally occurring neoplasms. Cystic keratinizing epitheliomas (squamous cysts) and nonkeratinizing epitheliomas have been described only in the rat lung, and naturally occurring cases are extremely rare. Pulmonary neuroendocrine tumors have been reported only after administration of carcinogens (Blair 1974; Schüller et al. 1988), and only in the Syrian hamster have they been studied by immunohistochemical or ultrastructural investigations. The model for induction of neuroendocrine lung tumors in the hamster, however, has not been confirmed (Witschi and Schüller 1991).

In addition to epithelially derived tumors, any of the vascular, connective, supporting, and nerve tissues of the respiratory tract can conceivably give rise to primary tumors. Therefore mesenchymal tumors and other tumors such as malignant schwannomas may occur in the respiratory tract. All these neoplasms are named according to the apparent cell of origin. Another category are undifferentiated tumors, which should be divided if possible into "not otherwise specified carcinomas and sarcomas."

In addition to primary tumors, metastases may occur in the lung and are in fact found here more frequently than primary pulmonary tumors.

**Table 14.** Classification and occurrence of primary pulmonary tumors in laboratory rodents

| Histological tumor types | Rat | Mouse | Syrian hamster |
|---|---|---|---|
| Papilloma, bronchial/bronchiolar | + | + | + |
| Adenocarcinoma, bronchial/bronchiolar | + | + | + |
| Adenoma, bronchioloalveolar | + | + | + |
| Carcinoma, bronchioloalveolar | + | + | + |
| Epithelioma, cystic keratinizing | + | − | − |
| Epithelioma, nonkeratinizing | + | ? | ? |
| Carcinoma, squamous cell | + | + | + |
| Carcinoma, Adenosquamous | + | + | + |
| Tumor, neuroendocrine, malignant[a] | + | ? | + |
| Undifferentiated tumors | | | |
| Carcinoma, not otherwise specified | + | + | + |
| Sarcoma, not otherwise specified | + | + | + |
| Mesenchymal tumors | + | + | + |

[a]Neuroendocrine lung tumors have been described in literature in treated animals only. In both rats and hamsters their experimental induction still needs to be confirmed.

## Gross Appearance

Primary neoplasms in the lungs of rodents are often seen at the pleural or cut surface. Smooth, white to grayish or yellow-brownish, solitary or multiple, spherical or irregular nodules may be visible. Small tumors may not be detected with the unaided eye, but larger ones are often elevated above the pleural surface and can fill much of the thorax. The consistency of the tumors is firm to soft. Whereas bronchioloalveolar tumors frequently show a glistening smooth cut surface, or in the case of necrosis cavities filled with reddish-brown hemorrhagic material, the cut surface of squamous cell tumors is often drier, firmer, and more granular or, in the case of extensive central keratinization and necrosis, partly soft and cystic with yellowish or reddish-brown contents.

The most common gross pattern of pulmonary tumor metastases is that of multifocal, well-circumscribed lesions that vary in size from small miliary nodules to large nodular masses. Another picture is that of diffuse infiltration of the lung which may be caused by systemic tumors such as malignant lymphomas. Pleural effusion may occur in association with malignant primary and secondary pulmonary tumors.

The presence of one larger lesion, possibly with smaller satellites, requires careful macroscopic and microscopic examination of all organs and tissues to provide the best chance to differentiate between a metastasis and a primary pulmonary tumor.

## Descriptions

### Papilloma, Bronchial/Bronchiolar

*Synonyms.* Papilloma of the bronchus; bronchial squamous cell papilloma; bronchiogenic papilloma; bronchial adenoma; bronchial papillary adenoma; papillary adenoma arising in a bronchiole; bronchogenic adenoma; bronchial adenomatoid tumor; mucoepidermoid papilloma; papillary polyp; adenomatous polyp.

*Species.* Papillomas of the distal bronchi or bronchioles rarely occur in rats. They are more frequently observed in mice and Syrian hamsters.

*Microscopic Features.* Papillomas in general undergo exophytic growth. In rare cases tumors may grow beneath the mucosal surface ("inverted" or "endophytic" papilloma). Papillomas are characterized by papillary structures composed of peripheral epithelial cells resting on a vascularized connective tissue stalk (Fig. 209). The basement membrane is intact. The bronchial or bronchiolar lumen may be partly or, rarely, completely obstructed. There may be growth by expansion into alveolar parenchyma. Proliferating cells can migrate into the alveolar parenchyma either at the end of a terminal bronchiole or through pores in its wall. Sometimes papillomas are composed of

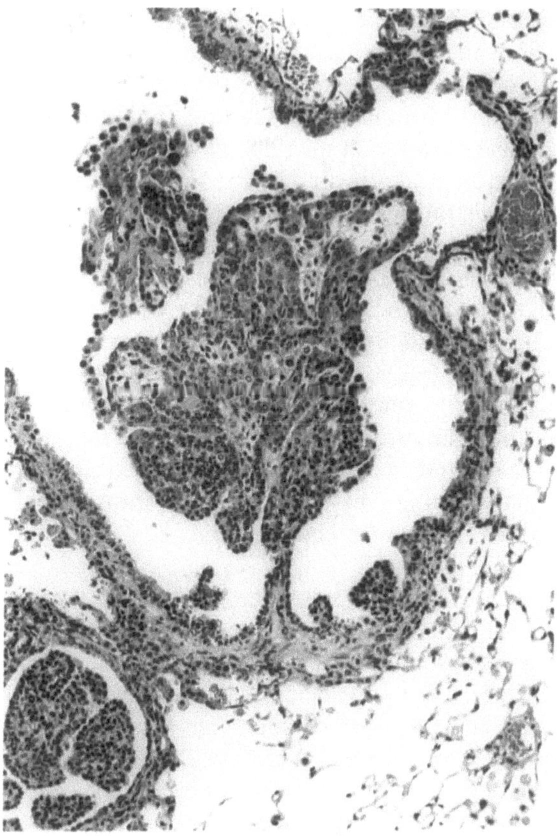

**Fig. 209.** Papilloma, bronchiolar, bronchiolus, NMRI mouse. Partial obstruction of the bronchiolar lumen by a papilloma of respiratory epithelial type. H&E, ×130

transitional epithelial or mucous cells. Mitotic figures are rare and when present are limited to the basal layers of the epithelium.

*Papilloma, Respiratory Epithelial Type.* The surface epithelium of respiratory epithelial type papillomas consists of cuboidal or columnar cells.

*Papilloma, Squamous Cell Type.* Squamous cell papillomas are covered by squamous cells which may contain only keratohyalin granules, but occasionally they produce excessive amounts of keratin.

*Papilloma, Mixed Type.* These papillomas have a surface covered by various proportions of squamous and cuboidal or columnar respiratory epithelium. Well-differentiated mucous cells are sometimes seen in the intermediate layers.

*Comment.* Bronchial papillomas lined by uniform cuboidal to columnar cells and those crowded papillary structures that mimic a glandular pattern are sometimes referred to as bronchial adenomas. In mice the morphological structure of respiratory epithelial type papillomas originating in bronchioles may be identical to bronchioloalveolar adenomas with papillary growth pattern originating in the lung parenchyma. In Syrian hamsters adenomas are occasionally observed in the lung which are composed of mucus-producing cylindrical cells on branched delicate connective tissue septa, which probably originated in the epithelium of a large bronchus (Pour 1983).

*Ultrastructure.* In mice the bronchial papillomas arising in peripheral bronchioles have ultrastructural features of Clara cells (Kauffman 1981). Clara cell features may also be found in papillary adenomas arising from bronchioles and alveolar ducts (Sato and Kauffman 1980). These exophytic papillary tumors may be classified as papillomas of the bronchi or bronchioles.

## Adenoma, Bronchioloalveolar, Lung

*Synonyms.* Pulmonary adenoma, alveologenic adenoma, type II cell adenoma.

*Species.* Rat, mouse, Syrian hamster.

*Microscopic Features.* At low magnification there are well circumscribed areas of high epithelial cell density, usually with strongly convex borders. The underlying alveolar architecture is obscured to various degrees. They are sharply demarcated from the surrounding tissue (Fig. 210). The neoplastic epithelial cells are relatively uniform.

In rats and Syrian hamsters bronchioloalveolar adenomas may have an alveolar, papillary, solid, tubular, or mixed growth pattern. In mice solid, alveolar, papillary, and mixed growth patterns have been described. The alveolar growth pattern is characterized by glandular structures composed of cuboidal or columnar cells which enclose a central lumen. There is only slight cellular atypia. Nuclei are often ovoid. Tumors with solid growth pattern are composed of uniform cells with moderate amounts of cytoplasm and ill-defined borders. The nuclei are round and of variable size. Papillary growth is characterized by prominent papillary fronds. Elongated lumina or prominent tubular profiles represent the tubular growth pattern. Tumors of mixed type contain different growth patterns in the same neoplasms. In bronchioloalveolar adenomas mitotic figures are mostly rare or absent. Small foci of mild atypia may be present. In these foci cells tend to have a higher degree of pleomorphism, and the number of mitoses is slightly increased. Occasionally bronchioloalveolar adenomas extend into adjacent bronchioles.

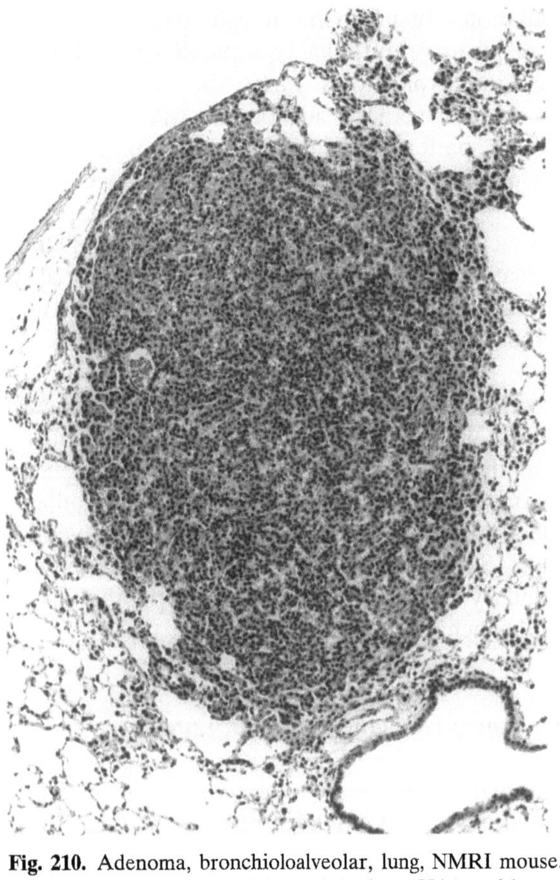

**Fig. 210.** Adenoma, bronchioloalveolar, lung, NMRI mouse. Nodular growth in the periphery of the lung. H&E, ×85

*Comment.* Although ultrastructural and histochemical evaluations can sometimes distinguish between tumors of bronchiolar (Clara cell) origin and alveolar type II cell origin, this is not always possible. This, and the uncertainty of differentiation by routine histology, is why the classification "bronchioloalveolar" is retained. Clear differentiation between bronchioloalveolar hyperplasia and bronchioloalveolar adenoma, as well as between bronchioloalveolar adenoma and bronchioloalveolar carcinoma, is sometimes arbitrary. Because bronchioloalveolar adenomas can develop from bronchioloalveolar hyperplasia, and transitional stages may be observed, there is no way of definitively separating borderline proliferations into hyperplasia versus adenoma.

In mice papillary neoplasms are more frequently associated with malignant features than are solid neoplasms (Rehm et al. 1988; Dixon et al. 1991). The histological growth patterns vary between the different strains (Gunning et al. 1991; Thaete et al. 1991). The histological growth pattern and the number and size of induced tumors depend on the age of the mice when a carcinogen is administered (Anderson and Budinger 1981; Branstetter et al. 1988; Branstetter and Moseley 1991). Compression of the surrounding lung parenchyma is present as an artifact in immersion-fixed lung but is not a significant feature in lungs fixed at near normal volume by intratracheal infusion of fixative (Dungworth et al. 1992).

*Ultrastructure.* The presence of small, lamellated osmiophilic bodies in the cytoplasm indicates that the active proliferating cells in the neoplasms have characteristics of alveolar type II cells, which may be the cell of origin of adenomas arising in the alveoli (Sato and Kauffman 1980; Reznik-Schüller et al. 1981; Reznik-Schüller and Reznik 1982; Rehm et al. 1989; Dixon et al. 1991).

In nitrosamine-treated Syrian hamsters osmiophilic lamellar bodies have also been found in induced tumors which derived from bronchial or bronchiolar Clara cells (Schüller 1987). Presence of Clara cells may suggest a bronchiologenic tumor origin.

*Differential Diagnosis.* In contrast to bronchioloalveolar adenomas, bronchioloalveolar hyperplasias are less well defined, segmental (cone-shaped) lesions with apex at terminal bronchiole. They are composed of single layers of epithelial cells lining the alveolar ducts and alveoli distal to bronchioles without significant distortion of pulmonary architecture unless they are accompanied by scarring and/or inflammation. In hyperplastic lesions prominent papillary proliferations or complete filling of alveoli by epithelial cells are generally absent. If signs of malignancy, such as frequent mitoses, and/or cellular atypia, invasion into surrounding tissues or beyond the visceral pleura, lymphatics, vessels, and/or bronchi, and/or metastases are present, the tumors must be classified as bronchioloalveolar carcinomas.

## Epithelioma, Cystic Keratinizing, Lung

*Synonyms.* Tumor, squamous cell, keratinizing, cystic, benign, squamous cyst.

*Species.* This tumor type has been observed in only rats and not in Syrian hamsters or mice. Naturally occurring cases are seen only incidentally. After inhalation of aerosols containing particles higher incidences are frequent.

*Microscopic Features.* Cystic keratinizing epitheliomas are formed by a sharply demarcated, mostly highly keratinized squamous epithelium. In the center of the tumor mass are usually large amounts of keratin and necrotic tumor tissue (Fig. 211). The epithelium may be flattened to a thin layer of squamous cells, especially adjacent to pleura or interstitium surrounding bronchioles and vessels. Growth occurs mostly by peripheral extension into the alveolar spaces (Fig. 212).

▶

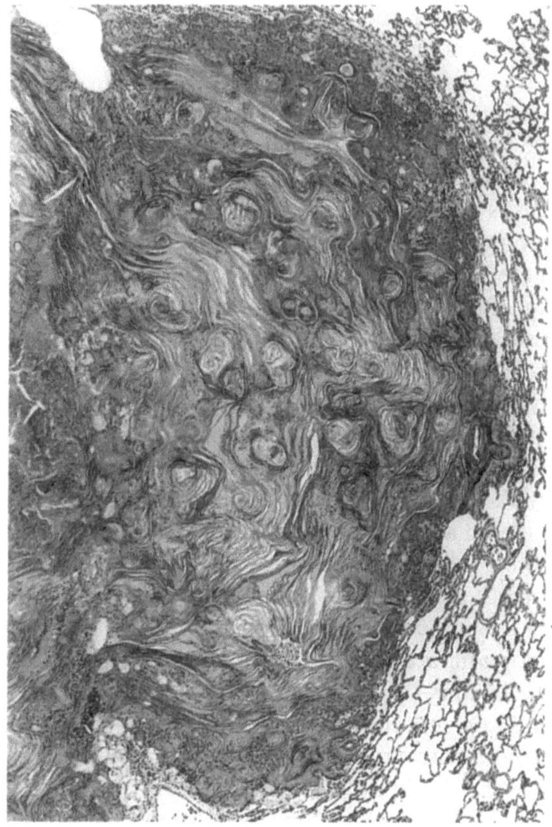

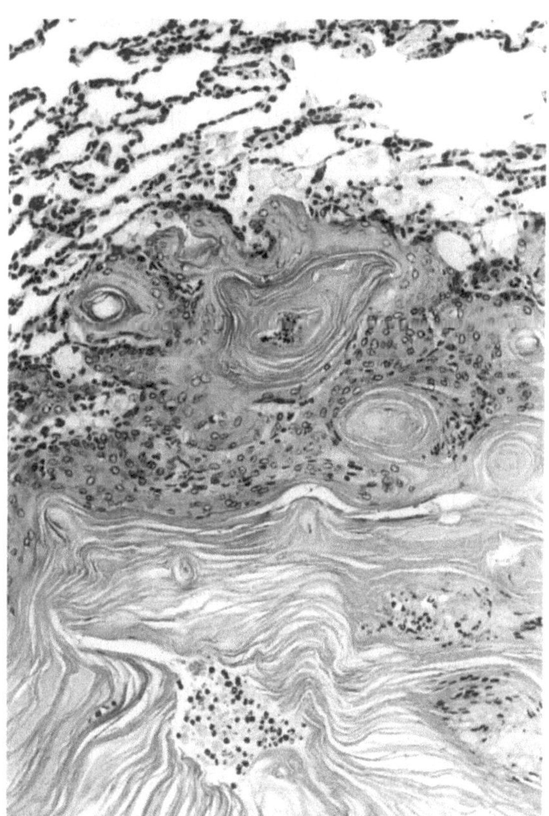

**Fig. 211.** (*above*) Epithelioma, cystic keratinizing, lung, rat. Keratin filling the central parts of the tumor. H&E, ×30

**Fig. 212.** (*below*) Epithelioma, cystic, keratinizing, lung, rat. Higher magnification, periphery of the tumor in Fig. 211. H&E, ×145

Mitoses are rarely seen and then only in the basal cell layers of the epithelium.

*Comment.* In the literature many different names are found for these benign cystic tumors, ranging from squamous or epidermal cysts (Boorman and Eustis 1990; Schwartz et al. 1991) to inverted papilloma to squamous cell carcinoma. Currently there is debate about the exact nature of the squamous cell proliferation. Because of the location and pattern of growth within the pulmonary parenchyma it does not appear to be simply hyperplasia, and across a variety of experimental studies there is a continuum from the benign cystic lesion to invasive squamous cell carcinomas (Mohr and Dungworth 1988; Mohr et al. 1990a; Kittel et al. 1993; Emura and DaCosta 1993). Main points of evidence indicating active centrifugal growth and presence of cells having some degree of regulatory defect consistent with benign neoplasia are that the growth of the cysts is predominantly by peripheral infiltration and the presence of cell clusters on the periphery of some tumors with up to four mitotic figures per high-power field. In experimental studies the growth of the cystic lesions occurs after a long lag period, and this strongly favors the need for one or more additional events before cystic growth is manifest (Dungworth et al. 1994).
Clear differentiation between epithelioma and well-differentiated squamous cell carcinoma is sometimes arbitrary, as it is between exaggerated squamous cell metaplasia and cystic keratinizing epithelioma.

*Ultrastructure.* Desmosomes are a major feature of squamous cells, although not as frequent as in normal squamous epithelia. Characteristic ultrastructural features include also the presence of short tonofilament bundles. In the cytoplasm polyribosomes and mitochondria are numerous. Cell nuclei are unimorphous with irregular distribution of heterochromatin and presence of some perichromatin granules. Frequent nuclear pores are found. Intercellular spaces are comparatively small. The intercellular junctions include desmosomes. Basal laminae are present between squamous cells and stroma (Nolte 1991).

*Differential Diagnosis.* In contrast to cystic keratinizing epitheliomas, squamous cell metaplasia tends to be multifocal. Metaplasias are small in size and preserve the normal pulmonary architecture. If the normal pulmonary architecture is distorted by a squamous cell proliferation, but there is evidence of neither malignancy nor keratinization, the diagnosis of benign nonkeratinizing epithelioma should be made. In the case of malignant behavior, which may be expressed in destruction of the basement membrane, cellular atypia and disorientation, frequent mitoses, invasion (into the interstitium, vessels, or pleural surfaces), and/or distant metastasis the tumors must be classified as squamous cell carcinomas.

## Epithelioma, Nonkeratinizing, Lung

*Synonyms.* Tumor, squamous cell, nonkeratinizing, benign epithelioma.

*Species.* In the rat the nonkeratinizing epithelioma is separated from the cystic keratinizing epithelioma because, although rare, it appears as a distinct entity and has a malignant counterpart. In mice and Syrian hamsters naturally occurring epitheliomas have not yet been described.

*Microscopic Features.* At low magnification nonkeratinizing epitheliomas are small, nodular lesions caused by filling of alveoli by squamous cells (Fig. 213). The cells towards the periphery of the involved alveoli have small, round to oval nuclei and little cytoplasm (basaloid appearance). The centrally located cells tend to have more abundant, finely granular eosinophilic cytoplasm and inconspicuous intercellular bridges. Mitoses are rarely seen. There is little or no evidence of keratinization.

*Ultrastructure.* Results of electron microscopic examinations of pulmonary nonkeratinizing epitheliomas have not been published to date.

*Differential Diagnosis.* In contrast to epitheliomas, squamous cell metaplasias tend to be multifocal, are small in size, and conform with the normal pulmonary architecture. Benign squamous cell tumors with large amounts of keratin and necrotic tumor cells in the center of the mass should be classified as cystic keratinizing epitheliomas. In the case of malignant behavior the tumors are classified as squamous cell carcinomas.

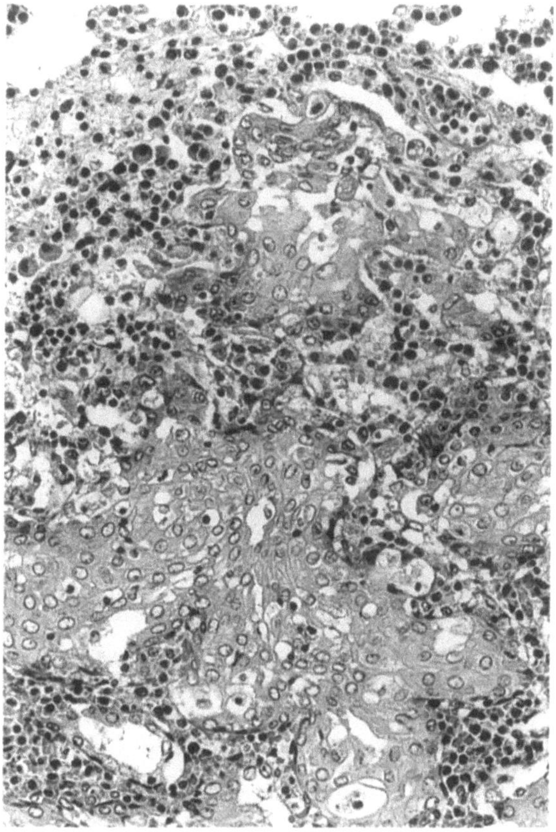

**Fig. 213.** Epithelioma, nonkeratinizing, lung, rat. Alveoli filled by masses of squamous cells and monocytes/macrophages. H&E, ×210

## Adenocarcinoma, Bronchial

*Synonyms.* Bronchiolar carcinoma, bronchial carcinoma, bronchogenic adenocarcinoma, bronchial adenocarcinoma, bronchial papillary carcinoma.

*Species.* Spontaneous malignant adenomatous neoplasms originating from bronchioles are uncommon in rodents. In rats and mice they can be induced by administration of carcinogens or by radiation.

*Microscopic Features.* The neoplasms clearly arise in the distal bronchi or bronchioles. The majority of bronchial carcinomas are exophytic masses composed of epithelial cells and connective tissue stroma but show evidence of invasion of the basement membrane or adjacent pulmonary structures.

*Adenocarcinoma, Bronchial, Papillary.* This is the most common type of bronchial adenocarcinoma. As their benign counterparts, the malignant neoplasms are mostly characterized by papillary structures composed of peripheral epithelial cells resting on a vascularized soft tissue stalk. The peripheral cells are cuboidal to columnar.

*Differential Diagnosis.* In mice bronchioloalveolar adenomas and carcinomas are nodular lesions which may have an alveolar, solid, papillary or mixed growth. The structure differs from that of bronchial papillary adenocarcinomas, which have a predominantly exophytic papillary growth. Whereas in bronchioloalveolar adenomas of mice pulmonary type II cell antigen can be demonstrated (Ward and Rehm 1990; Ward et al. 1985), in bronchial papillomas and papillary carcinomas Clara cell antigen is found (Rehm et al. 1991b).

## Carcinoma, Bronchioloalveolar, Lung

*Synonyms.* Adenocarcinoma, alveolar cell carcinoma, type II cell carcinoma, bronchioloalveolar adenocarcinoma.

*Species.* Rat, mouse, Syrian hamster.

*Microscopic Features.* As their benign counterparts, bronchioloalveolar carcinomas have a peripheral location in the lung. The neoplasms grow irregularly and are poorly circumscribed. They can occupy an entire pulmonary lobe. The tumors cause architectural distortion of the lung parenchyma. The tumor cells vary in appearance and organization from one region to another. In some cases the cytoplasm contains secretion granules of varying sizes. Mitotic activity is generally increased. Bronchioloalveolar carcinomas may have an alveolar (acinar), papillary, tubular, solid, or mixed growth pattern. The alveolar (acinar) growth pattern is represented by glandular structures composed of cuboidal to columnar cells which enclose a central lumen (Fig. 214). The papillary growth pattern is made up of cuboidal to tall columnar epithelium with papillary projections into the lumina (Figs. 215, 216). A tubular growth pattern contains prominent elongated profiles in section. The solid growth pattern consists of rounded cells without spaces between them. In the mixed growth pattern glandular, papillary, and solid areas in the same neoplasms are detected (Figs. 217, 218). Less well-differentiated tumors

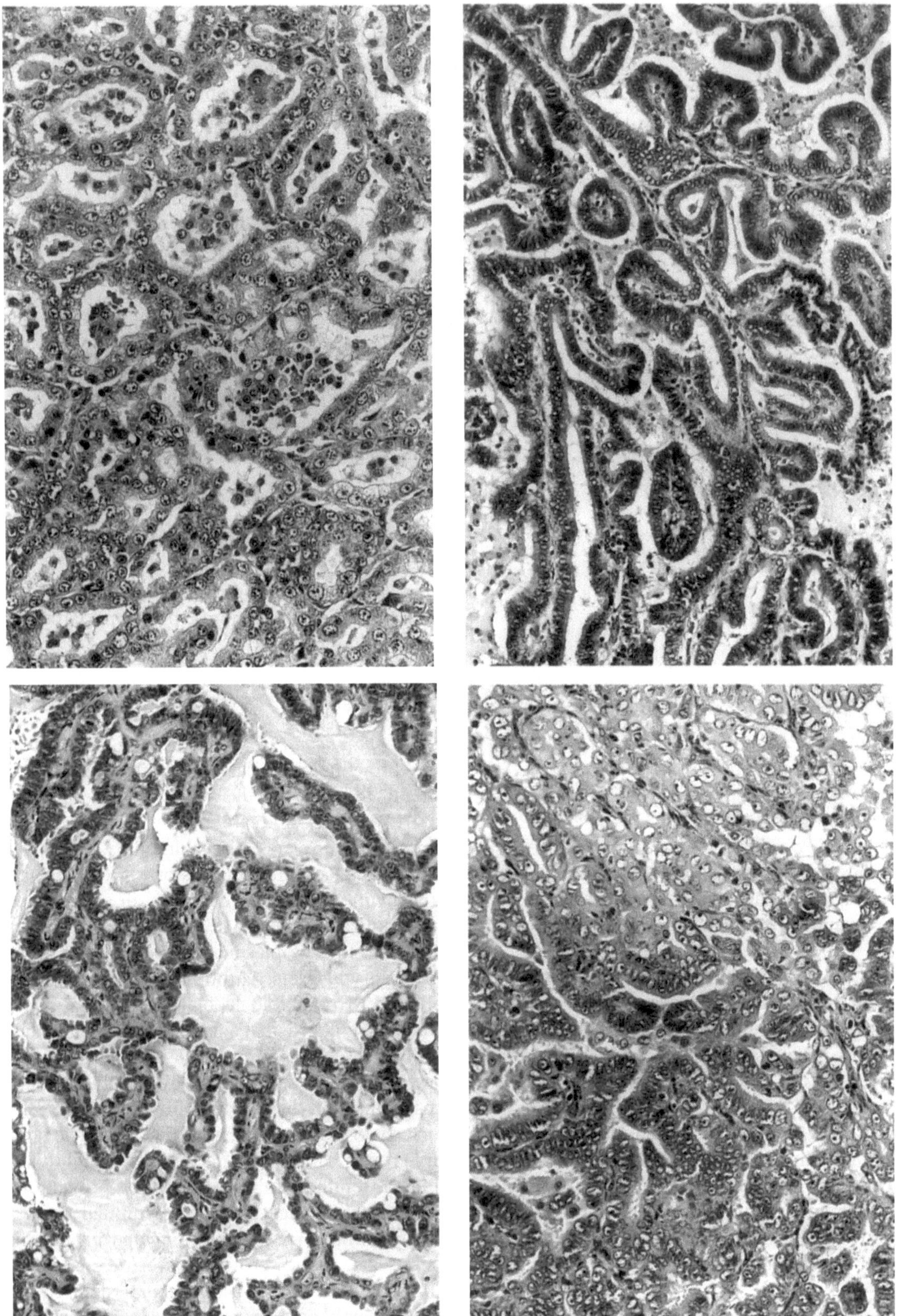

may have pleomorphic and spindle-shaped tumor cells (Figs. 219–221). Occasionally a scirrhous response is present, usually in induced neoplasms. Areas of squamous cell metaplasia may be found within a tumor. In rare cases abundant mucus production is evident (Yang and Grice 1965). Malignant behavior may be occasionally indicated by such features as invasive growth into the interstitium, lymphatics, vessels, bronchi, and pleural surfaces, or distant metastasis.

*Ultrastructure.* In rats and mice the cytoplasm of bronchioloalveolar carcinomas contains numerous small, lamellated osmiophilic bodies indicating proliferation of type II pneumocytes (Reznik-Schüller et al. 1981; Reznik-Schüller and Reznik 1982; Rehm et al. 1989; Belinsky et al. 1990). In $^{210}$Po-induced adenocarcinomas of Syrian hamsters Clara cells have been identified (Kennedy et al. 1977).

*Differential Diagnosis.* In contrast to bronchioloalveolar carcinomas, bronchioloalveolar adenomas are mostly well-circumscribed, rounded nodules with regular alveolar, papillary or solid pattern formed by uniform cells lacking significant atypia or mitoses. Bronchioloalveolar adenomas do not have malignant characteristics such as are manifested by invasive growth into the interstitium, lymphatics, vessels, or beyond the visceral pleura. If these unequivocal signs of malignancy are missing, clear differentiation between bronchioloalveolar adenoma and carcinoma is sometimes arbitrary.

If the tumors comprise significant amounts of both malignant glandular and squamous cell portions, they justify being classified as adenosquamous carcinomas.

In contrast to bronchioloalveolar carcinomas with mucus production, where immature goblet cells and multilayering are common features, mucous cell (goblet cell) metaplasia is composed of single layers of mature goblet cells lining mucus-filled spaces (Dungworth et al. 1992; Kittel et al. 1994).

Metastases to the lung from an adenocarcinoma, primary at another organ site, must be distinguished from bronchioloalveolar carcinomas. Metastases in the lung are mostly perivascular, multifocal, and usually closely resemble the histological and cellular pattern of the original primary tumor.

◀

**Fig. 214.** (*upper left*) Carcinoma, bronchioloalveolar, lung, rat. Alveolar growth pattern. H&E, ×230

**Fig. 215.** (*upper right*) Carcinoma, bronchioloalveolar, lung, rat. Papillary growth pattern. H&E, ×145

**Fig. 216.** (*lower left*) Carcinoma, bronchioloalveolar, lung, Syrian hamster. Papillary structures with columnar cells. H&E, ×120

**Fig. 217.** (*lower right*) Carcinoma, bronchioloalveolar, lung, rat. Mixed growth pattern. Note many mitotic figures. H&E, ×230

## Carcinoma, Squamous Cell

*Synonym.* Epidermoid carcinoma.

*Species.* Naturally occurring squamous cell carcinomas are detected occasionally in rats but are extremely rare in mice and Syrian hamsters.

*Microscopic Features.* Squamous cell carcinomas are composed of solid, often branching cords or masses of cells with various degrees of anaplasia (Fig. 222). The tumor cells are irregular in shape and size. They are large and polygonal or flattened and stratified. The cytoplasm is eosinophilic and granular to hyalinized due to the high keratin content. Cells may contain only keratohyalin granules, form keratin pearls, or be highly keratinized. Intercellular bridging may be prominent. The tumors may invade the pleura, vessels, bronchi, and surrounding lung parenchyma. Frequently there is marked scirrhous response to the growth of the tumor.

*Carcinoma, Squamous Cell, Keratinizing.* The amount of keratin ranges from small to abundant. Squamous cell carcinomas with a large central mass of keratin and necrotic tumor tissue appear to arise by malignant transformation in the walls of cystic keratinizing epitheliomas.

*Carcinoma, Squamous Cell, Nonkeratinizing.* These tumors are represented by nodules or small masses composed of nonkeratinizing squamous cells resembling greatly enlarged basal cells (Fig. 223). The preexisting alveolar architecture might still be evident. The cells have cytological features of malignancy (atypia, disorganization, and increased mitotic figures), but stromal or vascular invasion is not always evident.

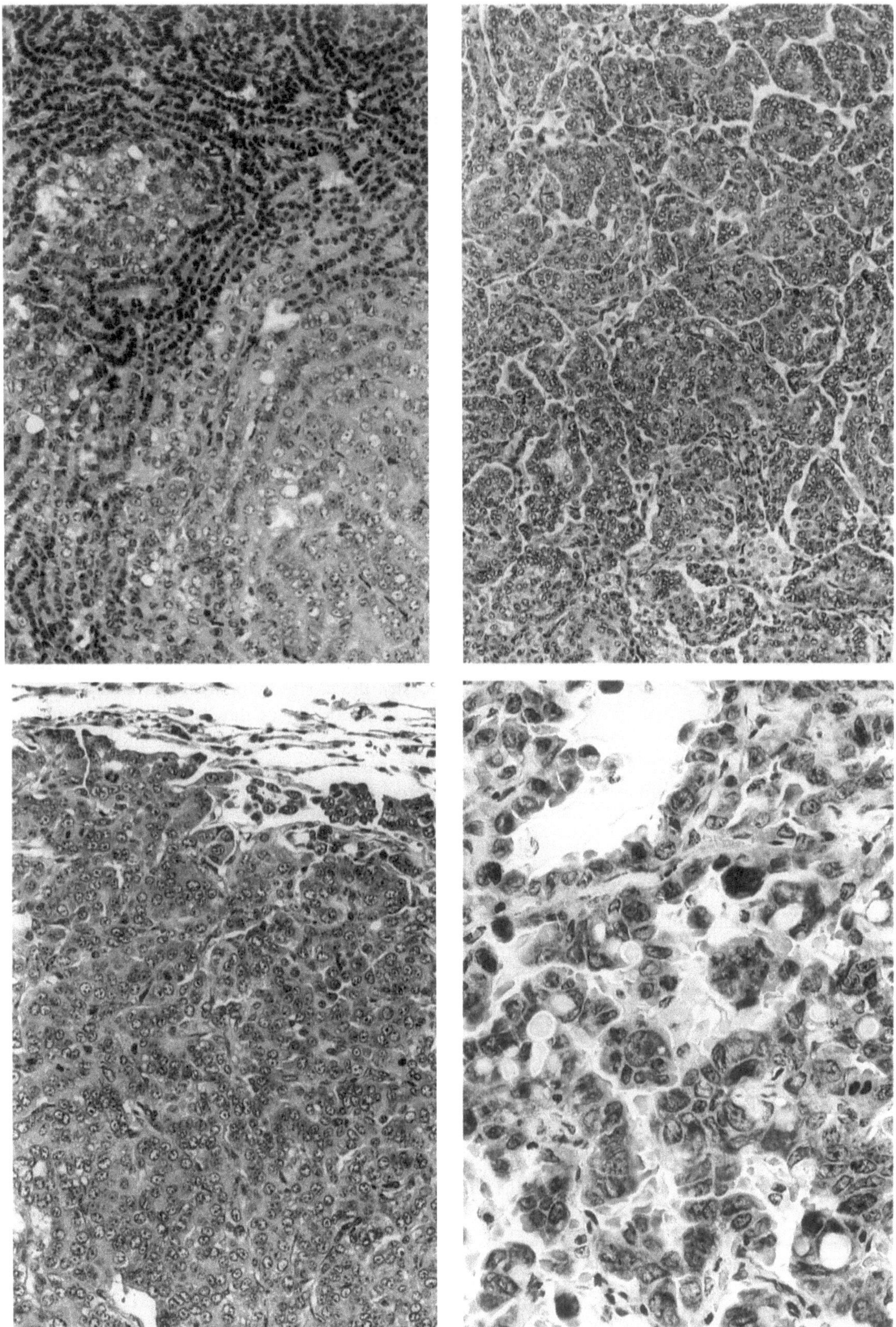

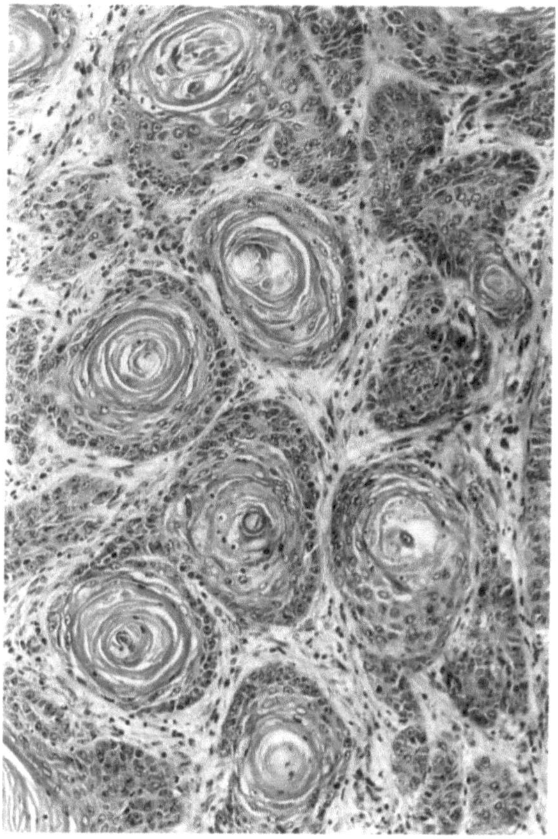

**Fig. 222.** Carcinoma, squamous cell, lung, rat. Tumor cell nests distributed in a fibrous tissue stroma. H&E, ×145

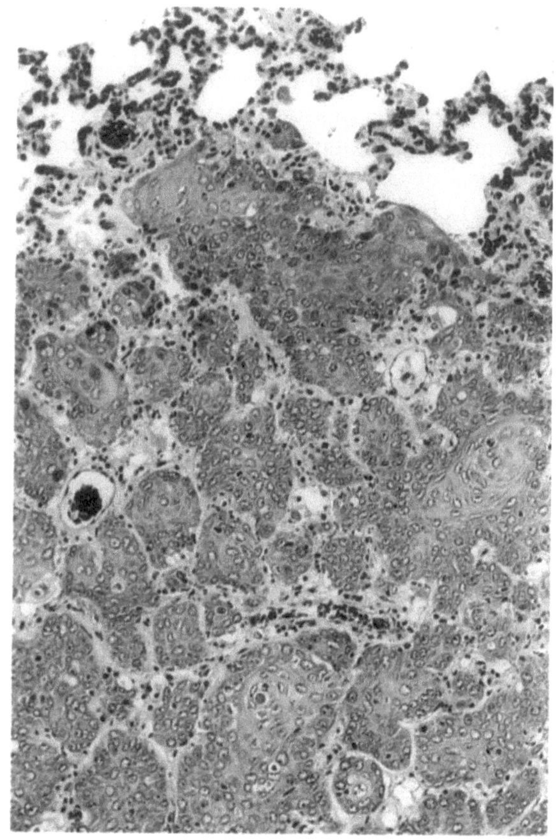

**Fig. 223.** Carcinoma, squamous cell, lung, Syrian hamster. Islands of nonkeratinized tumor cells. H&E, ×145

◄

**Fig. 218.** (*upper left*) Carcinoma, bronchioloalveolar, lung, rat. Mixed growth pattern. H&E, ×230

**Fig. 219.** (*upper right*) Carcinoma, bronchioloalveolar, lung, NMRI mouse. Less well-differentiated tumor. H&E, ×230

**Fig. 220.** (*lower left*) Carcinoma, bronchioloalveolar, lung, NMRI mouse. Pleomorphic cells invading the lung parenchyma. H&E, ×230

**Fig. 221.** (*lower right*) Carcinoma, bronchioloalveolar, lung, Syrian hamster. Area of poorly differentiated pleomorphic cells. H&E, ×300

*Comment.* Metastases to or invasion in the mediastinum are quite common features. Differentiation between epitheliomas and well-differentiated squamous cell carcinomas is sometimes arbitrary. In treated rats and Syrian hamsters the amount of keratin varies between small to abundant, whereas in mice squamous cell carcinomas usually produce only small amounts of keratin. Carcinomas containing many small basophilic cells resembling basal cells of the upper respiratory tract, which have been described in mice (Lijinsky and Reuber 1988), should be classified as squamous cell carcinomas.

*Ultrastructure.* Electron microscopy has been performed only on induced tumors. Characteristic ultrastructural features include the presence of tonofilament bundles and desmosomes. According to the degree of epithelial differentiation, tonofilament bundles are frequent and well developed, but in more anaplastic squamous cell carcinomas they are sparse and disarrayed. In the cytoplasm polyribosomes are numerous. Mitochondria tend to be sparse, and the rough endoplasmic reticulum is generally poorly developed. Cell nuclei are polymorphous with multiple nucleoli (Nolte 1991). In Syrian hamsters the presence of tonofilament bundles has been described as well as the presence of areas with dense-cored granules, the ultrastructural characteristic of neuroendocrine cells (Pour and Reznik-Schüller 1985).

*Differential Diagnosis.* In contrast to squamous cell carcinomas, squamous cell metaplasias preserve the normal pulmonary architecture and are small in size. Metaplastic lesions for the most part are multifocal. Squamous cell tumors devoid of any signs of cytological (atypia, disorganization, mitoses) or behavioral (invasion) features of malignancy may be classified as nonkeratinizing or cystic keratinizing epitheliomas, according to the amount of keratinization.

## Carcinoma, Adenosquamous

*Species.* Adenosquamous carcinomas are observed in rats, mice, and Syrian hamsters. The mucoepidermoid type develops mainly in the hamster, but in rats and mice the tumors mostly have a mixture of squamous and nonsecretary cuboidal to columnar cells (Dungworth et al. 1992; Dungworth et al., in preparation). The induction of a mucoepidermoid (adenosquamous) carcinoma in the rat is described as well (Nolte et al. 1995).

*Microscopic Features.* Adenosquamous carcinomas are characterized by significant amounts of both malignant squamous and glandular portions (Fig. 224). The squamous components of the tumors may be keratinized.

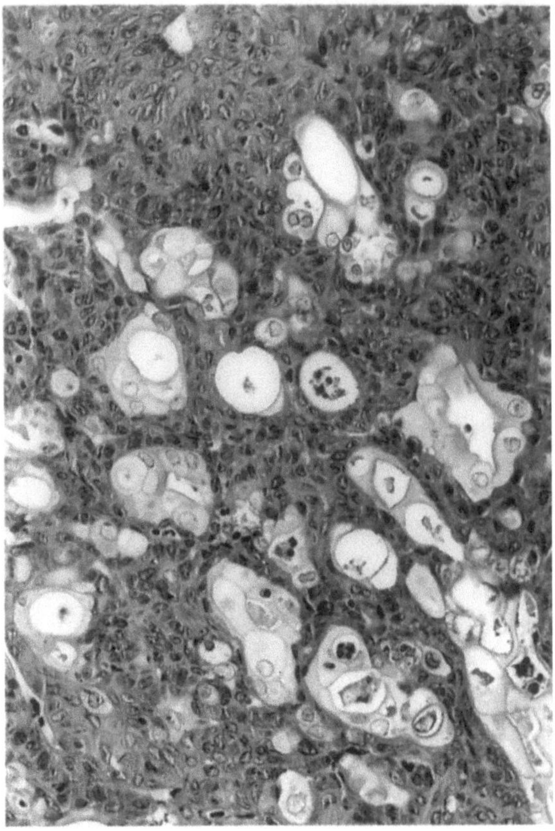

**Fig. 224.** Carcinoma, adenosquamous, lung, Syrian hamster. Tumor consisting of glandular structures and slightly keratinized squamous cells. H&E, ×230

*Carcinoma, Adenosquamous, Mucoepidermoid Type.* Tumors composed predominantly of epithelium with squamous and mucous cells in the same glandular structures are classified as mucoepidermoid carcinomas. This tumor subtype is formed by epithelial tumor cells enclosing a central lumen. The cells surrounding the lumen have all characteristics of mucous cells, and outer cell layers have features of epidermoid and basal cells. A variable number of intraepithelial cysts are filled with PAS-positive mucus substances. Mucous cells and squamous cells may also be easily distinguished by applying Kreyberg's stain.

*Comment.* The differentation between adenosquamous carcinoma and bronchioloalveolar carcinoma with squamous cell metaplasia is sometimes difficult, but in the absence of evidence of malignant characteristics in the squamous cell population a diagnosis of adenosquamous carcinoma should not be made. Conversion of cells to metaplastic and neoplastic cells may occur in the same tumor because this tumor type is assumed to develop from bronchioloalveolar carcinoma, presumably with clonal shifts to malignant squamous cell phenotype. Tumors composed predominantly of malignant squamous cells and only small numbers of cells with mucous cell characteristics should be classified as squamous cell carcinomas.

*Ultrastructure.* The tumors are composed of varying numbers of cells which ultrastructural studies reveal to have epidermoid features such as the presence of tonofilament bundles and cells which are mucus-secreting and are therefore considered to be glandular (McDowell 1987).

*Differential Diagnosis.* Bronchioloalveolar adenocarcinoma with squamous cell metaplasia has a large neoplastic glandular part with minor amounts of more regular squamous cells. Squamous cell carcinomas which may entrap bronchioles or alveoli lined by type II cells must also be distinguished. In these tumors the glandular component is composed of normal-appearing, nonneoplastic bronchiolar or type II alveolar cells entrapped and surrounded by cords of neoplastic squamous cells.

## Tumor, Neuroendocrine, Malignant

*Synonyms.* Small cell carcinoma, oat cell carcinoma, clear cell carcinoma, neuroendocrine carcinoma, carcinoid.

*Species.* Naturally occurring pulmonary neuroendocrine tumors have not been described in laboratory rodents in the literature up to now. Malignant neuroendocrine tumors of the lung have been reported to be induced in Syrian hamsters (Schüller et al. 1988) and rats (Blair 1974). Unfortunately the tumors in rats were not examined ultrastructurally or immunohistochemically, so that the diagnosis of neuroendocrine tumors in the lung needs additional verification for this species. Also, the induction of neuroendocrine tumors in hamster lungs has not been confirmed (Witschi and Schüller 1991).

*Microscopic Features.* The tumors may be located at all levels of the airways, including lobar and segmental bronchi as well as bronchiolar and alveolar areas. In hamsters the reported tumors have been highly cellular, with only occasionally glandular patterns. The cells are closely packed with little or no interstitial tissue. The arrangement of cells is generally highly irregular. Cells may be polygonal with distinct cell borders and abundant pale, finely granular cytoplasm. The chromatin of the basophilic nuclei may be marginated. Mitotic figures are often frequent. Squamous cell metaplasia may be observed. Argyrophilic neurosecretory granules in cytoplasm can be demonstrated by using Grimelius silver impregnation stain, but proper characterization requires the use of immunocytochemical and ultrastructural methods.

*Comment.* The description of microscopic diagnostic features of this tumor type is based on reports on such tumors induced in Syrian hamsters (Schüller et al. 1990). The tumors in Syrian hamsters do not have the oat cell type morphology typical of most small cell carcinomas in humans. Small cell carcinomas are common in humans and can be diagnosed in many cases by light microscopy. These tumors, which are composed of neuroendocrine cells, should therefore be regarded as malignant neuroendocrine tumors. The tumors contain immunoreactivity with calcitonin and bombesin. Neuroendocrine tumors of the larynx and trachea in the syrian hamster, have been demonstrated to contain, calcitonin, gene-related peptide, serotonin, and neuron-specific enolase (Ernst et al.; see p. 107, this volume).

*Ultrastructure.* Numerous dense-cored cytoplasmic granules, the ultrastructural hallmark of pulmonary neuroendocrine cells, should be demonstrable in all tumor cells by electron microscopy (Schüller et al. 1988). In Syrian hamsters nitrosamine-induced tumors contained dual differentiation into alveolar type II cells with lamellar bodies and neuroendocrine cells with dense-cored secretion granules (Schüller et al. 1990).

## Carcinoma, Not Otherwise Specified

*Synonyms.* Undifferentiated carcinoma, not otherwise specified carcinoma.

*Species.* Rat, mouse, Syrian hamster.

*Microscopic Features.* The term carcinoma, not otherwise specified, may be used for malignant epithelial tumors composed of small or large undifferentiated round cells, spindle cells, pleomorphic or anaplastic cells which cannot with certainty be classified by routine light microscopy under any other tumor category.

*Comment.* This term should be used only when no other is appropriate. In many instances some degree of cell differentiation can be revealed by histochemical, immunocytochemical, or electron microscopic methods.

## Mesenchymal and Nerve Tissue Tumors

*Species.* Rat, mouse, Syrian hamster.

*Microscopic Features.* The absence of epithelial components is essential to fully support the diagnosis of a primary mesenchymal neoplasm since some carcinomas may contain an extensive tumor stroma consisting of fibroblasts or other spindle cell components. Mesenchymal tumors are classified according to the apparent cell of origin. Microscopic features vary, because any of the vascular, connective, supporting, and nerve tissues of the respiratory tract conceivably can give rise to primary tumors.

Examples of mesenchymal tumors observed in the lung are hemangioma, hemangiosarcoma, fibroma, fibrosarcoma, leiomyoma, leiomyosarcoma and not otherwise specified/undifferentiated sarcoma. Malignant schwannomas (Bomhard 1992) and lipomas (Bomhard and Rinke 1994) are occasionally found in the lung of rodents.

All these tumors exhibit the same microscopic features as described for these lesions in other organs (Carlton et al. 1992).

*Comment.* There are only few reports of naturally occurring pulmonary mesenchymal neoplasms of laboratory animals in the literature. Most frequent in rats seem to be fibrosarcomas, leiomyomas, or leiomyosarcomas (Reznik 1983; Boorman and Eustis 1990). In rats primary pulmonary hemangiosarcomas are reported only as induced tumors (Hahn and Lundgren 1992).

## Metastases

*Secondary Neoplasms of the Lung.* Microscopically, metastatic tumors usually resemble the primary lesions, although they may be either better or less differentiated. Therefore metastases can easily mimic primary pulmonary tumors. In contrast to primary tumors, metastases are mostly perivascular and multifocal. Careful search may reveal tumor emboli in arteries and/or capillaries. The mere fact that metastases are found in the lung does not warrant the conclusion that this organ is not the primary site of the tumor. Especially in mice large primary adenocarcinomas of the lung tend to spread inside the organ via alveolar spaces and lymph vessels. In these cases, mostly in addition to one large tumor mass, many small tumor satellites or emboli are observed inside lymph vessels or growing into the parenchyma exhibiting the same growth pattern, and adenocarcinomas with similar growth pattern are not observed in other organs (see p. 234, this volume). In rats of the Fischer 344 strain large granular lymphocyte leukemia (malignant lymphoma) frequently involves the lung but cannot be considered as a primary lung neoplasm (Boorman and Eustis 1990). The spread of lymphomas in the lungs occurs characteristically around the bronchi, bronchioles, and vessels (Faccini et al. 1990). Relatively often metastases of osteosarcomas are also found in the lungs (Reznik 1983). In several strains of rats systemic histiocytic sarcoma (Kaspareit-Rittinghausen and Deerberg 1988; Carlton et al. 1992) are occasionally observed infiltrating the lung. Frequencies for metastases of rat are given in Table 19. Although the lung is a site of predilection for the establishment of metastases, they are relatively infrequent in most strains of rats (Rittinghausen et al. 1992). In various strains of mice malignant lymphomas and histiocytic sarcomas also affect the lungs relatively frequently (Sheldon and Greenman 1979), and metastases of osteosarcomas may often be observed (Frith et al. 1981). Furthermore, mammary gland tumors are often reported to metastasize to the lungs (Sass and Liebelt 1985). In Syrian hamsters metastases of clear cell carcinomas (neuroendocrine cell tumors) of the larynx have been described (Pour 1983).

*Metastasis of Primary Lung Tumors.* For induced lung tumors it has been shown in rats that bronchioloalveolar carcinomas tend to metastasize more frequently than squamous cell carcinomas. The primary lung tumors and their metastases exhibit mainly the same histological features, but occasionally the metastases are less differentiated than their primaries (Kamino and Mohr 1993). Metastases are found most frequently in the regional lymph nodes, but organs all over the body may be affected (Reznik-Schüller and Reznik 1982; Kamino and Mohr 1993), with kidney as one preferential site for distant metastases (Maeda et al. 1986). In mice the regional lymph nodes, chest wall, heart, kidney, and liver have been reported as preferential sites (Stewart et al. 1979; Turusov et al. 1974). Additionally, metastases occurring incidentally in the testes, prostate, pancreas, and brain have been reported (Reznik 1981).

**Biological Features**

Pathogenesis and Histogenesis

*Bronchioloalveolar Adenoma and Carcinoma.* In rodents bronchioloalveolar adenomas and carcinomas are believed to originate from Clara cells and/or alveolar type II pneumocytes.

In Fischer 344 rats, however, electron microscopy has identified only features of alveolar type II cells in naturally occurring and induced peripherally located bronchioloalveolar carcinomas (Reznik-Schüller and Reznik 1982; Belinsky et al. 1990). Using immunocytochemical methods in addition, in most cells surfactant apoprotein antigen could be demonstrated, but some neoplasms also showed focally immunoreactivity to Clara cell antigen (Ohshima et al. 1985).

These neoplasms in mice, based on immunohistochemical and/or ultrastructural investigations, are believed to originate from type II cells (Ward et al. 1985; Ward and Rehm 1990; Rehm et al. 1988, 1991a; Belinsky et al. 1992), but some authors conclude from their ultrastructural and/or histochemical investigations the possibility of an alternate origin from Clara cells (Kauffman et al. 1979; Kauffman and Sato 1985; Beer and Malkinson 1985; Thaete et al. 1987; Thaete and Malkinson 1990, 1991; Gunning et al. 1991, 1992; Dixon et al. 1991). One probable reason for these different opinions is that the phenotypic differences between Clara and type II alveolar epithelial cells becomes blurred during neoplastic transformation. It is also possible that clonal variations develop among the neoplastic population involving the extent to which Clara or type II cell phenotype is expressed.

In Syrian hamsters chemically induced adenomatous tumors in the bronchioloalveolar region have been investigated ultrastructurally. These neoplasms consist of a mixture of cells, some of which have the morphology of Clara cells, alveolar type II cells, neuroendocrine cells, or squamous cells (Schüller and McMahon 1985). Clara cells producing mature lamellar bodies have been observed as well (Reznik-Schüller 1976, 1977a, b; Ito 1985; Schüller et al. 1990). Immunocytochemical methods have demonstrated Clara cell antigen in bronchioloalveolar carcinomas of the hamster lung (Rehm et al. 1993). Ultrastructural evidence for type II cell derivation has also been found in pulmonary adenomas in Syrian hamsters (Ito et al. 1988).

*Adenosquamous Carcinoma.* Adenosquamous carcinomas in rat lungs are believed to develop from bronchioloalveolar adenocarcinomas, presumably with clonal shifts to malignant squamous cell phenotype (Dungworth et al. 1992). In Syrian hamsters there is evidence that such tumors may origin from pluripotent progenitor cells, which line the bronchi and bronchioles. Fully differentiated mucous cells or basal cells of the bronchial epithelium are being considered as a possible origin (Becci et al. 1978; McDowell 1987; McDowell and Trump 1983). Basal cells are known to give rise to squamous cells in the tracheal and bronchial epithelium of vitamin A deficient animals (McDowell et al. 1984).

*Squamous Cell Tumors.* Epitheliomas and squamous cell carcinomas originate from squamous cell metaplasia (transdifferentiation) of alveolar epithelium and/or Clara cells. Squamous cell metaplasia may occur in all locations of the airway tree, including type II cells (Adamson and Bowden 1979; Nolte et al. 1993), or fully differentiated mucous cells of the bronchi (Becci et al. 1978). Squamous cell carcinomas may develop directly from squamous cell metaplasia (Becci et al. 1978; Rehm et al. 1991b; Herbert et al. 1993) or arise by malignant transformation in the walls of cystic keratinizing epitheliomas. In Syrian hamsters chemically induced squamous cell carcinomas are found to arise from metaplasia of bronchiolar or bronchial Clara cells (Pour and Reznik-Schüller 1985) but in rats may originate from metaplasia of bronchial basal cells or bronchiolar nonciliated cells (Reznik-Schüller and Gregg 1981; Hahn 1985). In mice transdifferentiation of squamous epithelium from alveolar type II cells has been reported (Adamson and Bowden 1979). In Syrian hamsters the transition from squamous cell papilloma, which may occur in the bronchi, to squamous cell carcinoma has also been described (Mohr et al. 1995).

*Bronchial Papilloma.* Because this term combines a variety of benign lesions arising in the distal airways, different cells of origin are found.

**Table 15.** Prevalence of naturally occurring bronchioloalveolar tumors in lungs of various strains of rats: number of animals (*n*) and percentage with tumor (%)

| Strain | Study duration | Males | | Females | | Reference |
|---|---|---|---|---|---|---|
| | | *n* | % | *n* | % | |
| *F344* | | | | | | |
| F344 | 2 years | 1794 | 2.8 | 1754 | 1.7 | Goodman et al. (1979) |
| F344/DuCrj | 2 years | 296 | 7.5 | 297 | 4.7 | Maekawa et al. (1983a) |
| F344 | Life span | 529 | 2.3 | 529 | 1.3 | Solleveld et al. (1984) |
| F344 | 2 years | 2305 | 3.7 | 2354 | 2.3 | Haseman et al. (1984) |
| F344/Jcl | 2 years | 469 | 0.6 | 354 | 0.6 | Takaki et al. (1989) |
| F344 | 2 years | 1933 | 2.3 | 1974 | 1.1 | Haseman et al. (1990) |
| F344 | 2 years | 740 | – | 740 | 0.3 | Chandra and Frith (1992b) |
| *Sprague-Dawley* | | | | | | |
| Sprague-Dawley | 18 months | 179 | 1.7 | 181 | 0.6 | Prejean et al. (1973) |
| Sprague-Dawley | 2 years | 365 | 1.6 | 365 | 0.3 | Stula (1975) |
| Hap:(SD) | 24–29 months | 34 | 5.8 | – | – | Anver et al. (1982) |
| Sut:SDT | 2 years | 100 | 1.0 | 100 | 2.0 | Löhrke et al. (1982) |
| Sprague-Dawley | 2 years | 1340 | 0.4 | 1329 | 0.2 | Chandra et al. (1992) |
| Sprague-Dawley | 24–30 months | 1130 | 1.2 | 1076 | 0.4 | RITA (1995) |
| CD BR | 2 years | 880 | 0.5 | 877 | – | Compiled by Lang (1987a) |
| *Wistar* | | | | | | |
| Chbb:THOM(SPF) | 15–30 months | 600 | 1.2 | 600 | 0.6 | Ueberberg and Lützen (1979) |
| Han:WIST | Life span | 304 | 1.3 | 305 | 2.6 | Deerberg et al. (1980) |
| Wistar SPF Tox | 30 months | 192 | 0.5 | 192 | – | Kroes et al. (1981) |
| Slc:Wistar | 2 years | 98 | 8.0 | 100 | 3.0 | Maekawa et al. (1983b) |
| Wistar TNO/W.70 | 2 years | 962 | 0.1 | 968 | 0.2 | Bomhard et al. (1986) |
| BOR:WISW(SPF Cpb) | 32 months | 444 | 0.7 | 448 | 0.2 | Bomhard (1992) |
| Wistar | 24–31 months | 2147 | 1.0 | 2198 | 0.4 | RITA (1995) |
| BOR:WISW(SPF Cpb) | 2 years | 1256 | 0.3 | 1254 | <0.1 | Bomhard and Rinke (1994) |
| *Other strains* | | | | | | |
| Osborne-Mendel | 2 years | 975 | 0.5 | 970 | 0.2 | Goodman et al. (1980) |
| ACI/seg Hap BR | 24–40 months | 216 | 1.0 | – | – | Ward et al. (1983) |

RITA, Registry of Industrial Toxicology Animal-Data, Hanover, Germany.

In mice bronchial papillomas arising in peripheral bronchioles exhibit ultrastructural features of Clara cells (Kauffman 1981). Adenomas with papillary growth pattern arising from the bronchioles of mice and extending into the lung parenchyma have been shown also to have ultrastructural and histochemical features of Clara cells (Palmer 1985). Clara cell antigen has been detected immunocytochemically in chemically induced bronchial adenomatoid tumors of mice as well as in epidermoid tumors with central glandular portions (Rehm et al. 1991b).

**Table 16.** Prevalence of naturally occurring squamous cell tumors in lungs of various strains of rats: number of animals (*n*) and percentage with tumor (%)

| Strain | Study duration | Males | | Females | | Reference |
|---|---|---|---|---|---|---|
| | | *n* | % | *n* | % | |
| *F344* | | | | | | |
| F344 | 2 years | 1794 | – | 1754 | 0.1 | Goodman et al. (1979) |
| F344/DuCrj | 2 years | 296 | 0.3 | 297 | – | Maekawa et al. (1983a) |
| F344 | Life span | 529 | 0.6 | 529 | 0.2 | Solleveld et al. (1984) |
| F344/Jcl | 2 years | 469 | 0.2 | 354 | 0.3 | Takaki et al. (1989) |
| F344 | 2 years | 1933 | 0.2 | 1974 | – | Haseman et al. (1990) |
| *Sprague-Dawley* | | | | | | |
| SD-JCL | Life span | 108 | 0.9 | 128 | – | Morii and Fujii (1973) |
| SD-JCL | Life span | 77 | 1.3 | 73 | – | Muraoka et al. (1977) |
| Sut:SDT | 2 years | 100 | – | 100 | – | Löhrke et al. (1982) |
| Sprague-Dawley | 24–30 months | 1130 | – | 1076 | 0.3 | RITA (1995) |
| *Wistar* | | | | | | |
| Chbb:THOM(SPF) | 15–30 months | 600 | 1.3 | 600 | 0.8 | Ueberberg and Lützen (1979) |
| Wistar CPB | 18–30 months | 173 | 0.6 | 174 | – | Kroes et al. (1981) |
| Wistar TNO/W.70 | 2 years | 962 | 0.1 | 968 | – | Bomhard et al. (1986) |
| BOR:WISW(SPF Cpb) | 2 years | 1256 | <0.1 | 1254 | – | Bomhard and Rinke (1994) |
| *Other strains* | | | | | | |
| Osborne-Mendel | 2 years | 975 | 0.1 | 970 | – | Goodman et al. (1980) |

RITA, Registry of Industrial Toxicology Animal-Data, Hanover, Germany.

In rats bronchial or bronchiolar papillomas are believed to originate from respiratory epithelium with or without squamous cell metaplasia (Dungworth et al. 1992). Bronchial papillomas observed after inhalation of urban ambient air and consisting of nonciliated epithelial cells and fibrous stroma have been shown to contain cells with a positive immunoreaction to calcitonin. It has been suggested that these papillomas develop from hyperplasia of neuroendocrine cells, especially in rats (Ito et al. 1989).

In Syrian hamsters papillary projections of endocrine cells into bronchioles have been found after treatment with 4-nitroquinoline 1-oxide. The lesions are composed of argyrophilic nonciliated cells which stain positively for calcitonin (Ito et al. 1988). On the other hand, squamous cell papillomas which occur occasionally in the bronchi, develop from surface lining cells which have undergone squamous cell metaplasia (Mohr et al. 1995).

*Etiology.* The causes of primary pulmonary tumors arising spontaneously in the lungs of rodents is not known.

*Frequency.* Naturally occurring neoplasms of the lung are rare in rats, uncommon in Syrian hamsters, but quite frequent in a number of strains of mice.

Frequencies of bronchioloalveolar tumors in different strains of rats are depicted in Table 15; this Table combines bronchioloalveolar adenomas and carcinomas. Data on prevalence of pulmonary tumors in Sprague-Dawley and Wistar rats are also available from the data base of Registry of Industrial Toxicology Animal-Data in Hanover, Germany (Mohr et al. 1990a; Morawietz et al. 1990, 1992; Rittinghausen et al. 1992). Current data are also summarized in Tables 15–18. They support the observation that primary pulmonary tumors seem to be less common in Sprague-

**Table 17.** Prevalence of naturally occurring adenosquamous carcinomas in lungs of various strains of rats: number of animals (*n*) and percentage with tumor (%)

| Strain | Study duration | Males | | Females | | Reference |
|---|---|---|---|---|---|---|
| | | *n* | % | *n* | % | |
| *F344* | | | | | | |
| F344 | 2 years | 1794 | – | 1754 | – | Goodman et al. (1979) |
| F344/DuCrj | 2 years | 296 | 0.3 | 297 | – | Maekawa et al. (1983a) |
| F344 | Life span | 529 | – | 529 | – | Solleveld et al. (1984) |
| F344 | 2 years | 2305 | – | 2354 | – | Haseman et al. (1984) |
| F344 | 2 years | 1933 | – | 1974 | – | Haseman et al. (1990) |
| F344 | 2 years | 740 | – | 740 | – | Chandra and Frith (1992b) |
| *Sprague-Dawley* | | | | | | |
| Sprague-Dawley | 18 months | 179 | – | 181 | – | Prejean et al. (1973) |
| Sprague-Dawley | 2 years | 365 | – | 365 | – | Stula (1975) |
| Sprague-Dawley | 2 years | 1340 | – | 1329 | – | Chandra et al. (1992) |
| Sprague-Dawley | 24–30 months | 1130 | – | 1076 | 0.2 | RITA (1995) |
| *Wistar* | | | | | | |
| Chbb:THOM(SPF) | 15–30 months | 600 | – | 600 | – | Ueberberg and Lützen (1979) |
| Han:WIST | Life span | 304 | – | 305 | – | Deerberg et al. (1980) |
| Wistar SPF Tox | 30 months | 192 | – | 192 | – | Kroes et al. (1981) |
| Wistar TNO/W.70 | 2 years | 962 | – | 968 | – | Bomhard et al. (1986) |
| Wistar | 24–31 months | 2147 | 0.1 | 2198 | – | RITA (1995) |
| *Other strains* | | | | | | |
| Osborne-Mendel | 2 years | 975 | – | 970 | – | Goodman et al. (1980) |
| ACI/seg Hap BR | 24–40 months | 216 | – | – | – | Ward et al. (1983) |

RITA, Registry of Industrial Toxicology Animal-Data, Hanover, Germany.

Dawley and Wistar than in F344 rats. Frequencies of squamous lung tumors, benign and malignant, for varous strains of rat may be seen in Table 16. The frequencies are for the most part lower than for bronchioloalveolar tumors. Incidences for adenosquamous carcinomas in the rat lung are given in Table 17. Primary mesenchymal neoplasms of the rat lung are extremely rare (Schwartz et al. 1991). Metastases or direct invasion of soft tissue neoplasms are more frequently observed in the rodent lung. Frequencies for secondary lung tumors are given in Table 19 (see p. 234, this volume).

Table 18 contains a list of lung tumor frequencies, mainly bronchioloalveolar tumors, in common strains of mice. Benign and malignant tumors are combined here because of the varying criteria for classification used by the different authors.

Tables 14–19, especially those for the bronchioloalveolar tumors, indicate that the naturally occurring tumor rates in male mice and rats are higher than in female mice and rats.

*Syrian Hamsters.* For Syrian hamsters only few incidence data are available. The incidence of naturally occurring lung tumors in the Syrian hamster is estimated to be not more than 0.1%–0.2% (Pour et al. 1976, 1979; Pour 1983; Mohr and Ketkar 1980; Mohr 1982; Mohr et al. 1995).

**Table 18.** Prevalence of naturally occurring pulmonary tumors in lungs of various strains of mice: number of animals (*n*) and percentage with tumor (%)

| Strain | Study duration | Males | | Females | | Reference |
|---|---|---|---|---|---|---|
| | | *n* | % | *n* | % | |
| *Strain A* | | | | | | |
| A | 20 months | 23 | 78.0 | 20 | 75.0 | Stoner and Shimkin (1982) |
| A | 22 months | 14 | 86.0 | – | – | Dixon et al. (1991) |
| *Swiss/ICR Swiss/CD-1* | | | | | | |
| CD-1 HaM/ICR | 2 years | 99 | 23.8 | 102 | 32.6 | Homburger et al. (1975) |
| CD-1 | 2 years | 480 | 19.8 | 481 | 20.2 | Compiled by Lang (1987) |
| CD-1 | 18–23 months | 1232 | 22.0 | 1240 | 17.0 | Sher et al. (1982) |
| CD-1 | 2 years | 891 | 33.0 | 890 | 27.0 | Maita et al. (1988) |
| Swiss | Life span | 100 | 23.0 | 100 | 21.0 | Toth and Shimizu (1974) |
| ICR Swiss | 19 months | 50 | 12.0 | 50 | – | Rao et al. (1988) |
| ICR Swiss | 22 months | 250 | 24.0 | 250 | 17.0 | Rao et al. (1988) |
| ICR Swiss | 19–24 months | 300 | 18.0 | 300 | 14.0 | Rao et al. (1988) |
| ICR Swiss | 25 months | 270 | 23.0 | 270 | 16.0 | Rao et al. (1988) |
| ICR Swiss | 25 months | 50 | 21.0 | 50 | 19.0 | Rao et al. (1988) |
| ICR Swiss | 25 months | 400 | 32.0 | 400 | 27.0 | Rao et al. (1988) |
| CD-1 | 2 years | 725 | 21.8 | 725 | 13.8 | Chandra and Frith (1992a) |
| *BALB/c* | | | | | | |
| BALB/c | 18 months | – | – | 554 | 20.3 | Sheldon and Greenman (1979) |
| BALB/c | 24 months | – | – | 762 | 36.6 | Sheldon and Greenman (1979) |
| BALB/c | 33 months | – | – | 102 | 52.4 | Sheldon and Greenman (1979) |
| BALB/c | 2 years | – | – | 762 | 34.9 | Heath et al. (1982) |
| BALB/c | 2 years | 791 | 51.8 | 12579 | 36.4 | Compiled by Frith (1987) |
| BALB/c | 2 years | – | – | 760 | 37.0 | Rao et al. (1988) |
| *NMRI* | | | | | | |
| Han:NMRI | Life span | – | – | 150 | 39.0 | Rehm et al. (1985) |
| NMRI | 24–34 months | 203 | 33.1 | 122 | 20.6 | Bomhard and Mohr (1989) |
| *C57Bl* | | | | | | |
| C57Bl/10ScSn | Life span | 39 | – | 35 | 2.9 | Smith et al. (1973) |
| C57Bl/6 | 16–23 months | 214 | 6.1 | 216 | 2.8 | Frith et al. (1983) |
| C57Bl/10J | 25 months | 50 | 3.0 | 50 | 3.0 | Rao et al. (1988) |
| C57Bl/6 | 2 years | 447 | 8.7 | 1227 | 2.5 | Compiled by Frith (1987) |
| $B6C3F_1$ | | | | | | |
| $B6C3F_1$ | 2 years | 2543 | 12.7 | 2522 | 4.4 | Ward et al. (1979) |
| $B6C3HF_1$ | 20–24 months | 425 | 13.0 | 426 | 2.0 | Sher et al. (1982) |
| $B6C3HF_1$ | 20–23 months | 321 | 8.0 | 342 | 4.0 | Sher et al. (1982) |
| $B6C3F_1$ | 16–23 months | 188 | 42.0 | 219 | 28.3 | Frith et al. (1983) |
| $B6C3F_1$ | 2 years | 1780 | 17.0 | 1777 | 6.9 | Haseman et al. (1985) |
| $B6C3F_1$ | 2 years | 244 | 13.9 | 246 | 5.3 | Tamano et al. (1988) |
| $B6C3F_1$ | 25–26 months | 320 | 13.0 | 320 | 6.0 | Rao et al. (1988) |
| $B6C3F_1$ | 25–26 months | 900 | 17.0 | 900 | 7.0 | Rao et al. (1988) |
| $B6C3F_1$ | 2 years | 2084 | 19.1 | 2079 | 7.3 | Dixon and Maronpot (1991) |
| $B6C3F_1$ | 2 years | 200 | 10.5 | 200 | 11.5 | Chandra and Frith (1992c) |
| *Other strains* | | | | | | |
| DBA/2J | Life span | 67 | – | 51 | – | Smith et al. (1973) |
| CBA/J | Life span | 17 | – | 33 | – | Smith et al. (1973) |
| LP/J | Life span | 77 | 5.2 | 51 | 3.9 | Smith et al. (1973) |
| C3H | Life span | 29 | 6.9 | – | – | Smith et al. (1973) |
| C3H.K | Life span | 25 | – | – | – | Smith et al. (1973) |
| 129/J | Life span | 41 | – | 95 | 1.1 | Smith et al. (1973) |

**Table 19.** Primary tumors with frequently occurring metastases in the lung of rats (data from Registry of Industrial Toxicology Animal-Data, Hanover, Germany, 1995)

| Organ (primary site) | Lesion type | Animals with metastasizing tumors | | Animals with metastases in the lung | |
|---|---|---|---|---|---|
| | | *n* | % | *n* | % |
| *Sprague Dawley, Males* | | 1130 | | | |
| Bone, NOS | Osteosarcoma | 3 | 0.3 | 3 | 0.3 |
| Hematopoietic tissue | Leukemia | 10 | 0.9 | 4 | 0.4 |
| Hematopoietic tissue | Lymphoma, malignant | 28 | 2.5 | 13 | 1.2 |
| Mononuclear phagocytic tissue | Sarcoma, histiocytic | 32 | 2.8 | 19 | 1.7 |
| *Sprague Dawley, Females* | | 1076 | | | |
| Hematopoietic tissue | Lymphoma, malignant | 20 | 1.9 | 9 | 0.8 |
| Mammary gland | Adenocarcinoma | 12 | 1.1 | 12 | 1.1 |
| *Wistar, Males* | | 2147 | | | |
| Adrenal gland | Adenocarcinoma, cortical | 5 | 0.2 | 5 | 0.2 |
| Hematopoietic tissue | Lymphoma, malignant | 58 | 2.7 | 34 | 1.6 |
| Mononuclear phagocytic tissue | Sarcoma, histiocytic | 37 | 1.7 | 26 | 1.2 |
| *Wistar, Females* | | 2198 | | | |
| Hematopoietic tissue | Lymphoma, malignant | 32 | 1.5 | 16 | 0.7 |
| Mammary gland | Adenocarcinoma | 15 | 0.7 | 12 | 0.5 |
| Mononuclear phagocytic tissue | Sarcoma, histiocytic | 18 | 0.8 | 8 | 0.4 |
| Thyroid gland | Carcinoma, C cell | 5 | 0.2 | 4 | 0.2 |
| Uterus | Adenocarcinoma | 28 | 1.3 | 15 | 0.7 |

## Comparison with Other Species

In laboratory rodents, especially in rats and mice, naturally occurring tumors of the lower respiratory tract are mostly peripheral neoplasms occurring in the bronchioloalveolar region. This is also true for domestic animals (Moulton 1978; Dungworth 1985). In humans lung tumors of the bronchioloalveolar type in the periphery are considerably less common than centrally located carcinomas of the hilar region. The majority of human pulmonary tumors are squamous cell carcinomas originating in segmental or lobar bronchi (Addis 1988). Centrally arising malignant neuroendocrine tumors are also common (Addis 1988). These occur naturally only in the trachea and larynx of Syrian hamsters (Ernst et al.; see p. 107, this volume).

*Acknowledgements.* The authors are most grateful to Dr. J. Woicke (Bristol-Myers Squibb, Regensburg) for providing slides, and would like to thank Mr. Marcel Tauscher and Mr. Frank Müller for their photographic assistance.

## References

Adamson IYR, Bowden DH (1979) Bleomycin-induced injury and metaplasia of alveolar type 2 cells. Relationship of cellular responses to drug presence in the lung. Am J Pathol 96:531–544

Addis BJ (1988) Pathology of lung cancer. In: Hoogstraten B, Addis BJ, Hansen HH, Martini N, Spiro SG (eds) UICC series. Current treatment of cancer. Lung tumors: lung, mediastinum, pleura, and chest wall. Springer, Berlin Heidelberg New York, pp 17–36

Anderson LM, Budinger JM (1981) Qualitative histological differences between transplacentally-induced lung tumors in young and aging mice. Cancer Lett 11:285–293

Anver MR, Cohen BJ, Lattuada CP, Foster SJ (1982) Age-associated lesions in barrier-reared male Sprague-Dawley rats: a comparison between Hap:(SD) and Crl:COBS[R]CD[R](SD) stocks. Exp Aging Res 8:3–23

Becci PJ, McDowell EM, Trump BF (1978) The respiratory epithelium. IV. Histogenesis of epidermoid metaplasia and carcinoma in situ in the hamster. J Natl Cancer Inst 61:577–586

Beer DG, Malkinson AM (1985) Genetic influence on type 2 or Clara cell origin of pulmonary adenomas in urethan-treated mice. J Natl Cancer Inst 75:963–969

Belinsky SA, Foley JF, White CM, Anderson MW, Maronpot RR (1990) Dose-response relationship between O6-methylguanine formation in Clara cells and induction of pulmonary neoplasia in the rat by 4(methylnitrosamino)-1-(3-pyridyl)-1-butanone. Cancer Res 50:3772–3780

Belinsky SA, Devereux TR, Foley JF, Maronpot RR, Anderson MW (1992) Role of the alveolar type II cell in the development and progression of pulmonary tumors induced by 4-(methylnitrosamino)-1-(3-pyridyl)-1-butanone in the A/J mouse. Cancer Res 52:3164–3173

Blair WH (1974) Chemical induction of lung carcinomas in rats. In: Karbe E, Park JF (eds) Experimental lung cancer: international symposium on experimental lung cancer-carcinogenesis and bioassay. Springer, Berlin Heidelberg New York, pp 199–206

Bomhard E (1992) Frequency of spontaneous tumors in Wistar rats in 30-months studies. Exp Toxicol Pathol 44:381–392

Bomhard E, Mohr U (1989) Spontaneous tumours in NMRI mice from carcinogenicity studies. Exp Pathol 36:129–145

Bomhard E, Rinke M (1994) Frequency of spontaneous tumours in Wistar rats in 2-year studies. Exp Toxicol Pathol 46:17–29

Bomhard E, Karbe E, Loeser E (1986) Spontaneous tumors of 2000 Wistar TNO/W.70 rats in two-year carcinogenicity studies. J Environ Pathol Toxicol Oncol 7:35–52

Boorman GA, Eustis SL (1990) Lung. In: Boorman GA, Eustis SL, Elwell MR, Montgomery CA, MacKenzie WF (eds) Pathology of the Fischer rat: reference and atlas. Academic, San Diego, pp 339–367

Branstetter DG, Moseley PP (1991) Effect of lung development on the histological pattern of lung tumors induced by ethylnitrosourea in the C3HeB/FeJ mouse. Exp Lung Res 17:169–179

Branstetter DG, Stoner GD, Budd C, Conran PB, Goldblatt PJ (1988) Effect of gestational development of lung tumor size and morphology in the mouse. Cancer Res 48:379–386

Carlton WW, Ernst H, Faccini JM, Greaves P, Krinke GJ, Long PH, Maekawa A, Newsholme SJ, Weisse G (1992) Soft tissue and musculoskeletal system. In: Mohr U, Capen CC, Dungworth DL, Griesemer RA, Ito N, Turusov VS (eds) International classification of rodent tumors, part 1: the rat. IARC Sci Publ 122:1–62

Chandra M, Frith CH (1992a) Spontaneous neoplasms in aged CD-1 mice. Toxicol Lett 61:67–74

Chandra M, Frith CH (1992b) Spontaneous neoplasms in aged control Fischer 344 rats. Cancer Lett 62:49–56

Chandra M, Frith CH (1992c) Spontaneous neoplasms in $B6C3F_1$ mice. Toxicol Lett 60:91–98

Chandra M, Riley MGI, Johnson DE (1992) Spontaneous neoplasms in aged Sprague-Dawley rats. Arch Toxicol 66:496–502

Deerberg F, Rapp K, Pittermann W, Rehm S (1980) Zum Tumorspektrum der Han:WIST Ratte. Z Versuchstierkd 22:267–280

Dixon D, Maronpot RR (1991) Histomorphologic features of spontaneous and chemically-induced pulmonary neoplasms in $B6C3F_1$ mice and Fischer 344 rats. Toxicol Pathol 19:540–556

Dixon D, Horton J, Haseman JK, Talley F, Greenwell A, Nettesheim P, Hook GE, Maronpot RR (1991) Histomorphology and ultrastructure of spontaneous pulmonary neoplasms in strain A mice. Exp Lung Res 17:131–155

Dungworth DL (1985) The respiratory system. In: Jubb KVF, Kennedy PC, Palmer N (eds) Pathology of domestic animals, 3rd edn. Academic, Orlando, pp 413–556

Dungworth DL, Hahn FF, Hayashi Y, Keenan K, Mohr U, Rittinghausen S, Schwartz L (1992) Respiratory system. In: Mohr U, Capen CC, Dungworth DL, Griesemer RA, Ito N, Turusov VS (eds) International classification of rodent tumours, part I: the rat. IARC Sci Publ 122:1–57

Dungworth DL, Mohr U, Heinrich U, Ernst H, Kittel B (1994) Pathologic effects of inhaled particles in rat lungs: associations between inflammatory and neoplastic processes. In: Mohr U, Dungworth DL, Mauderly JL, Oberdörster G (eds) Toxic and carcinogenic effects of solid particles in the respiratory tract. International Life Sciences Institute, Washington DC, pp 75–98

Dungworth DL, Harkema J, Hayashi Y, Kittel B, Lewis D, Miller R, Mohr U, Morgan K, Rehm S, Rittinghausen S, Schwartz L, Slayter M. Respiratory system and mesothelium. In: Mohr U, Capen CC, Dungworth DL, Griesemer RA, Hardisty J, Ito N, Long P, Turusov VS (eds) International classification of rodent tumours, part II: the mouse. IARC Sci Publ (in preparation)

Emura M, DaCosta C (1993) In vitro investigation on proliferative cystic keratinizing squamous lesions in the rat lung. Exp Toxicol Pathol 45:189–195

Faccini JM, Abbott DP, Paulus GJJ (1990) Respiratory tract. Mouse histopathology. Elsevier, Amsterdam New York, pp 48–63

Frith CH (1987) Incidence of neoplastic and nonneoplastic lesions in several strains of mice. Toxicology Pathology Associates, Little Rock, pp 1–57

Frith CH, Littlefield NA, Umholtz R (1981) Incidence of pulmonary metastases for various neoplasms in BALB/cStCrlfC3H/Nctr female mice fed N-2-fluorenylacetamide. J Natl Cancer Inst 66:703–712

Frith CH, Highman B, Burger GT, Sheldon WD (1983) Spontaneous lesions in virgin and retired breeder BALB/c and C57BL/6 mice. Lab Anim Sci 33:273–286

Goodman DG, Ward JM, Squire RA, Chu KC, Linhart MS (1979) Neoplastic and nonneoplastic lesions in aging F344 rats. Toxicol Appl Pharmacol 48:237–248

Goodman DG, Ward JM, Squire RA, Paxton MB, Reichardt WD, Chu KC, Linhart MS (1980) Neoplastic and nonneoplastic lesions in aging Osborne-Mendel rats. Toxicol Appl Pharmacol 55:433–447

Gunning WT, Castonguay A, Goldblatt PJ, Stoner GD (1991) Strain A/J mouse lung adenoma growth patterns vary when induced by different carcinogens. Toxicol Pathol 19:168–175

Gunning WT, Goldblatt PJ, Stoner GD (1992) Keratin expression in chemically induced mouse lung adenomas. Am J Pathol 140:109–118

Hahn FF (1985) Radiation-induced squamous cell carcinoma, lung of rodents. In: Jones TC, Mohr U, Hunt RD (eds) Monographs on pathology of laboratory animals. Respiratory system. Springer, Berlin Heidelberg New York, pp 127–133

Hahn FF, Lundgren DL (1992) Pulmonary neoplasms in rats that inhaled cerium-144 dioxide. Toxicol Pathol 20:169–178

Haseman JK, Huff J, Boorman GA (1984) Use of historical control data in carcinogenicity studies in rodents. Toxicol Pathol 12:126–135

Haseman JK, Huff JE, Rao GN, Arnold JE, Boorman GA, McConnell EE (1985) Neoplasms observed in untreated and corn oil gavage control groups of F344/N rats and (C57BL/6N × C3H/HeN)$F_1$ ($B6C3F_1$) mice. J Natl Cancer Inst 75:975–984

Haseman JK, Arnold J, Eustis SL (1990) Tumor incidences in Fischer 344 rats: NTP historical data. In: Boorman GA,

Eustis SL, Elwell MR, Montgomery CA, MacKenzie WF (eds) Pathology of the Fischer rat. Academic, San Diego, pp 555–564

Heath JE, Frith CH, Wang PM (1982) A morphologic classification and incidence of alveolar-bronchiolar neoplasms in BALB/c female mice. Lab Anim Sci 32:638–647

Herbert RA, Gillett NA, Rebar AH, Lundgren DL, Hoover MD, Chang IY, Carlton WW, Hahn FF (1993) Sequential analysis of the pathogenesis of plutonium-induced pulmonary neoplasms in the rat: morphology, morphometry, and cytokinetics. Radiat Res 134:29–42

Homburger F, Russfield AB, Weisburger JH, Lim S, Chak SP, Weisburger EK (1975) Aging changes in CD-1 HaM/ICR mice reared under standard laboratory conditions. J Natl Cancer Inst 55:37–45

Ito T (1985) An ultrastructural study of the acute effects of 4-nitroquinoline 1-oxide on the hamster lung. Exp Mol Pathol 42:220–233

Ito T, Kitamura H, Inayama Y, Kanisawa M (1988) Pulmonary adenoma and endocrine cell hyperplasia in Syrian golden hamster treated with 4-nitroquinoline 1-oxide. Acta Pathol Jpn 38:1097–1104

Ito T, Ikemi Y, Kitamura H, Ogawa T, Kanisawa M (1989) Production of bronchial papilloma with calcitonin-like immunoreactivity in rats exposed to urban ambient air. Exp Pathol 36:89–96

Kamino K, Mohr U (1993) Frequency of metastasis depending on histologic type of primary lung carcinoma in rats. J Exp Anim Sci 35:161–165

Kaspareit-Rittinghausen J, Deerberg F (1988) High frequency of spontaneous histiocytic sarcomas in BDII/Han rats. J Comp Pathol 99:299–307

Kauffman SL (1981) Histogenesis of the papillary Clara cell adenoma. Am J Pathol 103:174–180

Kauffman SL, Sato T (1985) Bronchiolar adenoma, lung, mouse. In: Jones TC, Mohr U, Hunt RD (eds) Monographs on pathology of laboratory animals. Respiratory system. Springer, Berlin Heidelberg New York, pp 107–111

Kauffman SL, Alexander L, Sass L (1979) Histologic and ultrastructural features of the Clara cell adenoma of the mouse lung. Lab Invest 40:708–716

Kennedy AR, McGandy RB, Little JB (1977) Histochemical, light and electron microscopic study of polonium-210 induced peripheral tumors in hamster lungs: evidence implicating the Clara cell as the cell of origin. Eur J Cancer 13:1325–1340

Kittel B, Ernst H, Dungworth DL, Rittinghausen S, Nolte T, Kamino K, Stuart B, Lake SG, Cardesa A, Morawietz G, Mohr U (1993) Morphological comparison between benign keratinizing cystic squamous cell tumours of the lung and squamous lesions of the skin in rats. Exp Toxicol Pathol 45:257–267

Kittel B, Dungworth DL, Mohr U (1994) Goblet cell metaplasia in the peripheral lung tissue of rats after chronic exposure to particles. In: Mohr U, Dungworth DL, Mauderly JL, Oberdörster G (eds) Toxic and carcinogenic effects of solid particles in the respiratory tract. International Life Sciences Institute, Washington DC, pp 545–548

Kroes R, Garbis-Berkvens JM, de Vries T, van Nesselrooy HJ (1981) Histopathological profile of a Wistar rat stock including a survey of the literature. J Gerontol 36:259–279

Lang PL (1987a) Spontaneous neoplastic lesions in the Crl:CD BR rat. Technical publication. Charles River Laboratories, Wilmington, pp 1–13

Lang PL (1987b) Spontaneous neoplastic lesions in the Crl:CD-1 (ICR)BR mouse. Technical publication. Charles River Laboratories, Wilmington, pp 1–13

Lijinsky W, Reuber MD (1988) Neoplasms of the skin and other organs observed in Swiss mice treated with nitrosoalkylureas. J Cancer Res Clin Oncol 114:245–249

Löhrke H, Hesse B, Goerttler K (1982) Spontaneous tumours in male and female specified pathogen-free Sprague-Dawley rats (outbred stock Sut:SDT). Z Versuchstierkd 24:225–230

Maeda T, Izumi K, Otsuka H, Manabe Y, Kinouchi T, Ohnishi Y (1986) Induction of squamous cell carcinoma in the rat lung by 1,6-dinitropyrene. J Natl Cancer Inst 76:693–701

Maekawa A, Kurokawa Y, Takahashi M, Kokubo T, Ogiu T, Onodera H, Tanigawa H, Ohno Y, Furukawa F, Hayashi Y (1983a) Spontaneous tumors in F-344/DuCrj rats. Gann 74:365–372

Maekawa A, Onodera H, Tanigawa H, Furuta K, Kodama T, Horiuchi S, Hayashi Y (1983b) Neoplastic and non-neoplastic lesions in aging Slc:Wistar rats. J Toxicol Sci 8:279–290

Maita K, Hirano M, Harada T, Mitsumori K, Yoshida A, Takahashi K, Nakashima N, Kitazawa T, Enomoto A, Iniu K, Shirasu Y (1988) Mortality, major cause of moribundity, and spontaneous tumors in CD-1 mice. Toxicol Pathol 16:340–349

McDowell EM (1987) Bronchogenic carcinomas. In: McDowell EM (ed) Lung carcinomas. Churchill Livingstone, Edinburgh, pp 255–285

McDowell EM, Trump BF (1983) Histogenesis of preneoplastic and neoplastic lesions in tracheobronchial epithelium. Surv Synth Path Res 2:235–279

McDowell EM, Keenan KP, Huang M (1984) Effects of vitamin A-deprivation on hamster tracheal epithelium. A quantitative morphologic study. Virchows Arch B Cell Pathol 45:197–219U (1982) Tumours of the respiratory tract. In: Turusov VS, Della Porta G, Hollander CF, Mohr U, Shabad LM, Sobin LH, Stanton MF (eds) Pathology of tumours in laboratory animals, vol III: tumours of the hamster. IARC Sci Publ 34:115–130

Mohr U, Ketkar M (1980) Animal model of human disease: Bronchogenic spontaneous carcinoma of the lung. Am J Pathol 99:521–524

Mohr U, Dungworth DL (1988) Relevance to humans of experimentally induced pulmonary tumors in rats and hamsters. In: Mohr U, Dungworth DL, Kimmerle G, Lewkowsky J, McClellan R, Stöber W (eds) Inhalation toxicology: the design and interpretation of inhalation studies and their use in risk assessment. Springer, Berlin Heidelberg New York, pp 209–232

Mohr U, Bader R, Ernst H, Ettlin RA, Gembardt C, Harleman JH, Hartig F, Jahn W, Kaliner G, Karbe E, Kaufmann W, Krieg K, Krinke G, Kuttler K, Landes C, Mettler F, Morawietz G, Notman J, Puschner H, Qureshi S, Reznik G, Rittinghausen S, Tuch K, Urwyler H, Weisse G, Weisse I, Zehnder J (1990a) Tumor Registry Data Base: suggestions for a systematized nomenclature of pre-neoplastic and neoplastic lesions in rats. Exp Pathol 38:1–18

Mohr U, Rittinghausen S, Takenaka S, Ernst H, Dungworth DL, Pylev LN (1990b) Pathology of tumours in laboratory animals. Tumours of the lower respiratory tract and pleura in the rat. In: Turusov VS, Mohr U (eds) Pathology of tumours in laborat ory animals, vol I: tumours of the rat, 2nd edn. IARC Sci Publ 99:275–299

Mohr U, Emura M, Dungworth DL, Ernst H (1995) Tumours of the lower respiratory tract. In: Mohr U (ed) Pathology of tumours in laboratory animals. III. Tumours of the hamster. IARC Sci Publ (in press)

Morawietz G, Rittinghausen S, Mohr U (1990) Tumor registry data base: advantages using a systematized nomenclature. Schweiz Arch Tierheilkd 132:448–449

Morawietz G, Rittinghausen S, Mohr U (1992) RITA-Registry of Industrial Toxicology Animal-Data progress of the working group. Exp Toxicol Pathol 44:301–309

Morii S, Fujii T (1973) Spontaneous tumors in Sprague-Dawley JCL rats (authors' translation). Jikken Dobutsu (Jpn) 22:127–138

Moulton JE (1978) Tumors of the respiratory system. In: Moulton JE (ed) Tumors in domestic animals, 2nd edn. University of California Press, Berkeley, Los Angeles, pp 205–239

Muraoka Y, Itoh M, Yamashita F, Hayashi Y (1977) Spontaneous tumors in aged SD-JCL rats. Jikken Dobutsu (Jpn) 26:13–22

Nolte T (1991) Histogenese und Validierung von Plattenepitheltumoren der Lunge nach Partikel- und Karzinogenexposition bei der Ratte. Medical veterinary dissertation, Tierärztliche Hochschule Hannover

Nolte T, Thiedemann KU, Dungworth DL, Ernst H, Paulini I, Heinrich U, Dasenbrock C, Peters L, Überschär S, Mohr U (1993) Morphology and histogenesis of squamous cell metaplasia of the rat lung after chronic exposure to a pyrolized pitch condensate and/or carbon black, or to combinations of pyrolized pitch condensate, carbon black and irritant gases. Exp Toxicol Pathol 45:135–144

Nolte T, Dungworth DL, Ernst H, Kittel B, Rittinghausen S, Mohr U (1995) Chemically induced pulmonary mucoepidermoid carcinoma in a female Wistar rat. Exp Toxicol Pathol (in press)

Ohshima M, Ward JM, Singh G, Katyal SL (1985) Immunocytochemical and morphological evidence for the origin of N-nitrosomethylurea-induced and naturally occurring primary lung tumors in F344/NCr rats. Cancer Res 45:2785–2792

Palmer KC (1985) Clara cell adenomas of the mouse lung. Interaction with alveolar type 2 cells. Am J Pathol 120:455–463

Pour PM (1983) Spontaneous respiratory tract tumors in Syrian hamsters. In: Reznik-Schüller HM (ed) Comparative respiratory tract carcinogenesis, vol I: spontaneous respiratory tract carcinogenesis. CRC, Boca Raton, pp 131–170

Pour PM, Reznik-Schüller HM (1985) Squamous cell carcinoma, lung, Syrian hamster. In: Jones TC, Mohr U, Hunt RD (eds) Monographs on pathology of laboratory animals. Respiratory system. Springer, Berlin Heidelberg New York, pp 117–123

Pour PM, Mohr U, Cardesa A, Althoff J, Kmoch N (1976) Spontaneous tumors and common diseases in two colonies of Syrian hamsters. II. Respiratory tract and digestive system. J Natl Cancer Inst 56:937–948

Pour PM, Althoff J, Salmasi SZ, Stepan K (1979) Spontaneous tumors and common diseases in three types of hamsters. J Natl Cancer Inst 63:797–811

Prejean JD, Peckham JC, Casey AE, Griswold DP, Weisburger EK, Weisburger JH (1973) Spontaneous tumors in Sprague-Dawley rats and Swiss mice. Cancer Res 33:2768-2773

Rao GN, Birnbaum LS, Collins JJ, Tennant RW, Skow LC (1988) Mouse strains for chemical carcinogenicity studies: overview of a workshop. Fund Appl Toxicol 10:385–394

Rehm S, Rapp KG, Deerberg F (1985) Influence of food restriction and body fat on life span and tumour incidence in female outbred Han:NMRI mice and two sublines. Z Versuchstierkd 27:249–283

Rehm S, Ward JM, ten Have-Opbroek AAW, Anderson LM, Singh G, Katyal SL, Rice JM (1988) Mouse papillary lung tumors transplacentally induced by N-nitrosoethylurea: evidence for alveolar type II cell origin by comparative light microscopic, ultrastructural, and immunohistochemical studies. Cancer Res 48:148–160

Rehm S, Takahashi M, Ward JM, Singh G, Katyal SL, Henneman JR (1989) Immunohistochemical demonstration of Clara cell antigen in lung tumors of bronchiolar origin induced by N-nitrosodiethylamine in Syrian golden hamsters. Am J Pathol 134:79–87

Rehm S, Devor DE, Henneman JR, Ward JM (1991a) Origin of spontaneous and transplacentally induced mouse lung tumors from alveolar type II cells. Exp Lung Res 17:181–195

Rehm S, Lijinsky W, Singh G, Katyal SL (1991b) Mouse bronchiolar cell carcinogenesis. Histologic characterization and expression of Clara cell antigen in lesions induced by N-nitrosobis-(2-chloroethyl) ureas. Am J Pathol 139:413–422

Rehm S, Lijinsky W, Thomas RG, Kasprzak BH (1993) Clara cell antigen in normal and migratory dysplastic Clara cells, and bronchioloalveolar carcinoma of Syrian hamsters induced by N-nitrosomethyl-n-heptylamine. Virchows Arch B Cell Pathol 64:181–190

Rehm S, Ward JM, Sass B (1994) Tumours of the lungs. In: Mohr U, Turusov VS (eds) Pathology of tumours in laboratory animals, vol II: tumours of the mouse, 2nd edn. IARC Sci Publ 111:325–355

Reznik G (1981) Unusual sites of lung tumor metastases in $B6C3F_1$ mice and F344 rats. Anticancer Res 1:159–162

Reznik G (1983) Spontaneous primary and secondary lung tumors in the rat. In: Reznik-Schüller HM (ed) Comparative respiratory tract carcinogenesis, vol 1: spontaneous respiratory tract carcinogenesis. CRC, Boca Raton, pp 95–116

Reznik-Schüller HM (1976) Ultrastructural alterations of nonciliated cells after nitrosamine treatment and their significance for pulmonary carcinogenesis. Am J Pathol 85:549–554

Reznik-Schüller HM (1977a) Sequential morphologic alterations in the bronchial epithelium of Syrian golden hamsters during N-nitrosomorpholine-induced pulmonary tumorigenesis. Am J Pathol 89:59–66

Reznik-Schüller HM (1977b) Ultrastructural alterations of APUD cells during nitrosamine-induced lung carcinogenesis. J Pathol 121:79–82

Reznik-Schüller HM, Gregg M (1981) Pathogenesis of lung tumors induced by N-nitrosoheptamethylene-imine in F344 rats. Virchows Arch A Pathol Anat Histopathol 393:333–343

Reznik-Schüller HM, Reznik G (1982) Morphology of spontaneous and induced tumors in the bronchioloalveolar region of F344 rats. Anticancer Res 2:53–57

Reznik-Schüller HM, Hague PH, Creasia DA (1981) Ultrastructure of pulmonary tumors induced in rats by N-nitrosomethylurethane. J Toxicol Environ Health 8:501–506

Rittinghausen S, Dungworth DL, Ernst H, Mohr U (1992) Primary pulmonary tumors. In: Mohr U, Dungworth DL, Capen CC (eds) Pathobiology of the aging rat, vol 1. Interna-

tional Life Sciences Institute, Washington DC, pp 161–172
Sass B, Liebelt AG (1985) Metastatic tumors, lung, mouse. In: Jones TC, Mohr U, Hunt RD (eds) Monographs on pathology of laboratory animals. Respiratory system. Springer, Berlin Heidelberg New York, pp 138–159
Sato T, Kauffman SL (1980) A scanning electron microscopic study of the Type II and Clara cell adenoma of the mouse lung. Lab Invest 43:28–36
Schüller HM (1987) Experimental carcinogenesis in the peripheral lung. In: McDowell EM (ed) Lung carcinomas. Churchill Livingstone, Edinburgh, pp 243–254
Schüller HM, McMahon JB (1985) Inhibition of N-nitrosodiethylamine-induced respiratory tract carcinogenesis by piperonylbutoxide in hamsters. Cancer Res 45:2807–2812
Schüller HM, Becker KL, Witschi HP (1988) An animal model for neuroendocrine lung cancer. Carcinogenesis 9:293–296
Schüller HM, Witschi HP, Nylen E, Joshi PA, Correa E, Becker KL (1990) Pathobiology of lung tumors induced in hamsters by 4-(methylnitrosamino)-1-(3-pyridyl)-1-butanone and the modulating effect of hyperoxia. Cancer Res 50:1960–1965
Schwartz LW, Hahn FF, Keenan KP, Keenan CM, Brown HR, Mann PC (1991) Proliferative lesions of the rat respiratory tract, R-1. Guides for toxicologic pathology. STP/ARP/AFIP, Washington DC, pp 1–26
Sheldon WG, Greenman DL (1979) Spontaneous lesions in control BALB/c female mice. J Exp Pathol Toxicol 3:155–167
Sher SP, Jensen RD, Bokelman DL (1982) Spontaneous tumors in control F344 and Charles River-CD rats and Charles River CD-1 and B6C3HF$_1$ mice. Toxicol Lett 11:103–110
Smith GS, Walford RL, Mickey MR (1973) Lifespan and incidence of cancer and other diseases in selected long-lived inbred mice and their F$_1$ hybrids. J Natl Cancer Inst 50:1195–1213
Solleveld HA, Haseman JK, McConnell EE (1984) Natural history of body weight gain, survival, and neoplasia in the F344 rat. J Natl Cancer Inst 72:929–940
Stewart HL, Dunn TB, Snell KC, Deringer MK (1979) Tumours of the respiratory tract. In: Turusov VS, Della Porta G, Hollander CF, Mohr U, Shabad LM, Sobin LH, Stanton MF (eds) Pathology of tumors in laboratory animals, vol II: tumors of the mouse. IARC Sci Publ 23:251–287
Stoner GD, Shimkin MB (1982) Strain A mouse lung tumor bioassay. J Am Coll Toxicol 1:145–169
Stula EF (1975) Naturally occurring pulmonary tumors of epithelial origin in Charles River-CD rats. Bull Soc Pharmacol Environ Pathol 3:3–11
Takaki Y, Kitamura S, Uekusa T, Honma S, Aze Y, Wakabayashi K, Kuwabara N, Fukuda Y (1989) Spontaneous tumors in F-344/Jcl rats. J Toxicol Sci 14:181–195
Tamano S, Hagiwara A, Shibata MA, Kurata Y, Fukushima S, Ito N (1988) Spontaneous tumors in aging (C57BL/6N × C3H/HeN)F$_1$ (B6C3F$_1$) mice. Toxicol Pathol 16:321–326
Thaete LG, Malkinson AM (1990) Differential staining of normal and neoplastic mouse lung epithelia by succinate dehydrogenase histochemistry. Cancer Lett 52:219–227
Thaete LG, Malkinson AM (1991) Cells of origin of primary pulmonary neoplasms in mice: morphologic and histochemical studies. Exp Lung Res 17:219–228
Thaete LG, Gunning WT, Stoner GD, Malkinson AM (1987) Cellular derivation of lung tumors in sensitive and resistant strains of mice: results at 28 and 56 weeks after urethan treatment. J Natl Cancer Inst 78:743–749
Thaete LG, Nesbitt MN, Malkinson AM (1991) Lung adenoma structure among inbred strains of mice: the pulmonary adenoma histologic type (Pah) genes. Cancer Lett 61:15–20
Toth B, Shimizu H (1974) 1-Carbamyl- 2-phenylhydrazine tumorigenesis in Swiss mice. Morphology of lung adenomas. J Natl Cancer Inst 52:241–251
Turusov VS, Breslow NE, Tomatis L (1974) Frequency and organ distribution of lung tumor metastases in CF-1 mice. J Natl Cancer Inst 52:225–232
Ueberberg H, Lützen L (1979) The spontaneous rate of tumours in the laboratory rat: strain Chbb:THOM(SPF). Arzneimittelforschung 29:1876–1879
Ward JM, Rehm S (1990) Applications of immunohistochemistry in rodent tumor pathology. Exp Pathol 40:301–312
Ward JM, Goodman DG, Squire RA, Chu KC, Linhart MS (1979) Neoplastic and nonneoplastic lesions in aging (C57BL/6N × C3H/HeN)F$_1$ (B6C3F$_1$) mice. J Natl Cancer Inst 63:849–854
Ward JM, Hamlin MH II, Ackerman LJ, Lattuada CP, Longfellow DG, Cameron TP (1983) Age-related neoplastic and degenerative lesions in aging male virgin and ex-breeder ACI/segHapBR rats. J Gerontol 38:538–548
Ward JM, Singh G, Katyal SL, Anderson LM, Kovatch RM (1985) Immunocytochemical localization of the surfactant apoprotein and Clara cell antigen in chemically induced and naturally occuring pulmonary neoplasms of mice. Am J Pathol 118:493–499
Witschi H, Schüller HM (1991) Diffuse and continuous cell proliferation enhances radiation-induced tumorigenesis in hamster lung. Cancer Lett 60:193–197
Yang YH, Grice HC (1965) Mucinous bronchiolar carcinoma of the rat lung – a case report. J Comp Med Vet Sci 29:15–17

# Squamous Cell Carcinoma, Lung, Rat

Gary A. Boorman and Rick Hailey

*Synonyms.* Epidermoid carcinoma, lung; carcinoma, squamous cell

## Gross Appearance

Squamous cell carcinomas induced in the rat lung by polycyclic hydrocarbons are seen grossly as solid masses containing central areas of friable material (keratin; Shabad and Pylev 1970). The gross appearance of spontaneous squamous cell carcinoma of the rat lung has not been described in the literature. When carcinogen pellets are deposited in the lung, squamous cell carcinomas often arise at the site of deposition. A site predilection for the naturally occurring squamous cell carcinoma of the rat lung has not been reported. These pulmonary neoplasms may be quite large (Fig. 225).

## Microscopic Features

Spontaneous squamous cell carcinomas of the lung of the F344 rat are morphologically similar to those occurring in the skin and forestomach (Boorman and Eustis 1990). Some contain abundant keratin (Fig. 226), whereas others contain very little keratin (Fig. 227; Mohr 1992). Squamous cell carcinomas may be fairly well differentiated (Figs. 227, 228) with expansive growth, or they may be anaplastic and invasive (Fig. 229). Local invasion is more common although metastases are infrequent and are usually seen in the mediastinal tissue (Fig. 230), hilar lymph nodes, and rarely the kidney. Similar morphological characteristics are found in induced squamous cell carcinomas, but they may be more anaplastic. A scirrhous response (Kuschner and Laskin 1970; Shabad and Pylev 1970) with neoplastic cells separated by collagen fibers is a common feature (Fig. 231). Some induced squamous cell carcinomas are reported to contain both well-differentiated squamous epithelium and areas of atypical pleomorphic cells which have hyperchromatic nuclei and numerous mitotic figures (Shabad and Pylev 1970).

## Ultrastructure

A description of the ultrastructural features of spontaneous squamous cell carcinoma of the rat lung was not found in a review of the literature. In squamous cell carcinoma induced in the lung of the rat by *N*-nitrosoheptamethyleneimine or radioactive particles, ultrastructural features include the formation of tonofilaments, and interdigitating cell membranes connected by desmosomes (Reznik-Schüller and Gregg 1981; Herbert et al. 1994).

## Differential Diagnosis

Squamous cell carcinoma must be differentiated from keratinizing squamous cyst which is occa-

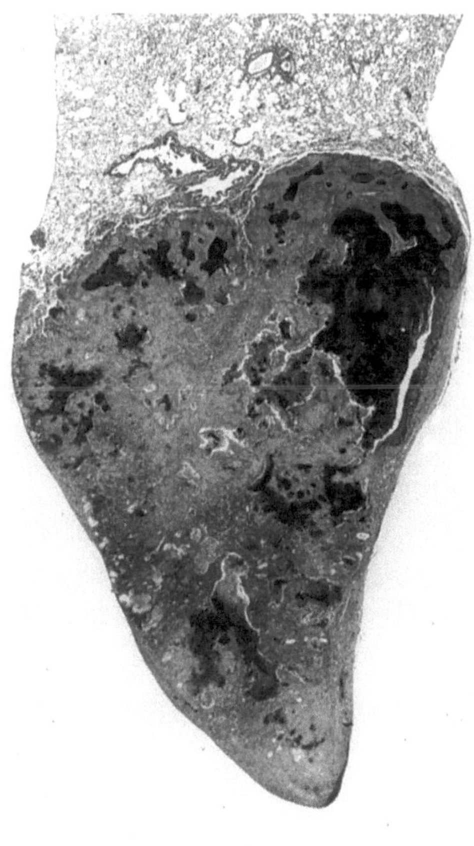

**Fig. 225.** Squamous cell carcinoma in the lung of a female F344/N rat exposed to 6 mg/m³ talc for 2 years. H&E, ×14

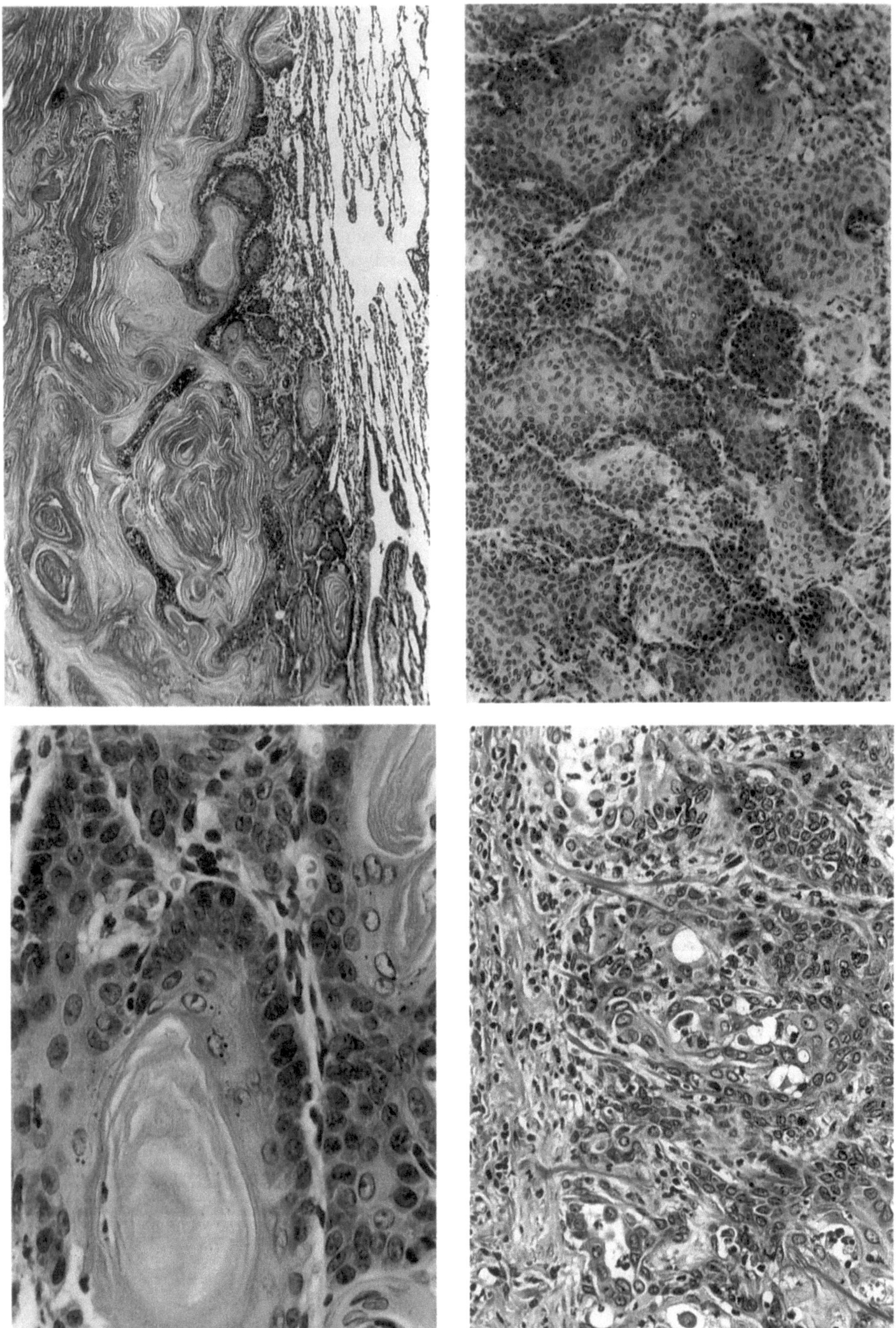

**Fig. 226.** (*upper left*) Squamous cell carcinoma, rat lung. Note abundant keratin production. H&E, ×80

**Fig. 227.** (*upper right*) Squamous cell carcinoma, rat lung. Note little cellular atypia and minimal keratin production. H&E, ×160

**Fig. 228.** (*lower left*) Squamous cell carcinoma, rat lung. Orderly progression of differentiation is evident from basal layer to central area of keratin. H&E, ×300

**Fig. 229.** (*lower right*) Squamous cell carcinoma in the lung of a untreated male F344/N rat at 2 years of age. There is marked atypia of individual cells with a prominent scirrhous response and a moderate inflammatory infiltrate. H&E, ×110

◄

sionally observed in the lung as an incidental lesion (Boorman and Eustis 1990). These keratinizing squamous cysts may be also seen after exposure to inert materials such as talc (NTP 1993), titanium dioxide (Lee et al. 1985), or aramid fibrils (Lee et al. 1988; Carlton 1994). The cyst consists of a wall of keratinized, stratified squamous epithelium with a central keratin filled lumen (Carlton 1994). The epithelium of the cyst wall is well differentiated without atypia, dysplasia, or invasive growth (Fig. 232). Very early squamous cell carcinoma may appear similar to a keratinizing squamous cyst and may in fact arise from a cyst. The same criteria used for the differentiation between squamous cell carcinoma and benign lesions in the forestomach and skin may also be used in the lung. Thus cellular atypia, dysplasia, mitotic activity, and extension of the squamous cells through the basement membrane are important criteria. Squamous cells that penetrate the basement membrane often incite a scirrhous response and an inflammatory reaction. Because both squamous cell carcinomas and keratinizing squamous cysts arise after exposure to inert dusts, the differential diagnoses, relationship, and pathogenesis of both lesions are of intense interest.

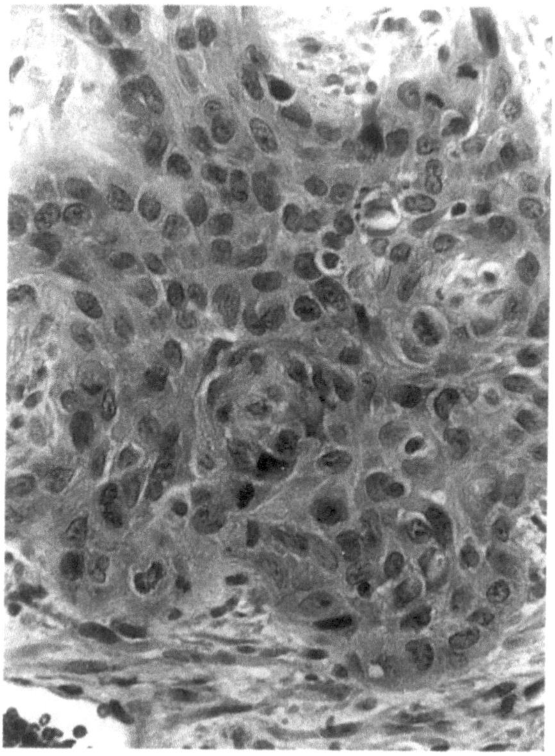

**Fig. 230.** Metastasis of pulmonary squamous cell carcinoma to mediastinum. Cells are less differentiated and mitotic figures are frequent. H&E, ×350

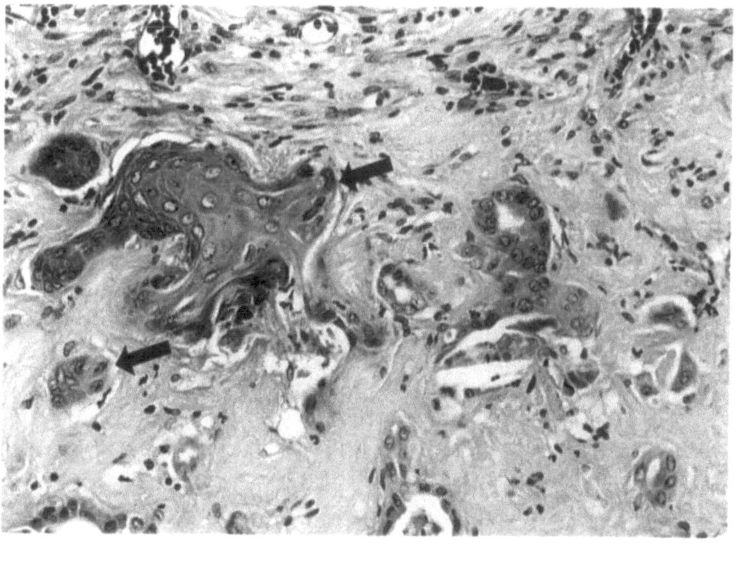

**Fig. 231.** Squamous cell carcinoma in the lung of a male F344/N rat exposed to nickel oxide by inhalation for 2 years. There is a dense scirrhous response surrounding islands of dysplastic squamous epithelial cells (*arrows*). H&E, ×225

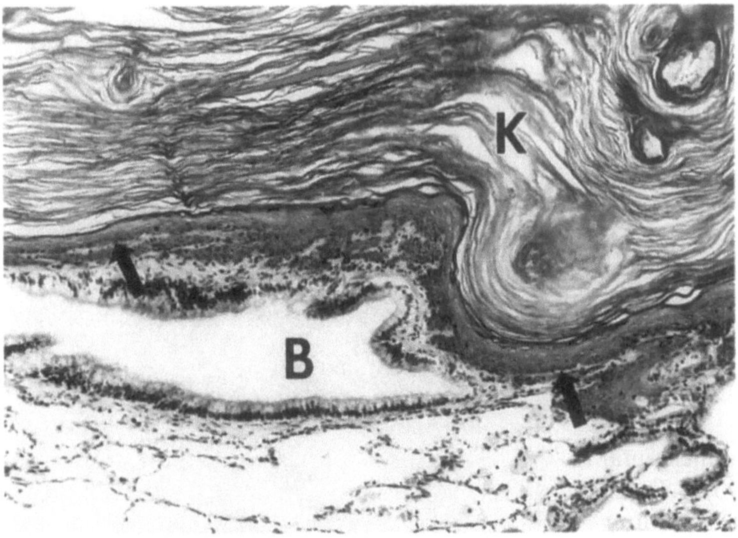


**Fig. 232.** Squamous keratinizing cyst in the lung of a male F344/N rat exposed to 18 mg/$m^3$ talc for 2 years. Abundant keratin (*K*) surrounded by well-differentiated squamous cells (*arrows*) is seen. *B*, Small bronchus. H&E, ×110

## Biological Features

The biological behavior of spontaneous squamous cell carcinomas of the lung in the rat is not well known because these neoplasms are uncommon and thus infrequently available for study. Induced squamous cell carcinomas of the rat appear to begin with basal cell hyperplasia in the airways, followed by squamous metaplasia and then squamous cell carcinoma (Reznik-Schüller and Gregg 1981). Squamous cell carcinomas in the rat lung induced by coal tar pitch also appear to derive from hyperplasia of bronchiolo-alveolar epithelium, progressing through stages of squamous metaplasia and/or dysplasia to carcinoma (Chang et al. 1992). Several studies on squamous cell carcinoma induced in the rat lung by radiation also undergo progressive stages from squamous metaplasia to carcinoma (Kuschner and Laskin 1970). When radioactive particulate material is deposited in the lung, squamous cell carcinomas arise in focal areas of scarring (Herbert et al. 1994).

Squamous cell carcinoma in the rat lung may be produced by implantation of pellets containing a variety of carcinogens (Deutsch-Wenzel et al. 1983; Mohr et al. 1990; Horikawa et al. 1991; Chang et al. 1992). Dinitrofluoranthene and benzo(a)pyrene when implanted into the rat lung cause neoplasms, most of which are squamous cell carcinomas (Horikawa et al. 1991), while 1,6-dinitropyrene induces mostly undifferentiated neoplasms (Iwagawa et al. 1989). Wistar rats given a single inhalation exposure to $^{239}PUO_2$ develop malignant lung tumors, which are predominately squamous cell carcinomas (Sanders et al. 1993). Cerium 144 dioxide by inhalation in F344 rats induces a high percentage of squamous cell carcinomas of the lung (Hahn and Lundgren 1992). Radiation-induced squamous cell carcinomas of the lung occur with a higher incidence and have a more malignant behavior than those induced by heavy loads of inert particulate material (Hahn and Lundgren 1992; National Toxicology Program 1993). See p. 213 this volume.

Most rat lung carcinogens induce epithelial hyperplasia. With some carcinogens bundles of tonofilaments are later found in the hyperplastic epithelium, suggesting squamous differentiation (metaplasia). Squamous cell carcinomas arise within these metaplastic areas (Reznik-Schüller and Gregg 1981). In the rat lung squamous cell carcinomas express cytokeratin which cross-reacts with human cytokeratins. Expression of cytokeratins in these neoplasms is an indication of the degree of differentiation (Kal et al. 1993).

In studies of point mutations in rat lung neoplasms, G → A transition mutations in codon 12 of the K-*ras* protooncogene, were found in 6/24 (25%) rat lung neoplasms induced by *N*-nitrosobis(2-oxopropyl) amine. The incidence of point mutations was significantly higher in squamous cell carcinomas (5/7; 71%) than in adenocarcinomas (1/17; 6%). This suggests that the mutational activation of K-*ras* is associated with a differential growth advantage in these two histologically distinct types of lung neoplasms. Mutations in codons 13 or 61 of the K-*ras*

**Table 20.** Naturally occurring squamous cell carcinoma in the rat lung

| Strain | Age[a] | Incidence[b] males | Females | Reference |
|---|---|---|---|---|
| Wistar | 124 weeks | 1/472 (0.2) | 0/457 | Kroes et al. (1981) |
| Osborne-Mendel | 126 weeks | 1/975 (0.1) | 0/970 | Goodman et al. (1980) |
| F344 | 116 weeks | 3/2305 (0.1) | 0/2356 | Haseman et al. (1984) |
| F344 | 112 weeks | 4/3877 (0.1) | 1/3919 (0.02) | Haseman et al. (1990) |
| F344 | Life span | 3/529 (0.6) | 1/529 (0.2) | Solleveld et al. (1984) |

[a] All reports include animals dying spontaneously: age given is the age at time of death.
[b] Incidence equals no. of animals with squamous cell carcinoma/animals at risk (%).

protooncogene were not found (Ohgaki et al. 1993).

Squamous cell carcinomas in the lung appear to be uncommon tumors in most rat strains. In a review of the literature most articles on naturally occurring, pulmonary neoplasms of various rat strains reported no squamous cell carcinoma. A few reports, which included a large number of rats, did contain one or more squamous cell carcinomas of the lung, as shown in Table 20. There is no evidence in these series of articles of any strain differences in the incidence of squamous cell carcinoma of the lung.

## Comparison with Other Species

In contrast to the rat, squamous cell carcinoma is the most frequent histological type of lung cancer in humans (Rothschild et al. 1982; WHO 1982). Induced squamous cell carcinomas in the rat are reported to have biological features analogous to those in man, tending to metastasize to the hilar lymph nodes and kidneys (Kuschner and Laskin 1970). Human patients with squamous cell carcinoma of the lung, in which there is overexpression of proteins encoded by the oncogenes c-*fos*, c-*jun*, and c-*erbBl*, have a significantly shorter survival time. This suggests that these genes may play an important role in the development of the human neoplasm (Volm et al. 1993). In rat lung neoplasms p53 expression is uncommon. However, in humans both in dysplasias (Sundaresan et al. 1992) and related squamous cell carcinomas p53 protein is expressed. The expression of p53 protein in nearly all dysplasias suggests that this could be an early event in the development of a squamous cell carcinoma of the lung in humans (Nuorva et al. 1993). Most squamous cell carcinomas in humans appear to arise from bronchial epithelium. Occasionally a squamous cell carcinoma arises in the wall of a squamous cyst (Usui et al. 1991).

In humans naturally occurring squamous cell carcinoma of the lung arise in the hilar region and is thus more centrally located than other types of lung neoplasms, which may arise in the peripheral lung (WHO 1982). Squamous metaplasia of the respiratory epithelium precedes or may be a "precondition" for squamous cell carcinoma in man (Grundmann 1983).

Squamous cell carcinomas are very uncommon in the mouse lung (Dixon and Maronpot 1991). Benzo(a)pyrene induces these neoplasms in the lung of mice (Schulte et al. 1994). In contrast to other induced mouse lung neoplasms, which are weakly antigenic (Yuhas et al. 1975), squamous cell carcinomas induced in the lung of the rat are capable of stimulating both cellular and humoral immunity (Jamasbi et al. 1978). In the dog and cat squamous cell carcinomas account for 6% and 12% of neoplasms of the lung, respectively (Moulton et al. 1981).

## References

Boorman GA, Eustis SL (1990) Chapter 21 Lung. In: Boorman GA, Eustis SL, Elwell MR, Montgomery CA, MacKenzie WF (eds) Pathology of the Fischer rat: reference and atlas. Academic, San Diego, pp 339–367

Carlton WW (1994) Proliferative keratin cyst; a lesion in the lungs of rats following chronic exposure to para-aramid fibrils. Fund Appl Toxicol 23:304–307

Chang F, Wang L, Zhao Q, Zhu Q, Wu Y, Chen C, Syrjanen S, Syrjanen K (1992) Investigation on the carcinogenic effects of coal tar pitch in rat respiratory tract by intratracheal instillations. Carcinogenesis 13:233–239

Deutsch-Wenzel RP, Brune H, Grimmer G, Dettbarn G, Misfeld J (1983) Experimental studies in rat lungs on the carcinogenicity and dose-response relationship of eight frequently occurring environmental polycyclic aromatic hydrocarbons. J Natl Cancer Inst 71:539–544

Dixon D, Maronpot RR (1991) Histomorphologic features of spontaneous and chemically-induced pulmonary neoplasms in B6C3Fl mice and Fischer 344 rats. Toxicol Pathol 19:540–546

Goodman DG, Ward JM, Squire RA, Paxton MB, Reichardt WD, Chu KC, Linhart MS (1980) Neoplastic and non-neoplastic lesions in aging Osborne-Mendel rats. Toxicol Appl Pharmacol 55:433–447

Grundmann E (1983) Classification and clinical consequences of precancerous lesions in the digestive and respiratory tracts. Acta Pathol Jpn 33:195–217

Hahn FF, Lundgren DL (1992) Pulmonary neoplasms in rats that inhaled cerium-144 dioxide. Toxicol Pathol 20:169–178

Haseman JK, Huff JE, Boorman GA (1984) Use of historical control data in carcinogenicity studies in rodents. Toxicol Pathol 12:126–135

Haseman JK, Eustis SL, Arnold J (1990) Tumor incidences in Fischer 344 rats: NTP historical data. In: Boorman GA, Eustis SL, Elwell MR, Montgomery CA, MacKenzie WF (eds) Pathology of the Fischer rat, chap 35. Academic, San Diego, pp 339–367

Herbert RA, Stegelmeier BS, Gillett NA, Rebar AH, Carlton WW, Singh G, Hahn FF (1994) Plutonium-induced proliferative lesions and pulmonary epithelial neoplasms in the rat: immunohistochemical and ultrastructural evidence for their origin from type II pneumocytes. Vet Pathol 31:366–374

Horikawa K, Sera N, Otofuji T, Murakami K, Tokiwa H, Iwagawa M, Izumi K, Otsuka H (1991) Pulmonary carcinogenicity of 3,9- and 3,7-dinitrofluoranthene 3-nitrofluoranthene and benzo[a]pyrene in F344 rats. Carcinogenesis 12:1003–1007

Iwagawa M, Maeda T, Izumi K, Otsuka H, Nishifuji K, Ohnishi Y, Aoki S (1989) Comparative dose-response study on the pulmonary carcinogenicity of 1,6-dinitropyrene and benzo[a]pyrene in F344 rats. Carcinogeneses 10:1285–1290

Jamasbi R, Nettesheim JP, Kennel SJ (1978) Demonstration of cellular and humoral immunity to transplantable carcinomas derived from the respiratory tract of rats. Cancer Res 38:261–267

Kal HB, van Berkel AH, Broers JL, Klein JC, Mijnheere EP, Roholl PJ, Zurcher C, Ramaekers FC (1993) Cytokeratins expressed in experimental rat bronchial carcinomas. Int J Cancer 53:506–513

Kroes RJ, Garbis-Berkvens JM, de Vries T, van Nesselrooy HJ (1981) Histopathological profile of a Wistar rat stock including a survey of the literature. J Gerontol 36:259–279

Kuschner M, Laskin S (1970) Pulmonary epithelial tumors and tumor-like proliferations in the rat. In: Nettesheim P, Hanna MG, Deatherage JW (eds) Morphology of experimental respiratory carcinogenesis. USAEC, Oak Ridge, pp 203–226 (AEC symposium series 21)

Lee KP, Kelly DP, O'Neal FO, Stadler JC, Kennedy GL Jr (1988) Lung response to ultrafine Kevlar aramid synthetic fibrils following 2-year inhalation exposure in rats. Fundam Appl Toxicol 11:1–20

Lee KP, Trochimowicz HJ, Reinhardt CF (1985) Pulmonary response of rats exposed to titanium dioxide ($TiO_2$) by inhalation for two years. Toxicol Appl Pharmacol 79:179–192

Mohr U (1992) International classification of rodent tumours. I. The rat. 1. Respiratory system. IARC, Lyon (IARC scientific publications no 122)

Mohr U, Rittinghausen S, Takenaka S, Ernst H, Dungworth DL, Pylev LN (1990) Tumours of the lower respiratory tract and pleura in the rat. In: Turusov V, Mohr U (eds) Pathology of tumours in laboratory animals, 2nd edn. IARC Scientific Publications, Lyon, pp 275–299

Moulton JE, von Tscharner C, Schneider R (1981) Classification of lung carcinomas in the dog and cat. Vet Pathol 18:513–528

National Toxicology Program (NTP) (1993) Toxicology and carcinogenesis studies of talc (CAS NO 14807-96-6) in F344/N rats and B6C3Fl mice (inhalation studies). Research Triangle Park NC, US Department of Health and Human Services Public Health Service National Institutes of Health (NTP technical report no 421)

Nuorva K, Soini Y, Kamel D, Autio-Harmainen H, Risteli L, Risteli J, Vahakangas K, Paakko (1993) Concurrent p53 expression in bronchial dysplasias and squamous cell lung carcinomas. Am J Pathol 142:725–732

Ohgaki H, Furukawa F, Takahashi M, Kleihues P (1993) *K-ras* mutations are frequent in pulmonary squamous cell carcinomas but not in adenocarcinomas of WBN/Kob rats induced by N-nitrosobis(2oxopropyl)amine. Carcinogenesis 14:1471–1473

Reznik-Schüller HM, Gregg M (1981) Pathogenesis of lung tumors induced by n-nitrosoheptamethyleneimine in F344 rats. Virchows Arch (Pathol Anat) 393:333–343

Rothschild H, Buechner H, Welsh R, Vial LJ, Weinberg R (1982) Histologic typing of lung cancer in Louisiana. Cancer 49:1874–1877

Sanders CL, Lauhala KE, McDonald KE (1993) Lifespan studies in rats exposed to $^{239}PUO_2$ aerosol III survival and lung tumours. Int J Radiat Biol 64:417–430

Schulte A, Ernst H, Peters L, Heinrich U (1994) Induction of squamous cell carcinomas in the mouse lung after long-term inhalation of polycyclic aromatic hydrocarbon-rich exhausts. Exp Toxicol Pathol 45:415–421

Shabad LM, Pylev LN (1970) Morphological lesions in rat lungs induced by polycyclic hydrocarbons. In: Nettesheim P, Hanna MG, Deatherage JW (eds) Morphology of experimental respiratory carcinogenesis. USAEC, Oak Ridge, pp 227–242 (AEC symposium series 21)

Solleveld HA, Haseman JK, McConnell EE (1984) Natural history of body weight gain, survival and neoplasia in the F344 rat. J Natl Cancer Inst 72:929–940

Sundaresan V, Ganly P, Hasleton P, Rudd R, Sinha G, Bleehen NM, Rabbitts P (1992) p53 and chromosome 3 abnormalities characteristic of malignant lung tumours are detectable in preinvasive lesions of the bronchus. Oncogene 7:1989–1997

Usui Y, Takabe K, Takayama S, Miura H, Kimula Y (1991) Minute squamous cell carcinoma arising in the wall of a congenital lung cyst. Chest 99:235–236

Volm M, Drings P, Wodrich W (1993) Prognostic significance of the expression of c-fos c-jun and c-erbB-l oncogene products in human squamous cell lung carcinomas. J Cancer Res Clin Oncol 119:507–510

World Health Organization (WHO) (1982) Histological typing of lung tumors. Neoplasma 29:111–123

Yuhas JM, Pazmiño NH, Wagner E (1975) Development of concomitant immunity in mice bearing the weakly immunogenic line 1 lung carcinoma. Cancer Res 35:237–241

# Radiation-Induced Squamous Cell Carcinoma, Lung, Rat

Fletcher F. Hahn

*Synonym.* Epidermoid carcinoma

## Gross Appearance

Squamous cell carcinomas usually appear as spherical or multilobulated nodules with circumscribed borders (Fig. 233). They are generally solitary, but occasionally several are found in one lung. Solitary nodules may be relatively large and occupy much of the thorax. There is no predilection for any one lung lobe. They are found in the parenchyma and are rarely oriented around major airways.

The nodules frequently are seen as gray-white through the pleura. The pleura may be elevated by the nodule in the deflated lung, but invasion of the pleura is infrequent. On the cut surface the nodules are dry, gray-white, and generally firm. In well-differentiated tumors the cut surface may be dry and caseous, the result of necrosis.

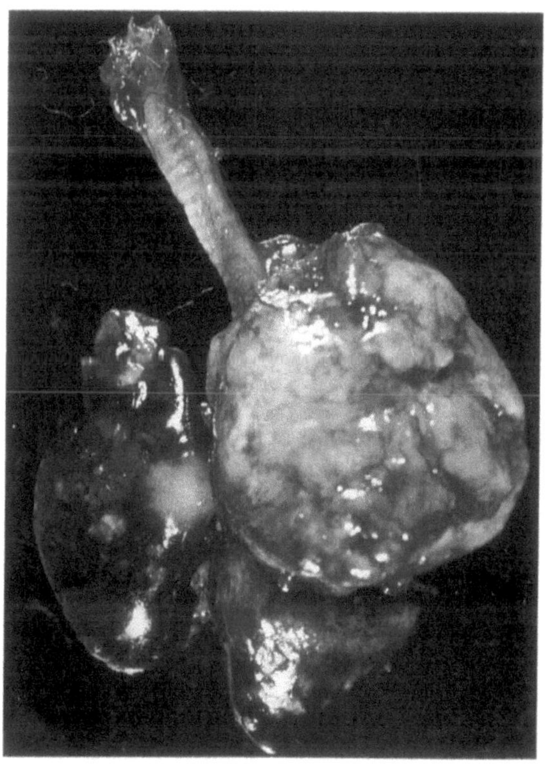

**Fig. 233.** Squamous cell carcinoma in the rat. Note spherical nature and circumscribed borders typical of these tumors. F344 rat 733 days after inhalation exposure to mixed transuranic oxides (plutonium/uranium), a mixture of alpha-emitting radionuclides

## Microscopic Features

A full range of squamous differentiation is expressed among the radiation-induced squamous cell carcinomas. The well-differentiated forms of squamous cell carcinoma are easily recognized by their resemblance to squamous epithelium and the keratinization of the more differentiated layers (Fig. 234). However, the basilar epithelium is dysplastic and contains foci of anaplastic cells (Fig. 234). Frequently these carcinomas are multiloculated, consisting of nests of readily identifiable squamous epithelium, keratohyalin, and epithelial pearls (Fig. 235). In some tumors abundant keratin debris accumulates in the epithelial nests. These well-differentiated tumors can grow to nearly occupy the entire lung lobe. In spite of their well-differentiated nature these tumors may invade blood vessels, including large muscular arteries (Fig. 236).

In the poorly differentiated forms of squamous cell carcinoma individual cells are keratinized, which makes them readily recognizable. Small nests of epithelial cells may be formed, but there is little resemblance to normally differentiated epithelium (Fig. 237). At the periphery of the nests there is usually a layer of large anaplastic cells that may have a small amount of eosinophilic cytoplasm. Toward the center of the nest the cells usually have more eosinophilic cytoplasm, indicative of individual cell keratinization (Fig. 237). On occasion the poorly differentiated tumors form a sheet of pleomorphic cells with a moderate amount of eosinophilic cytoplasm and polygonal nucleus with prominent nucleoli (Fig. 238). The cytoplasmic membrane is prominent, and intracellular bridges may be seen. Sometimes there is a fibrous stroma, but the tumors are usually not sclerosing. These tumors grow extensively within the lung and are locally invasive, but infrequently invade the pleura. Metastasis, when it occurs, is usually confined to the thorax and local lymph nodes. The invasiveness of these tumors is

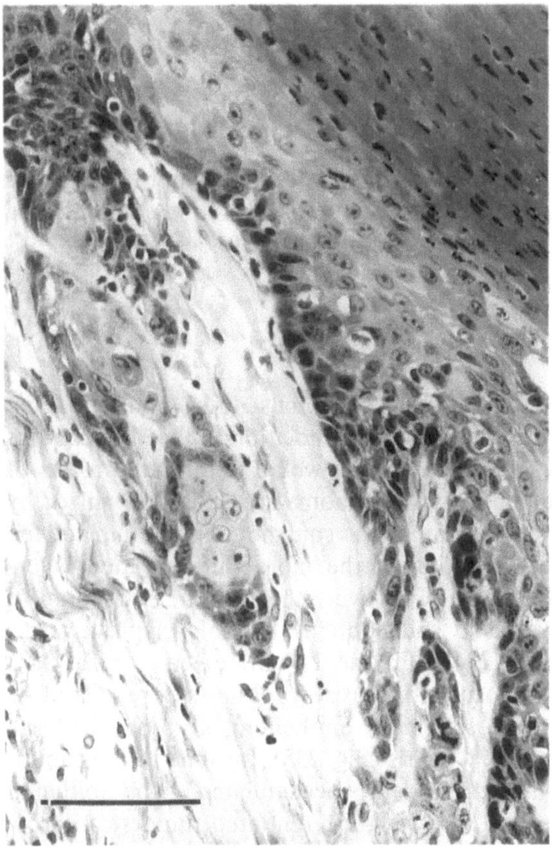

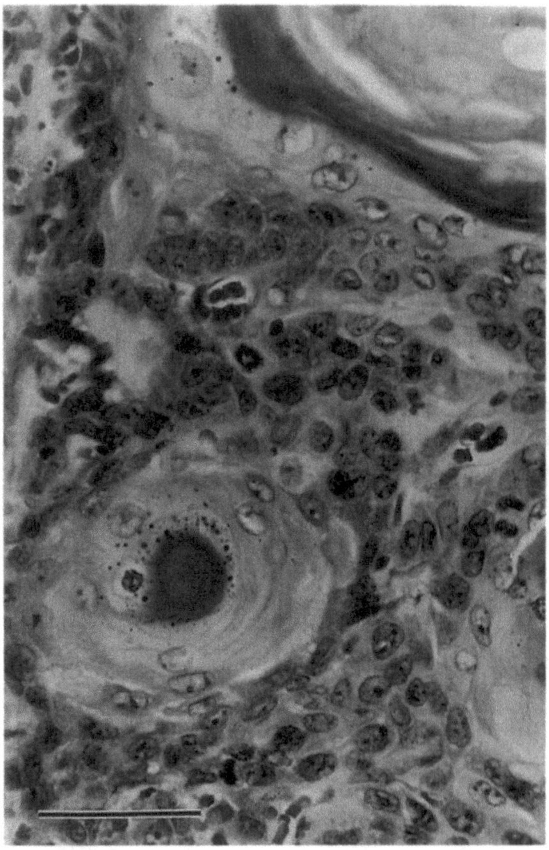

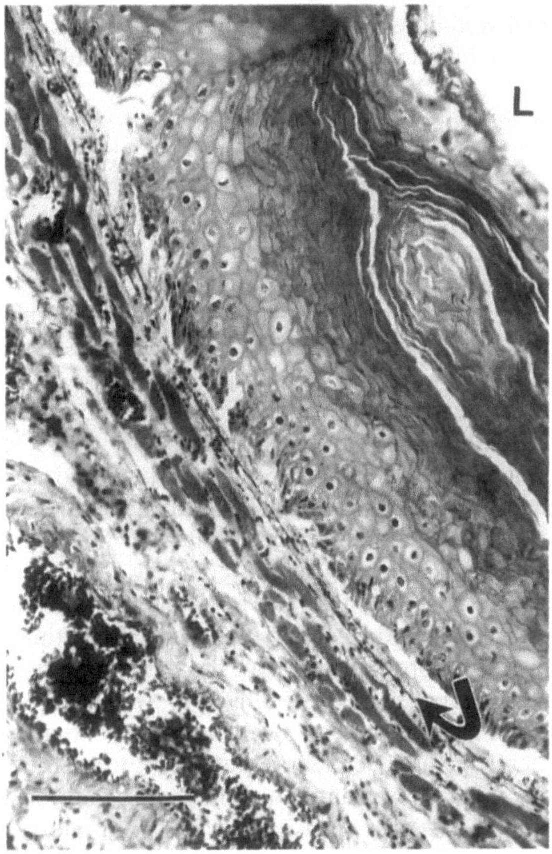
L

**Fig. 234.** (*upper left*) Well-differentiated squamous cell carcinoma in the lung of an F344 rat 588 days after inhalation exposure to a beta emitter, $^{144}CeO_2$. Tumor wall with dysplasia in basilar epithelial layer and invasion of underlying connective tissue. H&E, *bar*, 50 micra

**Fig. 235.** (*upper right*) Well-differentiated squamous cell carcinoma in the lung of an F344 rat 435 days after inhalation exposure to a beta emitter, $^{147}Pm$. Note nests of well-differentiated squamous epithelium among anaplastic squamous epithelium. H&E, *bar*, 50 micra

**Fig. 236.** (*below*) Growth of well-differentiated squamous cell carcinoma into large artery of an F344 rat 547 days after inhalation exposure to mixed transuranic oxides. *Arrow*, elastic lamina; *L*, arterial lumen. *Bar*, 100 micra. Elastic masson stain

◄

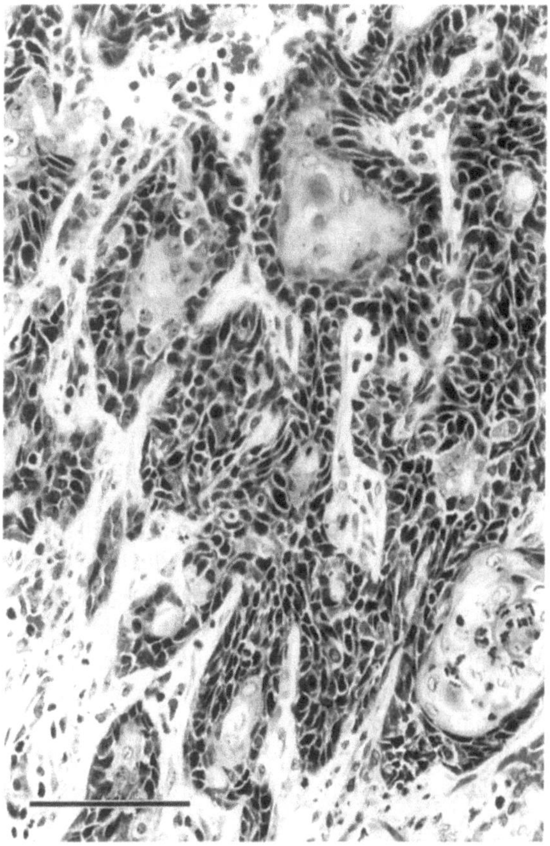

illustrated by their growth into pulmonary vessels and the mediastinum. Despite clear invasion of blood vessels, however, these tumors rarely develop metastases outside the thorax.

## Ultrastructure

The ultrastructure of these tumors has not been studied in rodents. However, ultrastructural characterization is not required for diagnosis because of the typical characteristic squamous cells in the vast majority of even the poorly differentiated tumors.

## Differential Diagnosis

On gross examination squamous cell carcinomas must be differentiated from other lung tumors and from abscesses. The poorly differentiated tumors may resemble pulmonary adenocarcinomas. The well-differentiated squamous cell carcinomas may grow by expansion and grossly appear as benign tumors or abscesses of the lung. Generally the cut

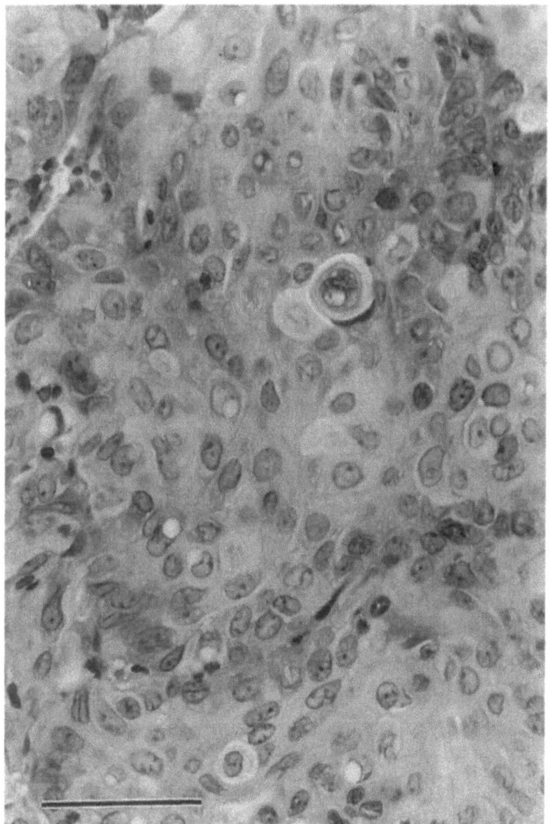

►

**Fig. 237.** Poorly differentiated squamous cell carcinoma in the lung of an F344 rat 557 days after inhalation exposure to mixed transuranic oxides. Small nests are present, with a distinct peripheral layer of cells and a central accumulation of a few large cells with abundant eosinophilic cytoplasm. H&E, *bar*, 50 micra

**Fig. 238.** Poorly differentiated squamous cell carcinoma in an F344 rat 486 days after inhalation exposure. Note sheet of pleomorphic cells with distinct cell membranes. H&E, *bar*, 50 micra

surface of the squamous cell carcinomas has a drier center with a lamellated gray appearance. Abscesses generally have a soft center with homogeneous appearance.

Microscopically, squamous cell carcinomas must be differentiated from squamous metaplasia, keratinizing squamous cysts, adenocarcinomas, and metastatic tumors. Metaplasia is usually associated with bronchioles and alveolar ducts but may extend to peripheral alveoli. Occasionally metaplasia occurs solely in the alveoli, usually in association with focal scars or accumulation of foreign particles. Metaplasia is well differentiated and usually conforms to the normal alveolar architecture of the lung. Keratinizing squamous cysts are nodules with a well-differentiated wall of squamous epithelium and a center filled with keratin debris. The component cells lack the features of anaplasia. The cysts grow by expansion and may attain a large size. Histologically, they resemble epidermal cysts with little papillary differentiation. Squamous cell carcinomas may originate from the wall of keratinizing cysts. Thickening, dysplasia, and anaplasia of the basilar layer are key features in the progression to carcinoma.

## Biological Features

The biological features of radiation-induced squamous cell carcinomas discussed here are based on studies of F344 rats exposed by inhalation to aerosols of cerium-144 dioxide, a beta-emitting radionuclide (Hahn and Lundgren 1992; Lundgren et al. 1992) or plutonium-239 dioxide, an alpha-emitting radionuclide. The squamous cell carcinomas induced are morphologically similar, regardless of radionuclide exposure.

Squamous cell carcinomas are generally seen only at the higher radiation doses (above an alpha dose of about 3.0 Gy and a beta dose of 170 Gy). A large fraction of the squamous cell carcinomas either cause death or are a major contributing factor in death, 70% with tumors induced by alpha-emitting radionuclides and 90% with those induced by beta-emitting radionuclides. Accordingly, the survival times are less than for rats with other types of lung tumors.

Because squamous cell carcinomas are generally found in rats with high radiation doses to the lung, radiation pneumonitis and focal alveolar septal fibrosis are frequent, particularly in rats that receive the alpha-emitting radionuclide. Accompanying the fibrosis is alveolar epithelial hyperplasia. In addition, lung tumors of other types are frequently found in the same rats that have squamous cell carcinomas.

Sanders and Dagle (1974) noted a direct correlation between the degree of inflammation and sclerosis around a radioactive particle and squamous metaplasia in surrounding tissue, frequently in subpleural regions. They envisioned progression from squamous metaplasia to squamous cell carcinoma.

The radiation-induced squamous cell carcinomas differ in many respects from the proliferative squamous lesions induced by diesel exhaust (Mauderly et al. 1987; Mohr et al. 1986), titanium dioxide (Lee et al. 1985), chromium dioxide (Lee et al. 1988), or paraaramid fibrils (Carlton 1994). Criteria for classifying proliferative squamous lesions in rat lungs have been outlined (Mohr et al. 1986). Criteria for proliferative keratin cysts have also been described (Carlton 1994). According to these criteria, most of the squamous tumors in diesel exhaust-exposed rats are benign keratinizing cysts that grow slowly by peripheral extension into air spaces and have a regular cytology with no atypia and few mitotic figures. A few low-grade carcinomas, which do not invade the pleura or mediastinum, are also induced. Squamous lung tumors induced by titanium dioxide and chromium dioxide have features of keratinizing cysts or low-grade squamous cell carcinomas. In none of these studies do squamous tumors invade vessels, the pleural cavity, or the mediastinum, nor do they metastasize.

The squamous cell carcinomas induced by inhaled $^{144}CeO_2$, on the other hand, are frequently invasive (>60%), and all exhibit some anaplasia. There does not appear to be a benign keratinizing cyst stage, although many tumors produce abundant keratin, even some of those that invade blood vessels.

In inhalation studies where benign keratinizing cysts of the lung are frequent, the rats have large lung burdens of the exposure material that are a factor in inducing squamous metaplasia (Lee et al. 1985; Carlton 1994). Such large quantities of particles are not a feature of inhalation studies with radioactive materials, where the absolute amount of compound deposited in the lung is in the microgram range. Radiation-induced squamous cell carcinomas of rats differ from those induced by heavy particle loads by their higher incidence, earlier occurrence, more malignant behavior, and possibly their pathogenesis.

**Table 21.** Comparison of squamous cell carcinoma characteristics in laboratory rodents and humans exposed to radionuclides internally deposited in the lung

| Characteristic | Rats[a] | Mice[b] | Syrian hamsters[c] | Dogs[d] | Humans[e] |
|---|---|---|---|---|---|
| Prevalence[f] | <1%–60% | 0%–10% | 2%–3% | 18% | 3% |
| Differentiation | Well | Moderate | Poor | Moderate | Poor |
| Metastasis | Infrequent | Rare | Rare | Infrequent | Frequent |
| Site of origin | Small airways, alveoli | Small airways, alveoli | Small airways, alveoli | Small airways alveoli | Large airways |

[a]Based on Hahn and Lundgren (1992).
[b]Based on Hahn et al. (1980).
[c]Based on Lundgren et al. (1982, 1983).
[d]Based on Tierney et al. (1994).
[e]Besed on data from uranium miners, Horacek et al. (1977); Kunz and Horacek (1979).
[f]Percentage of those at risk which have carcinoma.

## Comparison With Other Species

Squamous cell carcinomas of the lung of different species of laboratory rodents (Hahn et al. 1980; Lundgren et al. 1982, 1983; Hahn and Lundgren 1992) and of dogs (Tierney et al. 1994) are histologically similar. There are relative differences, however, in several characteristics, as noted in Table 21. More differences are apparent between squamous cell carcinomas in laboratory rodents and those in humans. Rarely are the tumors in laboratory rodents as poorly differentiated, aggressive, or metastasizing. In humans squamous cell carcinomas most frequently originate in major airways (Horacek et al. 1977; Kunz and Horacek 1979); this site of origin is rare in rodents. This difference may be related to differences in the site at which the radiation dose is delivered.

*Acknowledgements.* Research supported by the United States Department of Energy, Office of Health and Environmental Research, under Contract No. DE-AC04-76EV01013 and performed in facilities accredited by the American Association for the Accreditation of Laboratory Animal Care.

## References

Carlton WW (1994) "Proliferative keratin cyst," a lesion in the lungs of rats following chronic exposure to paraaramid fibules. Fundam Appl Toxicol 23:304–307

Hahn FF, Lundgren DL (1992) Pulmonary neoplasms in rats that inhaled cerium-144 dioxide. Toxicol Pathol 20:169–178

Hahn FF, Lundgren DL, McClellan RO (1980) Repeated inhalation exposure of mice to $^{144}CeO_2$. II. Biologic effects. Radiat Res 82:123–137

Horacek J, Placek V, Sevc J (1977) Histologic types of bronchogenic cancer in relation to different conditions of radiation exposure. Cancer 40:832–835

Kunz E, Sevc J, Place K V, Horacek J (1979) Lung cancer in man in relation to different time distribution of radiation exposure. Health Phys 36:699–706

Lee KP, Trochimowicz HJ, Reinhardt CF (1985) Pulmonary response of rats exposed to titanium dioxide ($TiO_2$) by inhalation for two years. Toxicol Appl Pharmacol 79:179–192

Lee KP, Ulrich CE, Geil RG, Trochimowicz HJ (1988) Effects of inhaled chromium dioxide dust on rats exposed for two years. Fundam Appl Toxicol 10:125–145

Lundgren DL, Hahn FF, McClellan RO (1982) Effects of single and repeated inhalation exposure of Syrian hamsters to aerosols of $^{144}CeO_2$. Radiat Res 90:374–394

Lundgren DL, Hahn FF, Rebar AH, McClellan RO (1983) Effects of the single or repeated inhalation exposure of Syrian hamsters to aerosols $^{239}PuO_2$. Int J Radiat Biol Relat Stud Phys Chem Med 43:1–18

Lundgren DL, Hahn FF, Diel JH (1992) Repeated inhalation exposure of rats to aerosols of $^{144}CeO_2$. Effects on survival and lung, liver and skeletal neoplasms. Radiat Res 132:325–333

Masse R (1980) Histogenesis of lung tumors induced in rats by inhalation of alpha emitters: an overview. In: Sanders CL, Cross FT, Dagle GE, Mahaffey JA (eds) Pulmonary toxicology of respirable particles. DOE Symp 53:498–521

Mauderly JL, Jones RK, Griffith WC, Henderson RF, McClellan RO (1987) Diesel exhaust is a pulmonary carcinogen in rats exposed chronically by inhalation. Fundam Appl Toxicol 9:208–221

Mohr U, Takemaka S, Dungworth DL (1986) Morphologic effects of inhaled diesel engine exhaust on lungs of rats: comparison with effects of coal oven flue gas mixed with pyrolized pitch. In: Ishinishi N, Koizumi A, McClellan RO, Stober W (eds) Carcinogenic and mutagenic effects of diesel engine exhaust. Elsevier/North Holland, Amsterdam, pp 459–470

Sanders CL, Dagle GE (1974) Studies of pulmonary carcinogenesis in rodents following inhalation of transuranic compounds. In: Karbe E, Park JF (eds) Experimental lung cancer: carcinogenesis and bioassays. Springer, Berlin Heidelberg New York, pp 422–429

Tierney LA, Hahn FF, Lachner JF (1994) p53, erbB2, and K-ras gene dysfunctions are rare in spontaneous and plutonium-239-induced canine lung neoplasia. Vet Pathol (submitted)

# Radiation-Induced Adenocarcinoma, Lung, Rat

Fletcher F. Hahn

*Synonyms.* Carcinoma, broncho-alveolar carcinoma, bronchiolo-alveolar carcinoma, alveolar-bronchiolar carcinoma

## Gross Appearance

Radiation-induced adenocarcinomas are found in the parenchymal portions of the lung. The gross appearance varies, dependent upon the histological pattern of the tumors. The adenocarcinomas with a papillary pattern may be very large, filling up an entire lung lobe with white lobulated masses (Fig. 239). The tumors with an alveolar pattern are usually smaller and more infiltrative, with an indistinct border. They are usually noted as nodules in the pulmonary parenchyma. Multiple tumors may be found, especially at higher radiation doses. Unlike squamous cell carcinomas, the center of large adenocarcinomas usually do not contain necrotic debris. The adenocar cinomas may invade the mediastinum or pleural cavity, creating a "seedy" appearance on the pleura or pericardium (Fig. 240). Very rarely do these tumors metastasize outside the thoracic cavity.

## Microscopic Features

Radiation-induced adenocarcinomas can generally be classified into three histological types; alveolar, papillary, and tubular patterns. Some tumors may have a mixture of patterns.

In the alveolar pattern the anaplastic cells grow along the alveolar septa, a feature that is prominent at the periphery of the tumor (Fig. 241). The tumor spreads by infiltration of surrounding structures, not by expansion as is seen with the papillary pattern. Some tumors invade bronchiolar walls, blood vessel walls, or lymphatics (Fig. 242); however, distant metastases are rare. The central portion of some tumors is compact and may be necrotic. The stroma generally has a fine collagenous appearance, contrasting with the dense fibrous tissue associated with inflammation. Individual tumor cells are rounded or low cuboidal in shape with moderate-sized round or oval nuclei and prominent nucleoli. These anaplastic cells may slough and fill the alveoli of the tumor.

In the papillary pattern cuboidal or columnar cells grow on papillary stalks of fibrous stroma that are usually delicate (Fig. 243). These tumors generally grow by expansion and may become large. Occasionally they invade small vessels or, more likely, the mediastinum or pleural cavity. Those that invade the cavity may cause seedy proliferations over the visceral and parietal pleura.

The tubular pattern is not seen frequently. The basic pattern is formed by nests or tubules of epithelial cells divided by a dense collagenous stroma (Fig. 244). The epithelial cells are large cuboidal cells, with a high nuclear to cytoplasmic ratio, oriented around a small lumen. These tumors appear to grow by expansion, compressing but rarely invading surrounding structures. Occasionally the tumor may have more anaplastic cells, less dense fibrous stroma, and invade surrounding structures (Fig. 245).

## Ultrastructural Features

The ultrastructural features of these three patterns of adenocarcinomas have not been studied in detail. Preliminary work has shown that ultrastructural characteristics of lung tumors have

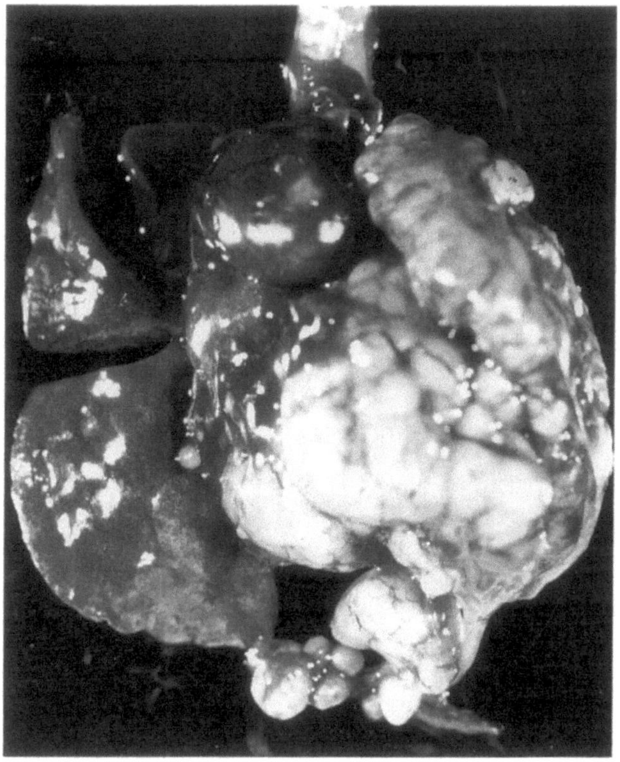

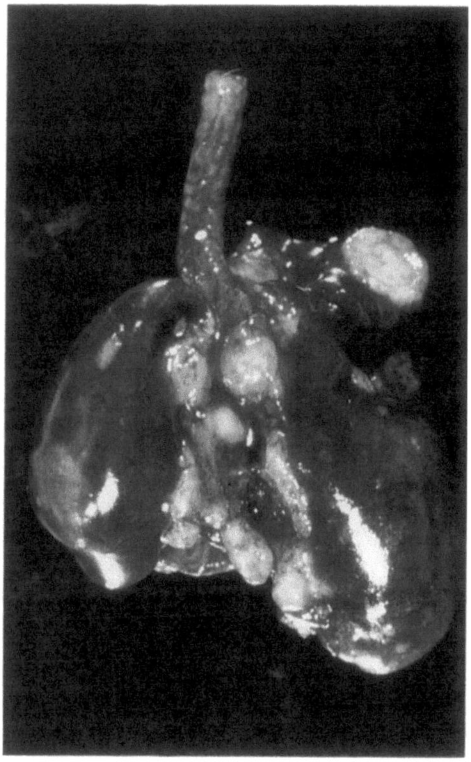

**Fig. 239.** (*left*) Adenocarcinoma, papillary pattern, fills the left lung of a rat that died 974 days after inhalation of $^{144}$Ce dioxide

**Fig. 240.** (*right*) Adenocarcinoma, alveolar pattern, invades the mediastinum of a rat that died 538 days after inhalation of $^{239}$Pu dioxide

improved diagnosis only for a few specific tumor types (Masse 1980). However, ultrastructural studies of plutonium-induced foci of epithelial hyperplasia and adenocarcinomas have shown similarity of the proliferative cells to type II cells of the lung (Herbert et al. 1994).

## Differential Diagnosis

Radiation-induced adenocarcinomas must be differentiated from squamous cell carcinomas, adenosquamous carcinomas, metastatic carcinomas, and adenomas of the lung as well as from the hyperplastic lesions that frequently occur in radiation-damaged lungs at high radiation doses. At the high doses tumors of different phenotypes may coexist in the same lung. Squamous cell carcinomas can be easily diagnosed since they almost always have well-differentiated squamous cells that are easily recognized histologically. Adenocarcinomas that are admixed with squamous cell carcinoma should be classified as adenosquamous carcinoma. This admixture occurs most often with the alveolar pattern of adenocarcinoma.

Adenosquamous carcinomas should not be confused with adenocarcinomas containing squamous metaplasia. Such metaplasia usually occurs with the papillary pattern, but this is infrequent.

Differentiation of adenocarcinoma from adenomas or other proliferative lesions is based on metastasis, which is rare, invasion, and cellular anaplasia. Invasion of the surrounding tissue by the tumor is a relatively frequent even but the invasive nature of the tumor varies with the tumor phenotype. Papillary adenocarcinomas expand, and the larger ones can invade airways or, more frequently, the pleura. Pleural invasion is frequently associated with invasion of the mediastinum and transpleural metastasis. Alveolar adenocarcinomas frequently invade bronchiolar walls or the walls of blood vessels or lymphatics. In spite of invasion of the blood vessels metastases are rare. In some cases tumors are classified as malignant based on anaplastic fea-

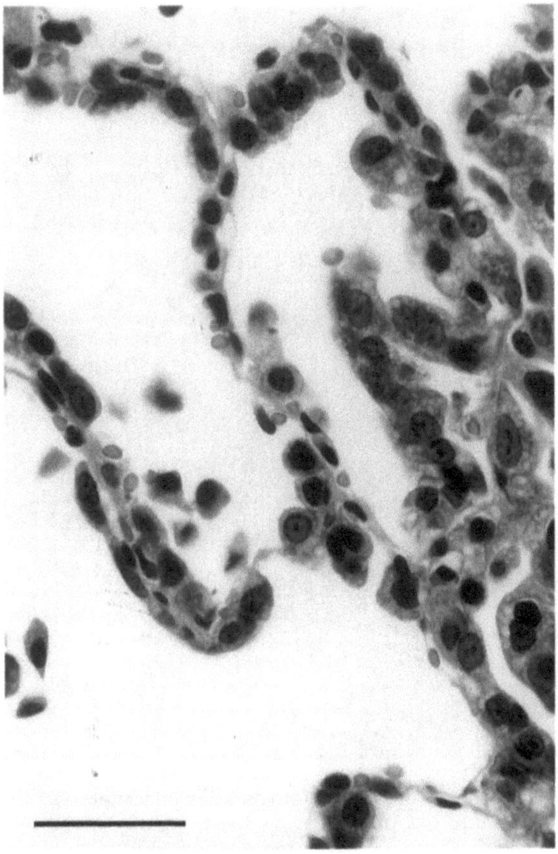

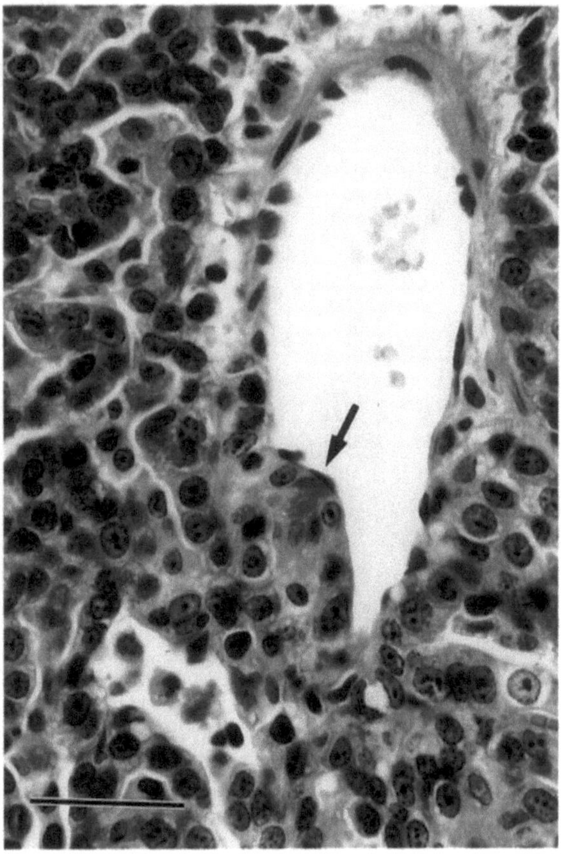

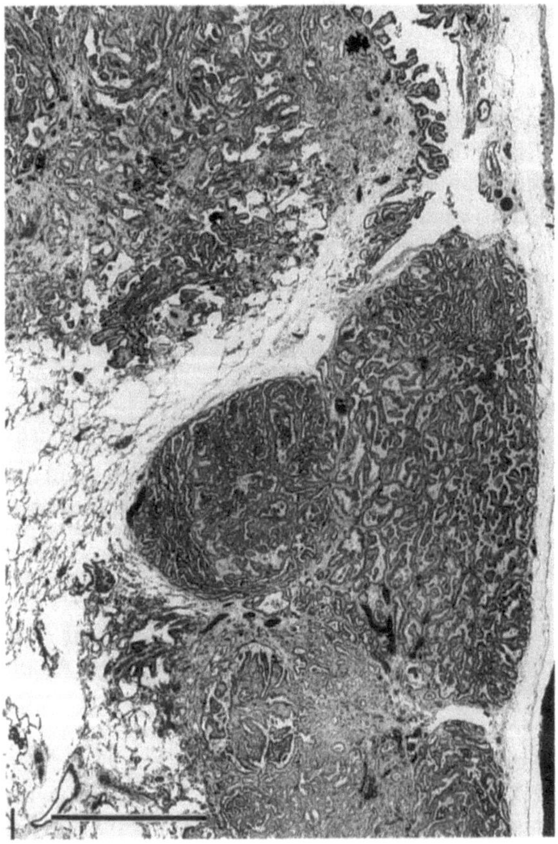

**Fig. 241.** (*upper left*) Anaplastic cells of an alveolar adenocarcinoma grow along the alveolar septa of an F344 rat 580 days after inhalation of $^{239}$Pu dioxide. H&E, *bar*, 33 micra

**Fig. 242.** (*upper right*) Invasion of a blood vessel (arrow) by the alveolar adenocarcinoma illustrated in Fig. 241. H&E, *bar*, 33 micra

**Fig. 243.** (*below*) Adenocarcinoma, papillary pattern in the lung of an F344 rat 889 days after inhalation of $^{239}PuO_2$ dioxide. H&E, *bar*, 70 micra
◀

tures similar to those seen in carcinomas where invasion has occurred.

Metastasis of carcinomas to the lung is not unusual. Frequent primary sites in F344 rats include mammary gland, ovary, uterus, adrenal, and liver. Multiple, solitary, similarly sized lesions of carcinoma, or those oriented around blood vessels, should be considered metastatic in origin.

## Biological Features

The biological features of radiation-induced adenocarcinomas discussed here are based on studies of F344 rats exposed by inhalation to aerosols of cerium-144 dioxide, a beta-emitting radionuclide (Hahn and Lundgren 1992; Lundgren et al. 1992), or plutonium-239 dioxide, an alpha-emitting radionuclide (Herbert et al. 1993; Lundgren et al. 1995). The types of adenocarcinomas induced are generally similar regardless of radionuclide.

The incidence of adenocarcinomas after radiation exposure is dependent on the radiation dose to the lung but is independent of gender. Adenocarcinomas of all types occur relatively late after exposure, a median of about 750 days with a range from about 510 to about 1100 days after exposure. At relatively high radiation doses about one-third of the adenocarcinomas are the cause of death, about one-third contribute to death, and about one-third are incidental to death. At

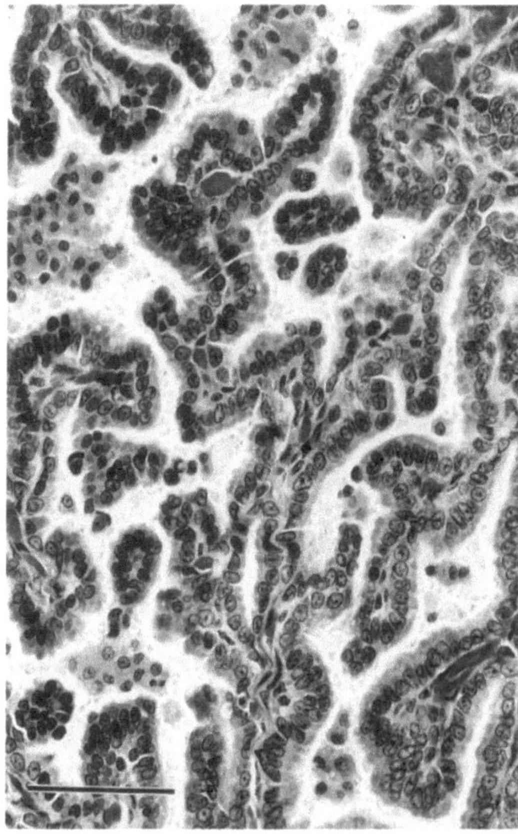

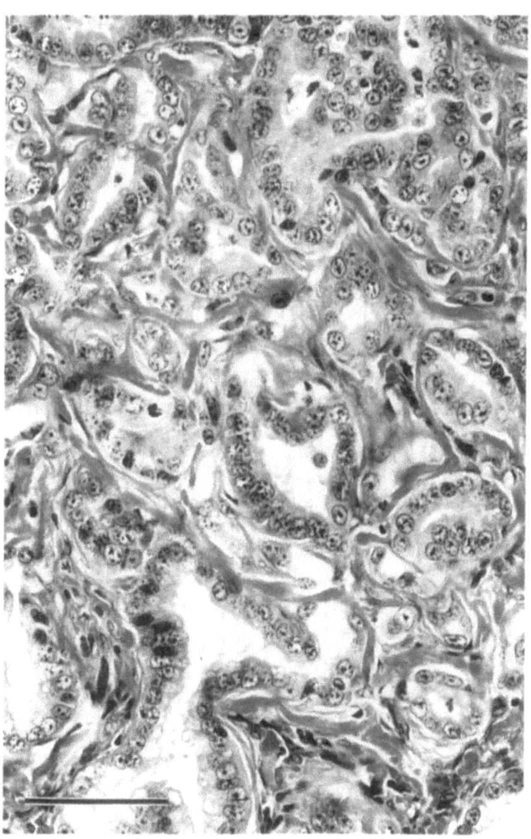

▶
**Fig. 244.** (*above*) Detail of papillary pattern (Fig. 243). Note proliferation of cuboidal cells with prominent nucleoli along a delicate papillary stroma. H&E, *bar*, 70 micra

**Fig. 245.** (*below*) Adenocarcinoma, tubular pattern in the lung of an F344 rat 581 days after inhalation of $^{238}$Pu dioxide and showing fibrous stroma separating tubules and nests of anaplastic cells. H&E, *bar*, 70 micra

**Table 22.** Comparison of adenocarcinoma characteristics in laboratory animals and humans exposed to radionuclides internally deposited in the lung

| Characteristic | Rats | Mice[a] | Syrian hamsters[b] | Dogs[c] | Man[d] |
|---|---|---|---|---|---|
| Adenocarcinomas as percentage total cancers | 45–75 | 50 | 85 | 66–90 | 12 |
| Morphological patterns | Alveolar papillary tubular | Papillary | Alveolar papillary tubular | Alveolar papillary | Tubular |
| Metastasis | Very rare | Very rare | Very rare | Rare | Common |
| Site of origin | Alveoli | Alveoli | Alveoli | Small airways alveoli | Airways |
| Cancer risk per unit dose | Moderate | High | Very low | Moderate | Moderate |

[a] Based on Hahn et al. (1980).
[b] Based o n Lundgren et al. (1982, 1983).
[c] Based on Hahn et al. (1994); Tierney et al. (1994).
[d] Based on NRC (1991).

lower doses the fraction of incidental tumors increases.

Plutonium-induced proliferative lesions and adenocarcinomas have been studied at intervals of killing of up to 450 days after inhalation exposure (Herbert et al. 1993). Maximal increases in alveolar and bronchiolar epithelial cell labeling with tritiated thymidine are seen at 30 days after exposure. Focal proliferative epithelial lesions develop by 180 days, but before the onset of pulmonary neoplasms. The volume density and epithelial surface area of the foci increase progressively between 180 and 450 days after exposure. Pulmonary neoplasms, including adenocarcinomas are initially seen at 308 days. Immunohistochemistry and transmission microscopy have been used to identify the proliferative lesions as containing type II alveolar cells and to identify most of the adenocarcinomas as containing type II cells. These findings have led to the conclusion that the cell of origin for most of the adenocarcinomas is the alveolar type II cell (Herbert et al. 1994).

## Comparison with Other Species

The radiation-induced adenocarcinomas are not strictly comparable among species (Table 22). Adenocarcinomas are the most frequently seen type in rats, dogs, and Syrian hamsters, although tumor type is somewhat dependent on radiation dose. The morphological patterns are also similar in these three species. Syrian hamsters differ from all species in their relative resistance to radiation-induced tumors, except in the case of intratracheal-instilled radionuclides. Mice differ from other species in their high incidence of pulmonary adenomas, both as spontaneous tumors and in response to irradiation. Humans also differ from the other species, primarily in the site of origin of the tumors and in the low incidence of adenocarcinomas in radiation-exposed populations. This difference may be due in part to the mode of exposure of the human populations, that is to radon and radon daughters which irradiate primarily the bronchial epithelium and to the high frequency of cigarette smoking in human populations with lung cancer.

*Acknowledgements.* Research supported by the United States Department of Energy, Office of Health and Environmental Research, under Contract No. DE-AC04-76EV01013 and performed in facilities accredited by the American Association for the Accreditation of Laboratory Animal Care.

## References

Hahn FF, Lundgren DL (1992) Pulmonary neoplasms in rats that inhaled cerium-144 dioxide. Toxicol Pathol 20:169–178

Hahn FF, Lundgren DL, McClellan RO (1980) Repeated inhalation exposure of mice to $^{144}CeO_2$. Biologic effects. Radiat Res 82:123–137

Hahn FF, Griffith WC, Hobbs CH, Muggenburg BA, Newton GJ, Boecker BB (1994) Biological effects of $^{91}Y$ in relatively insoluble particles inhaled by Beagle dogs. Ann Occup Hyg 38 [Suppl 1]:275–280

Herbert RA, Gillett NA, Rebar AH, Lundgren DL, Hoover MD, Chang IY, Carlton WW, Hahn FF (1993) Sequential analysis of the pathogenesis of plutonium-induced pulmonary neoplasms in the rat: morphology, morphometry, and cytokinetics. Radiat Res 134:29–42

Herbert RA, Stegelmeier BS, Gillett NA, Rebar AH, Carlton WW, Singh G, Hahn FF (1994) Plutonium-induced proliferative lesions and pulmonary epithelial neoplasms in the rat: immunohistochemical and ultrastructural evidence for their origin from type II pneumocytes. Vet Pathol 31:366–374

Lundgren DL, Hahn FF, McClellan RO (1982) Effects of single and repeated inhalation exposure of Syrian hamster to aerosols of $^{144}CeO_2$. Radiat Res 90:374–394

Lundgren DL, Hahn FF, Rebar AH, McClellan RO (1983) Effects of the single or repeated inhalation exposure of Syrian hamsters to aerosols of $^{239}PuO_2$. Int J Radiat Biol 43:1–18

Lundgren DL, Hahn FF, Diel JH (1992) Repeated inhalation exposure of rats to aerosols of $^{144}CeO_2$. II. Effects on survival and lung, liver, and skeletal neoplasms. Radiat Res 132:325–333

Lundgren DL, Haley PJ, Hahn FF, Diel JH, Griffith WC, Scott BR (1995) Pulmonary carcinogenicity of repeated inhalation exposure of rats to aerosols of $^{239}PuO_2$. Radiat Res 142:39–53

Masse R (1980) Histogenesis of lung tumors induced in rats by inhalation of alpha emitters: an overview. In: Sanders CI, Cross FT, Dagle GE, Mahaffey JA (eds) Pulmonary toxicology of respirable particles. Proceedings of the 9th Annual Hanford Life Sciences Symposium at Richland, Washington, 22–14 Oct 1979. DOE symposium series, 53 CONF-791002. Technical Information Centers, Oak Ridge, pp 498–521

National Research Council (NRC) (1991) Chapter 8. Cells of origin for lung cancer in comparative dosimetry of radon in mines and homes. Panel on dosimetric assumptions affecting the application of radon risk estimates. National Academy, Washington DC, pp 166–193

Tierney LA, Hahn FF, Lechner JF (1995) p53, erbB2, and K-ras gene dysfunctions are rare in spontaneous and plutonium-239-induced canine lung neoplasia. Radiat Res (submitted)

# Radiation-Induced Sarcomas, Lung, Rat

Fletcher F. Hahn

*Synonyms.* Radiation-induced hemangiosarcoma, fibrosarcomas

## Gross Appearance

Radiation-induced sarcomas include neoplasms with morphological patterns of hemangiosarcoma and fibrosarcoma. The hemangiosarcomas are moderately large, frequently occupying much of the affected lung lobe. The masses are hemorrhagic and friable. Since hemangiosarcomas are associated with high radiation doses, these tumors are frequently found in lungs with multiple tumors of varied morphological types. Fibrosarcomas occur less frequently than the hemangiosarcomas and appear grossly as firm, white masses.

## Microscopic Features

These hemangiosarcomas form irregular capillary or, more usually, cavernous sinuses. A key feature is spindle-shaped, anaplastic cells lining the vascular spaces (Fig. 246). The nuclei are flattened but plump with prominent nucleoli. Congestion of these vascular spaces is marked. Hemorrhage, hemoglobin crystals, hemosiderin, and alveolar macrophage hyperplasia are prominent in the tumor and surrounding alveoli. The volume of the blood present may account for much of the mass of the neoplasm. These tumors do not metastasize out of the lung and are usually associated with marked radiation pneumonitis and septal fibrosis. Some parts of the neoplasms may be solid with a proliferation of pleomorphic cells (Fig. 247).
The fibrosarcomas are readily recognized by their spindle cell pattern and collagen production (Fig. 248). These tumors tend to grow in the interstitium, along airways and blood vessels. They may invade large blood vessels but do not metastasize outside the thorax.

## Ultrastructure

The ultrastructure of these radiation-induced neoplasms in the rat has not been studied.

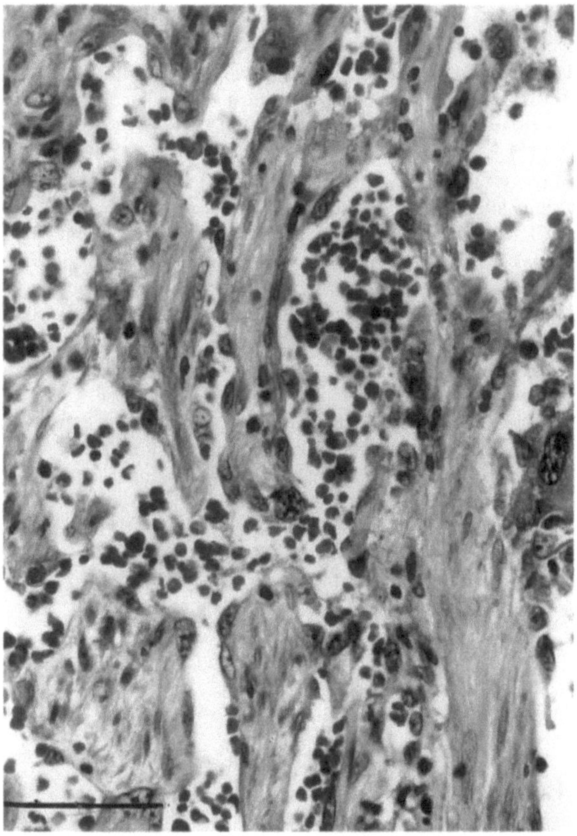

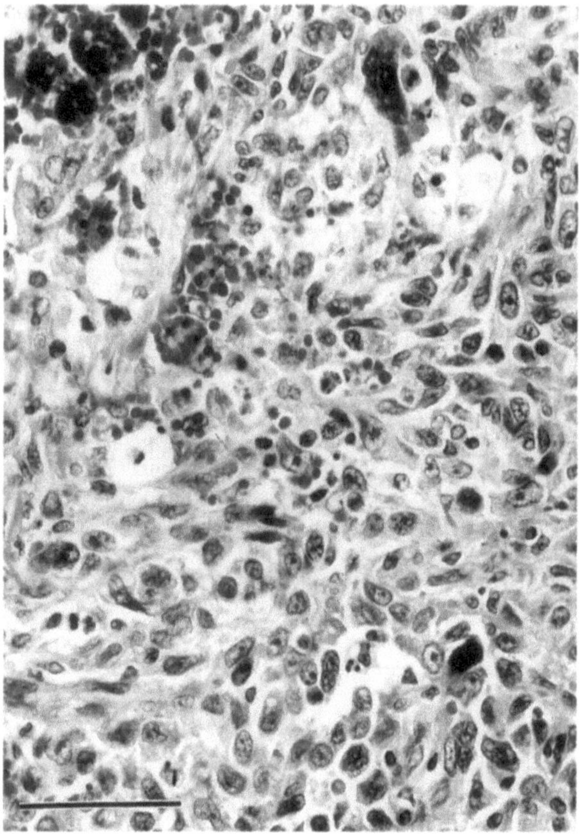

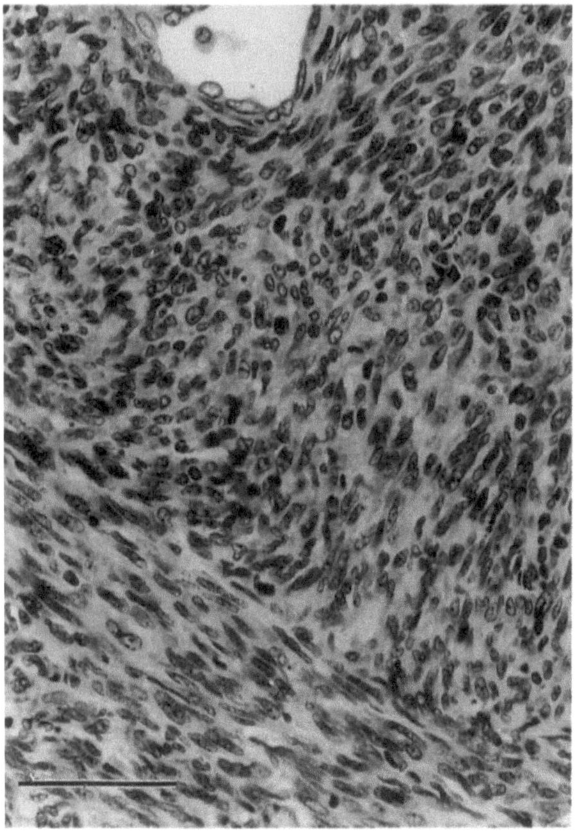

## Differential Diagnosis

The hemangiosarcomas must be differentiated from frankly organized hemorrhage that occasionally accompanies radiation pneumonitis. The hemorrhage may be recent or long-standing. Dysplastic-appearing cells, particularly alveolar type II cells, may be present as a result of high radiation doses to the tissues but are not believed to be part of a neoplasm. In addition, other neoplasms may be present, further confusing the histological appearance.

The histological appearance of the fibrosarcomas is relatively straightforward, with bundles and sheets of spindle shaped cells. The few fibrosarcomas noted have produced moderate amounts of collagen. Fibrosarcomas can be differentiated from leiomyosarcomas with trichrome stains, which show the presence of collagen but no smooth muscle cells.

Primary pulmonary sarcomas must be differentiated from metastases to the lung from another neoplasm in the body or arising elsewhere in the thorax. Metastases from mammary neoplasms, although not common, can be particularly confusing because of their frequent sarcomatous differentiation in the rat.

## Biological Features

Spontaneous primary hemangiosarcomas of the lung of rats have not been reported in the literature. They only occur in situations where very high radiation doses are delivered to the lung such as occurs with internally deposited radionuclides (Hahn and Lundgren 1992; Lundgren et al. 1995). For example, following inhalation exposure of F344 rats to $^{144}$Ce dioxide, pulmonary hemangiosarcomas are induced with an average dose to lung of 230 Gy which is about 100 times the dose required for an increased incidence of radiation-induced lung carcinoma. Doses higher than this frequently result in early death from acute effects. Beta-emitting radionuclides, such as $^{144}$Ce, induce relatively more hemangiosarcomas than alpha-emitting radionuclides, such as $^{239}$Pu. In addition, beta emitter induced hemangiosarcomas usually kill the rat (Lundgren et al. 1992). With alpha emitter induced hemangiosarcomas other lung tumors are frequently present that may kill the animal but at a later time in life than those induced by beta-emitting radionuclides (Lundgren et al. 1995).

So few fibrosarcomas have been noted in rats exposed to inhaled radionuclides that little can be said about their biological features. They do occur at lower radiation doses than hemangiosarcomas by a factor of 5–10 (Hahn and Lundgren 1992).

◄

**Fig. 246.** (*upper left*) Anaplastic cells lining vascular spaces (*arrows*) in a hemangiosarcoma of a rat 588 days after exposure to $^{147}$Pm. H&E, *bar*, 50 micra

**Fig. 247.** (*upper right*) Proliferation of pleomorphic anaplastic cells in a more solid portion of hemangiosarcoma. H&E, *bar*, 50 micra

**Fig. 248.** (*below*) Fibrosarcoma of the lung growing in the interstitium in a rat 404 days after inhalation exposure to $^{239}$Pu dioxide. Moderate amounts of collagen could be demonstrated with Masson's trichome stain. H&E, *bar*, 70 micra

## Comparison with Other Species

The radiation-induced hemangiosarcomas in rats have a striking resemblance histologically to those induced in mice (Hahn et al. 1980) and dogs (Hahn et al. 1973) by inhaled $^{144}$Ce dioxide. In all three species the neoplasms are characterized by irregular capillary or cavernous sinuses lined by spindle-shaped cells containing large nuclei with prominent nucleoli. Only in the dog, however, does the neoplasm metastasize out of the lung. Primary hemangiosarcomas of the lung are unreported in humans.

*Acknowledgements.* Research supported by the United States Department of Energy, Office of Health and Environmental Research, under Contract No. DE-AC04-76EV01013 and performed in facilities accredited by the American Association for the Accreditation of Laboratory Animal Care.

## References

Hahn FF, Lundgren DL (1992) Pulmonary neoplasms in rats that inhaled cerium-144 dioxide. Toxicol Pathol 20:169–178

Hahn FF, Benjamin SA, Boecker BB, Chiffelle TL, Hobbs CH, Jones RK, McClellan RO, Pickrell JA, Redman HC (1973) Primary pulmonary neoplasms in beagle dogs exposed to aerosols of $^{144}$Ce in fused-clay particles. J Natl Cancer Inst 50:675–698

Hahn FF, Lundgren DL, McClellan RO (1980) Repeated inhalation exposure of mice to $^{144}CeO_2$. II. Biologic effects. Radiat Res 82:123–137

Lundgren DL, Hahn FF, Diel JH (1992) Repeated inhalation exposure of rats to aerosols of $^{144}CeO_2$. II. Effects on survival and lung, liver, and skeletal neoplasms. Radiat Res 132:325–333

Lundgren DL, Haley PJ, Hahn FF, Diel JH, Griffith WC, Scott BR (1955) Pulmonary carcinogenicity of repeated inhalation exposure of rats to aerosols of $^{239}PuO_2$. Radiat Res 142:39–53

# Radiation-Induced Adenosquamous Carcinoma, Lung, Rat

Fletcher F. Hahn

*Synonyms.* Combined carcinoma, combined epidermoid and bronchiogenic adenocarcinoma, "mixed carcinoma"

## Gross Appearance

Radiation-induced adenosquamous carcinomas, in common with other carcinomas of the rat lung, are found in the parenchymal portions of the lung. The gross appearance of the smaller adenosquamous carcinomas is that of an indistinct nodule. Larger carcinomas may fill part or all of a lobe. The nodules are white or pale gray. On section the surface may be dry in keratinizing tumors; however, large keratin masses are usually not found.

## Microscopic Features

The morphological pattern of adenosquamous carcinoma is an admixture of squamous cell carcinomatous and adenocarcinomatous patterns (Fig. 249). One pattern may predominate in any given area of the tumor. The adenocarcinomatous differentiation may have a proliferation of anaplastic, low cuboidal cells either along a fine stroma in an alveolar pattern (Fig. 250) or along a fine papillary stroma forming a papillary pattern (Fig. 251). The squamous differentiation follows these patterns with individual keratinized cell or small foci of extracellular keratin. In areas where the squamous differentiation predominates epithelial nests or cords with well-differentiated squamous epithelium usually form. Abundant keratin with cyst formation is not a characteristic. The adenosquamous tumors grow by infiltration and infrequently invade blood vessels, lymphatics, and pleura. Either component of the carcinomas may invade. Admixtures occur most often with the alveolar phenotype of adenocarcinoma.

## Ultrastructure

The ultrastructure of these radiation-induced neoplasms in rats has not been studied in detail. However, an admixture of small mucous granules and squamous features within individual tumor cells has been described (Masse 1980). This phenotype expression is commonly found in human bronchogenic carcinomas examined with electron microscopy (McDowell et al. 1978).

## Differential Diagnosis

Adenosquamous carcinomas must be differentiated from squamous cell carcinomas and adenocarcinomas of all types. Since the adenosquamous pattern is a combination of the

▶

**Fig. 249.** (*upper left*) Overview of adenosquamous carcinoma in lung of an F344 rat 660 days after $^{239}PuO_2$ inhalation exposure showing squamous differentiation (**A**) and adenomatous differentiation (**B**). H&E, *bar*, 170 micra

**Fig. 250.** (*upper right*) Proliferation of anaplastic cuboidal cells and squamous cells (*arrow*) along alveolar septa in the adenosquamous carcinoma from Fig. 249. H&E, *bar*, 70 micra

**Fig. 251.** (*below*) Proliferation of anaplastic cuboidal cells adenosquamous cells along papillary projections in the adenosquamous carcinoma from Fig. 249. H&E, *bar*, 70 micra

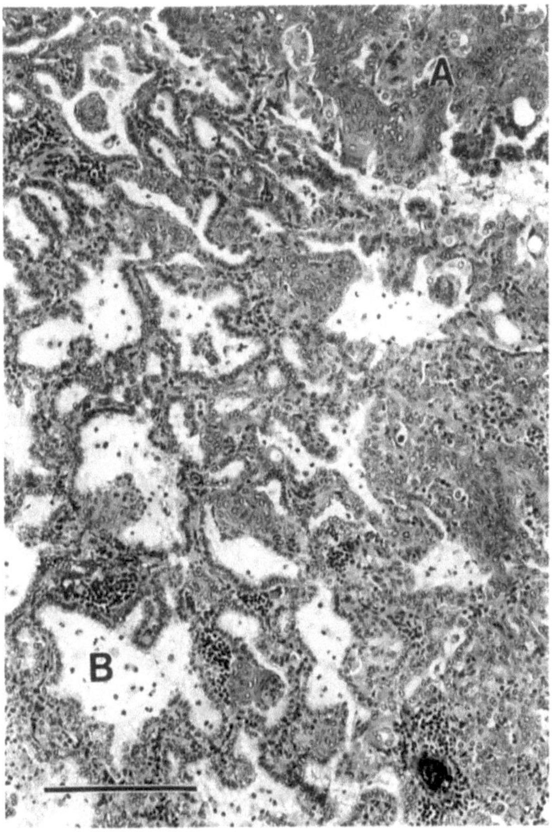
A
B

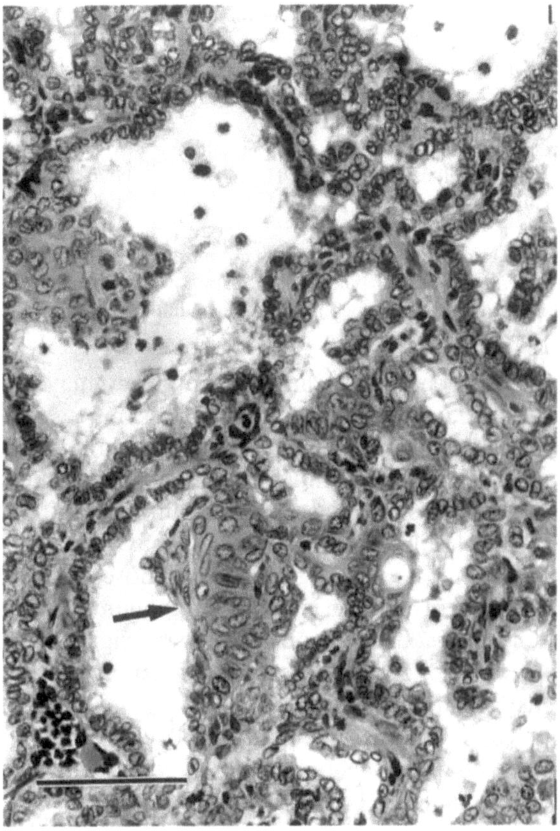

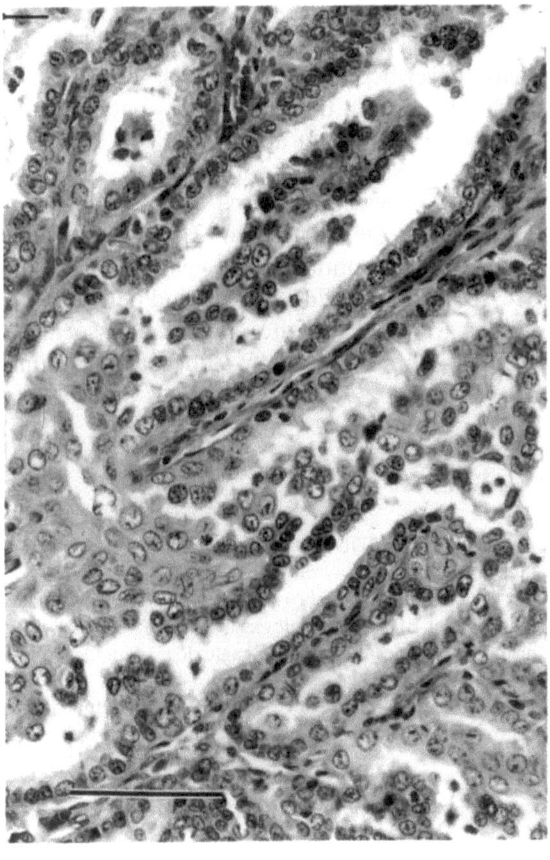

**Table 23.** Characteristics of major radiation-induced tumor types in the F344 rat

| Tumor type | Dose[a] | % Fatal[b] | Survival[c] |
|---|---|---|---|
| Adenosquamous carcinoma | Low | Intermediate ~50% | Intermediate |
| Adenocarcinoma | Intermediate | Low < 40% | Long |
| Squamous cell carcinoma | High | High > 70% | Short |
| Hemangiosarcoma | High | High > 80% | Short |

[a] Doses at which these tumor types are most frequently seen.
[b] Percentage of tumor types that are fatal.
[c] Life span of rats in which most of these tumor types are seen.

two other patterns, the differentiation may at times be problematical. To be classified as an adenosquamous carcinoma the tumor should have a true admixture of morphological patterns, not merely a collision of two separate tumors of different morphologies. Multiple tumors may occur, especially in rats with high radiation doses to the lung. The proportion of both components of an adenosquamous carcinoma should be significant, for example, 10%–20%, not just a few scattered cells or foci of cells.

Foci of squamous metaplastic cells can occur in adenocarcinomas should not be confused with adenosquamous carcinomas. The features of anaplasia and lack of differentiation should be used to identify a true neoplastic proliferation of squamous cells.

## Biological Features

Radiation-induced adenosquamous carcinomas have biological features that differ from those of squamous cell carcinomas or adenocarcinomas, based on studies of F344 rats that inhaled $^{144}$Ce dioxide (Hahn and Lundgren 1992; Lundgren et al. 1992) or $^{239}$Pu dioxide (Lundgren et al. 1995). These differences are the rationale for classifying radiation-induced adenosquamous carcinomas as a separate morphological pattern and not including them with squamous cell carcinomas or adenocarcinomas. Table 23 compares several important features among the major radiation-induced tumor types in the rat. The survival time of animals with adenosquamous carcinomas is shorter than that of rats with adenocarcinoma but about the same as that of rats with squamous cell carcinomas. The radiation dose to the lung for those rats with adenosquamous carcinomas is lower than the dose in rats with either squamous cell carcinoma or adenocarcinoma. The percentage of tumors that kill the animal or contribute to the death is high in those with squamous cell carcinoma and low in those with adenocarcinoma. Those with adenosquamous carcinoma are intermediate. These findings indicate that the adenosquamous carcinomas appear to be not only morphologically but also biologically different from the other types of radiation-induced cancers.

## Comparison with Other Species

Radiation-induced adenosquamous carcinomas have been described from a number of studies in rats exposed to plutonium or other alpha-emitting radionuclides (Masse 1980; Sanders 1973; Sanders et al. 1993). This morphological pattern is infrequently described in other species, but has been noted in dogs that inhaled beta-emitting radionuclides (Hahn et al. 1994).

*Acknowledgements.* Research supported by the United States Department of Energy, Office of Health and Environmental Research, under Contract No. DE-AC04-76EV01013 and performed in facilities accredited by the American Association for the Accreditation of Laboratory Animal Care.

## References

Hahn FF, Lundgren DL (1992) Pulmonary neoplasms in rats that inhaled cerium-144 dioxide. Toxicol Pathol 20:169–178

Hahn FF, Griffith WC, Hobbs CH, Muggenburg BA, Newton GJ, Boecker BB (1994) Biological effects of $^{91}$Y in relatively insoluble particles inhaled by Beagle dogs. Ann Occup Hyg 38 [Suppl 1]:275–280

Lundgren DL, Hahn FF, Diel JH (1992) Repeated inhalation exposure of rats to aerosols of $^{144}CeO_2$. II. Effects on survival and lung, liver, and skeletal neoplasms. Radiat Res 132:325–333

Lundgren DL, Haley PJ, Hahn FF, Diel JH, Griffith WC, Scott BR (1995) Pulmonary carcinogenicity of repeated inhalation

exposure of rats to aerosols of $^{239}PuO_2$. Radiat Res 142:39–53
Masse R (1980) Histogenesis of lung tumors induced in rats by inhalation of alpha emitters: an overview. In: Sanders CL, Cross FT, Dagle GE, Mahaffey JA (eds) Pulmonary toxicology of respirable particles. DOE Symp 53:498–521
McDowell E, McLaughlin JS, Merenyl DK, Kieffer RF, Harris CC, Trump BK (1978) The respiratory epithelium. V. Histogenesis of lung carcinoma in the human. J Natl Cancer Inst 61:587–606
Sanders CL (1973) Carcinogenicity of inhaled plutonium-238 in the rat. Radiat Res 56:540–553
Sanders CL, Lauhala KE, McDonald KE (1993) Lifespan studies in rats exposed to $^{239}PuO_2$ aerosol. III. Survival and lung tumours. Int J Radiat Biol 64:417–430

# Pleural Mesothelioma, Syrian Hamster

Antonio Cardesa and Josep A. Bombi

*Synonyms.* Malignant mesothelioma, mesothelial neoplasia

## Gross Appearance

Pleural mesotheliomas appear as whitish gray nodules, usually multiple, and of firm consistency. When initially detected, they form tiny masses less than 1 mm in diameter, which progressively grow and fuse together to form larger nodules and plaques measuring up to 5 mm at the widest point. The development of these nodules takes place from both the parietal and the visceral pleura, extending along and covering the pleural surfaces. The pleural cavity may be filled by the growth of the mesothelioma; nevertheless, even in advanced lesions, gross invasion of the lung parenchyma is generally not evident. In some mesotheliomas the pleural thickening may be particularly striking at the interlobular fissures. These lesions, when seen from the cut surface of the lung, may give a false impression of tumor invasion. Pleural effusions are occasionally present.

## Microscopic Features

Three main histological types of mesotheliomas are recognized: epithelioid, fusocellular, and mixed. The epithelioid mesotheliomas are made up of large polyhedral cells, with abundant amphophilic cytoplasm and sharply defined cell contours. Their nuclei are vesiculated, rounded to oval in shape, with the chromatin distributed principally adjacent to the nuclear membrane or attached to it. Epithelioid mesotheliomas frequently give rise to the development of papillary formations (Figs. 252, 253), which are supported by thin stalks of connective tissue. In other cases epithelioid mesotheliomas are manifested initially in nodular forms (Fig. 254). Occasionally the epithelioid type of mesothelioma has a tubular or glandlike arrangement of complex spaces which mimic the features of adenocarcinomas. In most instances it is possible to see how these tumor cells originate from the mesothelial covering (Fig. 255); in other cases they seem to develop from the submesothelial layer. Epithelioid mesotheliomas may grow in the form of wide sheets. In many areas these are composed of compactly arranged cells; in others the cells may be loosely attached to one another or even be devoid of intercellular cohesiveness. The nuclei of these cells may be eccentrically located, sometimes conferring upon them a plasmacytoid resemblance (Fig. 256).

The fusocellular type of mesothelioma is composed of cells with spindle-shaped cytoplasm, poorly defined cell contours, and oval nuclei elongated in the direction of the main cellular axis (Figs. 257, 258). Fusocellular mesotheliomas are able to form collagen, imitating the histological pattern of fibrosarcomas. This resemblance is occasionally striking since they may even adopt a herringbone structural arrangement. The cells frequently have atypical mitoses. Fusocellular mesotheliomas may also be arranged in intertwining or tangled strands, thus mimicking malignant fibrous histiocytomas.

Mesotheliomas of the mixed pattern have areas with characteristic epithelioid features alternating

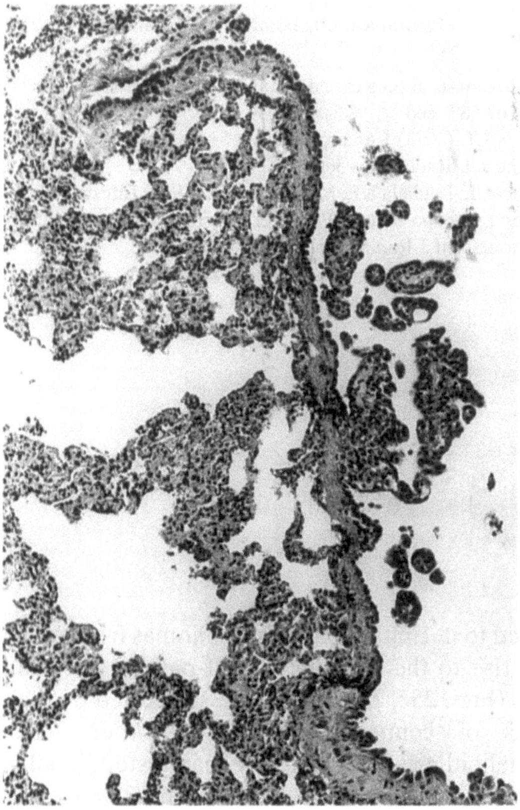

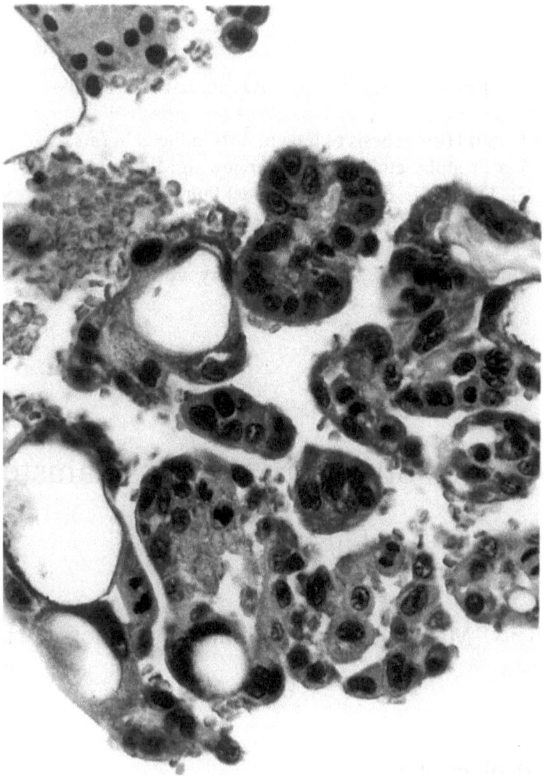

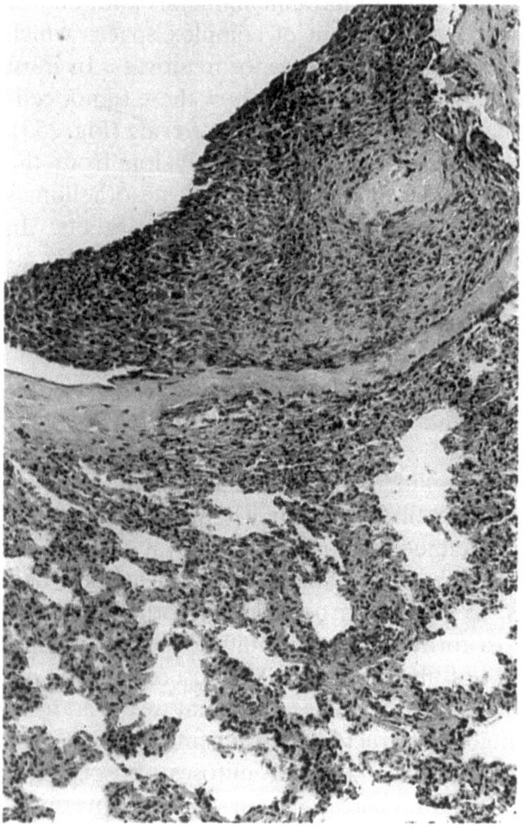

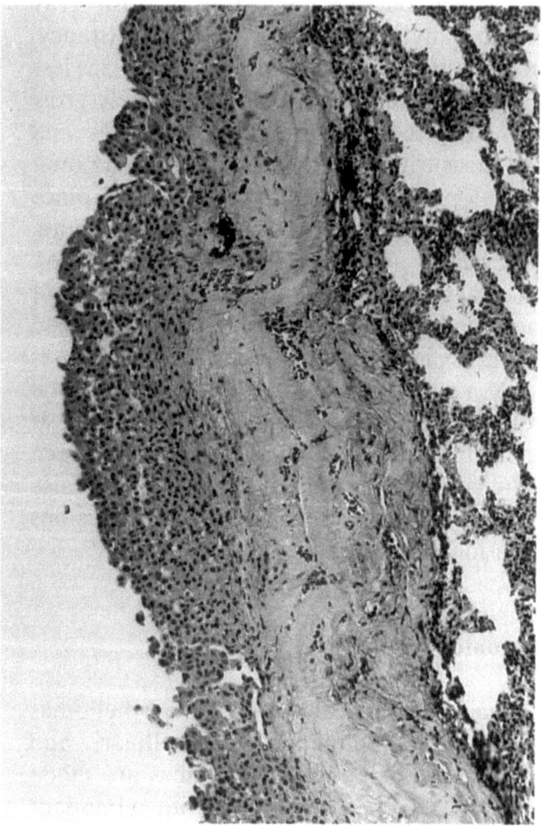

**Fig. 252.** (*upper left*) Papillary mesothelioma, Syrian hamster, at early stage of development, growing at the pleural surface. H&E, ×100

**Fig. 253.** (*upper right*) Papillary mesothelioma, Syrian hamster. Epithelioid cells with mitotic figures. H&E, ×400

**Fig. 254.** (*lower left*) Mesothelioma, hamster, attached to the pleural surface. H&E, ×100

**Fig. 255.** (*lower right*) Epithelioid mesothelioma, Syrian hamster, with spreading pattern. H&E, ×100

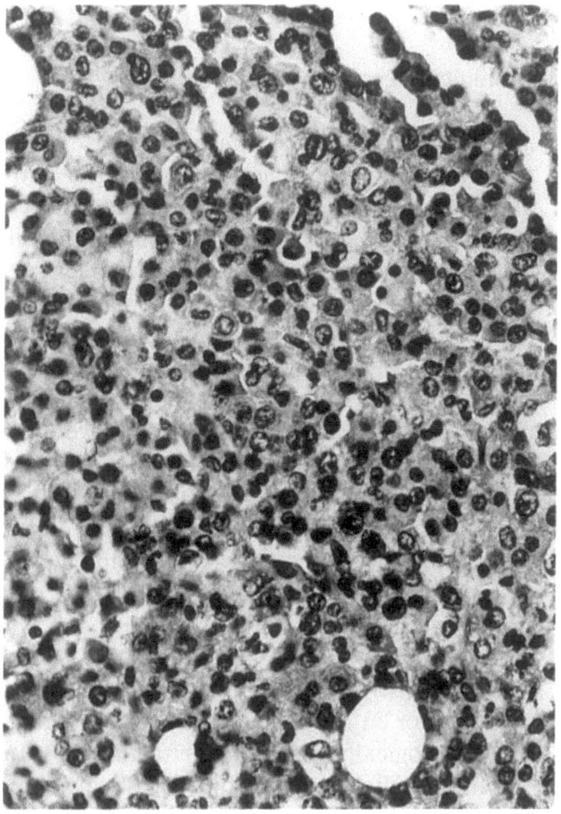

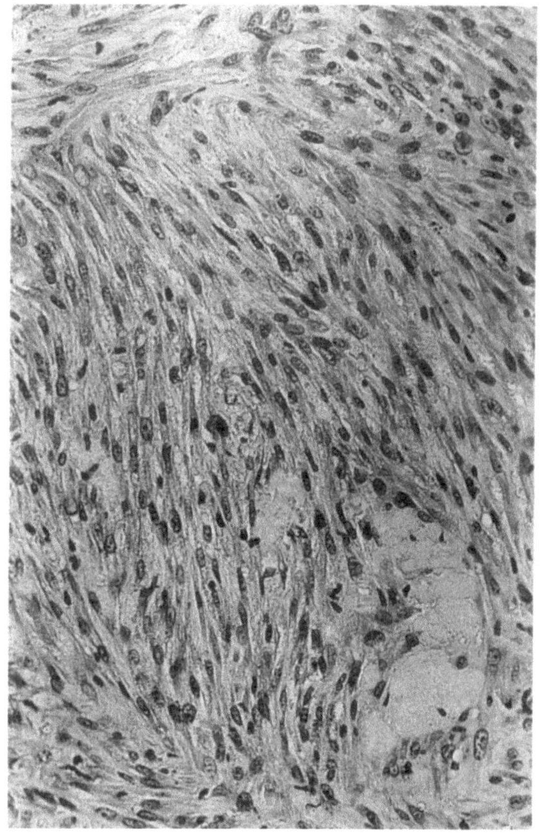

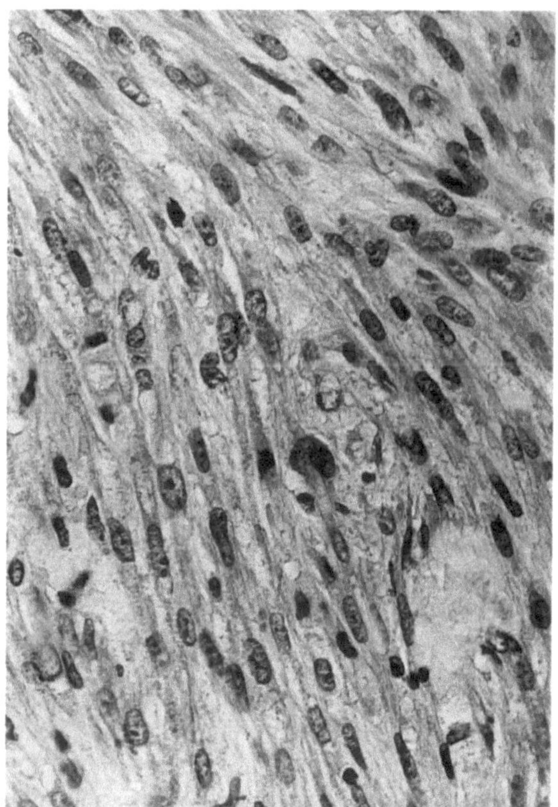

**Fig. 256.** (*upper left*) Epithelioid mesothelioma, Syrian hamster. Cells with eccentric nuclei and a lymphoplasmacytoid appearance. H&E, ×400

**Fig. 257.** (*upper right*) Fusocellular mesothelioma, Syrian hamster. Note cells with spindle-shaped cytoplasm imitating the pattern of fibrosarcoma. H&E, ×200

**Fig. 258.** (*below*) Fusocellular mesothelioma, Syrian hamster. Note spindle-shaped cells with nuclei elongated in the direction of the cellular axis. H&E, ×400

with other areas in which the fusocellular pattern is quite evident.

In the hamster the type of mesothelioma most commonly observed is epithelioid. These epithelioid cells are PAS positive, except after diastase digestion, and also positive for Alcian blue, but the color fades after treatment with hyaluronidase. The mesothelioma cells do not seem to contain mucin.

## Ultrastructure

The ultrastructural features of mesotheliomas have been reported in other laboratory rodents (Davis 1979; Kawai 1979), but we are not aware of reports on the transmission electron microscopy features of pleural mesotheliomas in the hamster. Mohr et al. (1984) examined by scanning electron microscopy pleural mesotheliomas in hamsters and found finding the presence of irregular and partly polypoid or papillary structures manifesting a coblestone relief consisting of polimorphic cells with a clear pleomorphism in the microvilli.

## Differential Diagnosis

The main differential diagnoses include neoplasias metastatic to the pleura, particularly carcinoma and sarcoma. In these instances the correct diagnosis should be based on finding a primary neoplasm with the histological features of the tumor found in the pleura. In distinguishing epithelioid mesotheliomas from metastatic carcinomas, the presence or absence of mucin in the pleural tumors is helpful because this substance is not produced by mesotheliomas. Another diagnosis to be considered is malignant lymphoma extending through the mediastinum, lung, and pleura. The epithelioid cells of mesothelioma, particularly when they lack cohesiveness, may adopt plasmacytoid features that may mimic a plasmacytoma or lymphoplasmacytic lymphoma. The absence of lymphoma in other organs should argue against that diagnosis. Finally, malignant mesotheliomas should not be confused with reactive fibrous pleural plaques, which are fibroblastic proliferations producing abundant collagen, usually in the vicinity of asbestos fibers.

## Biological Features

*Natural History*. Most mesotheliomas manifest their malignant behavior by superficial growth along the pleura. Invasion of the underlying chest wall or lung parenchyma is usually minimal or discrete in comparison to the tendency for intracavitary growth. A mesothelioma tends to fill the pleural cavities, resulting in considerable thickening and even fusion of both pleural surfaces. This may cause compression of lung parenchyma, which is accentuated by the development of pleural effusions. In advanced cases progressive invasion of mediastinum, pericardium, and diaphragm may occur. Lymphatic vascular invasion (Fig. 259), metastases to regional lymph nodes, or distant metastases should be regarded as exceptional findings.

*Pathogenesis*. Mesotheliomas are a well-recognized tumor entity, and epithelioid mesotheliomas are histologically quite similar to the cells lining the mesothelial surfaces. In spite of this, controversy exists with regard to their histogenesis. Some investigators maintain that they arise from cells of the mesothelial lining, others believe that they originate from the underlying submesothelial cells (Alvariez-Fernandez and Diez-Nau 1979; Cardesa et al. 1980). In the hamster, due to the paucity of studies, there is not yet enough information available to add to knowledge on this unsettled issue.

*Etiology*. Mesotheliomas are produced by exposure to different kinds of asbestos and glass fibers (Mohr et al. 1984; Adachi et al. 1991) and by treatment with virus (Rabson et al. 1960; Cicala et al. 1993).

*Frequency, Natural Occurrence, and Experimental Induction*. Mesotheliomas in the hamster are induced tumors. In a study of spontaneous tumors in two hamster colonies (Pour et al. 1976) no mesotheliomas were observed. Spontaneous mesotheliomas were not recorded in a wide review of the literature (Mohr 1982). Rabson et al. (1960) were able to induce mesotheliomas by treatment of hamsters with virus and asbestos. Smith et al. (1964, 1965) induced mesotheliomas by intrapleural injections of amosite into hamsters. Although Smith et al. (1970) induced pulmonary neoplasias and pleural mesotheliomas by the

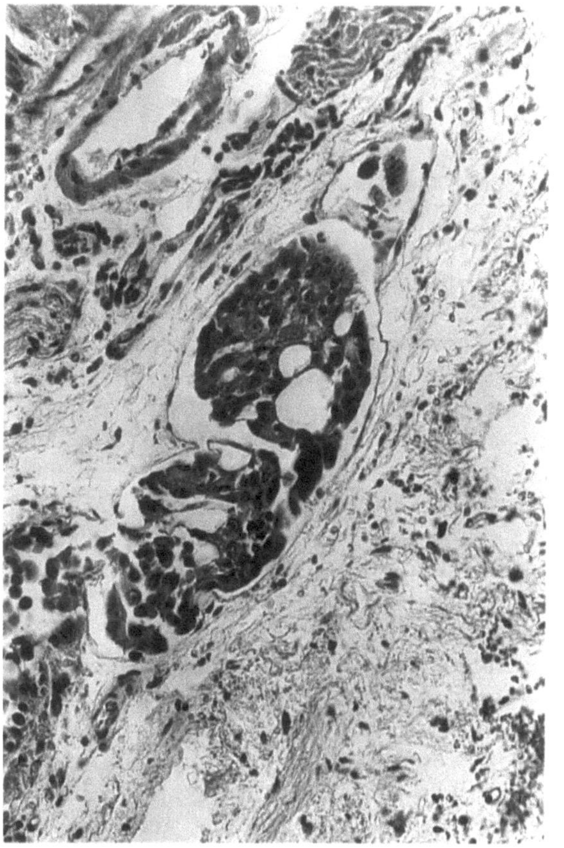

**Fig. 259.** Epithelioid mesothelioma, Syrian hamster. Tumor cells within lymphatic vessels. H&E, ×200

combined instillation of chrysotile and benzopyrene into the lower respiratory tract of hamsters, no tumors were found when the instillation was of chrysotile alone. Mohr et al. (1984) induced pleural mesotheliomas and some lung carcinomas in hamsters by intratracheal instillations of crocidolite and glass fibers. More recently Adachi et al. (1991) observed pleural mesotheliomas in hamsters by intratracheal administrations of fine man-made fibers. Recently Cicala et al. (1993) described the appearance of pleural and pericardial mesotheliomas in 100% of hamsters injected in their pleural cavity with wild-type SV40.

## Comparison with Similar Lesions in Human and Other Species

From the morphological standpoint, mesotheliomas induced in the hamster have striking gross as well as microscopic similarities with their counterparts in man (Brenner et al. 1982) and in other laboratory species (Pott et al. 1976).

## References


Adachi S, Takemoto K, Kimura K (1991) Tumorigenicity of fine man-made fibers after intratracheal administrations to hamsters. Environmental Res 54:52–73

Alvarez-Fernandez E, Diez-Nau MD (1979) Malignant fibrosarcomatous mesothelioma and benign pleural fibroma (localized fibrous mesothelioma) in tissue culture: a comparison of the in vitro pattern of growth in relation to the cell of origin. Cancer 43:1658–1663

Brenner J, Sordillo PP, Magill GB, Golbey RB (1982) Malignant mesothelioma of the pleura: review of 123 patients. Cancer 49:2431–2435

Cardesa A, Alvarez T, Pott F, Huth F, Mohr U Sept (1980) Morphological patterns of mesotheliomas produced by intraperitoneal exposure to various fibres. Abstracts XIIIth International Congress International Academy of Pathology, p 277

Cicala C, Pompetti F, Carbone M (1993) SV40 induces mesotheliomas in hamsters. Am J Pathol 142:1524–1533

Davis JM (1979) The histopathology and ultrastructure of pleural mesotheliomas produced in the rat by injections of crocidolite asbestos. Br J Exp Pathol 60:642–652

Kawai TO (1979) Histopathological studies on experimentally induced pulmonary, pleural and peritoneal neoplasms in mice by intraperitoneal injection of chrysotile asbestos and *N*-methyl-*N*-nitrosourethane. Acta Pathol Jpn 29:421–433

Mohr U (1982) Tumours of the respiratory tract. In: Turusov VS (ed) Pathology of tumours in laboratory animals, vol III, tumours of hamster. IARC Sci Publ no 34, Lyon, pp 115–145

Mohr U, Pott F, Vonnahme FJ (1984) Morphological aspects of mesotheliomas after intratracheal instillations of fibrous dusts in syrian golden hamsters. Exp Pathol 26:179–183

Pott F, Dolgner R, Friedrichs KH, Huth F (1976) L'effect oncongène des poussières fibreuses. Ann Anat Pathol (Paris) 21:237–246

Pour P, Mohr U, Cardesa A, Althoff J, Kmoch N (1976) Spontaneous tumors and common diseases in two colonies of Syrian hamsters. II. Respiratory tract and digestive system. JNCI 56:937–948

Rabson AS, Branigan WK, Legallais FY (1960) Lung tumors produced by intratracheal inoculation of polyoma virus in Syrian hamsters. JNCI 25:937–965

Smith WE, Miller L, Churg J, Selikoff IJ (1964) Pleural reaction and mesothelioma in hamsters injected with asbestos. Proc Am Assoc Cancer Res 5:9 (abstract no 234)

Smith WE, Miller L, Churg J et al. (1965) Mesotheliomas in hamsters following intrapleural injection of asbestos. J Mt Sinai Hosp 32:1–8

Smith WE, Miller L, Churg J (1970) An experimental model for study of carcinogenesis in the respiratory tract. In: Nettesheim P, Hanna MG, Deatherage JW (eds) Morphology of experimental respiratory carcinogensis. AEC symposium series no 21. USAEC, Division of Technical Information Extension, Oak Ridge

# Metastatic Tumors, Lung, Mouse

Annabel G. Liebelt

*Synonyms.* Secondary tumors of the lung; pulmonary metastases

Invasion and metastasis by neoplastic cells are the main causes of treatment failure, morbidity, and death in cancer patients. "By definition, every type of cancer described to date has the potential to metastasize at some time in its course, although for some tumors it may be a rare occurrence ..." (Liotta et al. 1991a). Metastatic tumors in laboratory animals have been reported since the turn of the century (Poste 1982; Sass and Liebelt 1985); these occur most often to the lungs. Tumors metastasize from primary spontaneous, induced, and transplanted tumors.

More recently the biology of metastasis in laboratory animals, particularly mice and rats, has been investigated using transplanted cells from cultured cell lines including cloned lines from primary and metastatic tumors. Human tumor cells transplanted into nude mice have been investigated for metastatic potential. Current studies are contributing knowledge regarding the molecular biology of metastasis regarding suppression or prevention of the spread of neoplastic cells.

## Gross Appearance

Metastatic tumors in the lungs of mice may be single or multiple and may occur in one or more lobes (Figs. 260–262). They may develop within the parenchyma of the lung or at the pleural surface. Orr et al. (1988) reported that passaged fibrosarcoma cells grow preferentially at the pleural surface of mouse lung; the site of growth is not related to the initial distribution of the injected tumor cells. They found a larger proportion of type I collagen at the pleura than the alveolar or bronchiolar regions. This finding is important since many experiments assess metastatic growths by counting nodules on intact gross specimens.

The appearance of metastatic tumors varies depending on the tissue of origin of the primary growth. Those from mammary tumors are usually soft and friable, grayish white, highly vascular, and usually elevate the surface; metastases of mammary tumors with extensive squamous metaplasia and/or keratinization may appear pearly white.

Secondary tumors from hepatocellular carcinomas are firm and pale brown gray. Malignant melanoma metastases are similar to the original tumor in being melanotic or amelanotic (Fig. 261). Metastases of primary tumors from cartilage or bone, on the other hand, are usually dense, firm to very hard, relatively avascular, white, and shiny. Although the lungs are involved with most lymphoreticular neoplasms, the lungs often do not contain grossly visible discrete nodules but rather a diffuse infiltrate of tumor cells in the entire lung causing a loss of normal pink color.

Pulmonary metastases have been evaluated with the dissecting microscope by examining serial or level sections of the lungs (Sass and Liebelt 1985). Consolandi et al. (1958) found pulmonary metastases macroscopically (confirmed microscopically) in 34% of the mice with mammary cancers; microscopic metastases were found in 46% of the apparently normal lungs. Another method outlines the tumors after injection of india ink into the trachea (Wexler 1966). The injection is followed by a wash in tap water and immersion in Fekete's solution (Fekete 1938), which allows viewing of the bleached lung tumors (Fig. 262).

## Microscopic Appearance

Although certain transplantable tumors of connective tissue metastasize to the lymph nodes, mouse mammary tumors metastasize to the lung primarily by the hematogenous route (Dunham and Stewart 1953; Sass and Liebelt 1985). With regard to mouse mammary cancer, "[T]rue metastases have never been found in the regional lymph nodes, in agreement with the results quoted by Ashburn (1937). Only 6 cases were dependent lymph nodes occupied by the tumor by contiguity invasion" (Consolandi et al. 1958). If true metastasis of spontaneous carcinoma to lymph nodes does occur in the mouse, it is not common. In this author's experience, mammary tumors may grow adjacent to salivary glands and lymph nodes but rarely invade these organs (Fig. 263).

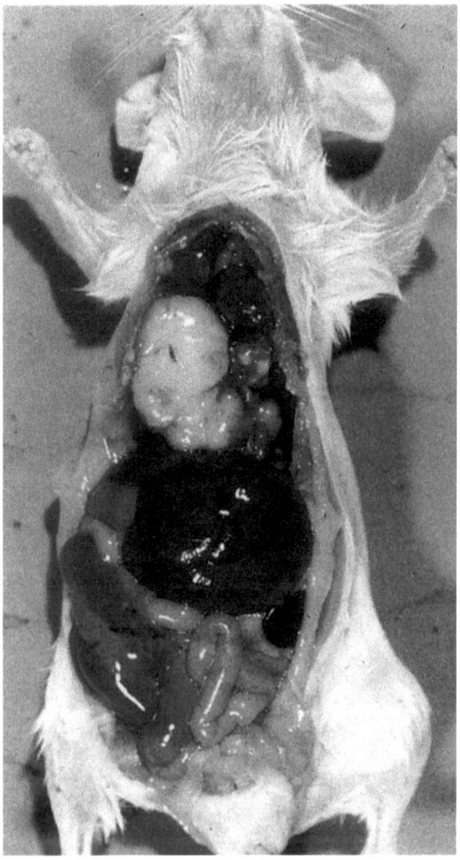

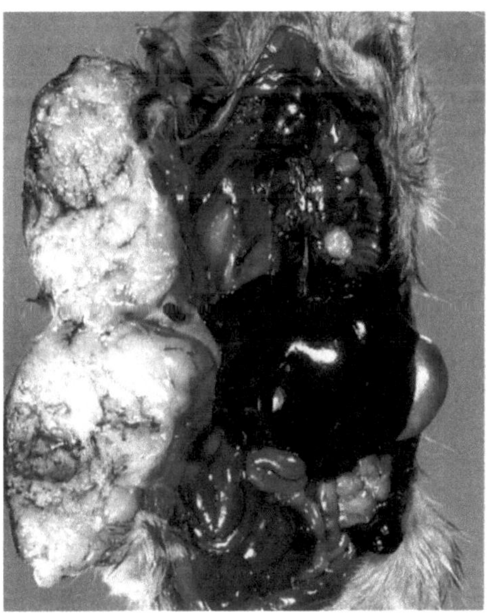

Fig. 260. (*above*) Large multinodular metastasis from spontaneous mammary carcinoma in lung of strain RIII female mouse. ×1.5

Fig. 261. (*below*) Pulmonary metastases from subcutaneous transplant of amelanotic melanoma in (BALB/c × DBA/$2_f$)$F_1$ hybrid mouse. This transplant line was derived by selection of an amelanotic portion from the melanotic transplant line. ×2

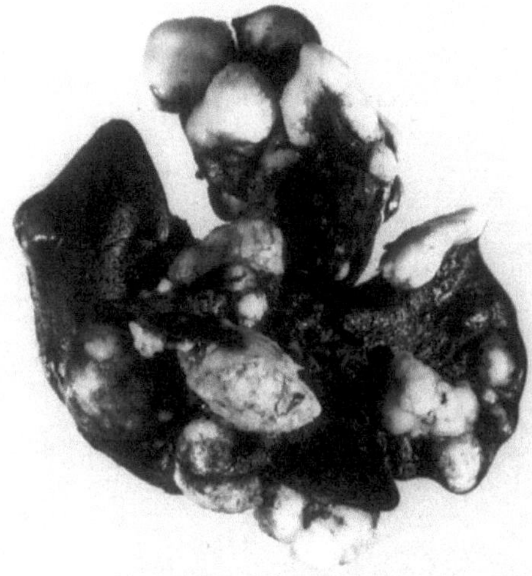

**Fig. 262.** Lungs of a strain RIII female mouse with pulmonary metastases from a mammary carcinoma. The lungs were distended with india ink; numerous pulmonary nodules are bleached white following exposure to Fekete's solution, ×2.5

The anatomic sites in which the tumor cells are found are: (a) intravascular in the pulmonary artery and peribronchial branches (Fig. 264) and in veins, and the cells may exist as emboli or thrombi (although Willis in 1973 suggested that they not be considered true metastases until the cells have penetrated the vessel walls), (b) intrabronchial and in any segment of the respiratory tree, and (c) parenchymal tissue, peribronchial capillary system and spaces in which the relationship to anatomic structures is not defined. Figure 265 illustrates cancer cells in the visceral pleura.

Tumor cells usually invade veins and are carried by the vena cava to the right heart and then by the pulmonary artery and its branches following the bronchial tree to end in the capillary plexus in the walls of the alveoli. Tumor cells enclosed by vessel walls are considered to be emboli either as single cells, clumps of cells, or fragments of a thrombus when they are nonadherent to vessel walls and are identifiable as thrombi when they are adherent to vessel walls. The thrombi may contain other blood elements such as leukocytes and thrombocytes. Once within the smaller arterial vessels, capillaries, interstitial tissue, lymphatic, alveolar, and bronchiolar spaces and walls, it may be difficult to identify precisely the origin of

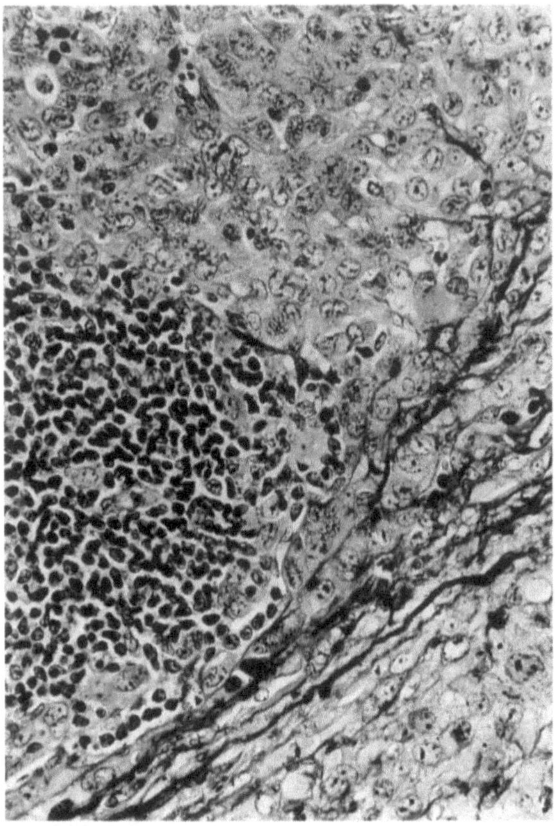

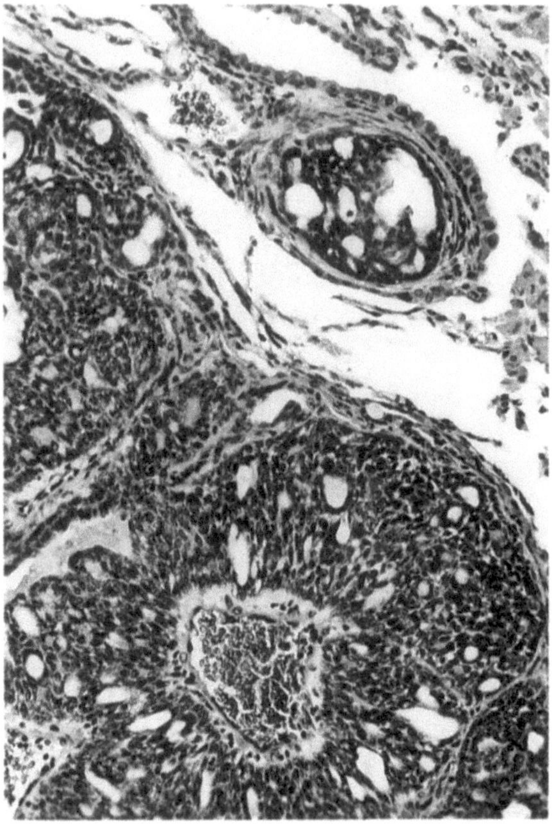

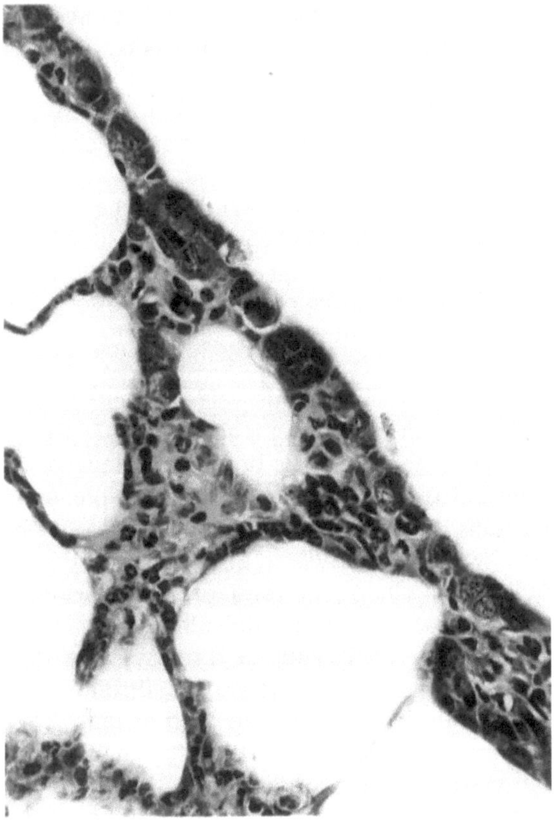

growth site due to distortion of the normal anatomic relationships. As the metastatic deposit grows, it compresses the surrounding tissues or extends into surrounding alveoli.

## Differential Diagnosis

Differential diagnoses include primary alveologenic carcinoma (type II alveolar epithelial cell), bronchiolar carcinoma (Clara cell), the rare squamous cell carcinoma, and adenomatosis, a proliferative inflammatory lesion. Spontaneous or induced primary alveologenic carcinomas may be deep within the lung and may elevate the surface of the lung and pleura. These tumors present "a uniform picture of closely packed columns of cuboidal and columnar cells supported by a sparse stroma of mature fibrous tissue" (Stewart et al. 1979). The cells are arranged in acini and may appear as solid, papillary, or glandular patterns. The silver stain for reticulin demonstrates a characteristic of epithelial growth. Differentiation of primary alveologenic carcinoma from pulmonary metastases from adenocarcinomas of the mammary gland or kidney, for example, must be considered.

The morphology of primary papillary lung tumors in some studies has indicated an origin from the bronchiolar Clara cells and not from the alveolar type II pneumocytes, whose morphology is more commonly of a solid pattern (Gunning et al. 1991). This conclusion is supported by electron microscopic studies in which the Clara cells are columnar and contain pleomorphic nuclei and cytoplasmic granules while the type II cells have the characteristic surfactant inclusion bodies.

Other studies employing light microscopic, ultrastructural, and immunohistochemical methods have concluded that papillary tumors, induced transplacentally by *N*-nitrosoethylurea in mice, constitute less well differentiated or poorly differentiated type II cell adenomas or carcinomas with fetal morphological and biochemical properties (Rehm et al. 1988). These investigators used a different chemical for induction (*N*-nitrosourea) and a different strain of mice (C3H, Swiss U6Ls1w). Still other studies (Rehm et al. 1991), using other chemicals [*N*-nitrosobis-(2-chloroethyl); *N*-nitroso-tris-bis-chloroethylurea; and *N*-nitroso-methyl-bis-chloroethylurea] for induction in Swiss mice, obtained tumors of bronchiolar cell origin. In these experiments the most common tumors were squamous cell carcinomas and adenosquamous carcinomas. These types in some instances would require differentiation from similar histological types metastatic from other organs, such as skin or mammary gland.

Lesions of adenomatosis, a nonneoplastic adenomatoid lesion, may appear grossly as grayish white areas near the pleural surface which is not elevated or may be deep within the lung. The overlying surface of the lung is indented due apparently to the atelectasis associated with the lesion. The histology of these lesions has been described (Horn et al. 1952; Snell and Stewart 1962; Stewart et al. 1979). Pulmonary adenomatosis in mice is a hyperplasia of alveolar epithelium on existing stroma without new acinar or papillary formation (Benirschke et al. 1978). There is no invasion of bronchi and no compression and no obstruction of blood vessels or bronchi; thus the architecture of the lungs otherwise is preserved. Within areas of adenomatosis arc spaces of varying sizes; the spaces and air sacs may contain cellular detritus (neutrophils, desquamated mucous cells, and degenerated cells), or mucus. Immunohistochemical staining for transferon growth factor-$B_1$($TGF$-$B_1$) of lungs of two mice with adenomatosis results in intracellulor immunoreactivity to anti-Pre TGF-B in the hyperplastic alveolar type II cells. Williams et al. (1993) suggested that the type II cells appear to be the sites of production and secretion of TGF-$B_1$.

Metastases from primary lung tumors, although rare, occur in lymph nodes, kidney, heart and along the diaphragm and chest wall (Stewart et al. 1979; Turusov et al. 1974). Some lung tumors spread to other parts of the lung (Matsuyama et al. 1969; Rehm et al. 1994).

Metastases from extrapulmonary primary or transplanted neoplasms are readily identified provided that they reproduce a histology similar to

◄

**Fig. 263.** (*upper left*) Lymph node, mouse, invaded by mammary carcinoma (*top*) from adjacent inguinal mammary gland (*bottom, left*). An $A_f$ mouse after having pituitary graft in anterior chamber of right eye. Mallory trichrome, ×400

**Fig. 264.** (*upper right*) Peribronchiolar blood vessel with adenocarcinoma and larger metastasis from a primary mammary tumor in a DBA/2 strain female breeder. H&E, ×200

**Fig. 265.** (*below*) Visceral pleura with metastatic cells from a transplantable gastric carcinoma in a CBA strain mouse. H&E, ×400

the original neoplasm. For example, metastases from yolk sac carcinomas or from fibrosarcomas closely resemble the primary tumors (Stewart et al. 1984), as seen in Fig. 266.

Mammary gland neoplasms and hepatocellular carcinoma, both of which occur frequently in certain strains of mice, commonly metastasize to the lungs. The morphology of the mammary gland neoplasms varies considerably between strains, within a strain, within a mouse, and within a tumor. Commonly, however, the metastatic lesions have the same predominant histological patterns as the parent tumors (Figs. 267–270). These may be alveolar or solid and may contain numerous cysts varying in size. Certain mammary gland carcinomas that have been carried in subcutaneous transplant for many years retain the morphology of the primary tumor. Secondary tumors from mammary gland neoplasms with extensive squamous metaplasia and keratinization including neoplasms classified as adenoacanthomas may be confused with metastases from squamous cell carcinomas originating in the skin (Figs. 271, 272). Similarly, differentiation must be made of metastatic squamous cell carcinomas originating from the forestomach (Fig. 273) and from the kidney (Fig. 274).

Hepatocellular carcinomas metastasize preferentially to the lung and may be found microscopically as tumor emboli or as larger nodules (Fig. 275). The secondary tumors may resemble the primary tumors that were trabecular or glandular, or they may appear solid. The morphology is not always correlated with the property of metastasis (Turusov and Takayama 1979). Metastases of hepatocellular carcinoma (Fig. 276) must be differentiated from metastases of adrenal cortical carcinomas (Fig. 277), which may have ceroid granules, and from those of diffuse solid type of granulosa cell tumors of the ovary. In secondary tumors from the endocrine organs the cells tend to be arranged in nests invested by a fine fibrovascular stroma. Some primary glomerulosa cell tumors of the ovary may have a tubular or

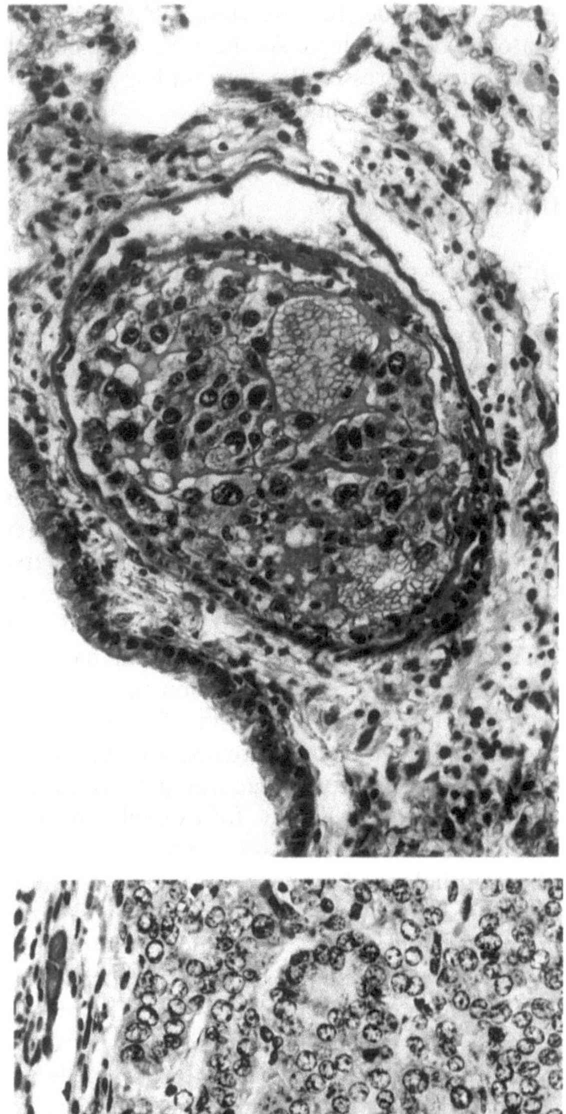

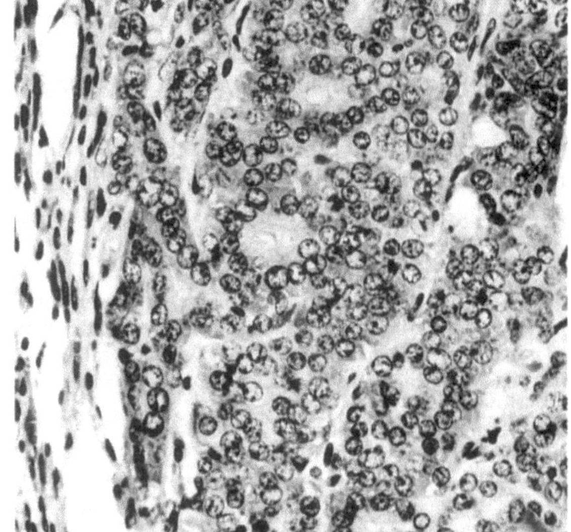

▶

**Fig. 266.** (*above*) Yolk sac carcinoma in a peribronchiolar blood vessel in the lung of an untreated $A_fB$ female mouse. Note the clusters and cords of cells of varying sizes, the basement membrane hyalin material and the bronchiolar epithelium. H&E, ×320

**Fig. 267.** (*below*) Mammary carcinoma of alveolar type (Dunn type A) in lung of A strain female mouse. H&E, ×400

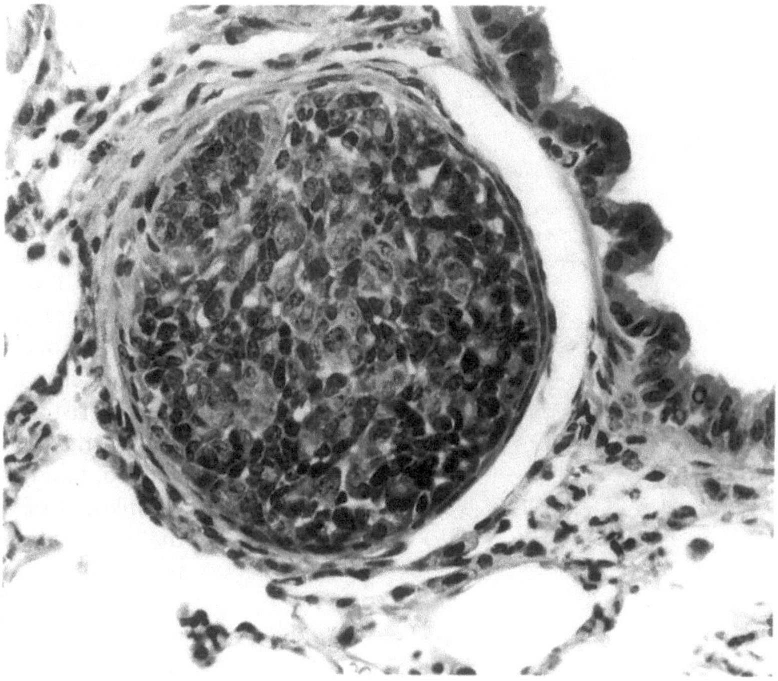

**Fig. 268.** (*above*) Small mammary carcinoma of solid type (Dunn type B) in peribronchial artery of untreated DBA/2 strain female mouse. H&E, ×400

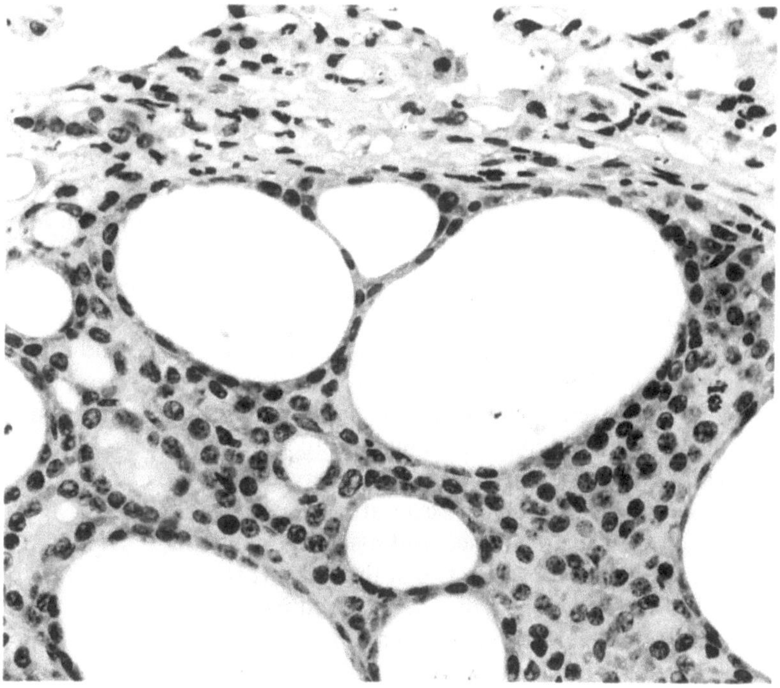

**Fig. 269.** (*below*) Mammary carcinoma of cystic type (Dunn type C) metastatic to lung of strain CBA mouse; female breeder. H&E, ×400

glomerular pattern, which differentiates them from the adrenal cortical carcinoma when metastatic to the lung. The rare primary hepatoblastoma differs from the hepatocellular carcinoma in that the cells stain deeply in H&E preparations, there may be spindle cells, rosettes and peculiar "organoids" formed by vascular channels surrounded by tumor cells. Hepatoblastomas are invariably found within or adjacent to hepatocellular carcinomas (Turusov and Takayama 1979). Hepatoblastomas metastatic to the lungs of CF-1 mice appeared as multiple nodules or multiple emboli and were similar in histology to the primary tumor.

Neoplasms of the reticular cell system, originally classified by Dunn in 1954, were recently reclassi-

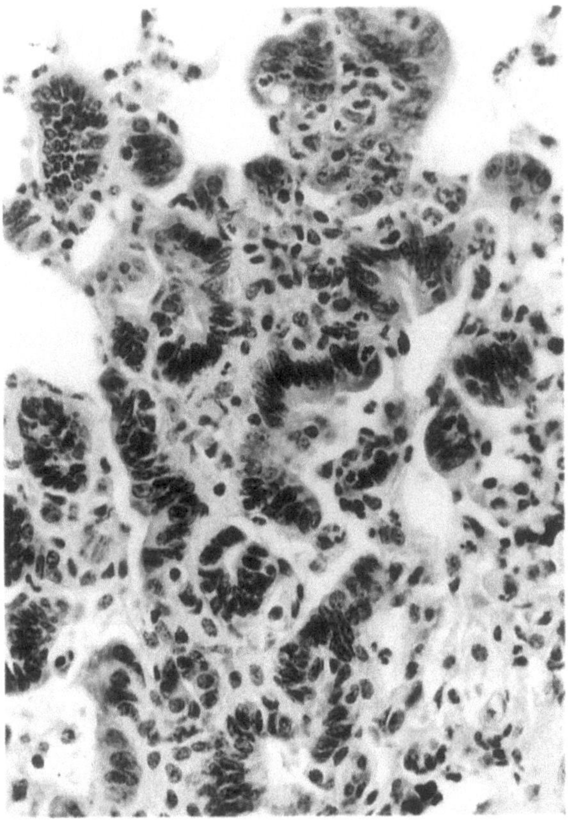

**Fig. 270.** Metastasis of comedo type of mammary carcinoma in DBA/$2_f$ strain female mouse that had been fed methylcholanthrene in olive oil. Note hyperchromasia of cells in capillaries and alveoli. H&E, ×400

fied by Pattengale (1990a,b) and by Fredrickson et al. (1995). These investigators combined morphological features with immunophenotypic and molecular data to characterize mouse lymphomas. In mice with immunoblastic lymphoma (composite lymphoma, reticulum cell neoplasm type B), nodules and foci of tumor tissue are present in organs of the reticular tissue and also in organs such as the kidneys, ovaries and in the lungs (Fig. 278). In the experience of Dr. T. Fredrickson (Registry of Experimental Cancers), pulmonary involvement is of two types. One type associated with leukemias is a diffuse stasis of cells within alveolar walls (Fig. 278). The other type is associated with lymphoblastic lymphomas and occurs as perivascular infiltrates encroaching on the pulmonary parenchyma and following the major vessels. A differential diagnosis must be made to distinguish these patterns of spread of hemopoietic neoplasms from peribronchial and perivascular cuffing due to proliferating macrophages and infiltration by lymphocytes following lesions of chronic pneumonia. Myeloid leukemia in advanced cases may infiltrate the lungs.

Histiocytic sarcomas (reticulum-cell sarcomas type A) occur frequently in some strains of mice. These tumors may originate in the liver or uterus in addition to hemopoietic organs such as spleen and mesenteric nodes (Frith 1990; Turusov 1994). The primary tumors are invasive and commonly spread to the lungs. Neither metastatic deposits nor primary tumors contain inflammatory cells, which aids in differential diagnosis from reticulum cell neoplasm type B. The neoplastic cells have the characteristics of histiocytes, may have vacuolated cytoplasm, sometimes resenble fibroblasts, and may contain multinucleated giant cells.

Neoplasms of the urinary system metastasize to the lungs in mice. Renal adenocarcinomas spread to the lungs, are composed of small, closely packed cells with indistinct borders which are arranged as nests and sheets (to be differentiated from adenocarcinomas arising in other organs). Two mice treated with 2-fluorenylacetamide developed transitional cell carcinomas in the urinary bladder that metastasized to the lungs (Frith et al. 1981; Sass and Liebelt 1985). These tumors also had squamous metaplasia. Figure 274 is a chemically induced squamous cell carcinoma from the kidney metastatic to the lung (see also Fig. 275, a renal carcinoma metastatic to the lung).

Malignant schwannomas, metastatic to the lung, consist almost wholly of Antoni type A tissue, namely interlacing parallel bundles and fibrils (Sass and Liebelt 1985). Lacking in some observed cases are other features of primary schwannoma, including pallisading of the nuclei, Verocay bod-

▶

**Fig. 271.** (*upper left*) Squamous cell carcinoma (nonkeratizing) from skin at anus, metastatic to lung of (C57BL × RIII) female mouse. One pituitary graft to the anterior chamber of the eye was given to the mouse earlier. H&E, ×400

**Fig. 272.** (*upper right*) Squamous cell carcinoma (keratinizing) from skin to right of nose metastatic to multiple sites in lungs of strain DBA/2 male breeder. Most of this lobe is filled with a mass of keratinized tissue. H&E, ×20

**Fig. 273.** (*lower left*) Squamous cell carcinoma metastatic to lungs from the forestomach of a female (DBA/2 ×C57BL/6) mouse that had received DMBA by gavage. H&E, ×400

**Fig. 274.** (*lower right*) Squamous cell carcinoma metastatic to the lungs from a renal carcinoma induced in a NON/Shi female mouse by *N*-buty-*N*-(4-hydroxybutyl) nitrosamine in the drinking water. Note subpleural growth in alveolar walls. H&E, ×400

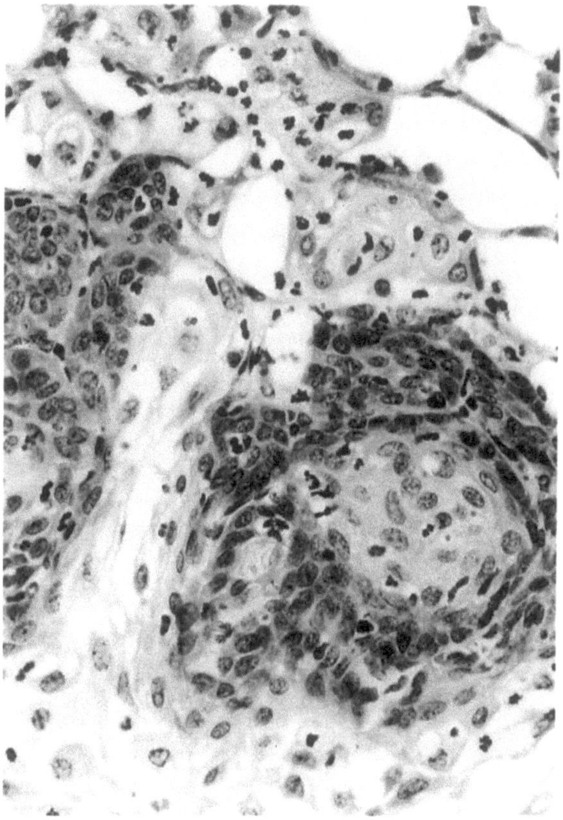

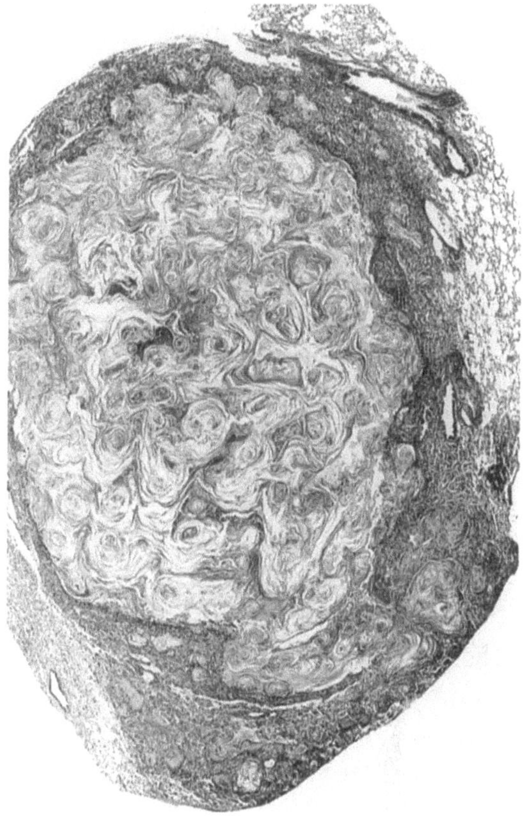

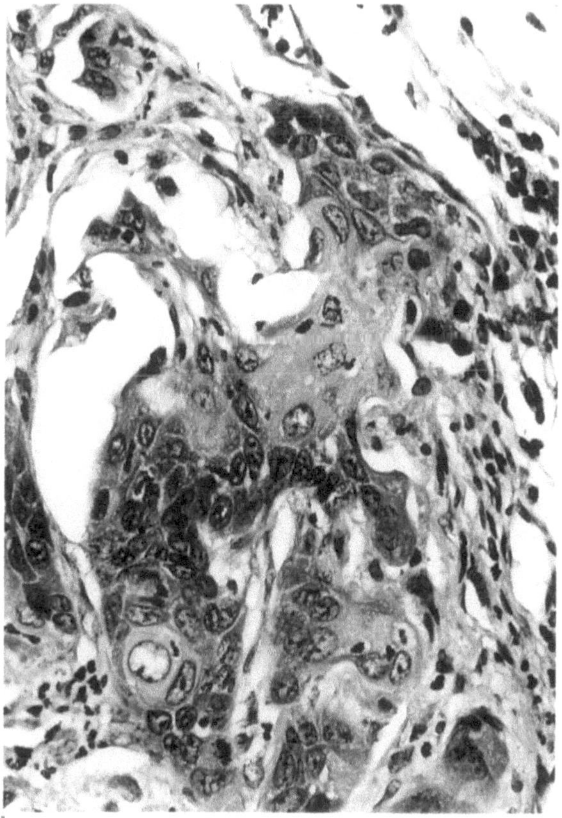

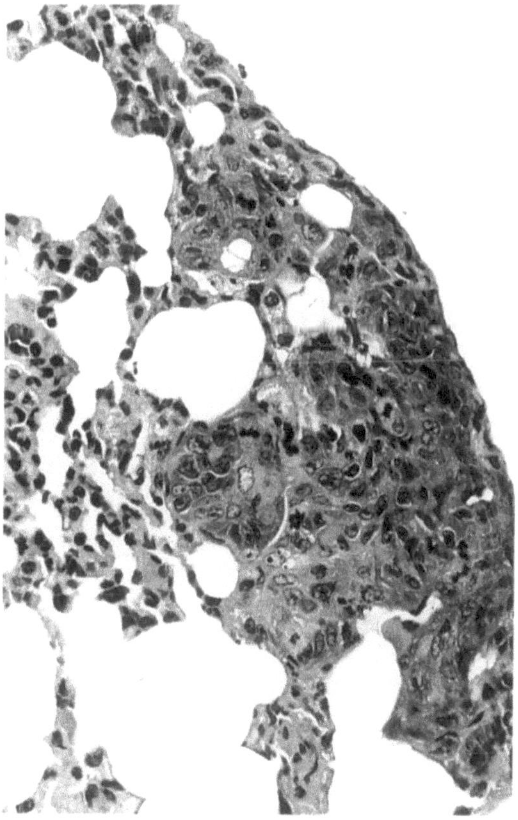

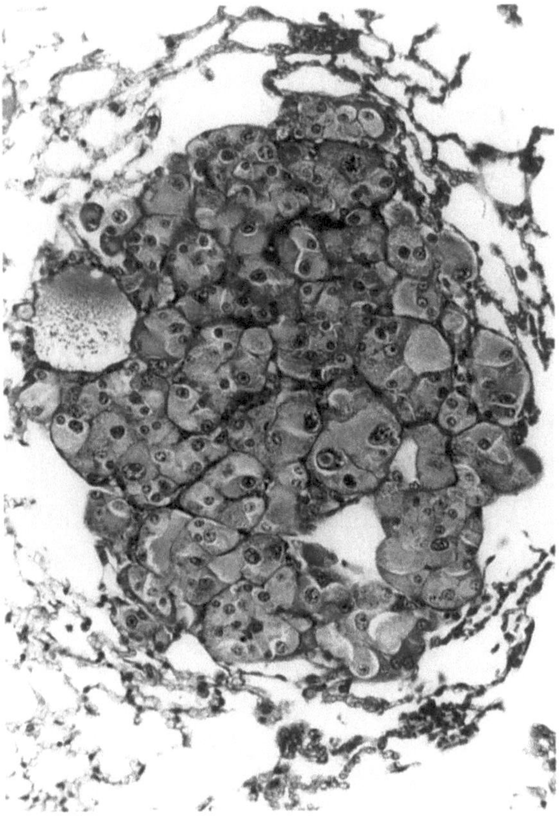

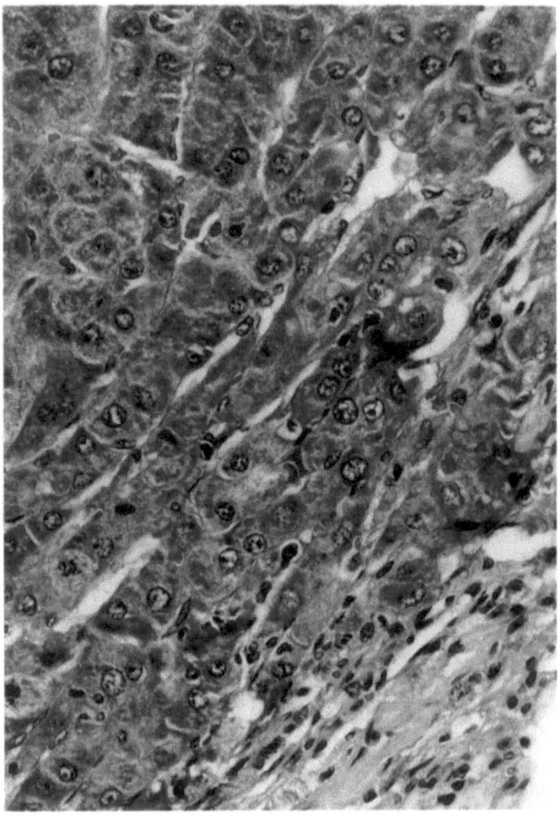

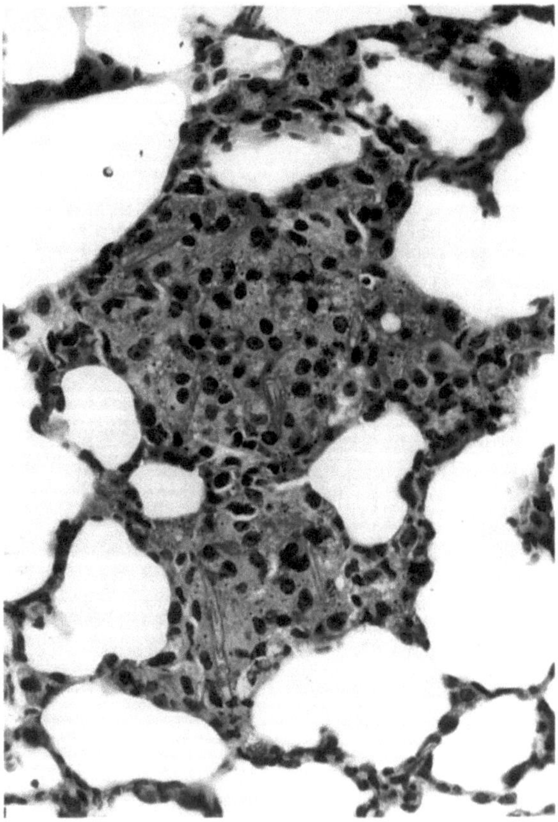

ies, cysts, and lipoid-containing pseudoxanthomatous cells. Pulmonary vessels may contain multiple and adherent thrombi.

Primary and transplanted osteosarcomas in mice metastasize to the lung, but there is no correlation between histological differentiation and the probability of metastasis (Luz et al. 1991). They may contain bone, osteoid and spindle cells, or undifferentiated cells (Fig. 279).

Tumors of the Harderian gland in mice are usually benign cystadenomas or adenocarcinomas of varying differentiation. Well-differentiated tumors may contain fat vacuoles (Fig. 280), while less well differentiated tumors may have a pleomorphic appearance. Tumors do not contain pigmented secretions. Malignant tumors, including transplanted tumors, metastasize to the lungs (Sheldon et al. 1983; Sheldon 1994).

Malignant fibrous histiocytomas and pleomorphic sarcomas show partial fibroblastic and histiocytic differentiation (with histiocytic enzymes) and may have myxomatous change and bizarre tumor giant cells. Many other tumors of the soft tissue may have eosinophilic globule cells or areas of rhabdomyosarcoma (Heider and Eustis 1994). It may be difficult with an H&E stain only to differentiate some sarcomas, fibrosarcomas, or malignant fibrous histiocytomas, particularly of the fibroblastic type.

Spontaneous and induced tumors of the skin originate in the epidermis, the skin appendages, connective tissue, and melanocytes. Although spontaneous skin tumors in mice are uncommon (fewer than 0.5%) tumors are readily inducible by many chemical carcinogens, UV light, and ionizing radiation (Klein-Szanto 1989). The epithelial tumors may be papillomas, keratoacanthomas, squamous cell carcinomas (Figs. 271, 272) which metastasize to lung and regional lymph nodes, occasional basal cell carcinoma, or tumors of the adnexa. Spontaneous melanotic tumors occur only rarely but can be produced by topical carcinogens (Kanno 1989). Klein-Szanto (1989) considers these tumors, which are morphologically similar to nevi and melanomas in humans, to be less aggressive and to metastasize rarely. Metastatic malignant melanomas were produced in C57BL/6 mice by DMBA and croton oil (Berkelhammer and Oxenhandler 1987).

The author has examined tumors in mice with transplantable melanomas from two different primary melanomas. Mouse 138, an irradiated (BALB/c × DBA/$2_f$)$F_1$ mouse developed a black tumor in the orbit (Liebelt and Liebelt 1967). Melanotic and melanotic lines were selected and produced metastases in the lungs and lymph nodes; these were pigmented or not pigmented, similar to the transplant in the same mouse (Figs. 261, 281).

A second melanoma that was examined arose spontaneously in the skin of the left hind limb of an untreated male ($A_f$ × $I^s$)$F_1$ hybrid mouse (M34964). Grossly the tumor was completely black, and histologically all cells were laden with pigment. During subcutaneous passage melanotic and amelanotic lines were selected. The original host had metastasis in the lumbar lymph node; a mouse in T-1 (M34965) had metastasis in the liver. In subsequent transplant generations the host mice had metastatic deposits in the lungs (Fig. 281), liver, kidney, axillary lymph nodes, and spleen. Transplants from a subcutaneous tumor in a mouse (M35200) in T-10 successfully transplanted into a mouse of the parent strain $A_f$, and pieces of spleen developed large melanotic tumors subcutaneously in two of seven mice. In addition, pigment-laden macrophages were found in many organs.

The established transplantable melanomas, such as B16, S91, and Harding-Passey lines, originated from spontaneous tumors. The B16 lines have been used extensively as the tumor cells of choice in studying the metastatic process (Fidler 1970, 1978; Fidler and Kripke 1977; Fidler and Nicholson 1976; Hart 1982).

◄

**Fig. 275.** (*upper left*) Lung, mouse, metastasis of renal adenocarcinoma that has compressed and invaded alveoli. Glands are absent. The tumor cells have sharply defined borders, abundant pale-staining cytoplasm, and excentrically placed, often multiple, nuclei. H&E, ×220

**Fig. 276.** (*upper right*) Hepatocellular carcinoma metastatic to lung in a C3H strain male mouse that had been injected intraperitoneally with urethane. H&E, ×400

**Fig. 277.** (*below*) Metastasis to lung from adrenal cortical carcinoma in an ovariectomized female mouse of the CE strain. H&E, ×400

## Ultrastructure

The ultrastructure of primary neoplasms in several organ systems in mice is described and illustrated in many publications, particularly in the ILSI Monographs on Pathology of Laboratory Animals. However, the literature contains few

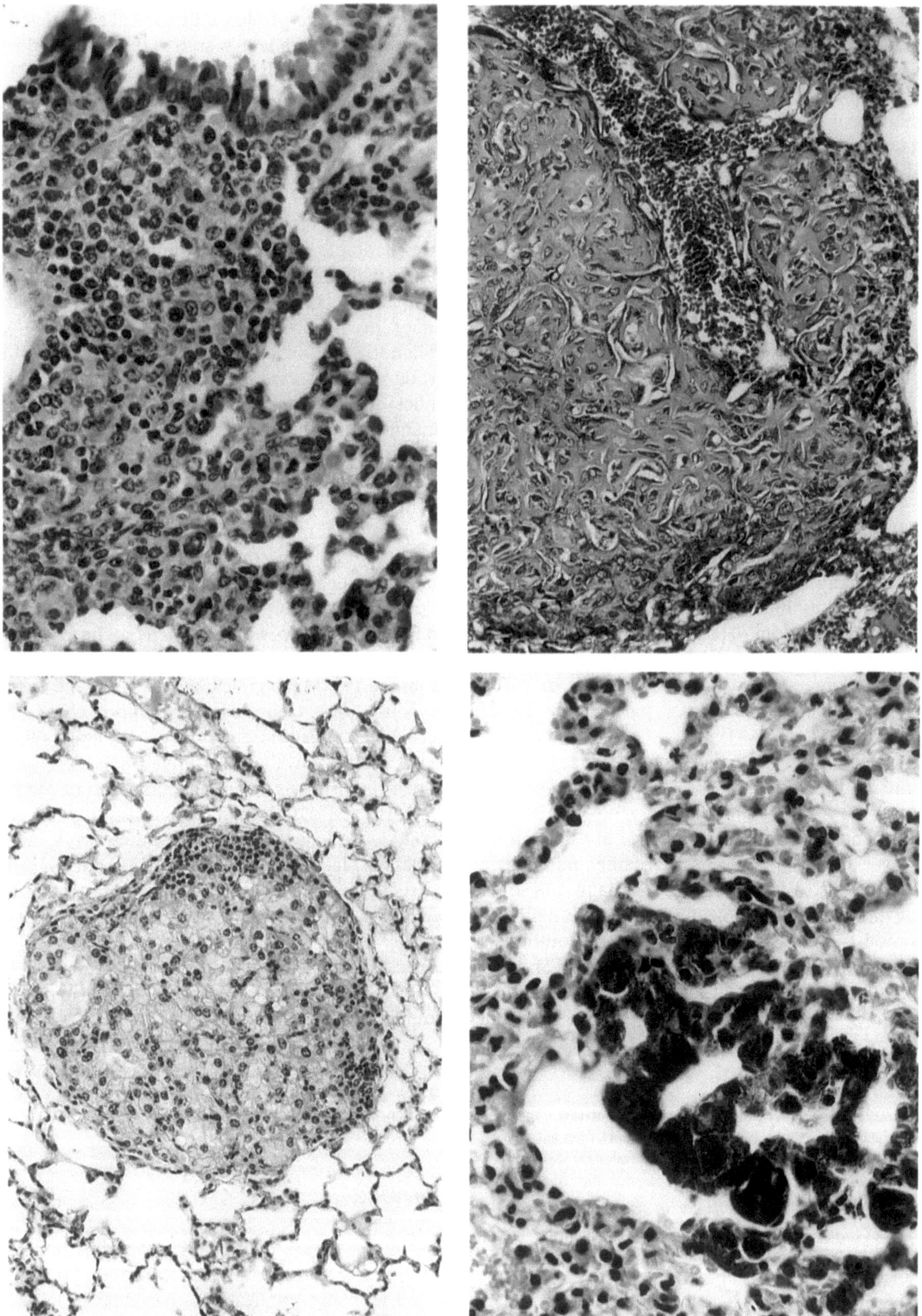

descriptions and illustrations of the ultrastructure of metastatic tumors.

Mammary tumor metastases in the lung examined by electron microscopic studies (Brooks 1970; Pitelka et al. 1980a, b). Brooks (1970) found that the mammary tumor cells in the lung were separated from the alveolar airspace by: (a) a thick basal lamina of the mammary tumor cell, (b) a loose connective tissue space containing fibroblasts and collagen fibrils, (c) the basal lamina of the alveolar epithelial cells, and (d) the alveolar air spaces themselves. "Where mammary tumor cells were seen within alveolar air spaces, the tumor cells shared the same basement membrane with extant alveolar lining cells."

The ultrastructure of primary and metastatic mammary tumors was compared by Pitelka et al. (1980a,b) with respect to epithelial cell junctions and basal lamina. No characteristic differences were found in the organization or ultrastructure of the mammary cells of the primary and metastatic tumors. On the other hand, the histology of the metastatic tumors was influenced to some degree by their relationship to surrounding lung tissue.

Hypertrophy of the basal lamina in both primary and metastatic mammary tumors is frequent; whorls of evenly spaced layers of basal lamina (a periodic structure) commonly developed in metastases but developed in only one primary tumor (Brooks 1970). Also, the disposition of the basal lamina is often abnormal, most significantly at the interface with pulmonary arteriolar endothelium and with pulmonary alveolar epithelium. When extravascular metastases invade the pulmonary alveolar air spaces, "the cells of the two epithelia share the same basal lamina and collaborate to form luminal tight junctions, showing that the tumor recognizes the pulmonary tissue as epithelial but not as nonmammary" (Pitelka et al. 1980b).

Luz et al. (1991), in an ultrastructural investigation, assessed the stage of cellular differentiation in richly cellular osteosarcomas. They illustrated a lung metastasis from an osteosarcoma; the area was bone forming with typical osteoblasts separated by partially mineralized trabeculae.

Liotta and Stetler-Stevenson (1989) in their studies of the metastatic cascade demonstrated the arrest and extravasation of circulating tumor cells in the capillaries of the lung, which is the target organ for the initiation of metastatic colonies of B16-F10 tumor cells. The illustrations show tumor cells in 3, 6, and 12 h and 2 weeks after IV inoculation. The cells at 3 hours in a capillary can directly embolize in the precapillary venules or may adhere to the endothelial luminal surface of arterioles. The endothelial cells retract, the tumor cells attach to the basement membrane, the endothelium extends over the tumor cell, the basement membrane dissolves, and tumor cells are extravasated and may then proliferate as such within an arteriole.

Tumor cells from three malignant lymphomas injected intravenously seeded to several organs, but only in the lungs were they confined to the capillaries. Electron microscopic observations elucidated that in the lung capillaries the endothelium was never injured (Dingemans 1973). More recently DeBruyn and Cho (1982) confirmed that the fully intact endothelial lining can and does permit the entry of malignant cells into the vascular lumen. This transcellular mode of entry into the circulation occurs through wide-lumened venules of the tumor which are formed during the angiogenic activity of the tumor cells.

◀

**Fig. 278.** (*upper left*) Lymphoma throughout the lungs of a (BALB/c × DBA/2)$F_1$ hybrid female mouse that had received a subcutaneous transplant of a piece of liver with lymphoma (2 months earlier; T-5 generation of a lymphoma line). H&E, ×400

**Fig. 279.** (*upper right*) Osteogenic sarcoma metastatic from the pelvic bone in a C57BL male mouse injected with polyoma virus. H&E, ×200

**Fig. 280.** (*lower left*) Harderian gland adenocarcinoma in lung of an NMRI strain female mouse that had received radiation. Many glandular cells contain single large fat vacuoles. H&E, ×220

**Fig. 281.** (*lower right*) Pigmented melanoma cells in alveolar walls of lung in an ($A_f \times I^s$) female mouse with the 10th generation of a subcutaneous transplant of a spontaneous melanoma. H&E, ×400

## Biological Features

*Frequency.* Tumors originating in the mammary gland and in the liver of mice either spontaneously or following treatment are more common than tumors of many other organs. Metastases to the lungs from these tumors have been reported by several investigators (Dunham and Stewart 1953; Frith et al. 1981; Sass and Liebelt 1985). The frequency may vary by strain, by experimental treatment, and by transplant passage (Liebelt et al. 1968). Long-term studies over the past several years with histological confirmation of tumors have provided information on metastases from the less commonly occurring tumors. Table 24 lists by system and organ, results of attempts to find metastases in certain types of tumors. Many of these studies have been described in the ILSI Monographs on Pathology of Laboratory Animals, first edition. No attempt was made to search anecdotal data from original papers. The frequency of lung metastases following the injection of tumor cells from cell culture lines is not included.

*Tumor Cell Heterogeneity.* Tumor cell heterogeneity refers to differences in morphology, immunogenicity, growth rate, metabolism, hormone receptors, pigment production, and sensitivity to environmental exogenous agents such as radiation and chemicals. Although not a new concept (originally hypothesized by Paget in 1889), the realization that neoplasms are biologically heterogeneous has gained wide acceptance (Fidler 1986). This heterogeneity exists in tumors in both experimental animals and man (Sugarbaker et al. 1982). "Studies in rodent systems have indicated that cancer metastases can be clonal in their origin and that different metastases can originate from different progenitor cells from the primary tumor" (Fidler 1986). This metastatic heterogeneity of tumor cells has many ramifications for studies of tumor biology in general and for studies of therapy in particular (Fidler 1986). Since the original observations of Fidler and Kripke in 1977, additional studies in that laboratory and in others (Fidler 1970, 1978; Fidler and Nicholson 1976; Kripke et al. 1978; Poste 1982; Hennings et al. 1986) using tumors from laboratory animals have developed methods to study the heterogeneity of human tumors that have been transplanted to nude mice.

*Preferential Site of Colonization.* Distant metastases in man occur in preferential organs and often in organs irrespective of the first organ encountered by the tumor cells (Nicholson 1988). For instance, malignant melanoma and breast cancer commonly metastasize to brain, bone, and liver instead of the lung. Even cancers such as lymphomas, which usually disseminate throughout the body, prefer to localize and grow in certain organs. Another concept is that cancers metastasize to a general site and then disseminate to other sites, unlike secondary involvement from hematopoietic malignancies. Metastasis to the spleen from solid tumors is considered rare and usually is detected only at autopsy. Edelman and Rotterdam (1990) reported a solitary splenic metastasis of an adenocarcinoma of the lung; the patient lacked metastatic disease elsewhere.

Paget in 1889 proposed the "seed and soil" hypothesis of selective colonization of certain ("preferential") organs by metastatic cells from some types of cancers. This hypothesis that the tumor cells, the seeds, find a suitable environment, the soil, in which to settle and grow, was somewhat controversial for many years but is now widely accepted and is being substantiated experimentally.

The soil may have factors that promote cell division resulting in growth. Also, there may be organ-specific growth factors such as transforming growth factor beta and tumor necrosis factor (Zetter 1990).

Recently several investigators have shown site-specific metastasis that is organ preference of metastatic cells; specific tumor cells interact with a compatible milieu provided by a particular organ environment. For example, Radinsky and Fidler (1992) concluded that organ-derived, perhaps organ-specific, paracrine growth factors stimulate the growth of receptive malignant cells (human colon carcinoma cells implanted in athymic nude mice) that posses the appropriate receptors.

The alternate hypothesis, also widely held, is that metastatic dissemination occurs by purely mechanical factors such as the anatomical structure of the blood and lymph vascular systems (Ewing 1928), that is, tumor cells in the blood circulation are trapped and lodged in the first capillary bed encountered, an occurrence which may explain the high number of neoplasms found in the lung. Nicholson (1988) concluded that some tumor cell properties for mechanical lodgement of circulating tumor cell emboli include (a) their release into the blood and lymph as cell clumps instead of single cells and (b) their ability to undergo homotypic (other tumor cells) and heterotypic (platelets, lymphocytes) adhesion during their transport to distant sites. Experimental studies with B16 melanoma cells support this conclusion.

The results of some clinical studies suggest that common regional metastatic involvements may be

**Table 24.** Pulmonary metastases from tumors in untreated mice

| Organ of origin | Diagnosis | Mice with metastasis/Mice with tumors | | Sex | Strain | Reference |
|---|---|---|---|---|---|---|
| | | *n* | % | | | |
| Liver | Hepatoma | | 1–2 | | | Slye et al. (1915) |
| | Hepatoma | 1/17 | 6 | M, F | CBA | Gorer (1940) |
| | Hepatoma | 1/97 | 1 | M | CF-1 | Turusov et al. (1973) |
| | Hepatoblastoma | 0/3 | 0 | M | CF-1 | Turusov et al. (1973) |
| | Hepatocellular carcinoma | 43/349 | 12 | F | $B6C3HF_1$ | Ward et al. (1979) |
| | | 7/58 | 12 | F | $B6C3HF_1$ | Ward et al. (1979) |
| | | 5/50 | 10 | M | $B6C3HF_1$ | National Toxicology Program (1982) |
| | | 0/50 | 0 | F | $B6C3HF_1$ | National Toxicology Program (1982) |
| Mammary gland | Carcinoma, NOS | 104/273 | 38 | | | Haaland (1911) |
| | | 26/68 | 40 | | | Murray (1908) |
| | | | 40 | | | Marsh (1927) |
| | | | 62[a] | | | Marsh (1929) |
| | | 123/314 | 39 | | | Marsh (1929) |
| | | 217/480 | 45 | | NIH white | Ashburn (1937) |
| | | Infrequent | | | AIBrA | van der Valk (1981) |
| | | | 16 | | BALB/cfC3H | van der Valk (1981) |
| | | 69/160 | 43 | | C3H, C3Hf BALB/cfC3H BALB/c NIV A, GR, and RIII | Pitelka et al. (1980a) |
| | | 78/464 | 17 | | RIII | Liebelt et al. (1968) |
| | | 39/80 | 49 | | C3H | Liebelt et al. (1968) |
| | | 65/169 | 39 | | A | Liebelt et al. (1968) |
| | | 16/78 | 20 | | DBA/2 | Liebelt et al. (1968) |
| | | 23/58 | 40 | | RIII/Imr (breeder) | Liebelt et al. (1981) |
| | | 18/61 | 30 | | RIII/Imr (virgin) | Liebelt et al. (1981) |
| | A, B, mixed AB | 40/51 | 78 | | BALB/cf/C3H/Cb/Se | Consolandi et al. (1958) |
| | | 16/28 | 57 | | RIII/Dm/Se | |
| | | 12/26 | 46 | | C3H/Cb/Se | Consolandi et al. (1958) |
| | Carcinoma, NOS | 12/19 | 63 | | BALB/cfC3H | Squartini and Bistocchi (1977) |
| | | 1/6 | 17 | | BALB/cfRIII | |
| Harderian gland | Adenocarcinoma | 3/30 | 10 | | BALB/c, C3H/He and C57BL/6J | Sheldon et al. (1983) |

NOS, Not otherwise specified.
[a] Following massage.

attributed to anatomical or mechanical considerations such as regional lymphatic drainage to lymph nodes, but that distant organ colonization occurs by cells that establish their own preferential site (Sugarbaker 1981). It appears likely that the two hypotheses of organ preference may not be mutually exclusive. Naturally occurring mammary tumors differ in their pulmonary colonization potentials after intravenous inoculation of cell suspensions using tumors from C3H/A$^{vy}$ and CBA/Lac strains of female mice. Tarin and Price (1981) and Tarin (1982) demonstrated that the pulmonary colonization potential of a given tumor is an intrinsic property of its constituent cells, and that the microenvironment of an organ can inhibit or permit expression of this intrinsic potential (Juacaba et al. 1989). Thus the degree and sites of colonization are the results of interaction between the tumor and organ-specific factors.

In the past several years a number of cell lines and sublines have been described that preferentially localize in and colonize specific organs (Poste 1982; Liotta and Stetler-Stevenson 1989; Nicholson 1988). In many cases target organ preference cannot be explained on an anatomical basis. As Liotta and Stetler-Stevenson point out, "Organ preference of metastatic colonization can be observed in some animal tumors that have not undergone purposeful selection". In other models organ selectivity has been experimentally amplified by sequential in vivo passage through the target organ.

*Cascade of Host-Tumor Interactions.* Metastatic dissemination of cancer is a highly selective, nonrandom process consisting of a cascade of linked, sequential steps involving multiple host-tumor interactions. Investigators have been focusing studies on one step at a time, utilizing the disciplines of cell biology, protein biochemistry, and molecular genetics (Carr and Orr 1983; Fidler and Nicholson 1987; Nicholson 1988; Liotta and Stetler-Stevenson 1989; Liotta et al. 1991a, b; Radinsky and Fidler 1992; Stracke and Liotta 1992).

The subpopulation of cancer cells that are successful in metastasizing (called "decathlon champions" by Fidler 1978) detach from the primary tumor, invade the surrounding tissue, penetrate into the blood or lymphatic vascular system, implant into the capillary beds of target organs, extravasate the target tissue, and proliferate at the secondary site to form a metastatic colony.

Cellular interactions at different stages of tumor dissemination may involve cell adhesion receptors such as fibronectin and laminin receptors. By this mechanism tumor cells may form emboli in the circulation and increase metastases in capillaries and then extravasate (Lotan 1987). At each step the cells must overcome immune cell killing (North and Nicholson 1987). Angiogenesis is a prerequisite for expansion of both the primary tumor and the metastatic colony (Liotta et al. 1991b). A very small percentage (<0.01%) of the circulating tumor cells succeed in establishing metastatic colonies (Liotta et al. 1974). During the interactions of the metastatic cells with the host cells, endocrine, autocrine, and paracrine factors may inhibit or stimulate tumor cell proliferation. Recently Radinsky and Fidler (1992) described mechanisms involving growth factors and their receptors of human colon carcinoma cells implanted into athymic nude mice. In addition to genetic changes in the tumor cells that lead to imbalance of growth regulation, there appears to be an imbalance of regulation of motility and proteolysis required for invasion and metastasis (Liotta and Schiffman 1988; Stracke and Liotta 1992). Also, negative regulation of proliferation, invasion, and metastasis includes the activity of tumor suppressor genes and metastasis progressor genes such as nm23 and of growth inhibitors and protease inhibitors.

*Other Factors.* Genetic factors such as species or strain of animal, hormonal factors such as breeding status (virgin female, breeder allowed to nurse, or breeder "force bred", e.g., no nursing and males left in cage) and viral factors such as the type of mammary tumor virus, type of carcinogenic treatment, and immune state of the mouse have all been shown to affect the ability of certain mouse tumors to metastasize to the lung (Sass and Liebelt 1985; Hart 1982). Opinions differ as to whether the histology or location of the primary tumor has effects on metastases. On the other hand, the incidences of pulmonary metastases of mammary cancers may be influenced by the number of primary tumors, the size and/or weight and the duration of the tumor, and the surgical ablation of a primary tumor which may lead to an extension of lifespan (Sass and Liebelt 1985; Sheldon et al. 1982). The value of using transplantable mouse tumor cells in therapeutic studies has been described by Rosenberg et al. (1985), who obtained inhibition of growth of established metastases following the administration of interleukin 2.

## Comparison with Other Species

Metastases of the more commonly occurring neoplasms in mice and rats have been observed more often than metastases in species not commonly used in the laboratory. Few authors have reported metastases from mammary cancers in rats, probably due to short periods of observation. Rats that live 2–3 years do develop metastatic tumors in the lungs and lymph nodes (Russo et al. 1990). The histology of the tumor does not affect consistently the ability to metastasize.

Chemically induced bladder carcinomas metastasize more frequently in mice than in rats (Boorman et al. 1994). Advanced cancer in the human does metastasize frequently, a fact which may be related to a prolongation of life span by treatment. Rat models of bladder cancer are particularly suitable for studying the etiology and pathogenesis since most tumors induced are papillary and superficial, although invasion of the underlying muscle is a late event. The invasion is of clinical concern in humans (Kunze and Chowaniec 1990).

Osteosarcomas frequently metastasize in cats and dogs. Induced osteosarcomas of the rat are similar histologically to those in dog and man and often metastasize (Sass and Liebelt 1985).

Hepatocellular tumors are uncommon in domestic animals and seldom metastasize to the lungs. Induced tumors in rats commonly metastasize to the lungs.

An extensive list of transplantable metastatic animal tumors by Poste in 1982 contains examples of tumors metastatic to lungs (and other organs) from mouse, rat, and rabbit. These are examples of so-called in vivo – in vitro tumor cell lines.

More detailed comparative aspects may be found in the IARC Series on Pathology of Tumours in Laboratory Animals and in the ILSI Monographs on Pathology of Laboratory Animals.

Acknowledgments. I thank Dr. Takashi Murai, Department of Pathology, Osaka City University Medical School, Japan, for the microscopic section for Fig. 274, Dr. Sabine Rehm, SmithKline Beecham Pharmaceuticals, King of Prussia, PA, for the microscopic section for Fig. 273, Ricardo Dreyfuss for excellent photography, and Dr. Umberto Saffiotti for editorial comments and assistance.

## References

Ashburn LL (1937) Spontaneous mammary tumors in mice. Factors influencing the incidence of metastases. US Publ Health Rep 52:915–929

Benirschke K, Garner FM, Jones TC (1978) Pathology of laboratory animals, vol II. Springer, Berlin Heidelberg New York, pp 1075–1082

Berkelhammer J, Oxenhandler RW (1987) Evaluation of premalignant and malignant lesions during the induction of mouse melanomas. Cancer Res 47:1251–1254

Boorman GA, Wood M, Fukushima S (1994) Tumours of the urinary bladder. In: Turusov VS, Mohr U (eds) Pathology of tumours in laboratory animals, vol 2. Tumours of the mouse, 2nd edn. IARC, Lyon, pp 383–407 (IARC scientific publication no 111)

Brooks RE (1970) Mouse mammary tumor metastases in lung: an electron microscopic study. Cancer Res 30:2156–2165

Carr I, Orr FW (1983) Invasion and metastasis. Can Med Assoc J 128:1164–1167

Consolandi G, Veronesi U, Briziarelli G (1958) Metastatic spread of mammary cancer: a comparative study in human beings and in mice. In: Severi L (ed) Proc of II International symposium on mammary cancer, 1957. Division of Cancer Research, Perugia, pp 791–804

De Bruyn PPH, Cho Y (1982) Vascular endothelial invasion via transcellular passage by malignant cells in the primary stage of metastases formation. J Ultrastruct Res 81:189–201

Dingemans KP (1973) Behavior of intravenously injected malignant lymphoma cells. A morphologic study. J Natl Cancer Inst 51:1883–1895

Dunham LJ, Stewart HL (1953) A survey of transplantable and transmissible tumors. J Natl Cancer Inst 13:1299–1377

Dunn TB (1954) Normal and pathologic anatomy of the reticular tissue in laboratory mice, with a classification and discussion of neoplasms. J Natl Cancer Inst 14:1281–1433

Edelman AS, Rotterdam H (1990) Solitary splenic metastasis of an adenocarcinoma of the lung. Am J Clin Pathol 94:326–328

Ewing J (1928) A treatise on tumors, 3rd edn. Saunders, Philadelphia

Fekete E (1938) A comparative morphological study of the mammary gland in a high and low tumor strain of mice. Am J Pathol 14:557–578 and 3 plates

Fidler IJ (1970) Metastasis: quantitative analysis of distribution and fate of tumor emboli labeled with $^{125}$I-5-iodo-2$^{1}$-deoxyuridine. J Natl Cancer Inst 45:773–782

Fidler IJ (1978) Tumor heterogeneity and the biology of cancer invasion and metastasis. Cancer Res 38:2651–2660

Fidler IJ (1986) Rationale and methods for use of nude mice to study the biology and therapy of human cancer metastasis. Cancer Metastasis Rev 5:29–49

Fidler IJ, Nicolson GL (1976) Brief communication: organ selectivity for implantation survival and growth of B16 melanoma variant tumor lines. J Natl Cancer Inst 57:1199–1202

Fidler IJ, Kripke ML (1977) Metastasis results from preexisting variant cells within a malignant tumor. Science 197:893–895

Fidler IJ, Nicholson GL (1987) The process of cancer invasion and metastasis. Cancer Bull 39: 126–131

Fredrickson TN, Hartley JW, Morse HC III, Chattopadhyay SK, Lennert K (1995) Classification of mouse lymphomas. In: Potter M, Melchers F (eds) Mechanisms in B-cell neoplasia 1994. Springer, Berlin Heidelberg New York, pp 109–116

Frith CH (1986) Transitional cell carcinoma, urinary tract, mouse. In: Jones TC, Mohr U, Hunt RD (eds) Monographs on pathology of laboratory animals. Urinary system. Springer, Berlin Heidelberg New York, pp 331–337

Frith CH (1990) Histiocytic sarcoma, mouse, In: Jones TC, Ward JM, Mohr U, Hunt RD (eds) Monographs on pathology of laboratory animals, hemopoietic system. Springer, Berlin Heidelberg New York, pp 58–65

Frith CH, Littlefield NA, Umholtz R (1981) Incidence of pulmonary metastases for various neoplasms in BALB/cStCrlfC3H/Nctr female fed N-2-fluorenylacetamide. J Natl Cancer Inst 66:703–712

Giddens WE Jr, Renne RA (1985) Hemangiosarcoma, nasal cavity, mouse. In: Jones TC, Mohr U, Hunt RD (eds) Monographs on pathology of laboratory animals. Respirtory system. Springer, Belin Heidelberg New York, pp 72–74

Gorer PA (1940) The incidence of tumours of the liver and other organs in a pure line of mice (Strong's CBA strain). J Pathol Bacteriol 50:17–24

Gunning WT, Castonguay A, Goldblatt PJ, Stoner GD (1991) Strain A/J mouse lung adenoma growth patterns vary when induced by different carcinogens. Toxicol Pathol 19:168–175

Haaland M (1911) Spontaneous tumours in mice. 4th sci rep. Imp cancer research fund. Taylor and Francis, London, pp 1–113

Hart IR (1982) The role of animal models in the study of experimental metastasis. In: Liotta LA, Hart IR (eds) Tumor invasion and metastasis. Nijhoff, Boston, pp 1–14

Heider K, Eustis SL (1994) Tumours of the soft tissues. In: Turusov V, Mohr U (eds) Pathology of tumours in laboratory animals, vol 2. Tumours of the mouse, 2nd edn. IARC, Lyon, pp 611–649 (IARC scientific publication no 111)

Hennings H, Spangler EF, Shores R, Mitchell P, Devor D, Shamsuddin AKM, Elgjo KM, Yuspa SH (1986) Malignant conversion and metastasis of mouse skin tumors: a comparison of SENCAR and CD-1 mice. Environ Health Perspect 68:69–74

Horn HA, Congden CC, Eschenbrenner AB, Andervont HB, Stewart HL (1952) Pulmonary adenomatosis in mice. JNCI 12:1297–1315

Juacaba SF, Horak E, Price JE, Tarin D (1989) Tumor cell dissemination patterns and metastasis of murine mammary carcinoma. Cancer Res 49:570–575

Kanno J (1989) Melanocytic tumors, skin mouse. In: Jones TC, Mohr U, Hunt RD (eds) Monographs on pathology of laboratory animals, Integument and mammary glands. Springer, Berlin Heidelberg New York, pp 63–70

Klein-Szanto AJP (1989) Pathology of human and experimental skin tumors. In: Conti CJ, Slaga TJ, Klein-Szanto AJP (eds) Skin tumors: experimental and clinical aspects. Raven, New York, pp 19–53

Kripke ML, Gruys E, Fidler IJ (1978) Metastatic heterogeneity of cells from an ultraviolet light-induced murine fibrosarcoma of recent origin. Cancer Res 38:2962–2967

Kunze E, Chowaniec J (1990) Tumours of the urinary bladder. In: Turusov VS, Mohr U (eds) Pathology of tumours in laboratory animals, vol 1. Tumours of the rat, 2nd edn. IARC, Lyon, pp 345–397 (IARC scientific publication no 79)

Liebelt AG, Liebelt RA (1967) Transplantation of tumors. In: Busch H (ed) Methods in cancer research, vol 1. Academic, New York, pp 143–240

Liebelt RA, Liebelt AG, Gulledge AA, Calvert J (1968) Autoregulation-normal organ and tissue homeostasis. In: The University of Texas MD Anderson Hospital and Tumor Institute at Houston (ed) The proliferation and spread of neoplastic cells. Williams and Wilkins, Baltimore, pp 733–768

Liebelt AG, Bailey C, Fu MM (1981) Mammary cancer in RIII mice-another look. AALAS Publ 103:81–83

Liotta LA, Schiffmann E (1988) Tumour motility factors. Cancer Surv 7:631–652

Liotta LA, Stetler-Stevenson WG (1989) Principles of molecular cell biology of cancer: cancer metastasis. In: DeVita VT Jr, Hellman S, Rosenberg SA (eds) Cancer: principles and practice of oncology, vol 1, 3rd edn. Lippincott, Philadelphia, pp 98–115

Liotta LA, Kleinerman J, Saidel GM (1974) Quantitative relationships of intravascular tumor cells, tumor vessels and pulmonary metastases following tumor implantation. Cancer Res 34: 997–1004

Liotta LA, Kohn E, Steeg PS, Stetler-Stevenson W (1991a) Molecular biology of metastasis. In: Broder S (ed) Molecular foundations of oncology. Williams and Wilkins, Baltimore, pp 57–81

Liotta LA, Steeg PS, Stetler-Stevenson WG (1991b) Cancer metastasis and angiogenesis: an imbalance of positive and negative regulation. Cell 64:327–336

Lotan R (1987) Cell adhesion receptors and cancer metastasis. Cancer Bull 39:156–162

Luz A, Gössner W, Murray AB (1991a) Osteosarcoma, spontaneous and radiation-induced, mouse. In: Jones TC, Mohr U, Hunt RD (eds) Monographs on pathology of laboratory animals. Cardiovascular and musculoskeletal systems. Springer, Berlin Heidelberg New York, pp 202–213

Marsh MC (1927) Tumor massage and metastases in mice. J Cancer Res 11:101–107

Marsh MC (1929) Spontaneous mammary cancer in mice. J Cancer Res 13:313–339

Matsuyama M, Suzuki H, Nakamura T (1969) Carcinogenesis in dd-I mice injected during suckling period with urethane, nitrogen mustard N-oxide, and nitroso-urethane. Br J Cancer 23:167–171

Murray JA (1908) Spontaneous cancer in the mouse; histology, metastasis, transplantability and the regulation of malignant new growth to spontaneously affected animals. 3rd sci rpt, Imp cancer res fund, London, pp 69–115

National Toxicology Program (1982) Carcinogenesis bioassay of di(2-ethylhexyl)adipate in F344 rats and B6C3F[1] mice. US Dept HHS, PHS, NIH, Washington DC (Technical report series 212)

Nicolson GL (1988) Organ specificity of tumor metastasis: role of preferential adhesion, invasion and growth of malignant cells at specific secondary sites. Cancer Metastasis Rev 7:143–188

North SM, Nicolson GL (1987) Host responses and tumor metastasis. In: Herberman RB, Wiltrout RH, Gorelik E (eds) Immune responses to metastases, vol 1. CRC, Boca Raton, pp 1–22

Orr FW, Young L, King GM, Adamson IYR (1988) Preferential growth of metastatic tumors at the pleural surface of mouse lung. Clin Exp Metastasis 6:221–232

Paget S (1989) The distribution of secondary growths in cancer of the breast (1889 classical article, Lancet 1:571–573). Cancer Metastasis Rev 8:98–101

Pattengale PK (1990a) Classification of mouse lymphoid neoplasms. In: Jones TC, Ward JM, Mohr U, Hunt RD (eds) Monographs on pathology of laboratory animals. Hemopoietic system. Springer, Berlin Heidelberg New York, pp 137–143

Pattengale PK (1990b) Follicular center cell lymphoma, mouse. In: Jones TC, Ward JM, Mohr U, Hunt RD (eds) Monographs on pathology of laboratory animals. Hemopoietic system. Springer, Berlin Heidelberg New York, pp 147–149

Pitelka DR, Hamamoto ST, Taggart BN (1980a) Epithelial cell junctions in primary and metastatic mammary tumors of mice. Cancer Res 40:1588–1599

Pitelka DR, Hamamoto ST, Taggart BN (1980b) Basal lamina and tissue recognition in malignant mammary tumors. Cancer Res 40:1600–1611

Poste G (1982) Experimental systems for analysis of the malignant phenotype. Cancer Metastasis Rev 1:141–199

Radinsky R, Fidler IJ (1992) Regulation of tumor cell growth at organ-specific metastases. In Vivo 6:325–331

Rehm S, Lijinsky W, Singh G, Katyal SL (1991) Mouse bronchiolar cell carcinogenesis. Histologic characterization and expression of Clara cell antigen in lesions induced by N-nitrosobis-(2-chloroethyl) ureas. Am J Pathol 139:413–422

Rehm S, Ward JM, Sass B (1994) Tumours of the lungs. In: Turusov V, Mohr U (eds) Pathology of tumours in laboratory animals, vol 2. Tumours of the mouse, 2nd edn. IARC, Lyon, pp 325–355 (IARC scientific publication no 111)

Rehm S, Ward JM, ten Have-Opbroek AW, Anderson LM, Singh G, Katyal SL, Rice JM (1988) Mouse papillary lung tumors transplacentally induced by N-nitrosoethylurea: evidence for alveolar type II cell orgin by comparative light microscopic, ultrastructural, and immunohistochemical studies. Cancer Res 48:148–160

Rosenberg SA, Mulé JJ, Spiess PJ, Reichert CH, Schwarz SL (1985) Regression of established pulmonary metastases and subcutaneous tumor mediated by the systemic administration of high-dose recombinant interleukin 2. J Exp Med 161:1169–1188

Russo I, Russo IH, Rogers AE, van Zwieten MJ, Gusterson B (1990) Tumours of the mammary gland. In: Turusov VS, Mohr U (eds) Pathology of tumours in laboratory animals, vol 1. Tumours of the rat, 2nd edn. IARC, Lyon, pp 47–78 (IARC scientific publication no 79)

Sass B (1986) Adenoma, adenocarcinoma, Kidney, mouse. In: Jones TC, Mohr U, Hunt RD (eds) Monographs on pathology of laboratory animals. Urinary system. Springer, Berlin Heidelberg New York, pp 87–101

Sass B, Liebelt AG (1985) Metastatic tumors, lung, mouse. In: Jones TC, Mohr U, Hunt RD (eds) Monographs on pathology of laboratory animals. Respiratory system. Springer, Berlin Heidelberg New York, pp 138–159

Sheldon W (1994) Tumours of the Harderian gland. In: Turusov V, Mohr U (eds) Pathology of tumours in laboratory animals, vol 2. Tumours of the mouse, 2nd edn. IARC, Lyon, pp 101–103 (IARC scientific publication no 111)

Sheldon WG, Owen K, Weed L, Kodell R (1982) Distribution of mammary gland neoplasms and factors influencing metastases in hybrid mice. Lab Anim Sci 32:166–168

Sheldon WG, Curtis M, Kodell RL, Weed L (1983) Primary Harderian gland neoplasms in mice. J Natl Cancer Inst 71:61–68

Slye M, Holmes HF, Wells HG (1915) Spontaneous tumors of the liver, associated frequency with other primary growths (mammary and lung). J Med Res 33:171–182

Snell KC, Stewart HL (1962) Pulmonary adenomatosis induced in DBA/2 mice by oral administration of dibenz[a,h]-anthracene. J Natl Cancer Inst 28:1043–1051

Squartini F, Bistocchi M (1977) Bioactivity of C3H and RIII mammary tumor viruses in virgin female BALB/c mice. J Natl Cancer Inst 58:1845–1847

Stewart HL, Dunn TB, Snell KC, Deringer MK (1979) Tumours of the respiratory tract. In: Turusov VS (ed) Pathology of tumours in laboratory animals, vol 2. Tumours of the mouse. IARC, Lyon, pp 251–287 (IARC scientific publication no 23)

Stewart HL, Sass B, Deringer MK, Dunn TB, Liotta LA, Togo S (1984) Pure yolk sac carcinoma of the mouse uterus: report of 8 cases. J Natl Cancer Inst 73:115–122

Stracke ML, Liotta LA (1992) Multi-step cascade of tumor cell metastasis. In Vivo 6:309–316

Sugarbaker EV (1981) Patterns of metastasis in human malignancies. Cancer Biol Rev 2:235–278

Sugarbaker EV, Weingrad DN, Roseman JM (1982) Observations on cancer metastasis in man. In: Liotta LA, Hart IR (eds) Tumor invasion and metastasis. Nijhoff, Boston, pp 427–465

Takahashi M, Migakawa Y (1989) Mast cell tumor, skin, mouse. In: Jones TC, Mohr U, Hunt RD (eds) Monographs on pathology of laboratory animals. Integument and mammary glands. Springer, Berlin Heidelberg New York, pp 112–117

Tarin D (1982) Investigations of the mechanisms of metastatic spread of naturally occurring neoplasms. Cancer Metastasis Rev 1:215–225

Tarin D, Price JE (1981) Influence of microenvironment and vascular anatomy on metastatic colonization potential of mammary tumors. Cancer Res 41:3604–3609

Turusov VS (1994) Histiocytic sarcoma. In: Turusov VS (ed) Pathology of tumors in laboratory animals, vol 2. Tumours of the mouse. IARC, Lyon, pp 671–680 (IARC scientific publication no 111)

Turusov VS, Takayama S (1979) Tumours of the liver. In: Turusov VS (ed) Pathology of tumours in laboratory animals, vol 2. Tumours of the mouse. IARC, Lyon, pp 193–233 (IARC scientific publication no 23)

Turusov VS, Deringer MK, Dunn TB, Stewart HL (1973) Malignant mouse liver tumors resembling human hepatoblastomas. J Natl Cancer Inst 51:1689–1695

Turusov VS, Breslow NE, Tomatis L (1974) Frequency and organ distribution of lung tumor metastases in CF-1 mice. J Natl Cancer Inst 52:225–232

van der Valk MA (1981) Survival, tumor incidence and gross pathology in 33 mouse strains. In: Hilgers J, Sluyser M (eds) Mammary tumors in the mouse. Elsevier, New York, chap 3

Ward JM, Goodman DG, Squire RA, Chu KC, Linhart MS (1979) Neoplastic and nonneoplastic lesions in aging (C57BL/6N × C3HHeNF$_1$) (B6C3F1) mice. J Natl Cancer Inst 63:849–854

Wexler H (1966) Accurate identification of experimental pulmonary metastases. J Natl Cancer Inst 36:641–645

Williams AO, Flanders KC, Saffiotti U (1993) Immunohistochemical localization of transforming growth factor-B$_1$ in rats with experimental silicosis, alveolar type II hyperplasia, and lung cancer. Am J Pathol 142:1831–1840

Willis RA (1973) The spread of tumours in the human body, 3rd edn. Butterworths, London

Zetter BR (1990) The cellular basis of site-specific tumor metastasis. New Engl J Med 322:605–612

# NONNEOPLASTIC LESIONS

## Bleomycin-Induced Injury, Mouse. A Model for Lung Injury

Drummond H. Bowden

### Gross Appearance

The gross appearance does not distinguish developing and established fibrotic lesions induced by bleomycin from injury caused by drugs or other chemicals. After a single intravenous dose fibrosis is multifocal, rarely confluent; diffuse lobular and lobar fibrosis follow endotracheal administration.

### Microscopic Features

The sequence of events induced by bleomycin is similar whatever the route of administration. What does vary is the speed of the response; intravenous and endotracheal injections induce pulmonary fibrosis in 2 weeks, twice weekly intraperitoneal injections in 4–8 weeks. Timing of the morphological events is most precise following a single intravenous injection. The following account describes the changes in Swiss albino mice given a single intravenous injection of bleomycin, 120 mg/kg.

The earliest detectable alteration is demonstrated by bronchoalveolar lavage. The number of cells obtained from controls is approximately $20 \times 10^4$, predominantly macrophages. Between one and three days after bleomycin the yield is more than doubled, and up to 10% are neutrophils.

In tissue sections of the lung, perivascular edema and endothelial swelling with vacuolation are observed at 5 days (Fig. 282). In some animals injury does not progress beyond endothelial swelling, interstitial edema, and a mild inflammatory infiltrate; these lesions are reversible.

The most critical event in the genesis of pulmonary injury is destruction of the alveolar type I epithelium. Damage to the epithelial barrier, though not directly visible by light microscopy, may be inferred from the presence of fibrin in the air sacs. Should capillary leakage be massive, the animal dies; if limited or multifocal the animal survives, but repair is accompanied by fibrosis.

With progression from injury to repair the inflammatory cellular response changes; initially it is predominantly macrophagic with some granulocytes; later an increase of lymphocytes and plasma cells is seen, particularly in perivascular spaces. As fibrosis develops, macrophages trapped in fibrosed segments of the lung become vacuolated; some binucleate and multinucleate forms are seen (Fig. 283).

The evolution of fibrosis is observed in two compartments of the lung, in fibrin-filled alveoli and in the interstitium. Proliferation of fibroblasts is most active between 10 and 14 days, and the laying down of collagen is progressive thereafter. Fibrosis, which is well established by 2–4 weeks, is most severe in subpleural areas and in perivascular and peribronchial spaces (Fig. 284).

The sequence of reparative events may be delineated precisely by [$^3$H]thymidine labeling of regenerating cells; endothelial regeneration is rapid with complete structural restoration; epithelial regeneration, on the other hand, is delayed and distorted. Necrosis of type I cells is followed as usual by division of type II cells, but instead of differentiating to reconstitute a thin barrier of type I cells, they persist and undergo a variety of metaplastic changes, including giant forms which almost fill the alveolus, ciliated cells, and keratinocytes. These changes are most pronounced after intraperitoneal injections given over a period of several weeks (Fig. 285).

### Ultrastructure

The earliest lesions observed with the electron microscope, endothelial blebbing and sub-

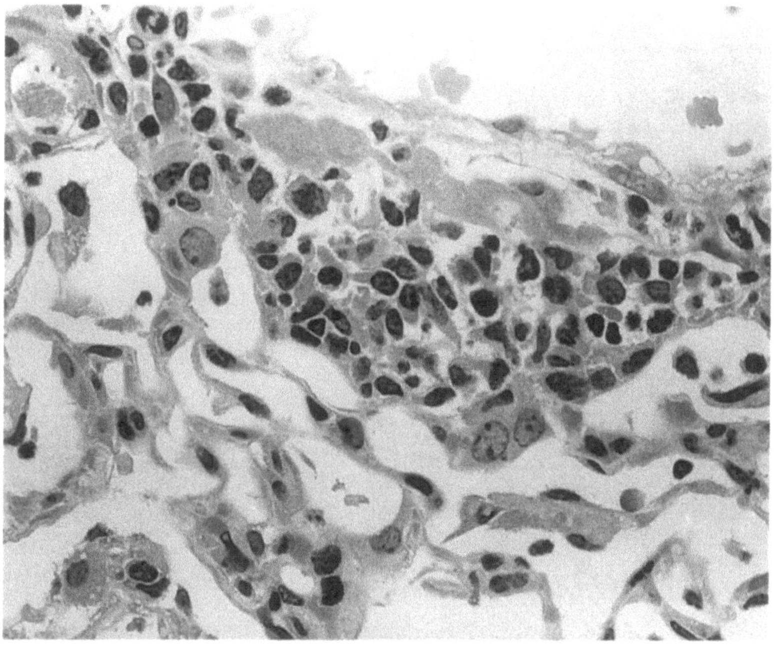

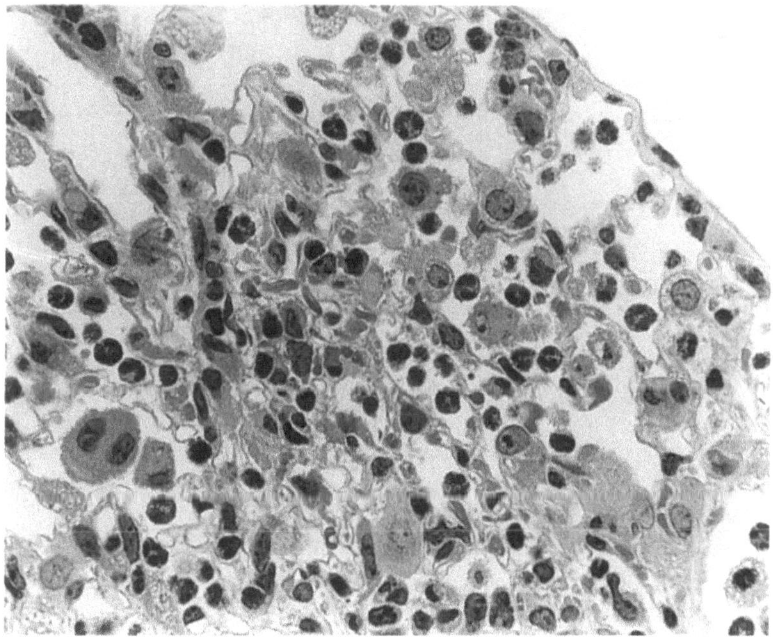

**Fig. 282.** (*above*) Lung, mouse. Vascular lesion 7 days after a single intravenous injection of bleomycin. There is endothelial vacuolation, subendothelial edema, and a perivascular cellular exudate, predominantly mononuclear. H&E, ×500

**Fig. 283.** (*below*) Lung mouse. Alveolar exudate 7 days after a single intravenous injection of bleomycin. The predominant cell is the macrophage; binucleate and multinucleate forms are not uncommon. H&E, ×500

endothelial edema, are present within 2 days of the injection (Fig. 286). Necrosis of type I alveolar cells, prominent between 7 and 10 days, is accompanied by exudation of fibrin into the air sacs (Fig. 287). Type II cells and bronchiolar cells show no evidence of injury. Regenerative activity is prompt, endothelial cells are rapidly replaced, and by 12 days many of the alveoli are lined by type II cells. In some alveoli these cells differentiate normally to type I cells; in other areas cuboidal cells persist, and metaplastic forms are seen (Fig. 288). Ultrastructural studies confirm the two components of the fibrotic response. In the early phase the intra-alveolar exudate becomes organized;

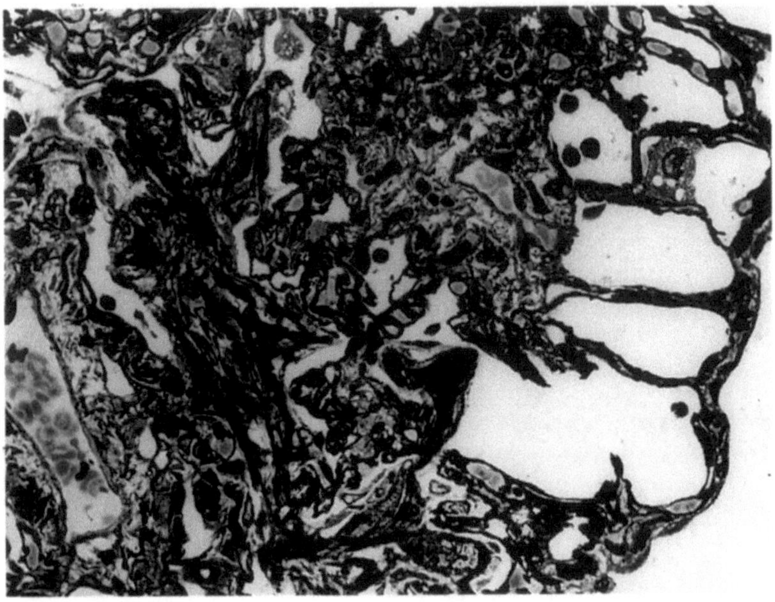

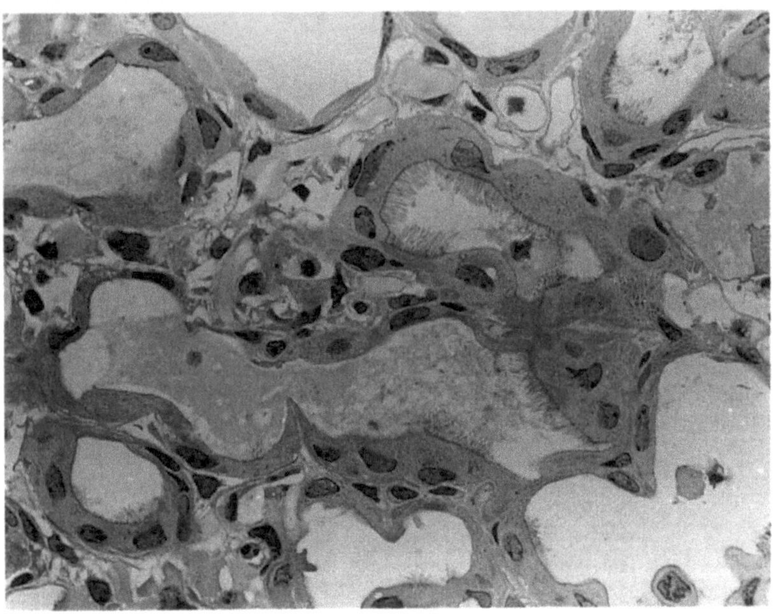

**Fig. 284.** (*above*) Lung mouse, after twice weekly intraperitoneal injection of bleomycin for 4 weeks. Dense bands of subpleural, interstitial collagen distort the normal architecture, producing a honeycomb pattern. Silver methenamine, ×350

**Fig. 285.** (*below*) Lung mouse, 12 weeks after twice weekly intraperitoneal injection of bleomycin. No normal alveoli are seen; many of the alveolar epithelial cells bear cilia. H&E, ×1000

these lesions tend to resolve. Interstitial fibrosis, which is progressive and irreversible, usually is associated with metaplastic changes in the alveolar epithelium.

## Differential Diagnosis

The pulmonary cells most susceptible to air-borne or blood-borne injury are type I epithelial cells and endothelial cells. Their response to injury by agents as diverse as viruses, oxidant gases, and blood-borne drugs is similar, varying of course with the dosage and duration of the insult. Rapid regeneration of both lining layers is the rule, with restitution of the thin air-blood barrier. Delayed or abnormal regeneration or failure to cover the surface "wound" is associated with proliferation of interstitial fibroblasts and the development of fibrosis. What distinguishes bleomycin-induced

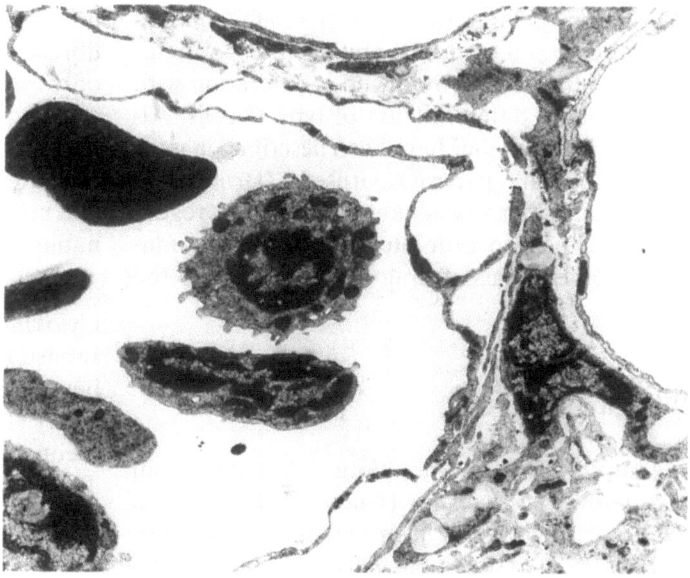

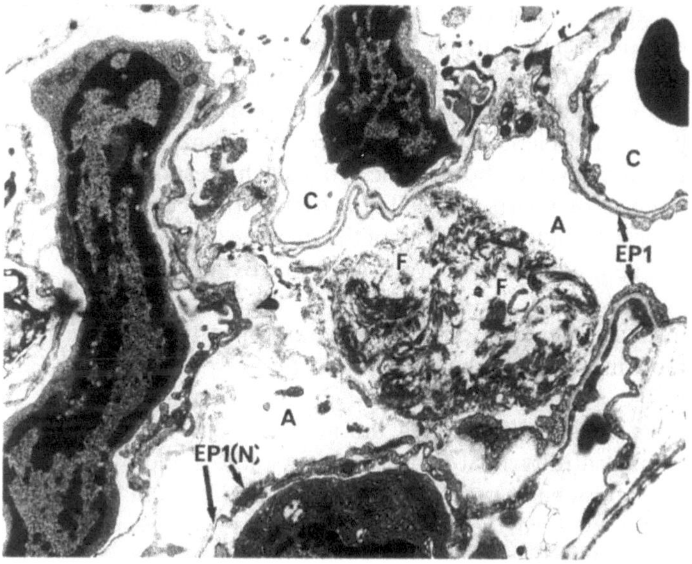


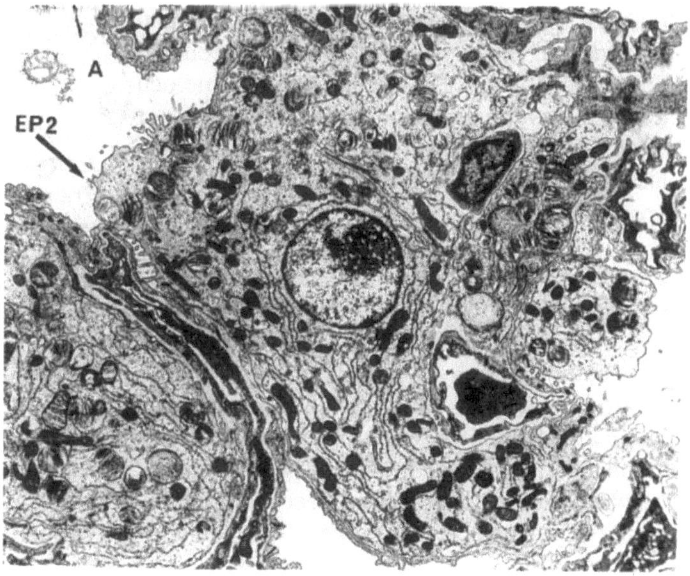


**Fig. 286.** (*above*) Lung mouse. Small pulmonary blood vessel 2 days after a single intravenous injection of bleomycin. There is severe cytoplasmic edema of the endothelial cells. TEM, ×8000

**Fig. 287.** (*middle*) Lung mouse. Alveolus 10 days after a single intravenous injection of bleomycin. Some of the type 1 cells (*EP1*) are intact; others (*EP1(N)*) have undergone focal necrosis allowing the exudation of fibrin (*F*) from the capillaries (*C*) into the alveolar lumen (*A*). TEM, ×6000

**Fig. 288.** (*below*) Lung mouse. Alveolus (*A*) 3 weeks after a single intravenous injection of bleomycin. A huge type II (*EP2*) epithelial cell occupies much of the alveolar lumen. TEM, ×6000

injury from other forms of drug-related pulmonary disease is the unusual epithelial response involving delayed and prolonged regeneration with inappropriate differentiation of type II cells. Although similar lesions have been described in mice infected with paramyxoviruses (Brownstein 1985), the pattern of abnormal epithelial regeneration associated with interstitial fibrosis is unusual in other forms of drug induced injury to the lung.

## Biological Features

Bleomycin is an antibiotic derived from *Streptomyces verticillatus* (Umezawa 1974). As a cytotoxic agent it has been particularly useful in the treatment of squamous cell carcinoma, testicular tumors, and lymphomas. Introduced largely because it has no major toxic effects on kidney or bone marrow, it soon became apparent that bleomycin injures the lung. In all cells, normal or neoplastic, bleomycin is degraded by an enzyme which cleaves carboxyamide groups. The responsiveness of a particular cell type to the drug seems to be related to the activity of this enzyme. Epidermal cells contain low levels of the inactivating enzyme so that bleomycin is able to reach the nucleus where it induces fragmentation of DNA, blocking or deranging synthesis of new DNA, RNA, and protein. These effects are most pronounced in cells entering the mitotic cycle. Following intratracheal administration, radiolabeled bleomycin binds rapidly to DNA; at 24h, less than 1% of the drug remains in the lung (Lazo and Pham 1984; Giri 1986). In vitro studies indicate breakage of DNA is dependent upon activation of bleomycin to an oxygenated iron-drug complex (Burger et al. 1981). The requirement for molecular oxygen may be a factor in the particular vulnerability of the lung and in the augmenting of bleomycin-induced pulmonary lesions by hyperoxia (Hay et al. 1987).

*Pathogenesis.* Adoption of the bleomycin model as a standard method for studying fibrogenic mechanisms has enhanced our understanding of the pathogenesis of pulmonary fibrosis. Bleomycin-induced injury to endothelial and epithelial cells allows plasma proteins, including complement, to reach the alveoli where interaction with macrophages initiates secretion of many of the cytokines responsible for launching inflammation and repair. The development of fibrosis is a complex process, involving not only cytokines and the immune system, but direct cell-to-cell interactions of fibroblasts with interstitial macrophages, epithelial cells, and endothelium. In all of these processes alveolar and interstitial macrophages play a central coordinating role.

*Cytokines.* Of the many cytokines secreted in response to bleomycin, transforming growth factor beta (TGFβ) is pivotal to the overall reaction to injury (Denholm and Rollins 1993). Intra-tracheal bleomycin induces a five- to sevenfold increase in TGFβ transcripts and stimulates DNA synthesis (Raghow et al. 1989). Added to cultured lung fibroblasts, bleomycin increases TGFβ mRNA, which, in turn, stimulates secretion of procollagens types I and III, each type derived from a distinct population of fibroblasts (Breen et al. 1992). This polypeptide growth factor has many functions: it stimulates recruitment of monocytes and fibroblasts and regulates macrophagic production of fibronectin, interleukin 1, tumor necrosis factor alpha (TNFα) and fibroblast growth factors; all are growth regulators (Wahl et al. 1990). In addition, TGFβ inhibits matrix-degrading enzymes and increases the levels of protease inhibitors (Edwards et al. 1987; Lund et al. 1987). The stimulatory and inhibitory activities of TGFβ and its derivative cytokines probably explain the doubling of the rate of collagen synthesis and the reduced collagen breakdown that occurs as bleomycin-induced fibrosis develops (Laurent and McAnulty 1983).

TNFα, secreted by macrophages, injures epithelial cells and enhances growth of cultured fibroblasts; systemic treatment with TNF antibody inhibits bleomycin-induced fibrosis in mice (Piguet et al. 1989; Vilcek et al. 1986).

*Cytokines* secreted by the alveolar macrophage are effective locally, but they cannot cross the intact epithelial barrier to reach the interstitial fibroblasts (Mangum et al. 1990). Other mechanisms, including direct communication between fibroblasts, macrophages, epithelium, and endothelium, must be invoked to explain the development of interstitial fibrosis.

*Interstitial Macrophages and Fibroblasts.* Macrophages and fibroblasts are intimately associated within the pulmonary interstitium. The importance of this relationship has been demonstrated in silicosis, where pulmonary fibrosis is induced by the interaction of silica particles with interstitial rather than alveolar macrophages (Bowden et al. 1989). Interstitial macrophages also appear to be essential to the development of bleomycin-induced fibrosis. TNFα production of alveolar and interstitial macrophages has been studied in two strains of mice, CBA/J, which is highly susceptible to bleomycin, and BALB/c, which is resistant to the drug (Phan and Kunkel 1992). In the resistant strain, bleomycin induces secretion of TNFα by alveolar macrophages only; in the susceptible strain TNFα production occurs in both alveolar and interstitial macrophages. These results suggest a dominant role for the interstitial macrophage in the induction of interstitial fibrosis. The production of transforming growth factor also varies in different strains; after bleomycin, TGFβ mRNA is elevated fivefold in C57B1/6 mice and depressed in BALB/c animals (Hoyt and Lazo 1988).

*Epithelial Cells and Fibroblasts.* While the interactive role of fibroblasts and macrophages is established, the epithelial-fibroblast control system is less well understood. The importance of this system in the developing lung is recognized (Adamson and King 1985), and there is increasing evidence that interruption of normal epithelial-fibroblast contacts during healing may favor unbridled proliferation of interstitial fibroblasts (Adamson et al. 1988, 1990). Although the nature of the intercellular messages has not been defined, undoubtedly they are influenced by the cytokine network. In the steady state, type II cells appear to inhibit the growth of fibroblasts possibly through the secretion of prostaglandin $E_2$, a known suppressor of fibroblast growth (Chauncey et al. 1988; Goldstein and Polgar 1982; Klein and Adamson 1989). The process may be augmented by TGFβ which not only stimulates fibroblasts but also inhibits DNA synthesis in epithelial cells (Howe et al. 1990).

*Endothelial Cells and Fibroblasts.* Pulmonary endothelial cells secrete several cytokines including TGFβ. Bleomycin stimulates cultured lung endothelial cells to produce TGFβ which in turn induces fibroblasts to secrete collagen (Phan et al. 1991).

*Immune Reactions.* An intact T cell system is essential to the development of fibrosis; when T cells are absent, as in the nude mouse or following thymectomy, fibrosis does not occur (Schrier et al. 1983b; Schrier and Phan 1987). In bleomycin-induced lung injury, lymphocytes infiltrate the lesions as collagen deposition begins, and the fibrotic response is suppressed by the administration of antilymphocyte globulin or steroids (Thrall et al. 1979; Phan et al. 1981). The divergent responses of different murine strains to bleomycin may also have an immune basis: "low responders" are converted to "high responders" by pretreatment with cyclophosphamide, which is cytotoxic to T-suppressor cells. An autoimmune mechanism has also been invoked; rats treated with bleomycin develop transient cellular sensitivity to type I collagen, the kinetics of the reaction matching the brief increase of collagen synthesis (Schrier et al. 1982).

*Frequency of Pulmonary Lesions.* The pulmonary response to bleomycin varies considerably in different strains; collagen production is high in C57BL/6, intermediate in DBA/2, and low in BALB/c (Schrier et al. 1983a). Possible reasons for these differences have been addressed. In the Swiss albino mouse, a sensitive strain, frequency and severity of pulmonary lesions are dose dependent. A single intravenous injection of bleomycin, 120 mg/kg, results in 50% mortality; survivors develop pulmonary fibrosis in 2–4 weeks. Twice weekly injections of bleomycin, 20 mg/kg, kill half the animals and induce fibrosis in the survivors within 4–8 weeks. Epithelial metaplasia is most pronounced in animals receiving intraperitoneal bleomycin for at least 8 weeks. Endotracheal bleomycin produces rapid and diffuse lesions in susceptible strains.

## Comparison with Other Species

The pulmonary toxicity of bleomycin varies considerably from species to species. In dogs, as little as 0.4 mg/kg induces pulmonary lesions whereas the corresponding dose in mice is 20 mg/kg by repeated intraperitoneal injection and 120 mg/kg given as a single intravenous injection (Table 25). In humans toxic effects are frequent when the drug is first introduced; later, as dosage is reduced, fewer pulmonary complications are observed. The occasional severe reaction to doses as small as

**Table 25.** Pulmonary toxicity of bleomycin

| Animal | Route of administration | Dose[a] | Reference |
|---|---|---|---|
| Mouse | | | |
| Swiss Albino | Intraperitoneal | 20 mg/kg twice daily | Adamson and Bowden (1974, 1979) |
| Swiss Albino | Intravenous | 120 mg/kg | Adamson and Bowden (1977, 1979) |
| Hamster | Intratracheal | 5 U/kg | Snider et al. (1978) |
| Dog | Intravenous | 0.4 mg/kg | Fleischman et al. (1971) |
| Baboon | Intramuscular | 1.5 U/kg twice weekly | McCullough et al. (1978) |
| Pheasant | Intravenous | 4.12 mg/kg twice weekly | Badrossian et al. (1977) |

[a] 1 mg is approximately 1 U bleomycin sulfate.

5 mg/kg suggests that individual susceptibility may be important in determining the response to bleomycin.

## References


Adamson IYR, Bowden DH (1974) The pathogenesis of bleomycin-induced pulmonary fibrosis in mice. Am J Pathol 77:185–198

Adamson IYR, Bowden DH (1977) Origin of ciliated alveolar epithelial cells in bleomycin-induced lung injury. Am J Pathol 87:569–580

Adamson IYR, Bowden DH (1979) Bleomycin-induced injury and metaplasia of alveolar type 2 cells. Relationship of cellular responses to drug presence in the lung. Am J Pathol 96:531–544

Adamson IYR, King G (1985) Epithelial-mesenchymal interactions in postnatal rat lung growth. Exp Lung Res 8:261–274

Adamson IYR, Young L, Bowden DH (1988) Relationship of alveolar epithelial injury and repair to the induction of pulmonary fibrosis. Am J Pathol 130:377–383

Adamson IYR, Hedgecock C, Bowden DH (1990) Epithelial cell-fibroblast interactions in lung injury and repair. Am J Pathol 137:385–392

Bedrossian CWM, Greenberg SD, Yawn DH, O'Neal RM (1977) Experimentally induced bleomycin sulfate pulmonary toxicity. Histopathologic and ultrastructural study in the pheasant. Arch Pathol Lab Med 101:248–254

Bowden DH, Hedgecock C, Adamson IYR (1989) Silica-induced pulmonary fibrosis involves the reaction of particles with interstitial rather than alveolar macrophages. J Pathol 158:73–80

Breen E, Shull S, Burne S, Absher M, Kelley J, Phan S, Cutroneo KR (1992) Bleomycin regulation of transforming growth factor-β mRNA in rat lung fibroblasts. Am J Respir Cell Mol Biol 6:146–152

Brownstein DG (1985) Sendai virus infection, lung, mouse and rat. In: Jones TC, Mohr U, Hunt RD (eds) Monographs on pathology of laboratory animals: respiratory system. Springer, Berlin Heidelberg New York, pp 194–203

Burger RM, Peisach J, Horwitz SB (1981) Activated bleomycin. A transient complex of drug, iron, and oxygen that degrades DNA. J Biol Chem 256:11636–11644

Chauncey JB, Peters-Golden M, Simon RH (1988) Arachidonic acid metabolism by rat alveolar epithelial cells. Lab Invest 58:133–140

Denholm EM, Rollins SM (1993) Expression and secretion of transforming growth factor-β by bleomycin-stimulated rat alveolar macrophages. Am J Physiol 264 (Lung Cell Mol Physiol 8):L36–L42

Edwards DR, Murphy G, Reynolds JJ, Whitham SE, Docherty AJP, Angel P, Heath JK (1987) Transforming growth factor β modulates the expression of collagenase and metalloproteinase inhibitor. EMBO J 6:1899–1904

Elson N, Szapiel S, Fulmer J, Crystal R (1977) Role of cell-mediated immunity in bleomycin-induced pulmonary fibrosis. Am Rev Respir Dis 115 [Suppl]:54 (abstract)

Fleischman RW, Baker JR, Thompson GR, Schaeppi UH, Ilievesky VR, Cooney DA, Davis RD (1971) Bleomycin-induced interstitial pneumonia. Thorax 26:675–682

Giri SN (1986) Pharmacokinetics, subcellular distribution and co-valent binding of [$^3$H] bleomycin in hamsters after endotracheal administration. Exp Mol Pathol 45:207–220

Goldstein R, Polgar P (1982) The effect and interaction of bradykinin and prostaglandins on protein and collagen production by lung fibroblasts. J Biol Chem 257:8630–8633

Hay JG, Haslam PL, Dewar A, Addis B, Turner-Warwick M, Laurent GJ (1987) Development of acute lung injury after the combination of intravenous bleomycin and exposure to hyperoxia in rats. Thorax 42:374–382

Howe PH, Draetta G, Leof EB (1990) Transforming growth factor β1 inhibition of $p34^{cdc2}$ phosphorylation and histone H1 kinase activity is associated with G1/S-phase growth arrest. Mol Cell Biol 11:1185–1194

Hoyt DG, Lazo JS (1988) Alterations in pulmonary mRNA encoding procollagens, fibronectin and transforming growth factor β precede bleomycin-induced pulmonary fibrosis in mice. J Pharmacol Exp Ther 246:765–771

Klein JH, Adamson IYR (1989) Fibroblast inhibition and prostaglandin secretion by alveolar epithelial cells exposed to silica. Lab Invest 60:808–813

Laurent G, McAnulty RJ (1983) Protein metabolism during bleomycin-induced pulmonary fibrosis in rabbits. Am Rev Respir Dis 128:82–88

Lazo JS, Pham ET (1984) Pulmonary fate of [$^3$H] bleomycin $A_2$ in mice. J Pharmacol Exp Ther 228:13–18
Lund LR, Riccio A, Andreasen PA, Nielsen LS, Kristensen P, Laiho M, Saksela O, Blasi F, Dano K (1987) Transforming growth factor-β is a strong and fast acting positive regulator of the level of type-1 plasminogen activator inhibitor mRNA in W1-38 human lung fibroblasts. EMBO J 6:1281–1286
Mangum JB, Everitt JI, Bonner JC, Moore LR, Brody AR (1990) Co-culture of primary pulmonary cells to model alveolar injury and translocation of proteins. In Vitro Cell Dev Biol 26:1135–1143
McCullough B, Schneider S, Greene ND, Johanson WG Jr (1978) Bleomycin-induced lung injury in baboons: alterations of cells and immunoglobulins recoverable by bronchoalveolar lavage. Lung 155:337–358
Phan SH, Kunkel SL (1992) Lung cytokine production in bleomycin-induced pulmonary fibrosis. Exp Lung Res 18:29–43
Phan SH, Thrall RS, Williams C (1981) Bleomycin-induced pulmonary fibrosis. Effects of steroid on lung collagen metabolism. Am Rev Respir Dis 124:428–434
Phan SH, Gharaee-Kermani M, Wolber F, Ryan US (1991) Stimulation of rat endothelial cell transforming growth factor-β production by bleomycin. J Clin Invest 87:148–154
Piguet PF, Collart MA, Grau GE, Kapanci Y, Vassalli P (1989) Tumor necrosis factor/cachectin plays a key role in bleomycin-induced pneumopathy and fibrosis. J Exp Med 170:655–663
Raghow R, Irish P, Kang AH (1989) Coordinate regulation of transforming growth factor β gene expression and cell proliferation in hamster lungs undergoing bleomycin-induced fibrosis. J Clin Invest 84:1836–1842
Schrier DJ, Phan SH (1987) Modulation of bleomycin-induced pulmonary fibrosis in the BALB/c mouse by cyclophosphamide- sensitive T cells. Am J Pathol 116:270–278
Schrier DJ, Phan SH, Ward PA (1982) Cellular sensitivity to collagen in bleomycin-treated rats. J Immunol 129:2156–2159
Schrier DJ, Kunkel RG, Phan SH (1983a) The role of strain variation in murine bleomycin-induced pulmonary fibrosis. Am Rev Respir Dis 127:63–66
Schrier DJ, Phan SH, McGarry BM (1983b) The effects of the nude (nu/nu) mutation on bleomycin-induced pulmonary fibrosis. Am Rev Respir Dis 127:614–617
Snider GL, Celli BR, Goldstein RH, O'Brien J, Lucey EG (1978) Chronic interstitial pulmonary fibrosis produced in hamsters by endotracheal bleomycin. Am Rev Respir Dis 117:289–297
Thrall RS, McCormick J, Jack R, Phan SH, Ward PA (1979) The effect of anti-lymphocyte globulin on the development of pulmonary fibrosis in the rat. Am Rev Respir Dis 119 [Suppl]:83
Umezawa H (1974) Chemistry and mechanism of action of bleomycin. Fed Proc 33:2296–2302
Vilcek J, Palombella VJ, Henrikson-De-Stephano D, Swenson C, Feinman R, Hirai M, Tsujimoto M (1986) Fibroblast growth enhancing activity of tumor necrosis factor and its relationship to other polypeptide growth factors. J Exp Med 163:632–643
Wahl SM, McCartney-Francis N, Dougherty EB, Dougherty SF (1990) Macrophage production of TGF-β and regulation by TGF-β. Ann NY Acad Sci 593:188–196

# Fibroblast Interactions with Epithelial Cells in Lung Injury and Repair

Drummond H. Bowden and Ian Y.R. Adamson

## Gross Appearance

*Acute Hyperoxia.* If adult mice are exposed to 90% oxygen for 6 days, either they die or, on return to air, they make a complete recovery with no sequelae. In those that die the lungs are hemorrhagic, solid, and airless (Adamson and Bowden 1974).

*Bleomycin.* A single intravenous injection of bleomycin (120 mg/kg) to mice induces multifocal fibrosis within three weeks (Adamson and Bowden 1979).

## Microscopic and Ultrastructural Features

The following measurements were made: radiographic indices for epithelial cells and fibroblasts, length of basal lamina for each type II cell, percentage of type II cells with continuous basement membrane; and number of contacts between epithelial and interstitial cells. The paper by Adamson et al. (1990) provides details of the techniques used.

*Normal Alveolus.* The alveolus is lined almost entirely by thin type I epithelial cells with type II cells at the corners. Type I cells have few foot processes, and their basal lamina is continuous. The foot processes of type II cells frequently penetrate the basement membrane, establishing contact with interstitial fibroblasts (Fig. 289).

*Hyperoxia.* Within the first 3 days of exposure to high concentrations of oxygen mice develop inter-

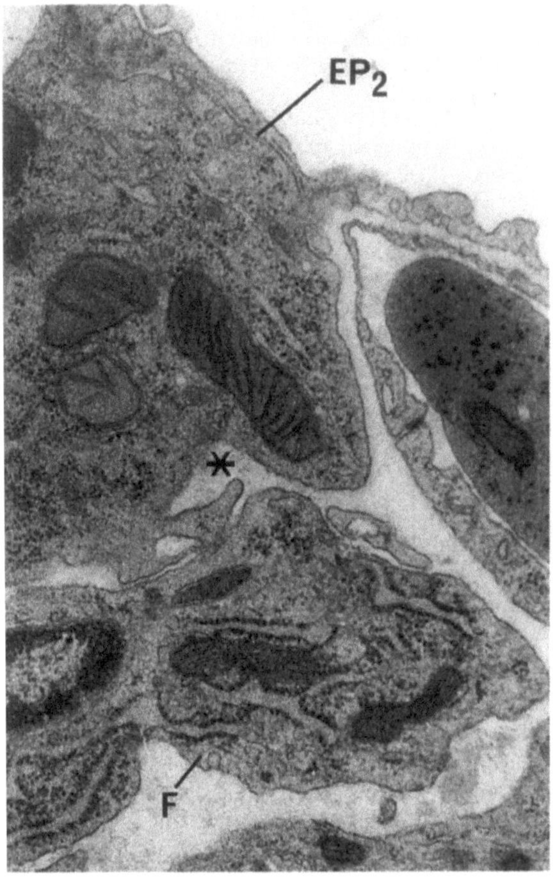


**Fig. 289.** Epithelial-fibroblast contact in normal mouse lung. At the base of a type II cell (*EP2*), a foot process (*) penetrates the basement membrane and appears to touch the underlying fibroblast (*F*). TEM, ×31 500. (From Adamson et al. 1990; by courtesy of the editor, copyright American Association of Pathologists)

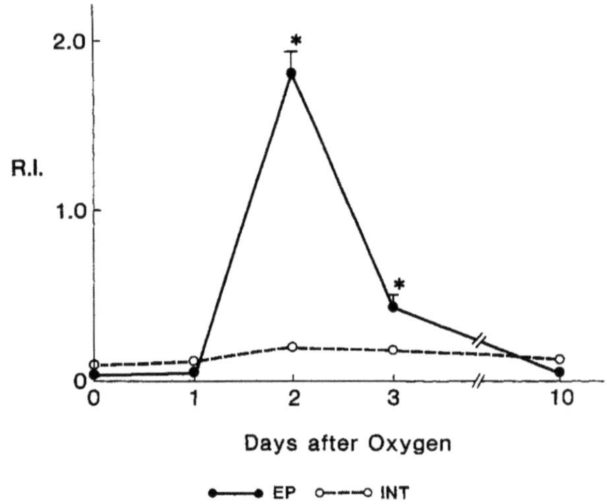


**Fig. 290.** Radiographic indices of type 2 epithelial cells (*EP*) and interstitial cells (*INT*) at various times after 6 days hyperoxia. *$p < 0.01$ greater than control. (From Adamson et al. 1990; by courtesy of the editor, copyright American Association of Pathologists)

**Table 26.** Type II cell measurements after hyperoxia

| Timer after 90% oxygen | Basal length (μM) | % Cells with continuous BM | EP-INT cell contacts/EP cell |
|---|---|---|---|
| No exposure | 13.5 ± 0.9 | 40.0 ± 3.1 | 0.48 ± 0.04 |
| 1 Day | 15.1 ± 1.3 | 55.4 ± 4.2 | 0.42 ± 0.03 |
| 2 Days | 15.8 ± 1.0* | 58.2 ± 4.0* | 0.50 ± 0.03 |
| 3 Days | 13.8 ± 1.1 | 28.7 ± 3.0** | 0.65 ± 0.04* |
| 10 Days | 13.7 ± 1.3 | 42.5 ± 2.5 | 0.51 ± 0.02 |

*$p < 0.01$, greater than control value; **$p < 0.01$, less than control value.

stitial edema; by 5 or 6 days focal necrosis of capillary endothelial, type I epithelial cells is observed, and the air-blood barrier becomes permeable to large molecular blood proteins. Focal intra-alveolar exudates of fibrin develop, concentrated mainly in centrilobular areas, and if the lesions are severe, the animals die. In the survivors alveolar lesions rapidly heal when the animals are allowed to breathe air (Adamson and Bowden 1974). The following description applies specifically to the recovery period.

On return to air there is a burst of mitotic activity, injured capillary endothelial cells are rapidly replaced and DNA synthesis by type II cells, measured by [$^3$H]thymidine labeling, peaks at 2 days and returns to normal at 3 days. Interstitial fibroblasts show no evidence of mitotic activity (Fig. 290).

Morphometry demonstrates that as type II cells proliferate they spread over the basement membrane covering the gaps left by necrotic type I cells. Accordingly, the basal length of the type II cells is increased during the first 2 days of recovery from hyperoxia (Table 26). At the time of maximal type II cell division the percentage of cells with a continuous basement membrane is higher than normal, thereby reducing the number of epithelial-interstitial cell contacts. By 3 days, when the mitotic peak has passed, fewer cells with a continuous basement are seen, and the transient gaps that appear in the lamina permit contact between type II epithelial cells and interstitial cells. The increased number of cell to cell contacts occurs at this time only, just as some of the type II cells differentiate to gas exchanging type I cells.

*Bleomycin.* A detailed description of the microscopic features of bleomycin induced fibrosis is provided elsewhere in this volume (p. 257). In contrast to recovery from hyperoxia, epithelial division is delayed and prolonged (5–14 days), while fibroblastic proliferation continues up to 3 weeks (Fig. 291). As in the oxygen model, necrosis of type I cells is followed by spreading of type II cells over the denuded basement membrane, a process that initially increases the basal length of the type II cells (Table 27). Subsequently clusters of type II cells are observed over areas of interstitial fibrosis; their foot processes often penetrate the basement membrane, some making direct contact with fibroblasts, others with collagen fibers (Figs. 292, 293).

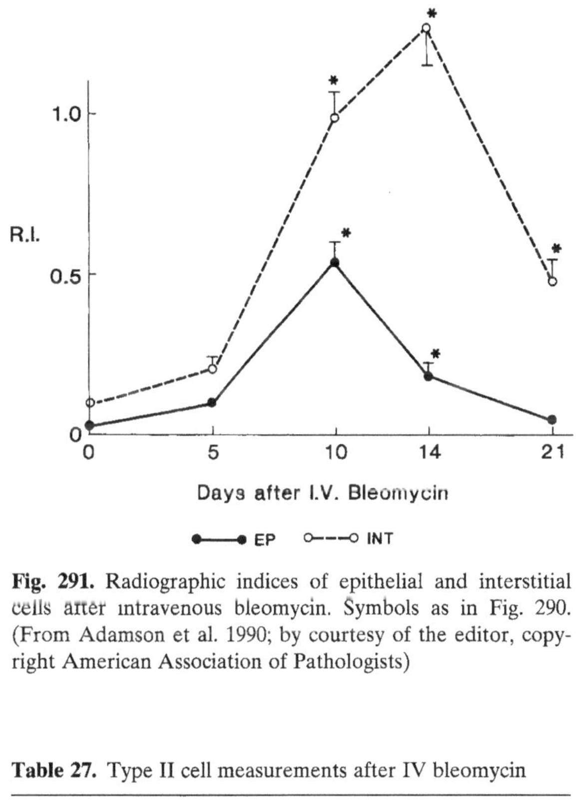


**Fig. 291.** Radiographic indices of epithelial and interstitial cells after intravenous bleomycin. Symbols as in Fig. 290. (From Adamson et al. 1990; by courtesy of the editor, copyright American Association of Pathologists)

**Table 27.** Type II cell measurements after IV bleomycin

| Time after injection | Basal length (μM) | % Cells with continuous BM | EP-INT cell contacts/EP cell |
|---|---|---|---|
| Control | 12.7 ± 1.4 | 42.5 ± 2.4 | 0.50 ± 0.05 |
| 5 Days | 17.0 ± 2.0* | 45.0 ± 2.8 | 0.50 ± 0.06 |
| 10 Days | 21.5 ± 2.1* | 42.2 ± 2.3 | 0.44 ± 0.04 |
| 14 Days | 18.3 ± 2.4* | 18.7 ± 1.1** | 0.85 ± 0.05* |
| 21 Days | 17.4 ± 1.9* | 40.7 ± 1.9 | 0.61 ± 0.04 |

*$p < 0.01$, greater than control value; **$p < 0.01$, less than control value.

## Biologicalal Features

*Pathogenesis.* One would anticipate that the lung with its vast surface area would be particularly vulnerable to gaseous and blood-borne agents. The reality is quite different; injury to the gas exchanging units is an unusual occurrence, their stability being reflected in the slow turnover rate of alveolar epithelial cells (Bowden 1983). The defenses of the lung protect the alveoli, and should they be injured by oxidant gases, viruses or blood-borne chemicals, repair usually is rapid. Endothelial cells proliferate to repopulate denuded capillaries; type II epithelial cells divide, spread to cover gaps created by necrotic type I cells, then differentiate to reconstitute a normal gas exchanging surface (Adamson and Bowden 1974). On occasion, depending upon the severity or chronicity of the injury, the outcome is less favorable, and fibrosis develops. The two models presented here depict the extremes of repair: complete healing with restitution of normal function (hyperoxia) and fibrosis with impairment of respiration and gas exchange (bleomycin). With minor modifications the changes described here may be transposed to most types of alveolar damage. The various methods available for the experimental induction of pulmonary fibrosis have been reviewed elsewhere (Bowden 1990).

Stability within the alveolus, so critical to normal respiration, is maintained by the coordinated interaction of epithelial and endothelial cells with mesenchymal cells and the extracellular matrix of the pulmonary interstitium. If this delicate balance is perturbed, alveolar injuries do not heal, and fibrosis develops. The situation is not unique to the lung; it occurs in the skin, the gut, and blood vessels. There is a difference, however; the alveolus has two "skins," endothelial and epithelial, both in close contact with fibroblasts. Fibrosis occurs when injured epithelial or endothelial surfaces are not rapidly covered by new cells.

The cells lining air sacs and capillaries sit on basement membranes largely composed of type IV collagen; deeper, are the mesenchymal cells including macrophages, fibroblasts, and mast cells. While it is customary to assign epithelial and mesenchymal cells to distinct compartments, they are by no means isolated. The basement membrane is not a continuous impenetrable barrier; there are gaps through which epithelial and endothelial cytoplasmic projections reach down to

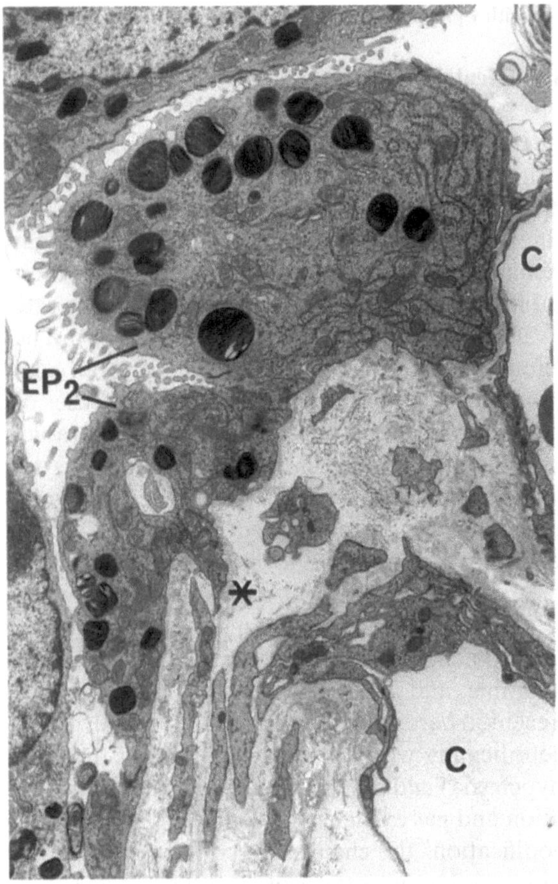


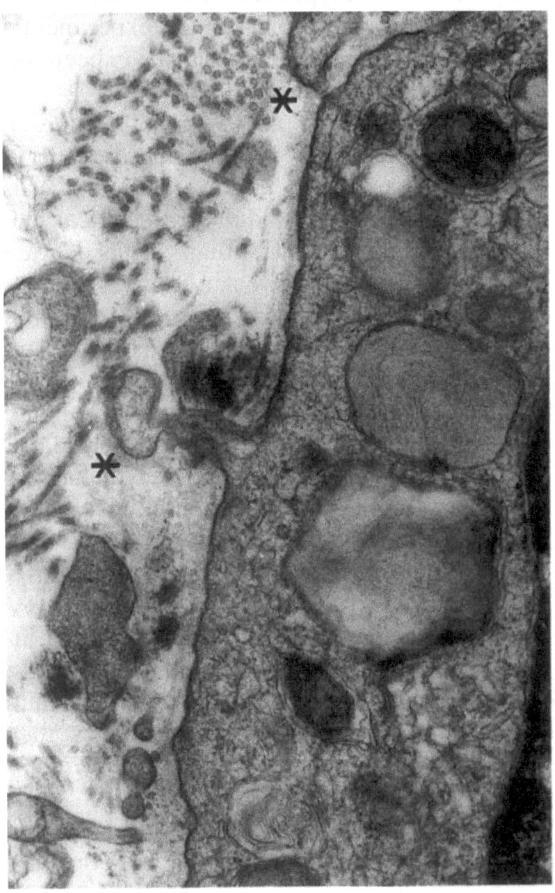


**Fig. 292.** (*above*) Alveolar wall 2 weeks after intravenous bleomycin is lined by type II cells lying on a fibrous interstitium. Occasional contacts with fibroblasts are seen (*). *C*, Capillary. TEM, ×6850. (From Adamson et al. 1990; by courtesy of the editor, copyright American Association of Pathologists)

**Fig. 293.** (*below*) Base of a type II cell 2 weeks after intravenous bleomycin. In fibrotic areas some foot processes penetrate the basement membrane and appear anchored to collagen. TEM, ×34 000. (From Adamson et al. 1990; by courtesy of the editor, copyright American Association of Pathologists)

make contact with the cells and the extracellular matrix of the interstitial compartment. The critical role of these connections has been demonstrated in the developing lung, where branching of the bronchial tree is dependent upon intimate contact between epithelial and mesenchymal cells. Later, as growth slows and differentiation begins, the number of close contacts between fibroblasts and type II cells increases, coinciding with the first appearance of lamellar bodies and the secretion of surfactant (Adamson and King 1986).

Direct cell-cell contacts may directly transmit signals involved in the control of epithelial cell division and/or differentiation. This pathway, described in several anatomic systems, has been given the title "juxtacrine intercellular signalling" (Zimmerman et al. 1993). It is thought that disruption of this communication network may have pathological sequelae. In the normal or steady state surface and mesenchymal cells are relatively quiescent. Following injury to the surface the balance between the two compartments is disturbed; destruction of epithelial or endothelial cells directly interrupts intercellular communication with fibroblasts and indirectly initiates the release of soluble growth factors and other cytokines.

The reciprocal relationship between type II cells and interstitial fibroblasts resembles a two-way highway with traffic passing in opposite directions; the vehicles are cytokines, chemical messengers operating between fibroblasts and epithelial cells (Piguet 1993). Many different cytokines are involved in this intercellular traffic; they may act alone or participate in cytokine networks (Kelley 1993). Type II cells secrete transforming growth factors alpha and beta (TGFα, TGFβ), cytokines that induce fibroblastic growth and the secretion of collagen in vivo (Piguet 1993; Fine and Goldstein 1987; Fine et al. 1990). In vitro these polypeptides may either stimulate or inhibit fibroblasts, a phenomenon that may be related to the heterogeneity of fibroblasts cultured from the lung (Jordana et al. 1988; Penney et al. 1992). Injured type II cells also secrete prostaglandin $E_2$ which inhibits fibroblastic growth (Klein and Adamson 1989), and as a reciprocal response fibroblasts secrete TGFβ, which inhibits epithelial proliferation (Howe et al. 1990). Fibroblasts also secrete a factor that promotes the growth of type II cells in vitro (Adamson et al. 1991). This factor probably is identical to the keratinocyte growth factor (KGF), a recently purified member of the fibroblast growth factor family that is secreted by fibroblasts and specifically enhances epithelial growth; when injected intratracheally to rats, keratinocyte growth factor promotes rapid proliferation of type II cells (Ulich et al. 1994).

Less is known about the role of endothelial cytokines in lung repair, most of our information being derived from studies of the vascular system (Reidy and Lindner 1992). In several test models endothelial damage induces proliferation of the underlying connective tissue cells, and it is reasonable to suppose that endothelial-derived cytokines affect healing and repair in much the same way as the products of type II cells.

In addition to the effects of locally secreted cytokines and direct cell-cell contact, the extracellular matrix (ECM) also participates in controlling and preserving the normal steady state and in determining the response of alveolar cells following injury. Thought originally to be an inert scaffold, the ECM is now seen as an active system, modifying cellular behavior and participating in the transmission of intercellular messages related to growth and differentiation. In the normal lung epithelial and endothelial cells rest on a basement membrane composed predominantly of type IV collagen. On this matrix cells tend to spread rather than divide, but if type IV basement membrane collagen is replaced by fibrillar type I or III collagen – as happens when repair is delayed and fibrosis ensues – the surface cells tend to divide rather than spread over the surface (Lwebuga-Mukasa et al. 1984; Madri and Williams 1983; Adamson et al. 1989). The effect of this is readily observed in established pulmonary fibrosis where rows of type II cells cover fibrosed areas. In addition to their structural proteins, the ECM also stores growth factors, a function that may explain the extraordinary success of products such as Matrigel, an isolated epithelial ECM, in supporting growth of various types of epithelial cells in culture (Vukicevic et al. 1992). Should the ECM be degraded, as it usually is during injury, fibroblast growth factors are released and are available for interaction with high, affinity receptors (Baird and Walicke 1989).

The stability of the ECM is dependent upon maintaining a balance between synthesis and breakdown, a process involving several enzymes, including a family of metalloproteinases (MMP). One of these proteases, MMPI, digests types I and III, the interstitial collagens; MMP2, on the other hand, specifically breaks down basement membrane type IV collagen (Woessner 1991). This enzyme digests the basement membrane during late fetal lung development, creating the gaps through which epithelial foot processes reach down to touch the fibroblasts; both epithelial cells and fibroblasts secrete this collagenase (Arden et al. 1993). A similar process probably accounts for the formation of the intercellular contacts that develop during normal and abnormal healing in the alveolus.

It is interesting to speculate that collagenases secreted by fibroblasts not only degrade the basement membrane but may release previously bound and stored growth factors, which may then stimulate growth of surviving cells in the immediate vicinity, thus promoting local repair. It has also been suggested that MMP2, secreted by interstitial cells, degrades epithelial basement membranes in human lung cancer, thereby facilitating spread of the tumor (Soini et al. 1993). If such matrix digestion also releases stored growth factors, tumor cells may be stimulated to multiply as well as migrate through the subepithelial tissue.

These combined processes reveal the complexity of interactions between epithelial cells and fibroblasts during lung development, healing, and neoplasia, a communication system involving direct cell-cell contact, stimulatory and inhibitory cytokines, and the secretion of proteolytic enzymes. These coordinated processes constitute a local mechanism that controls orderly growth and the repair of injuries; distorted by severe injury or neoplasia, the same mechanisms lead to fibrosis and enhance the growth and spread of tumors.

## References


Adamson IYR, Bowden DH (1974) The type 2 cell as progenitor of alveolar epithelial regeneration: a cytodynamic study in mice after exposure to oxygen. Lab Invest 30:35–42

Adamson IYR, Bowden DH (1979) Bleomycin-induced injury and metaplasia of alveolar type 2 cells. Relationship of cellular responses to drug presence in the lung. Am J Pathol 96:531–544

Adamson IYR, King GM (1986) Epithelial-interstitial cell interactions in fetal rat lung development accelerated by steroids. Lab Invest 55:145–152

Adamson IYR, King GM, Young L (1989) Influence of extracellular matrix and collagen components on alveolar type 2 cell morphology and function. In Vitro Cell Dev Biol 25:494–502

Adamson IYR, Hedgecock C, Bowden DH (1990) Epithelial cell fibroblast interactions in lung injury and repair. Am J Pathol 137:385–392

Adamson IYR, Young L, King GM (1991) Reciprocal epithelial: fibroblast interactions in the control of fetal and adult rat lung cells in culture. Exp Lung Res 17:821–835

Arden MG, Spearman MA, Adamson IYR (1993) Degradation of type IV collagen during the development of fetal rat lung. Am J Respir Cell Mol Biol 9:99–103

Baird A, Walicke PA (1989) Fibroblast growth factors. In: Waterfield MD (ed) Growth factors. Churchill Livingstone, New York, pp 438–452 (Br Med Bull 45[2])

Bowden DH (1983) Cell turnover in the lung. Am Rev Respir Dis 128:S46–S48

Bowden DH (1990) Experimental induction of pulmonary fibrosis. In: Gill J (ed) Lung biology in health and disease, vol 47. Microcopy and structural methods. Dekker, New York, pp 735–752

Fine F, Goldstein RH (1987) The effect of transforming growth factor β on cell proliferation and collagen formation by lung fibroblasts. J Biol Chem 262:3897–3902

Fine A, Poliks CF, Smith BD, Goldstein RH (1990) The accumulation of type 1 collagen mRNAs in human embryonic lung fibroblasts stimulated by transforming growth factor β. Connect Tissue Res 24:237–247

Howe PH, Cunningham MR, Leof EB (1990) Inhibition of mink lung epithelial cell proliferation by transforming growth factor-β is coupled through a pertussis-toxin sensitive substrate. Biochem J 266:537–543

Jordana M, Schulman J, McSharry C, Irving LB, Newhouse MT, Jordana G, Gauldie J (1988) Heterogeneous proliferative characteristics of human adult lung fibroblast lines and clonally derived fibroblasts from control and fibrotic tissue. Am Rev Respir Dis 137:579–584

Kelley J (1993) Transforming growth factor B. In: Kelley J (ed) Lung biology in health and disease, vol 61. Cytokines of the lung. Dekker, New York, pp 101–137

Klein JH, Adamson IYR (1989) Fibroblast inhibition and prostaglandin secretion by alveolar epithelial cells exposed to silica. Lab Invest 60:808–813

Lwebuga-Mukasa JS, Thulin G, Madri JA, Barrett C, Warshaw JB (1984) An acellular human amniotic membrane model for in vitro culture of type II pneumocytes: the role of the basement membrane in cell morphology and function. J Cell Physiol 121:215–225

Madri JA, Williams SK (1983) Capillary endothelial cell cultures: phenotypic modulation by matrix components. J Cell Biol 97:153–160

Penney DP, Keng PC, Derdak S, Phipps RP (1992) Morphological and functional characteristics of subpopulations of murine lung fibroblasts grown in vitro. Anat Rec 232:432–443

Piguet PF (1993) Cytokines involved in pulmonary fibrosis. Int Rev Exp Pathol 34B:173–181

Reidy MA, Linder V (1992) In: Simionescu N, Simionescu M (eds) Endothelial cell dysfunctions. Plenum, New York, pp 31–47

Soini Y, Paakko P, Autio-Haimaien H (1993) Genes of laminin β1 chain, alpha 1 (IV) chain of type IV collagen, and 72 kd type IV collagenase are mainly expressed by the stromal cells of lung carcinomas. Am J Pathol 142:1622–1630

Ulich TR, Yi ES, Langmuir K, Yin S, Blitz R, Morris CF, Housley RM, Pierce GF (1994) Keratinocyte growth factor is a growth factor for type II pneumocytes in vivo. J Clin Invest 93:1298–1306
Vukicevic S, Kleirman HK, Luyten FP, Roberts AB, Roche NS, Reddi AH (1992) Identification of multiple active growth factors in basement membrane Matrigel suggests caution in interpretation of cellular activity related to extracellular matrix components. Exp Cell Res 202:1–8
Woessner JF (1991) Matrix metalloproteinases and their inhibitors in connective tissue remodeling. FASEB J 5:2145–2154
Zimmerman GA, Lorant DE, McIntyre TM, Prescott SM (1993) Juxtacrine intercellular signaling: another way to do it. Am Respir Cell Mol Biol 9:573–577

# Fibroblast Interactions with Alveolar and Interstitial Macrophages. Models: Silicosis and Asbestosis in the Mouse

Drummond H. Bowden and Ian Y.R. Adamson

## Gross Appearance

The experiments described here were designed to study the interactions of macrophages and fibroblasts during the development of pulmonary fibrosis following a single intratracheal injection of 2 mg crystalline silica (particle diameter 0.3 μm), or 0.1 mg crocidolite asbestos fibers of two lengths: short fibers of less than 2.5 μm with a mean length 0.6 μm, and long fibers greater than 2.5 μm with a mean length 24.4 μm (Adamson and Bowden 1987a,b). With these models few if any gross changes are seen. Readers seeking detailed descriptions of the pathology of experimental asbestosis and silicosis are referred to the reviews of Wagner (1990) and of Wagner and Wagner (1990).

## Microscopic and Ultrastructural Features

The introduction of particles to the lung, by inhalation or injection, elicits an inflammatory response in the alveoli. With inert particles such as carbon a brief outpouring of neutrophils is followed by a more prolonged macrophagic response (Adamson and Bowden 1984). At a certain particulate load, which in the mouse is about $8 \times 10^{13}$ particles of carbon, the respiratory system becomes saturated, and beyond this point the number of alveolar macrophages does not increase further (Bowden 1987).

Overloading the alveolar macrophages with particles has two important consequences, decreased macrophagic mobility and increased transfer of particles to the interstitium. It has been calculated that when the volume of dust in each alveolar macrophage reaches 600 $\mu m^3$ movement toward the ciliated bronchiole is compromised, effectively terminating alveolar clearance (Morrow 1992). Decreased phagocytosis and clearance favors transepithelial transport of free particles from the alveolus to the interstitium (Adamson and Bowden 1981), and when the lung is overloaded in this way, dusts such as titanium, usually considered inert, may induce fibrosis (Lee et al. 1985; Mermelstein et al. 1991).

*Silica.* Following a single instillation of silica the neutrophilic response persists for several months. Initially, centripetal movement of particles and cells toward the terminal bronchiole produces a transient concentration of silica, neutrophils, and macrophages in centrilobular, areas where focal necrosis of type 1 cells is observed. This cell injury may be caused by the direct toxic action of silica on the epithelial cell membrane, by silica-induced spillage of neutrophil lysosomal enzymes or, as is more likely, by their combined effects (Bowden and Adamson 1984). Focal intra-alveolar exudates may become organized to form loose aggregates of collagen, but these lesions soon resolve. The other consequence to epithelial injury is more sinister; it facilitates the transfer of silica to the interstitium where toxic particles meet and are phagocytized by interstitial macrophages. This is a critical event in the development of silicotic granulomas and fibrosis (Bowden and Adamson 1984; Figs. 294–297).

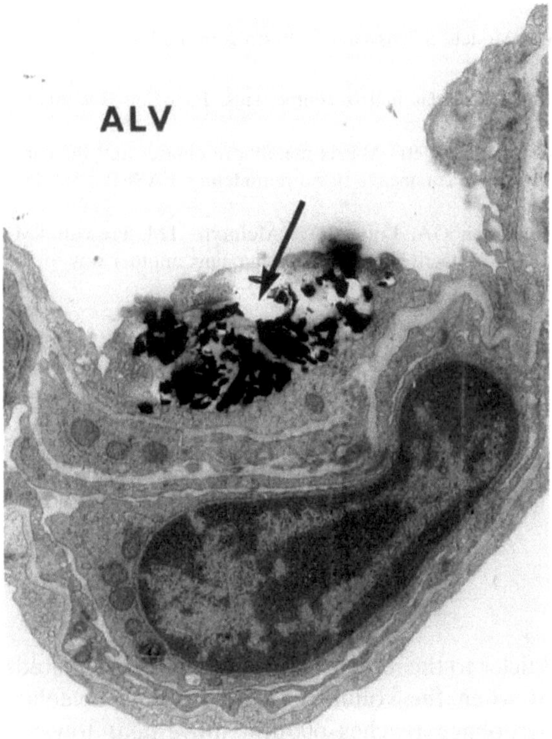


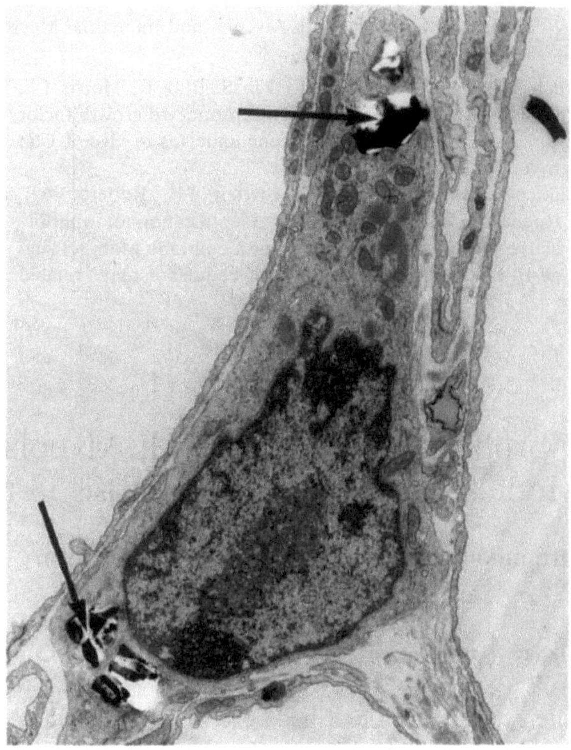

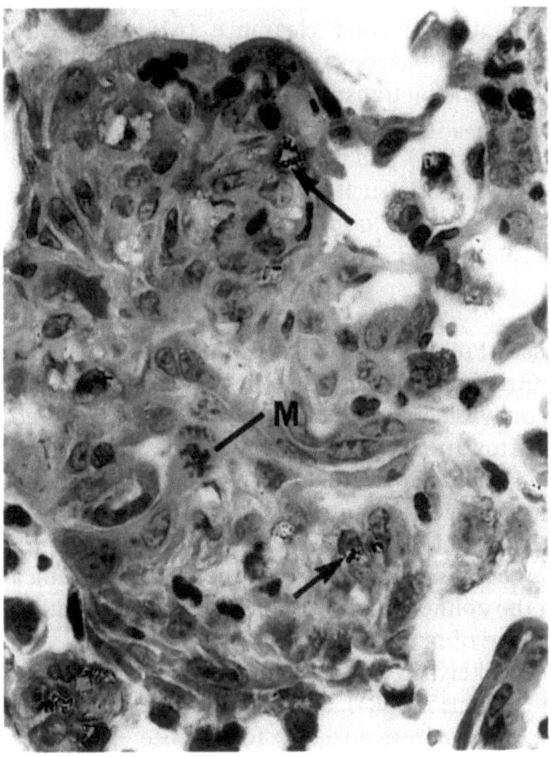


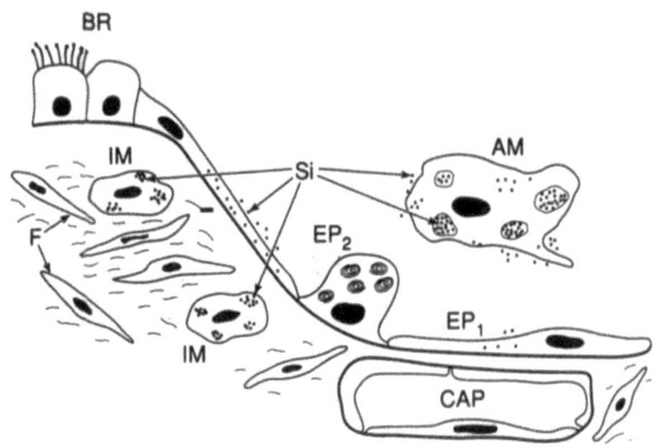


**Fig. 294.** (*upper left*) Alveolar wall, mouse lung, 3 days after intratracheal silica injection. Note particles within the cytoplasm of a type I epithelial cell (arrow). *ALV*, Alveolus. TEM, ×16000

**Fig. 295.** (*upper right*) Alveolar wall, mouse lung, 5 days after silica some particles are found within interstitial macrophages (*arrows*). ×11000

**Fig. 296.** (*lower left*) Mouse lung, 8 weeks after silica. Note a granuloma of mixed macrophages and fibroblasts. One macrophage is seen in mitosis (*M*), others contain silica (*arrows*) H&E, ×900. (From Bowden and Adamson 1984; by courtesy of the editor)

**Fig. 297.** (*lower right*) Summary cartoon of pulmonary response to silica. In the alveoli, particles (*Si*) are mostly phagocytized and cleared by alveolar macrophages (*AM*). Some free particles cross the type I epithelium (*EPI*) and are then phagocytized by interstitial macrophages (*IM*). Local proliferation of macrophages and fibroblasts (*F*) produces a granuloma. *BR*, Bronchiole; *CAP*, capillary; $EP_2$, type II epithelial cell

*Asbestos.* The pulmonary response to asbestos fibers varies with the length of the fibers. Alveolar deposition of fibers less than 2.5 μm in length provokes an acute inflammatory response mainly in the centrilobular zones. Within a few days almost all the short fibers have been engulfed by alveolar macrophages so that few are available to cross the epithelium to reach the interstitium (Fig. 298). Interstitial fibrosis is barely detectable in this model (Adamson and Bowden 1987a).

The reaction to longer fibers is different; they tend to be held up at bronchial and bronchiolar bifurcations where they initiate cell necrosis and penetrate the peribronchiolar connective tissue. Granulomas containing multinucleate giant cells develop in this location (Fig. 299), and as the proliferative phase passes, permanent fibrosis ensues (Adamson and Bowden 1987b).

## Differential Diagnosis

An inflammatory outpouring of neutrophils and macrophages into the alveoli is the common response to any particles reaching the air sacs. With nontoxic particles such as carbon the neutrophils soon disappear, and the size and duration of the macrophagic response, though dependent on the number of particles reaching the alveoli, is not prolonged (Bowden 1987). With silica,, a continuing inflammatory response is observed for up to 20 weeks, the persistence of neutrophils being reflected in high levels of lysosomal enzymes in lavaged fluids. Similar findings are reported for crocidolite asbestos (Adamson and Bowden 1984, 1986).

In contrast to the reaction induced by agents such as drugs, irradiation, or viruses, the fibrotic response to a single instillation of silica is multifocal, corresponding to the peribronchiolar location of the granulomas. If the administration of silica is

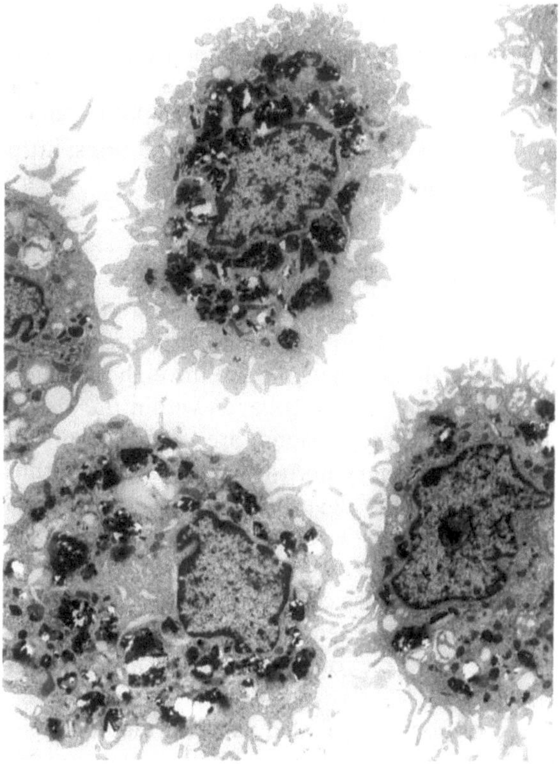

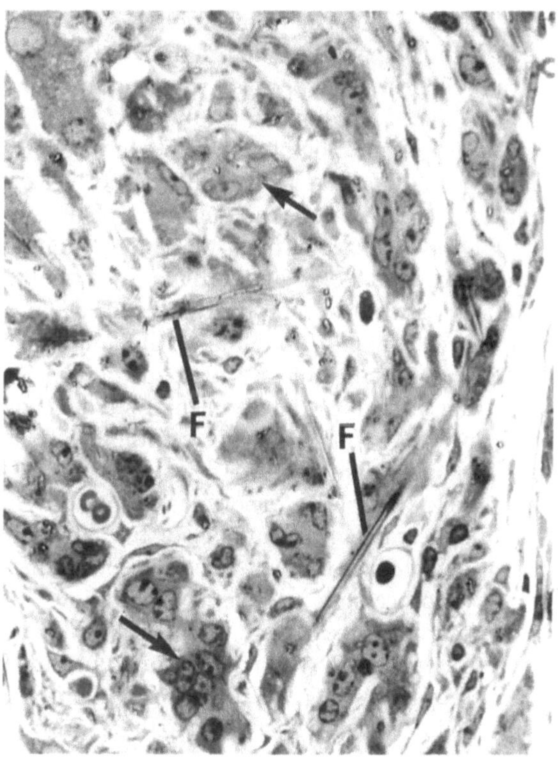


▶

**Fig. 298.** (*above*) Alveolar macrophages lavaged from mouse lung 1 week after injecting short crocidolite asbestos. Cells contain many phagocytized short fibers. H&E, ×4000. (From Adamson and Bowden 1987a; by courtesy of the editor)

**Fig. 299.** (*below*) Plastic section of mouse lung 8 weeks after instilling long crocidolite asbestos. A peribronchiolar granuloma contains several giant cells (*arrows*) and long asbestos fibers (*F*). ×1100. (From Adamson and Bowden 1987b; by courtesy of the editor)

continued, more particles cross the epithelium, some passing on to the hilar lymph nodes where they may induce silicotic granulomas. Interstitial fibrosis induced by long fibers of crocidolite asbestos is located close to bronchial bifurcations; little if any peripheral fibrosis is found.

## Biological Features

Fibroblasts reside in the pulmonary interstitium, and although they may migrate through damaged epithelium and secrete collagen within the alveolar lumen, these lesions are soon resolved. Chronic pulmonary fibrosis occurs largely within the interstitium, suggesting that the key to its pathogenesis is to be found here. In another chapter in this volume we describe how disruption of epithelial-fibroblast contacts stimulate growth of fibroblasts and the secretion of collagen. Here we examine the role of macrophages in initiating these events.

In the response to inhaled particles macrophages are key players. Following their initial contact with particles, alveolar macrophages secrete chemotactic polypeptides that initiate the inflammatory response. One of these, interleukin-8 (IL-8), is produced predominantly by macrophages. Expression of interleukin-8 can be induced by other cytokines, and it is also synthesized by pulmonary fibroblasts and epithelial cells (Kunkel et al. 1991). It is possible, then, that interaction of particles with alveolar and bronchial epithelial cells supplements macrophage-derived chemoattractants. Certainly the efflux of inflammatory cells is not limited to the alveoli; neutrophils and macrophages reach the bronchial lumen by squeezing between bronchial epithelial cells (Bowden and Adamson 1984).

The initial neutrophilic response is followed by a dramatic increase in the number of free alveolar and bronchial macrophages. This is accomplished by two processes, increased migration of monocytes and interstitial macrophages, and local proliferation of cells both in the interstitium and in the air sacs (Bowden 1987). However, there are limits to this adaptive response; if there are too many particles, or if the macrophagic response is inadequate, the system becomes overloaded (Morrow 1992; Adamson et al. 1989; Bowden et al. 1989). Under normal circumstances phagocytosis and clearance prevent the entry of inhaled particles into the interstitium. This defense mechanism, which protects the immune system from antigenic overload, probably explains the apparent lack of fibrogenicity of short asbestos fibers, few being available to cross the epithelial barrier. Long fibers, on the other hand, are held up at bronchial bifurcations where they injure and penetrate epithelium, reach the interstitium, and initiate the fibrotic process at this site (Adamson and Bowden 1987b).

Fibrosis is not induced directly by the interaction of particles and fibroblasts but indirectly through the activities of macrophages, which produce a variety of cytokines that may either stimulate or inhibit fibroblast growth and collagen production (Nathan 1987; Phan and Kunkel 1992; Piguet 1993). The most common cytokines identified in tissues and macrophages isolated from particle-induced fibrotic lungs are platelet derived growth factor, tumor necrosis factor alpha, and transforming growth factor beta; all have been associated with the induction of fibrosis in animals and humans (Fabisiak and Kelley 1993; Ulich 1993; Kelley 1993).

The majority of macrophage-fibroblast studies have utilized either isolated alveolar macrophages exposed to particles in vitro or cells lavaged from the lung as fibrosis develops. An on-going debate centers on whether polypeptides secreted by alveolar macrophages are able to stimulate distant interstitial fibroblasts. There is no convincing evidence that activated alveolar macrophages loaded with particles recross the epithelial barrier to enter the interstitial compartment, and the molecules of polypeptide growth factors secreted by these cells into the alveoli are too large to cross a normal epithelial barrier (Mangum et al. 1990). The question has been answered by demonstrating that free particles of quite considerable size are able to cross the epithelium without causing obvious injury (Adamson and Bowden 1981). When they reach the interstitium, they are phagocytosed by local macrophages which initiate the chain reaction that leads to fibrosis.

The predominance of fibrosis within the interstitium does not mean that alveolar macrophages are less efficient than their interstitial counterparts in producing fibroblast growth factors. Indeed, there is ample evidence that in response to silica both types of macrophage secrete these polypeptides (Adamson et al. 1991). Similarly, both long and short fibers of asbestos induce alveolar and interstitial macrophages to secrete fibroblastic growth factors. In vivo few short fibers reach the interstitium, and since cytokines secreted into the alveoli do not cross the epithelial barrier, fibrosis does not occur. Particle-induced interstitial pulmonary fibrosis occurs only when fibrogenic particles in sufficient number reach the interstitium where they are phagocytosed by interstitial macrophages. These cells, though somewhat different from alveolar macrophages, produce similar cytokines, including platelet derived growth factor, which accumulates in interstitial macrophages before the fibrotic process begins (Vignaud et al. 1991).

Collectively these studies suggest that direct macrophage fibroblast interaction within the pulmonary interstitium is the most likely and the most efficient method of cytokine transfer.

Furthermore, whereas clearance of particles and macrophages from the alveoli is rapid, elimination of particle-laden interstitial macrophages is very much slower. Some of these cells do cross the epithelium to reach the alveoli; others migrate through interstitial lymphatics to reach regional lymph nodes. The majority of these cells, however, often trapped in fibrotic nodules, remain in the interstitium where their continuing secretion of cytokines may perpetuate and extend the fibrotic process indefinitely.

## References


Adamson IYR, Bowden DH (1981) Dose response of the pulmonary macrophagic system to various particulates and its relationship to transepithelial passage of free particles. Exp Lung Res 2:165–175

Adamson IYR, Bowden DH (1984) Role of polymorphonuclear leukocytes in silica-induced pulmonary fibrosis. Am J Pathol 117:37–43

Adamson IYR, Bowden DH (1986) Crocidolite-induced pulmonary fibrosis in mice: cytokinetic and biochemical studies. Am J Pathol 122:261–267

Adamson IYR, Bowden DH (1987a) Response of mouse lung to crocidolite asbestos. I. Minimal fibrotic reaction to short fibers. J Pathol 152:99–107

Adamson IYR, Bowden DH (1987b) Response of mouse lung to crocidolite asbestos. II. Pulmonary fibrosis after long fibers. J Pathol 152:109–117

Adamson IYR, Letourneau HL, Bowden DH (1989) Enhanced macrophage fibroblast interactions in the pulmonary interstitium increases fibrosis after silica injection to monocute-depleted mice. Am J Pathol 134:411–418

Adamson IYR, Letourneau HL, Bowden DH (1991) Comparison of alveolar and interstitial macrophages in fibroblast stimulation after silica and long or short asbestos. Lab Invest 64:339–344

Bowden DH (1987) Macrophages, dust and pulmonary diseases. Exp Lung Res 12:89–107

Bowden DH, Adamson IYR (1984) The role of cell injury and the continuing inflammatory response in the generation of silicotic pulmonary fibrosis. J Pathol 144:149–161

Bowden DH, Hedgecock C, Adamson IYR (1989) Silica-induced pulmonary fibrosis involves the reaction of particles with interstitial rather than alveolar macrophages. J Pathol 158:73–80

Fabisiak JP, Kelley J (1993) Platelet derived growth factor. In: Kelley J (ed) Lung biology in health and disease, vol 61. Cytokines of the lung. Dekker, New York, pp 3–39

Kelley J (1993) Transforming growth factor-B. In: Kelley J (ed) Lung biology in health and disease, vol 61. Cytokines of the lung. Dekker, New York, pp 101–137

Kunkel SL, Standiford T, Kasahara K, Strieter RM (1991) Interleukin-8 (IL-8): the major neutrophil chemotactic factor in the lung. Exp Lung Res 17–23

Lee K, Trochimowicz HJ, Reinhardt CF (1985) Pulmonary response of rats exposed to titanium dioxide (TiO2) by inhalation for two years. Toxicol Appl Pharmacol 79:179–192

Mangum JB, Everitt JI, Bonner JC, et al (1990) Co-culture of primary pulmonary cells to model alveolar injury and translocation of proteins. In Vitro Cell Dev Biol 26:1135–1143

Mermelstein R, Kilpper RW, Morrow PE, Muhle H (1991) Lung overload, dosimetry of lung fibrosis and their implications on the respiratory dust standard. In: Proceedings inhaled particles VII. British Occupational Hygiene Society International Symposium, Edinburgh

Morrow PE (1992) Dust overloading of the lungs: update and appraisal. Toxicol Appl Pharmacol 113:1–12

Nathan CF (1987) Secretory products of macrophages. J Clin Invest 79:319–326

Phan SH, Kunkel SL (1992) Lung cytokine production in bleomycin induced pulmonary fibrosis. Exp Lung Res 18:29–43

Piguet PF (1993) Cytokines involved in pulmonary fibrosis. Int Rev Exp Pathol 34B:173–181

Ulich TR (1993) Tumor necrosis factor. In: Kelley J (ed) Lung biology in health and disease, vol 61. Cytokines of the lung. Dekker, New York, pp 307–332

Vignaud JM, Allam M, Martinet N, Pech M, Plenat F, Martinet Y (1991) Presence of platelet-derived growth factor in normal and fibrotic lung is specifically associated with interstitial macrophages while both interstitial macrophages and alveolar epithelial cells express the c-sis protooncogene (see comments). Am J Respir Cell Mol Biol 5:531–538

Wagner JC (1990) Experimental asbestosis. In: Gill J (ed) Lung biology in health and disease, vol 47: Microscopy and structural methods. Dekker, New York, pp 761–799

Wagner MM, Wagner JC (1990) Experimental silicosis. In: Gill J (ed) Lung biology in health and disease, vol 47. Microscopy and structural methods. Dekker, New York, pp 801–806

# Pulmonary Lipidosis, Rat

Yoichi Konishi and Ryuichi Higashiguchi

*Synonym.* Alveolar histiocytosis

## Gross Appearance

The weight of affected lungs (as a percentage of the body weight) does not differ significantly from lungs of control rats. The lungs are normal in color but contain multiple small (ca. 1–2 mm) white spots.

## Microscopic Features

Multiple focal lesions are present with alveoli filled with foamy cells (Fig. 300). Some of these cells are macrophages with abundant, lipid-laden cytoplasm, but others represent proliferation of type II pneumocytes in the alveolar walls (Fig. 301). In rare large lesions cholesterol crystals are present. Interstitial pneumonitis is not observed in the surrounding lung.

## Differential Diagnosis

Pulmonary lipidosis can be differentiated from lipid pneumonia. Animals generally do not die of pulmonary lipidosis but may succumb to lipid pneumonia. Grossly, the lesions of pulmonary lipidosis are small and sometimes difficult to recognize. Histologically, granulomatous changes observed in exogenous lipid pneumonia are not seen in pulmonary lipidosis. Endogenous lipid pneumonia is a form of chronic interstitial pneumonitis with the presence of foamy macrophages and proliferation of type II pneumocytes; pneumonitis is absent in pulmonary lipidosis. Accumulation of foamy cells is more prominent in endogenous lipid pneumonia and sometimes results in destruction of alveolar walls. In pulmonary lipidosis reactive foamy cells accumulate in the alveoli, but the alveolar wall is relatively well preserved, and giant cell reaction is seldom seen.

## Biological Features

Serum biochemistry values (Table 28) are elevated for total cholesterol, ester cholesterol, and beta-lipoprotein and decreased for high-density lipoprotein cholesterol in hypophysectomized rats. These abnormal values may be caused by general disturbance of lipid metabolism, resulting in pulmonary lipidosis.
Pulmonary lipidosis can be induced by anorectic drugs in laboratory animals (Lullmann-Rauch et al. 1972; Gaton and Wolman 1979); the lesions are reversible when administration of the drug is stopped. Myeloid bodies are commonly seen in foamy cells, suggesting that these cells could have originated from type II pneumocytes. Phospholipid accumulation in foamy cells may be related to increased acid phosphatase activity. Pulmonary lipidosis in hypophysectomized rats suggests that hormonal regulation by the hypophysis plays an important role in the development of this disease.

## Comparison of Lesions in Humans

Histologically the lesions are quite similar in animals and man. Epidemiological studies in Eastern Europe and Russia have shown that pulmonary lipidosis is observed in persons who have taken

**Table 28.** Serum biochemistry of nonoperated and hypophysectomized rats 55 weeks after the operation

| Treatment | TC | HDL-C | EC | TL | TG | PL | β-LP | NEFA |
|---|---|---|---|---|---|---|---|---|
| Nonoperated | 89.5 ± 3.5 | 13 ± 1 | 20 ± 1 | 348.5 ± 35.5 | 111 ± 26 | 177.5 ± 11.5 | 648 ± 2 | 797.5 ± 2.5 |
| Hypophysectomized | 148.5 ± 13.5 | 6.5 ± 0.5 | 137 ± 12 | 405.5 ± 47.5 | 91.5 ± 10.5 | 179.5 ± 0.5 | 1105 ± 18 | 633.0 ± 71.0 |

*TC*, Total cholesterol; *HDL-C*, high-density lipoprotein-cholesterol; *EC*, ester cholesterol; *TL*, total lipid; *TG*, triglyceride; *PL*, phospholipid; β-*LP*, beta-lipoprotein; *NEFA*, nonesterified fatty acid.

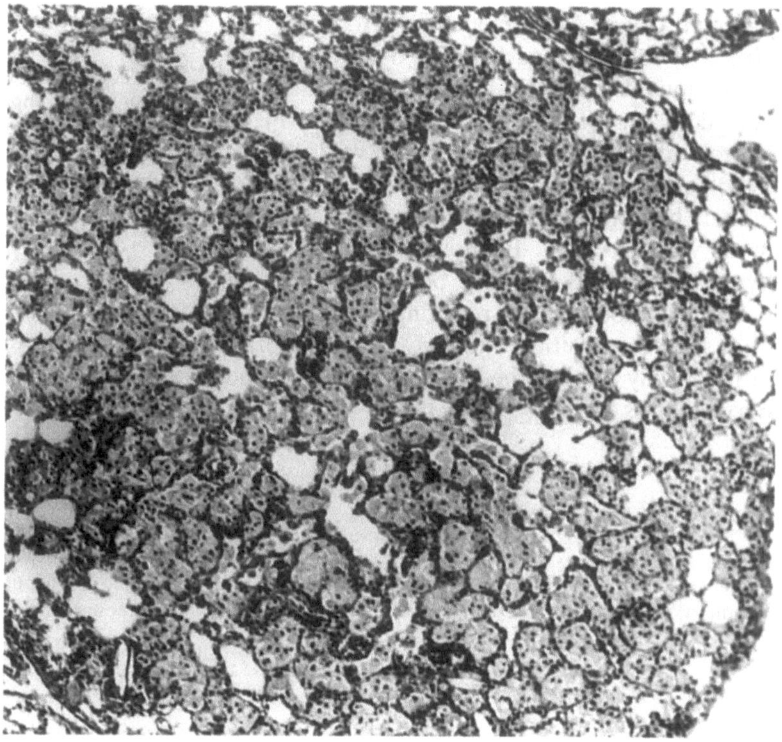

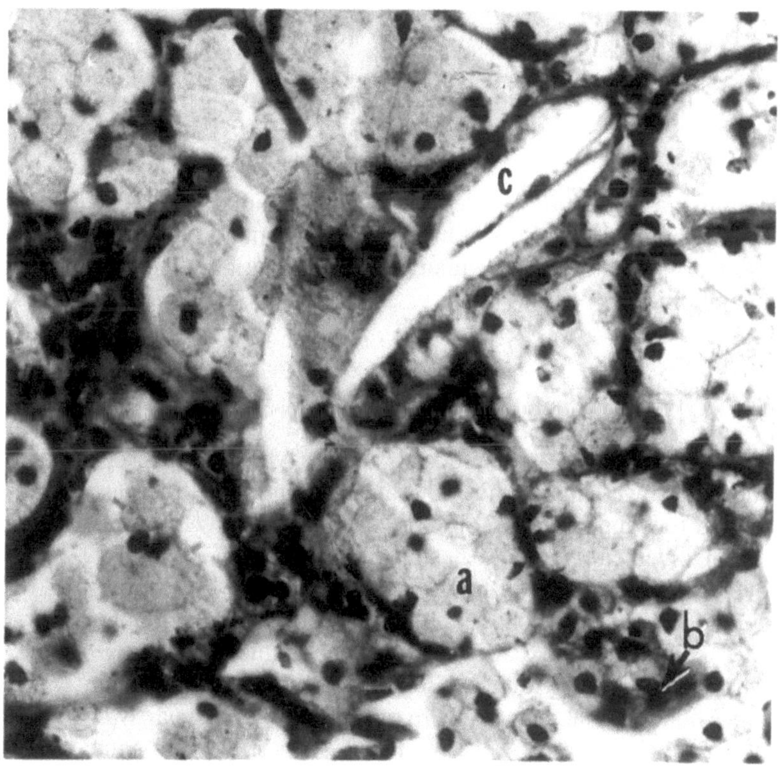


**Fig. 300.** (*above*) Pulmonary lipidosis, lung of hypophysectomized rat. Alveoli are filled with foamy cells and adjacent tissue is intact. H&E, ×40

**Fig. 301.** (*below*) Pulmonary lipidosis, lung of hypophysectomized rat. Alveoli are filled with lipid-containing foamy cells (*a*), type II pneumocytes (*b*), and rare cholesterol crystals (*c*). H&E, ×200

anorectic drugs (Amor et al. 1971; Homann 1974; Hruban et al. 1973; Mach 1972; Rivier et al. 1972; Ugriumova 1976). The anorectic drugs are reported to act on feeding centers located in the lateral hypothalamic area and ventromedial hypothalamic nucleus (Baker 1980). In man pulmonary hypertension frequently accompanies pulmonary lipidosis. Pulmonary lipidosis in hypohysectomized rats may be induced by their decreased food intake, resulting in changes in body lipid composition. Properly balanced intake of lipids may prevent the development of pulmonary lipidosis.

### References

Amor H, Schwingshacki H, Dienstl F (1971) Primary pulmonary hypertension. Presentation of 8 cases probably caused by use of an anorectic drug. Minerva Med 62:4623–4631

Baker CE Jr (ed) (1980) Physicians' desk reference. Medical Economic Company, Oradell

Gaton E, Wolman M (1979) Histochemical study on the pathogenesis of chlorocyclizine-induced pulmonary lipidosis. Histochemistry 63:203–207

Homann G (1974) Pulmonary hypertension following use of appetite depressants. Med Klin 69:211

Hruban Z, Slesers A, Aschenbrenner I (1973) Pulmonary intraalveolar histiocytosis induced by drugs. Toxicol Appl Pharmacol 26:72–85

Lullmann-Rauch R, Reil GH, Rossen E, Seiler KU (1972) The ultrastructure of rat lung changes induced by an anorectic drug (chlorphentermine). Virchows Arch (Cell Pathol) 11:167–181

Mach J (1972) Unusual increase in incidence of pulmonary hypertension. Vnitr Lek 18:194–196

Rivier JL, Jaeger M, Reymond C, et al (1972) Primary pulmonary arterial hypertension and appetite depressants. Arch Mal Coeur 65:787–796

Ugriumova MO (1976) Anorexic preparations and primary pulmonary hypertension. Ter Arkh 48(2):126–131

# Alveolar Lipoproteinosis, Rat

W. Weller

*Synonyms.* Alveolar proteinosis, endogenous lipid pneumonia, multifocal histiocytosis, desquamative pneumonia, desquamative interstitial pneumonia.

### Gross Appearance

The pleural surface of affected rats is quite typical. In initial stages small, white to grayish, round, elevated foci appear on lung surfaces (Fig. 302). If the involvement is minor, these foci can easily be overlooked. If the involvement is more extensive, a tendency toward confluence can be observed. The foci appear to expand and become confluent with greater age. In our test series two different types of additional changes were observed. In one of these the lesions were nodular, suggesting tumor (Fig. 303). The grayish white foci differed in size and were well separated from each other. In confluent lesions (the second type) single foci were not recognizable (Fig. 304); the affected lung surface was gray and slightly elevated in relief.

### Microscopic Features

The usual types of tissue changes in alveolar lipoproteinosis are presented in Figs. 305 and 306. Initially the lesions involve alveoli in focal areas (Fig. 305) but may become confluent. The alveoli are filled with a moderately dense granular mass, made up essentially of lipid-containing (foamy) macrophages.

Increased amounts of both protein and lipid are present (Beaver et al. 1963; Corrin and King 1969; Flodh et al. 1974; Gross and deTreville 1968; Heppleston 1967; Heppleston et al. 1970; Heppleston and Young 1972; Yang et al. 1966). At higher magnification (Fig. 305), the alveoli are seen to be filled with a partly eosinophilic, partly basophilic, PAS-positive, granular material. In some areas deposits of cholesterol crystals may be seen, usually engulfed by macrophages. These cells have dense, usually centrally placed nuclei and abundant foamy cytoplasm (Fig. 306).

In the center of larger foci the macrophages are often absent, but some shadowy single-cell struc-

**Fig. 302.** Lungs, alveolar lipoproteinosis, 12-month-old male Wistar rats

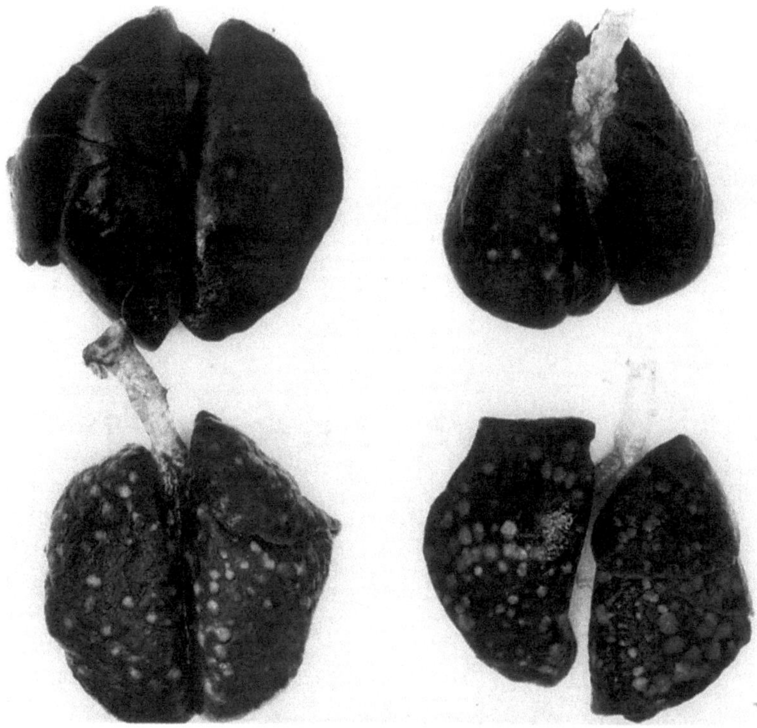

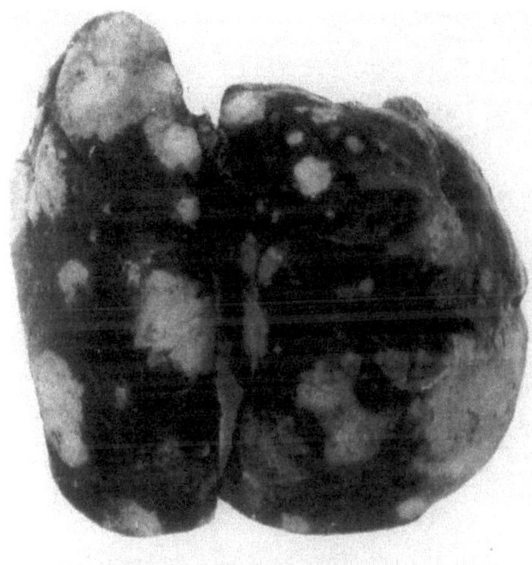

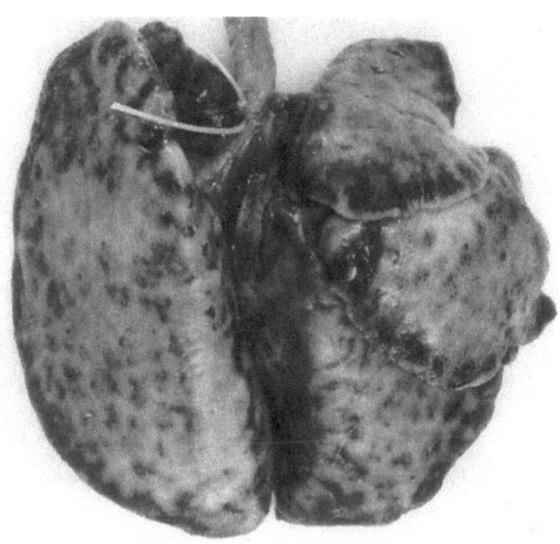

**Fig. 303.** (*above*) Lung, alveolar lipoproteinosis, confluent nodular lesions, 25-month-old Sprague-Dawley rat

**Fig. 304.** (*below*) Lung, 23-month-old Wistar rat. Alveolar lipoproteinosis, diffuse lesions

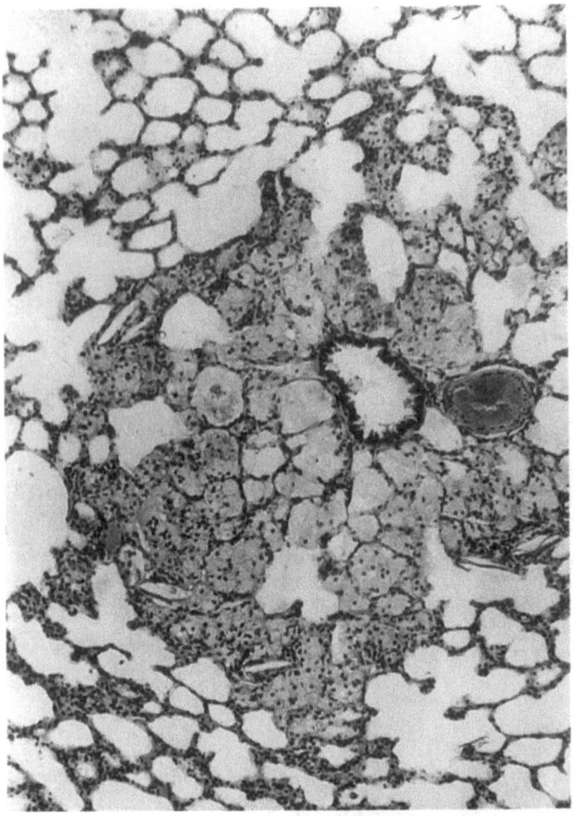

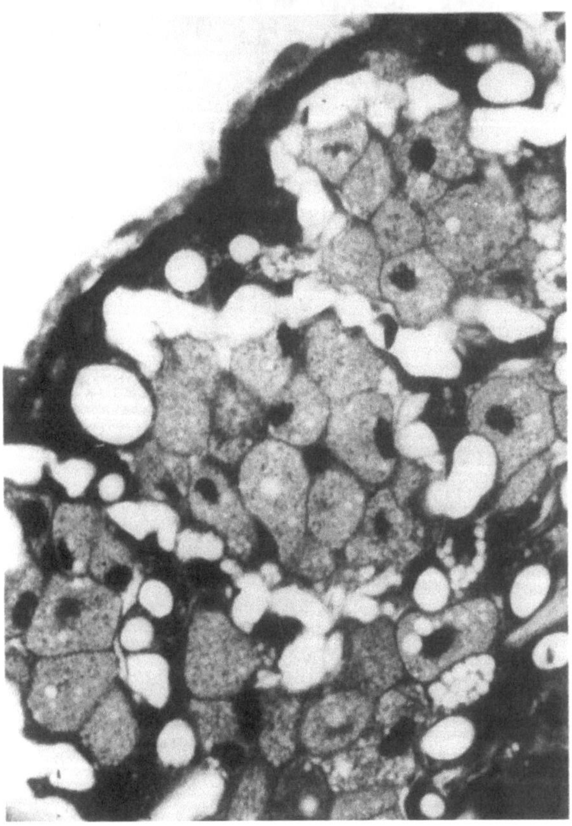

tures may be found. In the periphery of these larger foci, macrophages with foamy cytoplasm may be observed in varying numbers. The adjacent alveolar septa of the lung usually appear to be normal, but in some locations numerous cuboidal alveolar cells (type II pneumocytes) can be identified. In none of the animals are inflammatory infiltrates present in alveolar septa or in peribronchial tissue. Most of these foci in animals exposed to dust are free of dust and are generally distinct from zones of early fibrosis, which do contain dust particles.

Cholesterol granulomas with multinucleated giant cells have been described (Beaver et al. 1963; Corrin and King 1969; Gross and deTreville 1968; Pittermann 1973; Pittermann and Deerberg 1974; Weller et al. 1974, 1978; Yang et al. 1966). They are infrequent, however, and have no recognizable relationship to the degree of alveolar lipoproteinosis (Fig. 307).

## Enzyme Histochemical Findings

Our histochemical investigations have employed the following enzymes: hydrolases (acid and alkaline phsophatases, nonspecific esterase) and oxidoreductases (DPNH-/TPNH-diaphorase, α-glycerophosphate oxidase, succinic dehydrogenase).

In most type II pneumocytes enzyme activity was similar to that demonstrated in the same cells in histologically normal alveoli. In proliferating type II pneumocytes increased amounts of hydrolases and oxidoreductases were observed. This indicates elevated metabolic activity at the cellular level and is correlated with the electron microscropic findings of increased numbers of osmiophilic lamellar bodies in the cytoplasm. The greatest number of cells (macrophages) in the alveoli contained weak or nonreacting enzymes.

◀

**Fig. 305.** (*above*) Lung, rat, alveolar lipoproteinosis. Focal lesion with filled alveoli. H&E, ×25

**Fig. 306.** (*below*) Lung, rat, alveolar lipoproteinosis. Small focus of densely packed macrophages with foamy cytoplasm in alveoli. Methylene blue and basic fuchsin, ×630

**Ultrastructure**

Both light and electron microscopic findings in alveolar lipoproteinosis have been well described. The findings of the present study are not exceptional. Opinions differ, however, on the identity of the cells that fill the alveoli. Certain authors (Pittermann 1973), some with reservations (Heppleston et al. 1970; Heppleston and Young 1972), consider the cells in alveoli to be type II pneumocytes. In our study these cells were identified as macrophages. Our interpretation agrees with that of Heppleston et al. (1970). The very large, generally uninuclear macrophages that fill the alveoli contain relatively regular, large, round inclusions confined by a simple membrane. These inclusions are filled with layers of fine osmiophilic lamellae, often arranged concentrically. The cytoplasm of these cells appears only as a dark, narrow matrix between these lamellar particles. No other organelles have been identified. The nuclei are primarily located eccentrically and frequently appear to be indented by the inclusion bodies. The inclusion bodies are often adjacent to the cell membrane (Fig. 308). In addition to these round, intracytoplasmic particles, some cells also contain longitudinal and optically empty hollow spaces from which crystalline, needle-shaped deposits had been released during fixation and embedding.

The affected intraalveolar type II pneumocytes maintain their usual structures, although the osmiophilic lamellar bodies in these cells increase in number. Microvilli are present on the surface. Distinct finely granular deposits, in part consisting of fine osmiophilic lamellae, are present and are free in the alveolar lumen or, sometimes, located on the alveolar epithelium. Occasionally these deposits have a fine vesicular arrangement. The small residual alveolar lumen between pneumocytes and macrophages is in some sections filled with these deposits. In the surrounding regions focal increase of fibers is evident in the interstitium. Interstitial vessels are not changed.

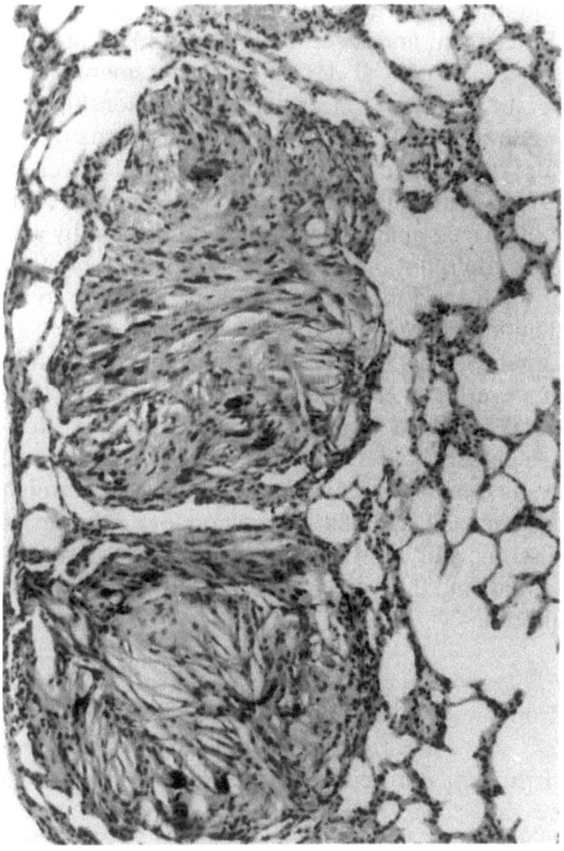

**Fig. 307.** Lung, rat. Subpleural cholesterol granulomas. H&E, ×25

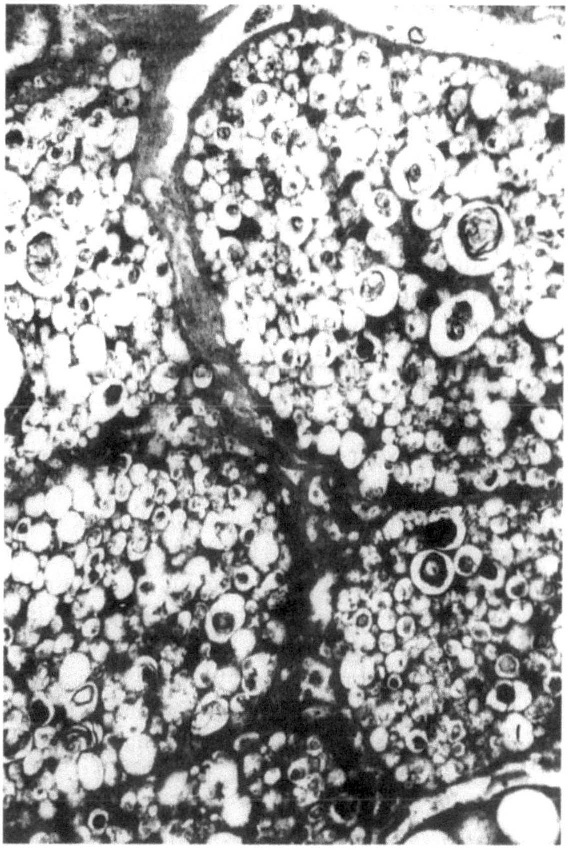

**Fig. 308.** Lung, rat, alveolar lipoproteinosis. Osmiophilic lamellar bodies in alveolar macrophages. TEM, ×5000

## Differential Diagnosis

The histological features of this disease are quite characteristic and usually provide the basis for precise diagnosis. The alveoli in small or large parts of the lung are filled with large lipid-laden cells. The presence of this lipid gives the cytoplasm a foamy appearance. The lesion is readily distinguished from infectious granulomas by the absence of other inflammatory exudate. In cryptococcosis and pneumocystosis, leukocyte response also may be minimal, but the organisms may be identified with special stains (Gomori's methenamine silver, Gridley's fungus stain, PAS).

## Biological Features

The existence of different terms for the same syndrome is due to the varying interpretations of the features observed by various investigators (see Brewer et al. 1969; Costello et al. 1975; Gaensler et al. 1966; Gough 1967; Liebow et al. 1965; Shortland et al. 1969; Weller 1976). In involved alveoli, protein-containing material is found which is believed to originate (Heppleston 1967) from decomposing macrophages. Surfactant and lamellar bodies may also contribute to the protein volume (Heppleston and Young 1972). The lipid volume in altered alveoli is of particular importance (Beaver et al. 1963; Corrin and King 1969; Flodh et al. 1974; Heppleston et al. 1970). The proportion of cholesterol, triglycerides, and especially phospholipids is distinctly increased. Therefore we suggest that this disease be named alveolar lipoproteinosis rather than alveolar proteinosis. The increased phospholipid proportion in alveolar lipoproteinosis suggests the interesting possibility of a relationship to the lung surfactant system (Corrin and King 1969; Heppleston et al. 1970; Heppleston and Young 1972). This disease may impair or invalidate animal experiments and thus be compared to chronic respiratory disease of conventional rats. On the basis of comparison of lesions in the lungs of both species, alveolar lipoproteinosis in rats may serve as a model for human alveolar lipoproteinosis.

*Natural History.* These changes in the lungs were first described in germ-free rats (Beaver et al. 1963). Subsequent reports described its appearance in both germ-free (Pittermann and Deerberg 1974) and specific-pathogen-free rats (Corrin and King 1969; Pittermann 1973; Weller 1977) and conventional rats (Kuhn et al. 1966; Yang et al. 1966).

*Morbidity.* The morbidity is quite variable and is significantly influenced by the age of the rats (Flodh et al. 1974). The percentage of animals with alveolar lipoproteinosis increases with age (Weller et al. 1978). According to Beaver et al. (1963), the percentage of animals with alveolar lipoproteinosis in different groups may vary between 0% and 97%. In published statistics the most frequent postmortem finding is alveolar lipoproteinosis (Pittermann and Deerberg 1974). Another report refers to frequencies as high as 20% (Yang et al. 1966).
In our tests the frequency in untreated control animals was as high as 55%. Postmortem findings in animals aged 12–15 months from different breeders revealed a frequency of alveolar lipoproteinosis between 40% and 90%. The earliest occurrences of the disease, as reported in three studies, were at 6 (Flodh et al. 1974), 11 (Pittermann and Deerberg 1974), and 15 months of age (Yang et al. 1966). Clear statements have not been made concerning the relationship between morbidity and strain of origin or sex of the rats: reports are even contradictory (Flodh et al. 1974; Weller et al. 1978; Yang et al. 1966). Although a comparison with completely healthy animals could not be made due to the small number of unaffected rats, mortality does not seem to be significantly influenced.
Organ weights in affected animals may be slightly or severely increased. In normal rats the lung weighs up to 1.5 g; rats with alveolar lipoproteinosis have lungs that weigh up to 4 g; and in dust-exposed animals the lungs may weigh as much as 18 g. In hilar lymph nodes neither macroscopic nor light microscopic changes are observed, and the weight of these lymph nodes is not altered.

*Etiology.* When the alveolar lipoproteinosis syndrome was first described (Beaver et al. 1963) during an investigation of germ-free rats, a cirrhogenic, protein-deficient diet was thought to be the cause. Subsequent reports postulated a causal influence of dust inhalation (Corrin and King 1969; Gross and deTreville 1968; Heppleston 1967; Heppleston et al. 1970; Heppleston and

Young 1972; Jennings et al. 1965). However, when alveolar lipoproteinosis also appeared in untreated rats kept under controlled conditions (Pittermann 1973; Pittermann and Deerberg 1974; Weller 1977; Weller et al. 1974; Yang et al. 1966), it was concluded that an independent lung disease was present in these rats (Weller et al. 1974, 1978). The pathogenesis of alveolar lipoproteinosis is not yet clarified. A variety of potential etiologies have been studied.

According to Gross and deTreville (1968) and Heppleston and Young (1972), a disturbance of the bronchial purification mechanism, an excessive production of alveolar macrophages, and a lack or insufficiency of autolytic enzymes can be regarded as the first stage in the pathogenesis. An excessive production of surfactant with an increased proportion of phospholipid, together with hyperreactivity of type II pneumocytes (Corrin and King 1969; Heppleston et al. 1970), has also been proposed. This suggestion is supported by the increased occurrence of free lamellar bodies in alveoli as well as phagocytized lamellar bodies in alveolar macrophages, a process which may be compared to a merocrine secretion passed from type II pneumocytes into the alveolar lumen (Hatasa and Nakamura 1965).

A pathological surfactant has also been described (Heppleston and Young 1972). Cholesterol, neutral fat, and cell decomposition products are able to deactivate normal surfactant. According to Felts (1965), glucose availability is important to lipometabolism in the lung. Furthermore, due to an increased capillary permeability the contents of alveoli have been regarded as transudates (Heppleston et al. 1970). In addition, an immunological disturbance has been suggested (Gray 1973).

The implications of the cholesterol granulomas (Beaver et al. 1963; Corrin and King 1969; Pittermann 1973; Pittermann and Deerberg 1974; Weller et al. 1974; Yang et al. 1966) need to be clarified. They are probably related to the increased cholesterol concentration in the abnormal lungs. However, only a small proportion of lungs with alveolar lipoproteinosis also contain cholesterol granulomas. According to Kluge (1959), cholesterol supplied intratracheally cannot be regarded as a cause of progressive cholesterol pneumonia. Flodh et al. (1974), however, found an increased number of foamy cells in lungs of rats that had been fed diets rich in cholesterol or triglyceride.

## Comparison with Other Species

Alveolar lipoproteinosis of rats is not only of importance in experimental animals but may also serve as a model for the human disease. The term "pulmonary alveolar proteinosis" was introduced by Rosen et al. (1958) for a human disease that had been previously unknown or misinterpreted. This disease is characterized by a recurring and/or progressive accumulation of phospholipid-containing material in the alveoli, but without inflammation. Patients suffer from an increasing dyspnea combined with cough and loss of weight; almost one-third eventually die of cardiorespiratory insufficiency following a protracted illness. Since the first description many other cases have been reported (Weller et al. 1978).

With respect to the comparability of lung changes found in humans and in rats, the following can be said: spontaneous alveolar lipoproteinosis in rats and alveolar lipoproteinosis in animals after dust inhalation do not differ significantly by light or electron microscopy or by enzyme histochemistry from that described for human patients.

Alveolar lipoproteinosis occurs not only in rats and man, but also in hamsters and guinea pigs (Gross and deTreville 1968).

## References


Beaver DL, Ashburn LL, McDaniel EG, Brown ND (1963) Lipid deposits in the lungs of germ-free animals. Arch Pathol 76:565–570

Brewer DB, Heath D, Asquith P (1969) Electron microscopy of desquamative interstitial pneumonia. J Pathol 97:317–323

Corrin B, King E (1969) Experimental endogenous lipid pneumonia and silicosis. J Pathol 97:325–330

Costello JF, Moriarty DC, Branthwaite MA, Turner-War wick M, Corrin B (1975) Diagnosis and management of alveolar proteinosis: the role of electron microscopy. Thorax 30:121–132

Felts JM (1965) Carbohydrate and lipid metabolism of lung tissue in vitro. Med Thorac 22:89–99

Flodh H, Magnusson G, Magnusson O (1974) Pulmonary foam cells in rats of different age. Z Versuchstierkd 16:299–312

Gaensler EA, Goff AM, Prowse CM (1966) Desquamative interstitial pneumonia. N Engl J Med 274:113–128

Gough J (1967) Silicosis and alveolar proteinosis: BMJ 1:629

Gray ES (1973) Autoimmunity in childhood pulmonary alveolar proteinosis. BMJ 4:296–297 (letter)

Gross P, deTreville RTP (1968) Alveolar proteinosis. Its experimental production in rodents. Arch Pathol 86:255–261

Hatasa K, Nakamura T (1965) Electron microscopic observations of lung alveolar epithelial cells of normal young mice

with special reference to formation and secretion of osmiophilic lamellar bodies. Z Zellforsch 68:266–277
Heppleston AG (1967) Atypical reaction to inhaled silica. Nature 213:199
Heppleston AG, Young AE (1972) Alveolar lipo-proteinosis: an ultrastructural comparison of the experimental and human forms. J Pathol 107:107–117
Heppleston AG, Wright NA, Stewart JA (1970) Experimental alveolar lipo-proteinosis following the inhalation of silica. J Pathol 101:293–307
Jennings IW, Gresham GA, Howard AN (1965) Pulmonary lipidosis in laboratory rats. J Reticuloendothel Soc 2:130–140
Kluge A (1959) Versuche zur Cholesterinpneumonie. In: Verhandlungen der Deutschen Gesellschaft für Pathologie. Fischer, Stuttgart, p 274
Kuhn C, Györkey F, Levine BE, Ramirez-Rivera J (1966) Pulmonary alveolar proteinosis. A study using enzyme histochemistry, electron microscopy, and surface tension measurement. Lab Invest 15:492–509
Liebow AA, Steer A, Billingsley JG (1965) Desquamative interstitial pneumonia. Am J Med 39:369–404
Pittermann W (1973) Pulmonale Alveolar-Proteinose bei alten SPF HAN: Sprague-Dawley-Ratten. XI. Scientific meeting of the Society for Laboratory Animal Science 9–12 May, Antwerp
Pittermann W, Deerberg F (1974) Erkrankungen bei keimfreien Ratten. Fortbildungslehrgang für Versuchstierkunde, 8–12 October 1973, Berlin. Institut für Versuchstierkunde und Versuchstierkrankheit, University of Berlin
Rosen SH, Castleman B, Liebow AA (1958) Pulmonary alveolar proteinosis. N Engl J Med 258:1123–1142
Shortland JR, Darke CS, Crane WA (1969) Electron microscopy of desquamative interstitial pneumonia. Thorax 24:192–208
Weller W (1976) Grundlagen der tierexperimentellen Pneumokonioseforschung. In: WT Ulmer, G Reichel (eds) Pneumokoniosen. Springer, Berlin Heidelberg New York, p 49 (Handbuch der inneren Medizin, vol 4/1)
Weller W (1977) Anthrakosilikose. Tierexperimentelle Forschung. Bergbau-Berufsgenossenschaft, Bochum
Weller W, Haacks H, Guzy JK, Heine W (1974) Silikoseentwicklung im Intraperitonealtest bei Verwendung von keimfreien, SPF- und konventionellen Ratten. Beitr Silikoseforsch 26:265–276
Weller W, Kissler W, Morgenroth K (1978) Alveolar-Lipoproteinose bei Ratten. Z Versuchstierkd 20:1–18
Yang YH, Yang CY, Grice HC (1966) Multifocal histiocytosis in the lungs of rats. J Pathol Bacteriol 92:559–561

# Fly Ash Pneumoconiosis, Hamster

Gerald E. Dagle and Alfred P. Wehner

*Synonyms.* Pneumoconiosis is the generic term for the presence of different dusts in the lung and the resultant lesions; anthracosis, the condition related to soot in the lungs, may include fly ash and/or other combustion products of fossil fuels (Sanders et al. 1980)

## Gross Appearance

The lungs are diffusely tan to gray, with black foci, typically 1–2mm in diameter, that tend to be distributed in subpleural areas (Fig. 309). Lung weights and volumes are increased after prolonged exposure.

## Microscopic Features

Dust, generally phagocytosed by alveolar macrophages, aggregates in alveoli throughout all lobes, with a predilection for peribronchiolar and subpleural areas (Fig. 310). An interestitial reaction, composed of thickened alveolar septa with prominent alveolar epithelial cells and collagenous stroma, is associated with the dust accumulation (Fig. 311). Bronchiolization (see "Bronchiolar/Alveolar Hyperplasia" p. 174), composed of proliferation of bronchiolar epithelium into alveolar ducts, is more pronounced in areas of peribronchiolar dust accumulation (Fig. 312). Vesicular emphysema occasionally occurs.

## Ultrastructure

The ultrastructural features of this lesion in hamsters have not been described.

## Differential Diagnosis

The lesions are associated with relatively high concentrations of dust in the lung. Definitive diag-

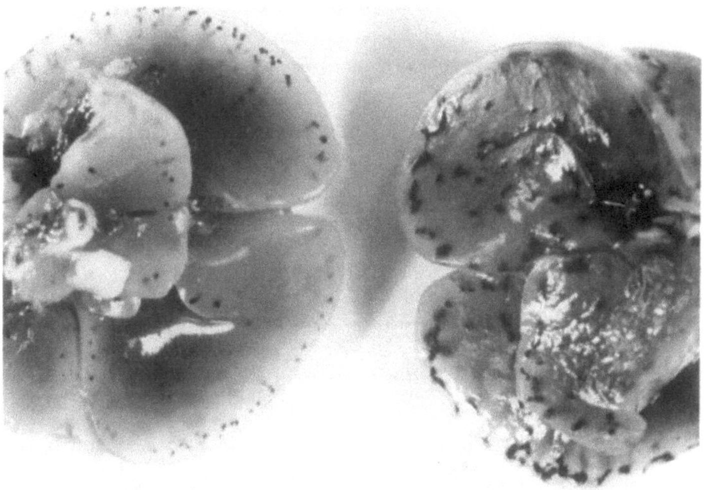


**Fig. 309.** Gross appearance of lungs from hamsters after 16 months of exposure to low (**A**) or high (**B**) concentrations of fly ash aerosol

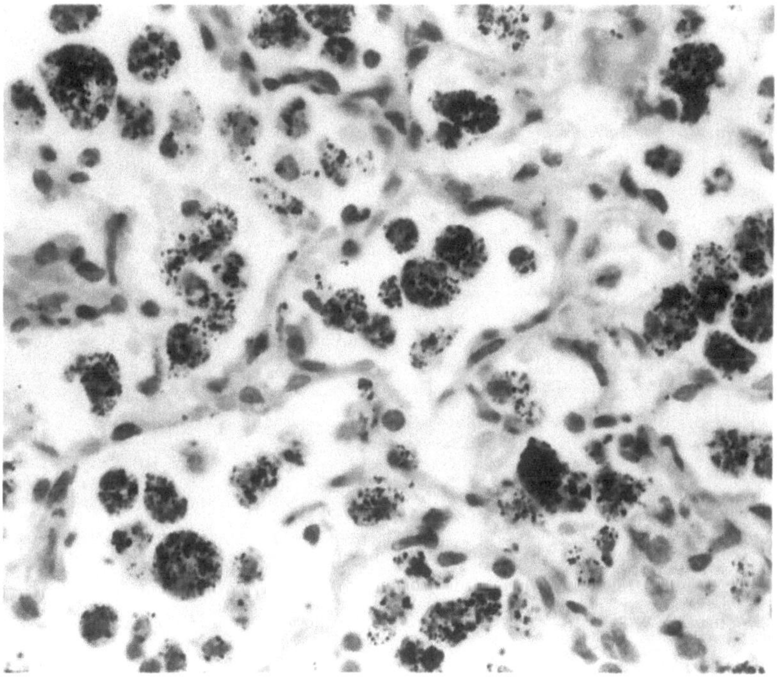

**Fig. 310.** Interstitial reaction in lung of hamster exposed to fly ash. H&E, ×486

nosis would depend upon X-ray or diffraction patterns from individual dust particles. Ferruginous bodies and multinucleated giant cells, as formed with asbestos, are lacking. The lesions also lack the interstitial fibrosis and alveolar proteinosis associated with silicosis. The epithelial proliferation of alveoli and bronchioles is limited to the immediate area of dust accumulation. Since prolonged exposure to high levels of dust is needed to produce the lesions, dust is always present in close association with lesions.

**Biological Features**

*Natural History.* The effects of inhaled fly ash were studied in the Syrian golden hamster exposed to 70 μg/l fly ash for 6 h/day, 5 days/week for up to 20 weeks (Wehner et al. 1981). Dust deposition increased with time and decreased with recovery. The interstitial reaction increased with time but did not diminish significantly after exposure stopped. Bronchiolization also increased with

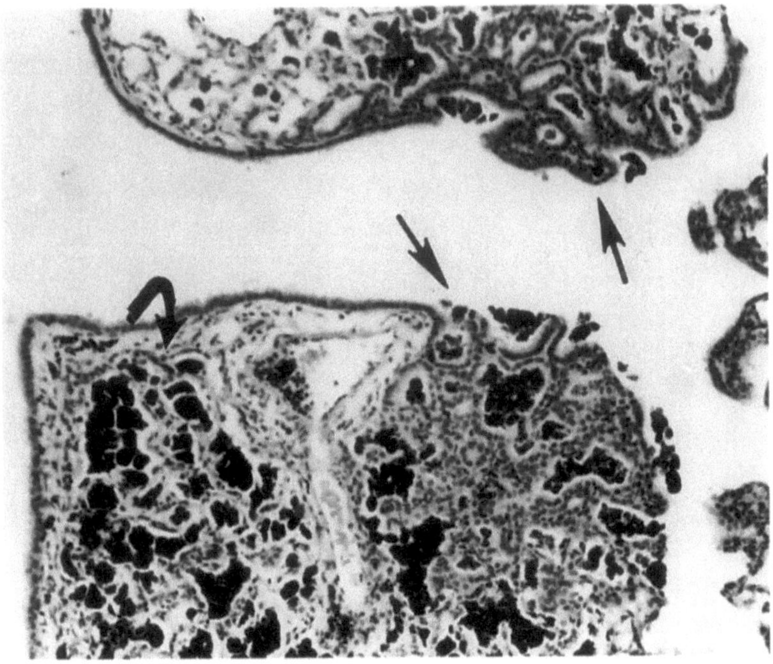

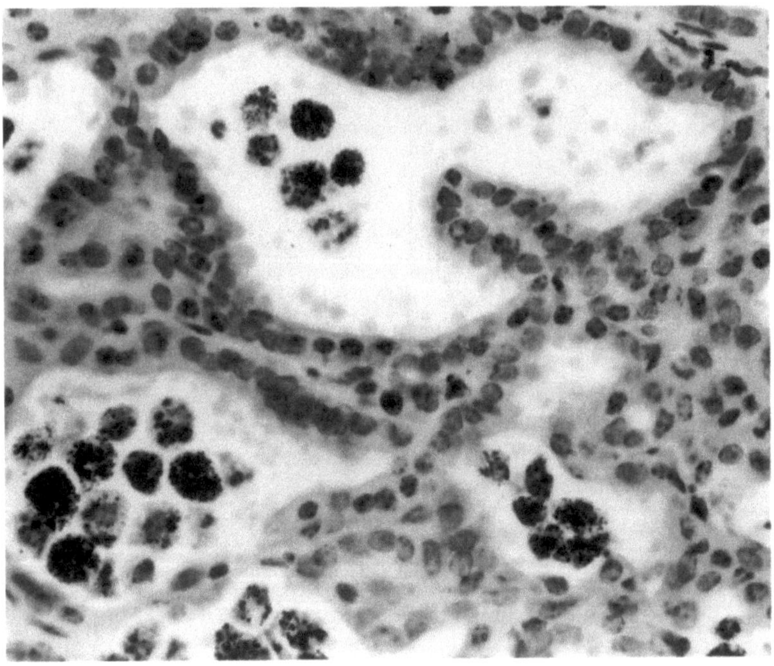

**Fig. 311.** (*above*) Bronchiolization (hyperplasia) (*straight arrows*) and interstitial reaction (*curved arrow*) in lung of hamster exposed to fly ash. H&E, ×120

**Fig. 312.** (*below*) Bronchiolization (hyperplasia) in lung of hamster exposed to fly ash. H&E, ×486

duration of treatment and occasionally progressed even after exposures ceased. Mortality for exposed animals was not higher than for controls (Wehner et al. 1981).

*Pathogenesis.* Dust is phagocytosed by alveolar macrophages; the release of enzymes from alveolar macrophages injures alveolar epithelium. This is followed by compensatory hyperplasia of alveolar and brochiolar epithelium and, if injury is severe, fibrosis (Sanders et al. 1980). Direct effects of fly ash minerals or absorbed materials on epithelium cannot, however, be ruled out. Dust is cleared from the lung by mucociliary

**Table 29.** Histological changes related to fly ash exposure of hamsters for 20 months

| Lung change observed | Exposure level (μg/l³) | Total no. of hamsters | No. of hamsters with lesions | Average severity of lesions[a] |
|---|---|---|---|---|
| Dust accumulation | 70 | 61 | 61 | 3.25[b] |
| | 17 | 62 | 62 | 2.29[bc] |
| | 0 | 55 | 0 | – |
| Interstitial reaction | 70 | 61 | 61 | 2.23[b] |
| | 17 | 62 | 56 | 1.39[bc] |
| | 0 | 55 | 4 | 1.00 |
| Bronchiolization | 70 | 61 | 44 | 1.45[b] |
| | 17 | 62 | 29 | 1.17[cd] |
| | 0 | 55 | 11 | 1.18 |

[a] Very slight (or very small amount) = 1, slight (or small amount) = 2, moderate = 3, marked = 4, severe = 5.
[b] Significantly different from sham-exposed controls, $p < 0.01$.
[c] Significantly different from 70 μg/l exposure level, $p < 0.01$.
[d] Significantly different from sham-exposed controls, $p < 0.05$.

escalator or accumulates in mediastinal lymph nodes.

*Etiology*. Fly ash consists of microcrystals and microspheroids of varying structure, size, and composition – in general. silicates and oxides of aluminum and other minerals that remain after complete combustion of coal. Various materials from the atmosphere may also adhere to the surfaces of the particles. Thus it is rather difficult to attribute to any specific component a given toxic/pathogenic effect observed after exposure to fly ash.

*Frequency*. Lesions observed in hamsters exposed to aerosols of fly ash for 6 h/day for 20 months are quantified in Table 29.

## Comparison with Other Species

Anthracosis, including that caused by fly ash, is regarded as an innocuous condition in humans (Spencer 1977). Studies of primates exposed to flay ash, at levels lower than those for hamsters in our study, demonstrated lesions "similar to that seen in any 'nuisance' dust" which were "not considered to be evidence of permanent pathological alteration" (MacFarland et al. 1968). Recently, however, it has been suggested that fly ash particles may act as carriers for toxic materials or may be fibrogenic per se in humans (Golden et al. 1982).

## References


Golden EB, Warnock ML, Hulett LD Jr, Churg AM (1982) Fly ash lung: a new pneumoconiosis? Am Rev Respir Dis 125:108–112

MacFarland HN, Ulrich CE, Martin A (1968) Chronic exposure of cynomolgus monkeys to fly ash. In: Walton WH (ed) Inhaled particles. Unwin, Surrey

Sanders CL, Cross FT, Dagle GE, Mahaffey JA (eds) (1980) Pulmonary toxicology of respirable particles. Proceedings: DOE symposium series. CONF-791002. National Technical Information Service, DOE, Oak Ridge

Spencer H (1977) Anthracosis. In: Spencer H (ed) Pathology of the lung, vol 1. Saunders, Philadelphia p 411

Wehner AP, Dagle GE, Milliman EM (1981) Chronic inhalation exposure of hamsters to nickel-enriched fly ash. Environ Res 26:195–216

# Asbestosis, Hamster

Gerald E. Dagle and Alfred P. Wehner

*Synonym.* Asbestos pneumoconiosis

## Gross Appearance

At higher exposure levels (23 μg/l) the lungs have a mottled appearance with slightly rusty-tan areas replacing the normal pink coloration. Lung weight tend to increase after prolonged exposure.

## Microscopic Features

Increased numbers of alveolar macrophages and ferruginous bodies are the principal lesions observed at lower exposure levels. The macrophages are distributed diffusely, with some aggregation in areas around respiratory bronchioles (Fig. 313). Those engulfing the ferruginous bodies are generally aggregated in alveoli and frequently form multinucleated giant cells (Fig. 314). The ferruginous bodies measure up to 20 μm long and 2 μm thick, are frequently curved, stain golden yellow with hematoxylin and eosin, and have a typical beaded appearance due to the hemosiderin deposited on the asbestos fibers. Numerous macrophages contain two or more ferruginous bodies. Portions of the ferruginous bodies frequently appear incompletely phagocytosed. Only rarely are ferruginous bodies seen outside of phagocytes.

A mild interstitial fibrosis occurs after 7 months of exposure (Wehner et al. 1975). This occurs in areas with aggregated alveolar macrophages and at high exposure levels is associated with lymphocytes and plasma cells (Fig. 315). Proliferation of alveolar and bronchiolar epithelium and cholesterol clefts occur only at very high exposure levels (Figs. 316 and 317). Occasionally alveoli in these hamsters develop vesicular emphysema.

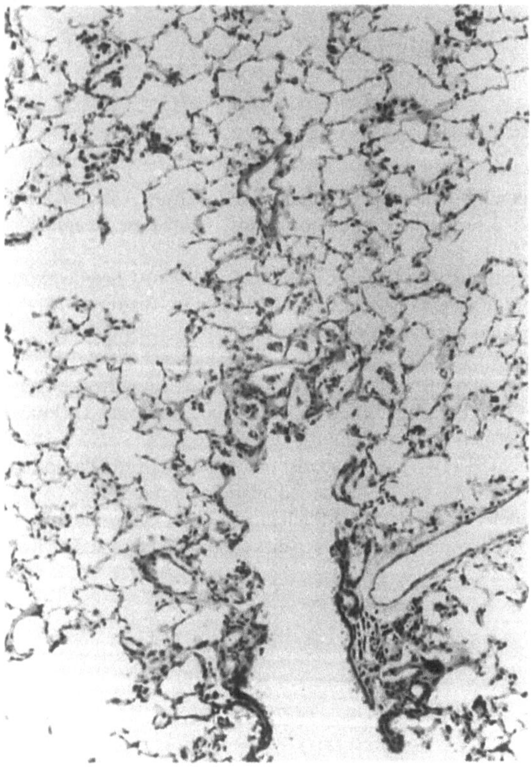

**Fig. 313.** Peribronchial distribution of macrophages and interstitial reaction after inhalation of asbestos. H&E, ×80

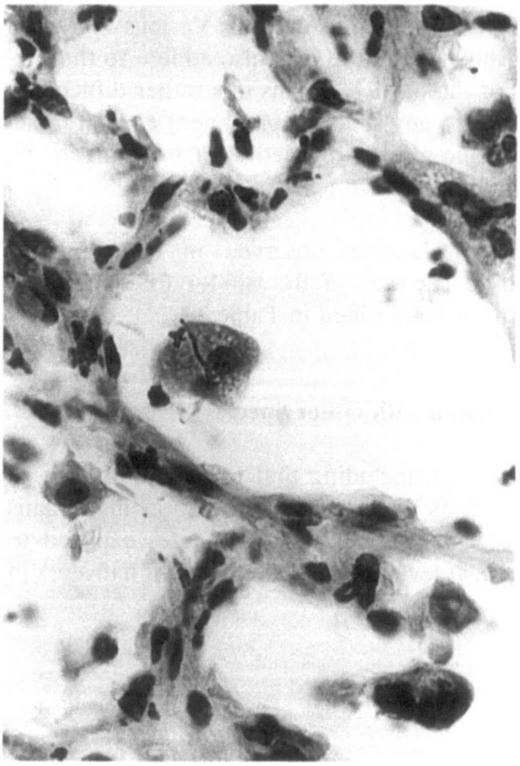

**Fig. 314.** Asbestos body in alveolar macrophage. H&E, ×512

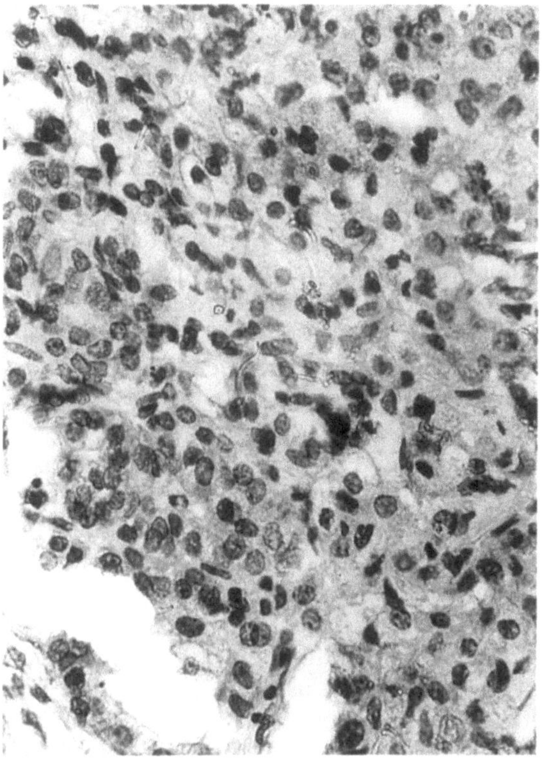

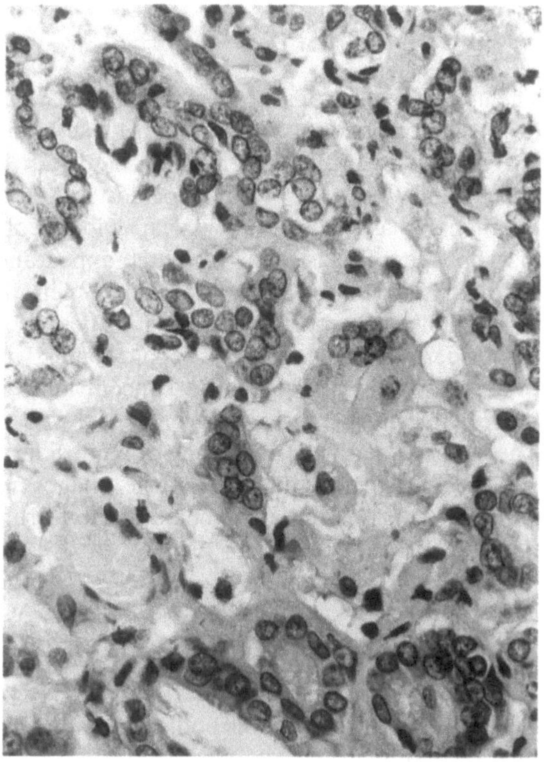

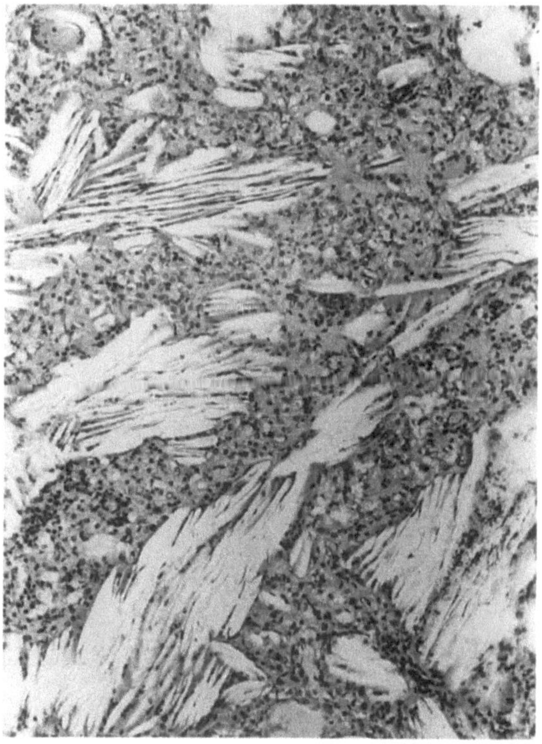

**Fig. 315.** (*upper left*) Diffuse granulomatous reaction with numerous asbestos bodies, after exposure to high levels of inhaled asbestos. H&E, ×320

**Fig. 316.** (*upper right*) Proliferation of bronchiolar epithelium associated with granulomatous reaction after exposure to high levels of inhaled asbestos. H&E, ×320

**Fig. 317.** (*below*) Cholesterol clefts associated with granulomatous reaction following high levels of inhaled asbestos. H&E, ×125

## Ultrastructure

The unique feature of asbestosis is the appearance of ferruginous bodies. Formation of these bodies has been previously described in hamsters by Suzuki and Churg (1969). Phagocytosis of small fragments of asbestos occurs primarily in alveolar macrophages. This is followed by the appearance of hemosiderin in the cytoplasm, then by intracellular transport of iron micelles from hemosiderin granules into the phagosomes with the asbestos fibers. Progressive concentration of the iron micelles occurs in the vicinity of the fibers. The central fiber, with its coating of hemosiderin, and the investing membranes of the phagosome are regarded as essential elements of the ferruginous body (Fig. 318).

## Differential Diagnosis

The presence of ferruginous bodies is characteristic of asbestosis in hamsters and serves to distinguish it from inflammatory lesions due to other causes.

## Biological Features

*Natural History*. Hamsters exposed to asbestos dust (approx. 25 μg/l) 7 h/day, 5 days/week for 11 months experienced respiratory distress which forced discontinuation of the exposures (Wehner et al. 1975, 1978). Body weight and survival time were significantly decreased at these high dosage levels.

*Pathogenesis*. Phagocytosis of inhaled asbestos fibers by alveolar macrophages is the initial event. This is followed by an influx of additional mature macrophages into alveoli, from which they are usually cleared by the mucociliary escalator. Those macrophages that have phagocytosed longer fibers tend to remain in the alveoli longer. Longer fibers are associated with more fibrosis. The macrophages have a significant role in fibrogenesis, perhaps through the regurgitation of

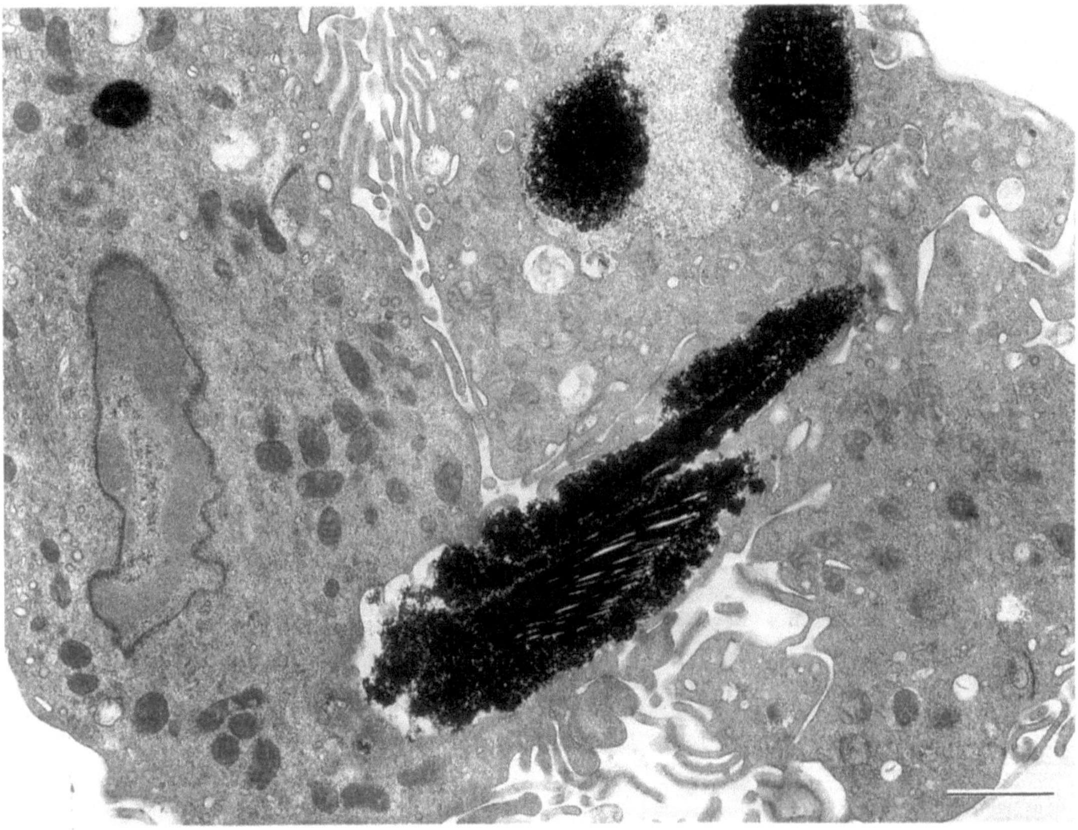

**Fig. 318.** Asbestos body after inhalation of an asbestos-cement mixture. *Bar*, 1 μm. TEM

lysosomal enzymes during phagocytosis, but the pathogenesis is unclear (Parkes 1982).

*Etiology.* Several forms of asbestos, chrysotile, crocidolite, amosite, and anthophylite are all capable of inducing asbestosis. Chrysotile was used to produce the lesions in hamsters described in this report.

*Frequency.* Alveolar macrophages and ferruginous bodies are present in lungs of animals exposed to asbestos. Asbestosis develops in all animals exposed to asbestos.

### Comparison with Other Species

Asbestosis in humans is characterized as bilateral, diffuse, interstitial pulmonary fibrosis and is found in persons occupationally exposed, thus affecting miners, insulators, and shipyard workers. The disease in man results in more severe, diffuse pulmonary fibrosis than is observed experimentally in hamsters. Other disorders considered to be related to asbestos exposure in humans, but not documented in hamsters, include hyaline plaques of parietal pleura, carcinoma of the lung, and skin corns (Parkes 1982). Asbestos-induced mesotheliomas of pleura and peritoneum in hamsters are discussed on p. 229. The Stanton hypothesis relates longer fiber length to increased carcinogenicity of asbestos (Harington 1981).

Asbestos inhalation in rats produces an initial increase in the number of alveolar macrophages, followed by diffuse interstitial pulmonary fibrosis with prominent hyperplasia of alveolar epithelial cells, several kinds of peripheral lung tumors (primarily adenomas, adenocarcinomas, and squamous cell carcinomas), and mesotheliomas (Wagner et al. 1974). Noteworthy differences in experimental lesions in the rat, compared to the hamster, are the absence of ferruginous bodies and the presence of malignant pulmonary tumors.

### References

Harington JS (1981) Fiber carcinogenesis: epidemiologic observations and the Stanton hypothesis. JNCI 67:977–989

Parkes WR (1982) Occupational lung disorders, 2nd edn. Butterworth, London

Suzuki Y, Churg J (1969) Structure and development of the asbestos body. Am J Pathol 55:79–107

Wagner JC, Berry G, Skidmore JW, Timbrell V (1974) The effects of the inhalation of asbestos in rats. Br J Cancer 29:252–269

Wehner AP, Busch RH, Olson RJ, Craig DK (1975) Chronic inhalation of asbestos and cigarette smoke by hamsters. Environ Res 10:368–383

Wehner AP, Dagle GE, Cannon WC, Buschbom RL (1978) Asbestos cement dust inhalation by hamsters. Environ Res 17:367–389

# Squamous Metaplasia, Lung, Rat

Thomas Nolte, Heinrich Ernst, and Donald L. Dungworth

*Synonyms.* Squamous cell metaplasia, metaplasia, squamous cell, epidermoid metaplasia

### Gross Appearance

Small lesions are generally not visible grossly. Larger lesions may appear as white pinpoint foci visible through the pleural surface. An opaque appearance extending over several millimeters may be observed from the pleural surface and cut surface of the largest lesions.

### Microscopic Features

Squamous metaplasia of the lung is a histologically well-defined lesion which can occur at all levels of the conducting airways and in the alveolar region. Small foci of squamous metaplasia are composed of a few cuboidal to polygonal cells with eosinophilic cytoplasm and large nuclei characterized by scant heterochromatin and one or two prominent nucleoli. The epithelium lacks any polarity (Fig. 319).

In larger foci of squamous metaplasia the stratified epithelium has the polar differentiation characteristic of typical squamous epithelium, for example, of the esophagus (Fig. 320). Depending on the site of origin, such lesions may occupy several alveoli or fill the lumen of a bronchus. Even in extensive squamous metaplasia extending over several pulmonary acini the preexisting structure of alveoli and conducting airways is still evident from the orientation of epithelial layers and keratin lamellae along unaffected interstitial septae (Fig. 321). The surrounding intact lung parenchyma may be unchanged or only slightly compressed (Mohr 1992). The cytoplasmic basophilia of keratinocytes is decreased in the larger foci of squamous metaplasia from the basal layer to the lumen, with corresponding increase in eosinophilia (Nolte et al. 1993). The nuclear cytoplasmic ratio decreases in the same direction (Nettesheim and Marchok 1983). The basal cell layers may be composed of typical prickle cells. A stratum granulosum is occasionally marked by deep basophilic keratohyalin granules. Foci of keratinized squamous metaplasia form well-developed keratin lamellae or, in cases of minor keratinization, ghost cells (Fig. 320). Cellular and nuclear polymorphism and mitotic figures are absent or inconspicuous (Mohr 1992).

Large foci of squamous metaplasia lacking any keratinization and polarity of the epithelium may also occur, but much less frequently than the keratinized variant (Fig. 322).

## Ultrastructure

The ultrastructural hallmarks of squamous metaplasia are abundant tonofilament bundles and desmosomes (McDowell et al. 1979; Espinoza et al. 1984). The tonofilament bundles are predominantly located in the perinuclear region (Figs. 323, 324) or inserted in desmosomes. The cytoplasm is rich in polyribosomes, indicating a high protein synthetic activity of these cells. Smooth and rough endoplasmic reticulum are sparse. Commonly, spiny-coated granules and mitochondria of the crista type are present. Cells with mitochondria as the dominating organelles may occur (Fig. 325). The nuclei are moderately polymorphic due to the presence of invaginations of the nuclear membranes. Sparse heterochromatin and a large number of nuclear pores are indicative of the high protein synthetic capacity of these cells. One or two large nucleoli, in most cases marginated, are present in each nucleus (Akagi et al. 1980; Nolte et al. 1993). Lateral cytoplasmic membranes of adjacent cells form numerous interdigitations (Fig. 325) or, in the case of prickle cells (Fig. 324), are connected by long cytoplasmic processes with small desmosomes (Nolte et al. 1993). Gap junctions represent a third form of connecting link between cells of squamous metaplasia (Akagi et al. 1980). Observed changes of the basement membrane in squamous metaplasia include focal duplication and thickening as well as focal thinning and absence or penetration by cytoplasmic processes of basally situated squamous cells (Akagi et al. 1980; Nolte et al. 1993).

In pulmonary squamous metaplasia dark epithelial cells may occur (Klein-Szanto et al. 1980a,b), which are characterized by intense electron-dense nuclear and cytoplasmic matrices (Raick 1973).

## Immunohistochemistry

In routinely processed lung tissue foci of squamous metaplasia react positively with broad spectrum anticytokeratin antibodies and with antibodies against specific high molecular cytokeratins, for example, CK 6, 11, or 13. The staining intensity with antibodies against specific cytokeratin fractions varies and is especially low in prickle cells (Nolte et al. 1993). Squamous metaplasia contains immunohistochemically detectable amounts of the placental form of glutathione S-transferase, a histochemical feature which distinguishes squamous metaplasia from bronchioloalveolar hyperplasia (Yamamoto et al. 1988).

## Differential Diagnosis

Minimal nonkeratinized squamous metaplasia may occasionally be difficult to differentiate from bronchioloalveolar hyperplasia. In contrast to bronchioloalveolar hyperplasia, squamous metaplasia is multilayered, and the cells are more eosinophilic, with large pale nuclei and prominent nucleoli. Large foci of keratinized squamous metaplasia must be distinguished from benign cystic keratinized squamous tumors (squamous cysts). In contrast to squamous metaplasia, the

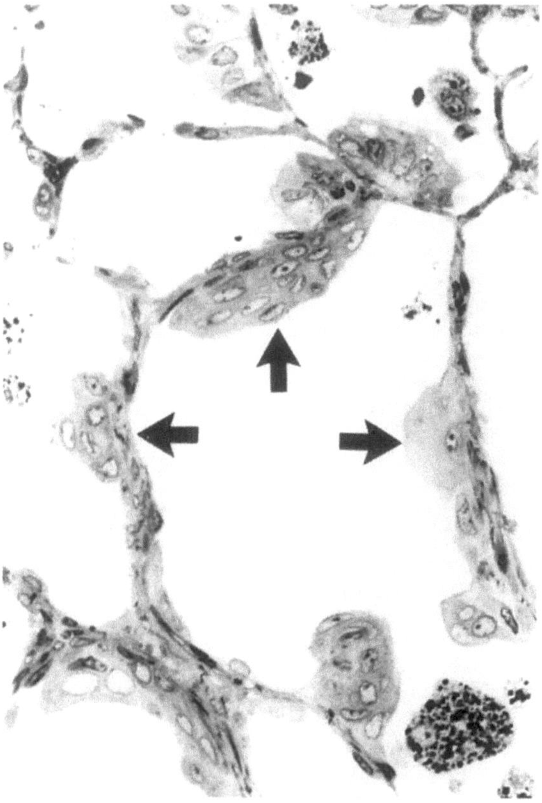

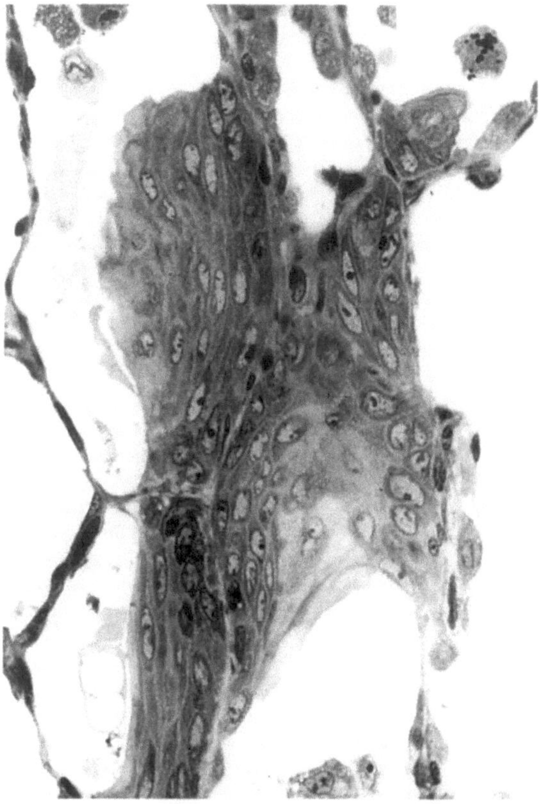

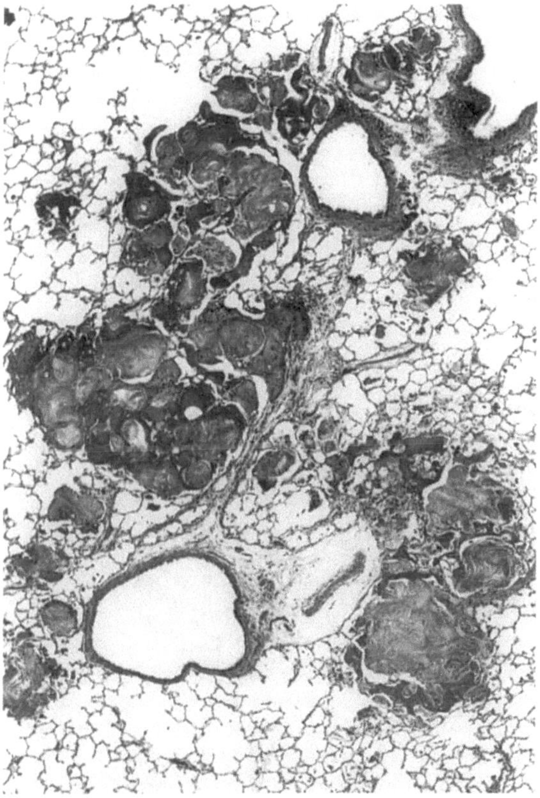

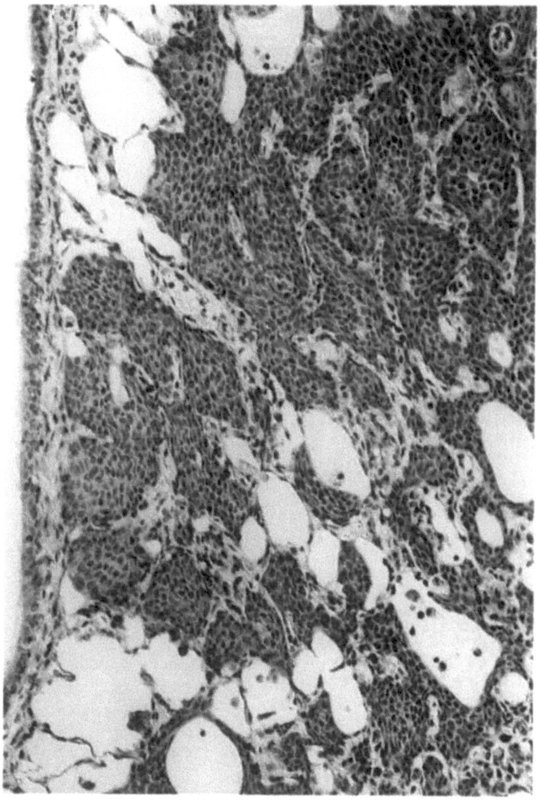

**Fig. 319.** (*upper left*) Lung, rat; small foci of alveolar squamous metaplasia (arrows). The epithelium lacks any polarity; note large pale nuclei with prominent nucleoli. Ito-Karnovsky, epon-embedded, Stevenel's blue, ×300

**Fig. 320.** (*upper right*) Lung, rat; focus of alveolar squamous metaplasia with polar differentiation of the epithelium; slight keratinization with desquamating ghost cells. Ito-Karnovsky, epon-embedded, Stevenel's blue, ×300

**Fig. 321.** (*lower left*) Lung, rat; exaggerated and well-keratinized squamous metaplasia. The alveolar architecture is not distorted. Adjacent unaffected pulmonary parenchyma is not compressed. H&E, ×30

**Fig. 322.** (*lower right*) Lung, rat; extensive nonkeratinized bronchioloalveolar squamous metaplasia

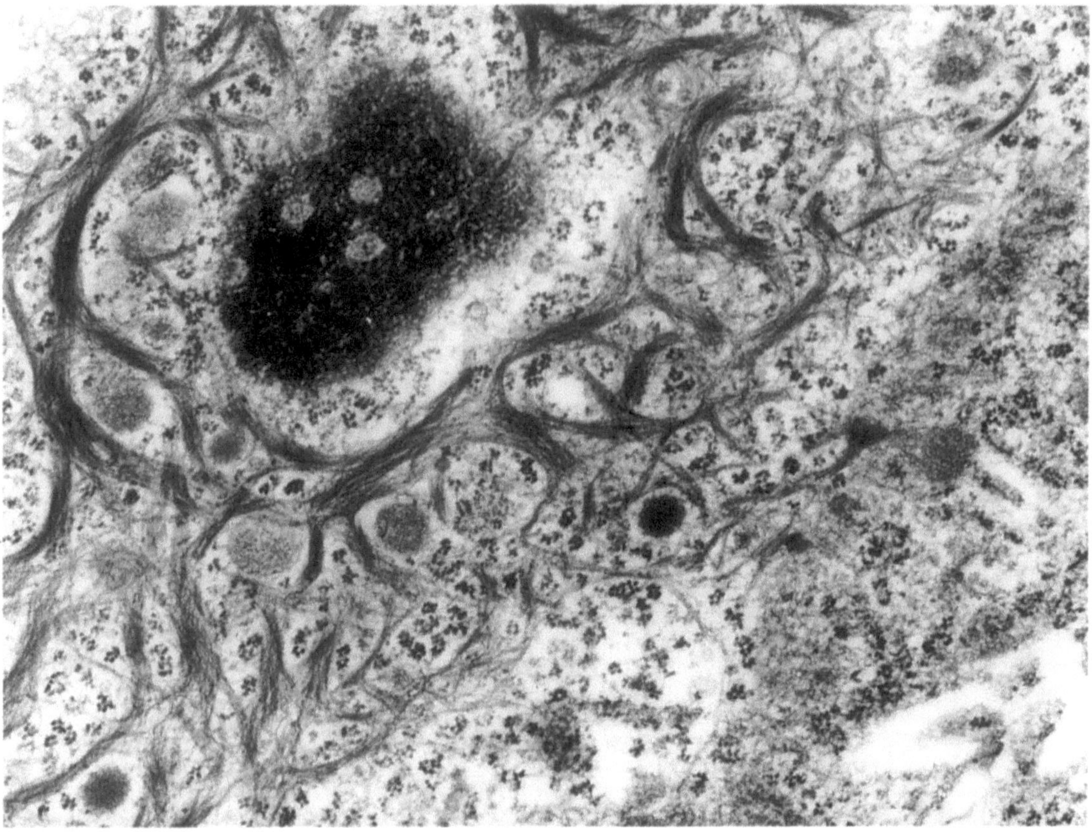

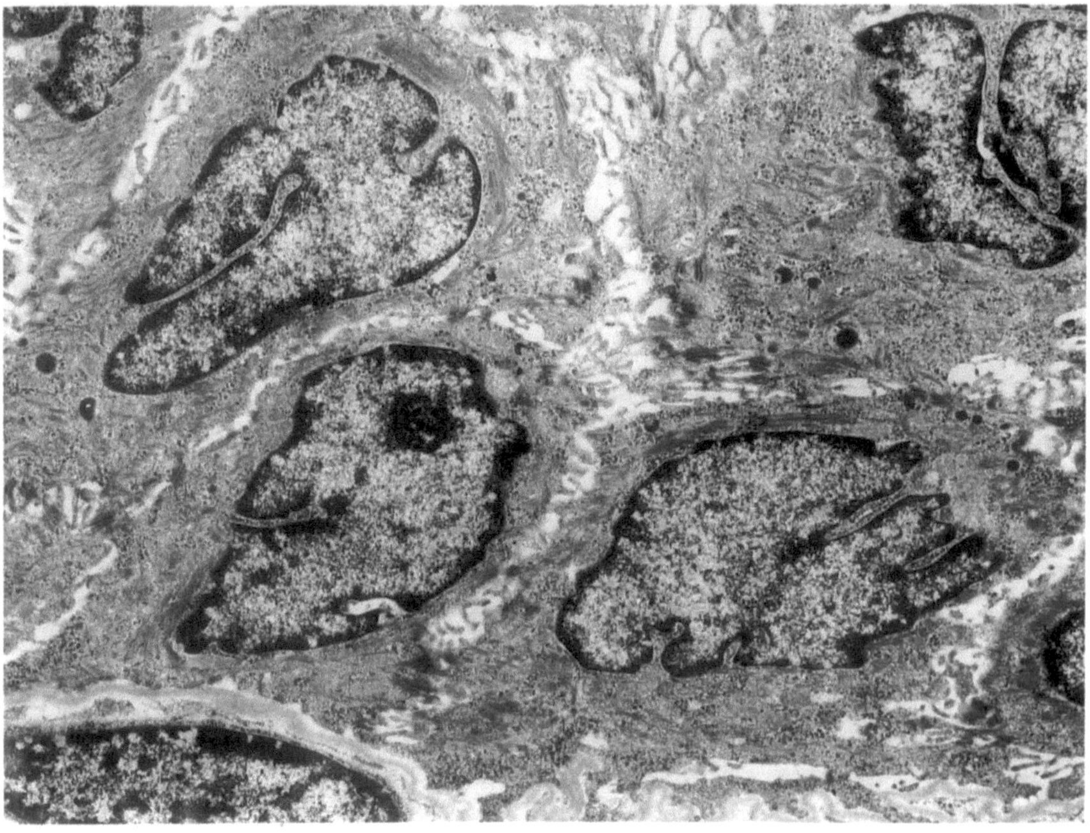

**Fig. 323.** (*above*) Lung, rat; cell of alveolar squamous metaplasia. Nucleus cut tangentially with pores visible. Numerous tonofilament bundles in perinuclear localization. Other prominent cytoplasmic organelles are polysomes and spiny coated granules. Ito-Karnovsky, epon-embedded, uranyl acetate and lead citrate, TEM, ×27500

**Fig. 324.** (*below*) Lung, rat; basal cells of a focus of alveolar squamous metaplasia. Wide intercellular spaces of neighbored cells are bridged by cytoplasmic processes and desmosomes. Moderate nuclear polymorphism. Basement membrane markedly folded. Ito-Karnovsky, epon-embedded, uranyl acetate and lead citrate, TEM, ×4400

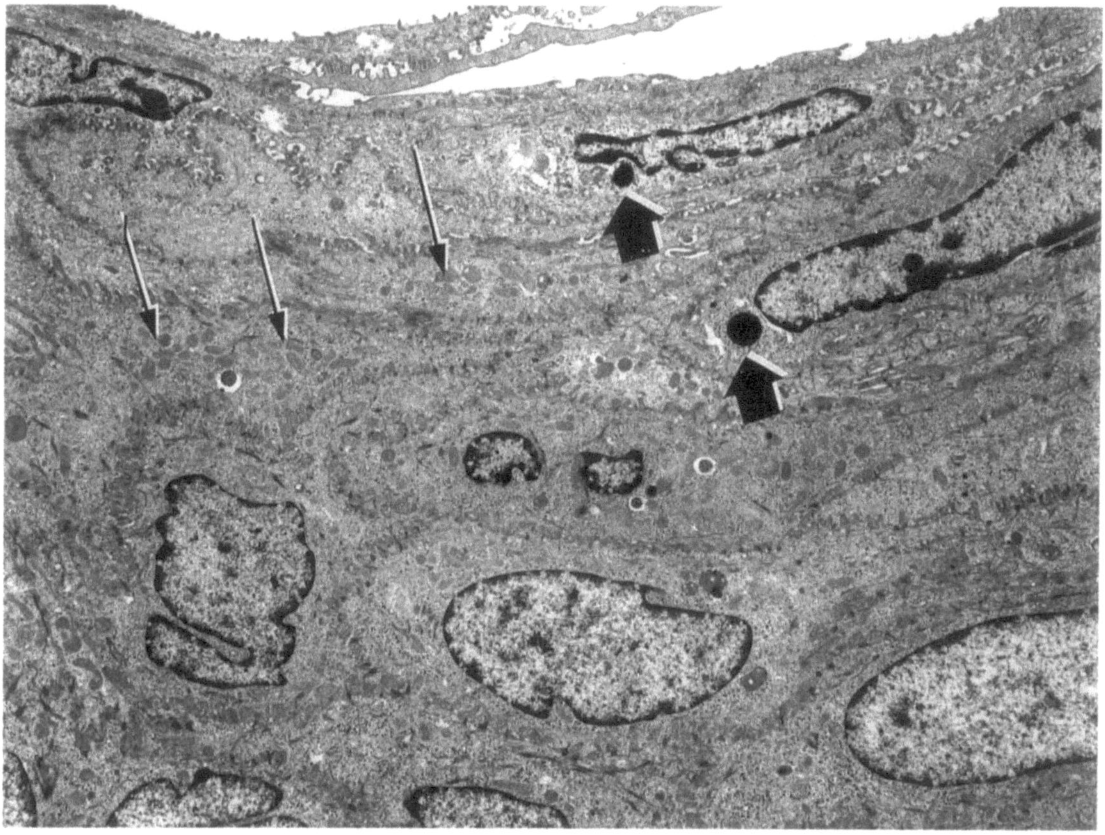

**Fig. 325.** Lung, rat; keratinized alveolar squamous metaplasia. Cytoplasmic membranes of neighboring cells are connected by numerous interdigitations and desmosomes. Mitochondria represent the dominating cytoplasmic organelles (*small arrows*). Note also deep electron dense keratohyaline granules (*thick arrows*). Nuclei with sparse heterochromatin. Ito-Karnovsky, epon-embedded, uranyl acetate and lead citrate, TEM, ×4400

latter form cystic nodules with peripherally growing squamous cells and with central keratinization and necrosis which effaces pulmonary parenchyma (Mohr 1992). Normal pulmonary architecture is also effaced in squamous cell carcinomas, which additionally have signs of malignancy such as cellular or nuclear atypia, frequent mitoses, invasive growth, and metastases (Mohr 1992).

As in the keratinized variant, the nonkeratinized squamous metaplasia can be differentiated from benign nonkeratinized squamous tumors by the distortion and loss of the alveolar architecture in case of the tumor.

## Biological Features

Squamous metaplasia, together with goblet cell metaplasia, are the most obvious forms of cellular adaptation to injury (Dungworth 1989). Squamous metaplasia tends to be associated with the more severe forms of injury, although there is variation according to toxicant (Buckley et al. 1984). Other than the role of vitamin A, little is known about the mechanisms responsible for signaling squamous as opposed to secretory metaplasia (Keenan 1987).

The histogenesis of squamous metaplasia depends on its site of origin. At any level of the airways it presumably develops from proliferating epithelial cells. Squamous metaplasia of the conducting airways induced by inhalation of carcinogens is believed to originate from focal basal cell hyperplasia (Reznik-Schüller and Gregg 1981). Squamous metaplasia of the alveolar region can develop from hyperplasia of type II alveolar epithelial cells (Adamson and Bowden 1979). It is likely that this transdifferentiation takes place via an undifferentiated cell type which ultrastructurally and immunohistochemically exhibits an early squamous phenotype (Nolte et al. 1993).

Whether metaplasia persists after withdrawal of an inhaled irritant seems to depend partly on duration of exposure. It can disappear after short-term exposures but appears to be more persistent after exposures in excess of several months (Dungworth et al. 1994). The full complexity of the situation concerning the roles of duration of exposure and nature of inciting agent in determining reversibility versus persistence or progression needs further exploration.

Foci of persistent squamous metaplasia of the bronchioloalveolar region can be regarded as preneoplastic precursor stages of squamous cell tumors of the rat lung (Kuschner and Laskin 1970; Schreiber et al. 1972; Mohr and Dungworth 1988). Similarities in morphology and immunohistochemical staining patterns for cytokeratins suggest that benign nonkeratinized squamous cell tumors may arise from nonkeratinized squamous cell metaplasia, and that benign cystic keratinized squamous cell tumors may develop from the keratinized counterpart of squamous cell metaplasia (Nolte et al. 1993).

Two types of bronchial squamous metaplasia exist which biologically behave in different ways (Akagi et al. 1980). Bronchial squamous foci induced by intrapulmonal administration of carcinogens consistently progress to bronchial squamous cell carcinomas. However, squamous metaplasia of the bronchial epithelium also commonly occurs in response to various types of chronic nonspecific injury. Such foci of squamous metaplasia rarely progress to carcinoma (Innes et al. 1967). Paradoxically they have a dysplastic appearance while those induced by carcinogens initially exhibit generally well-differentiated, mature squamous epithelium. The following morphological features are additionally described as characteristic for the reactive type of bronchial squamous metaplasia: cells bordering the surface sometimes possess differentiated features of either ciliated or mucous cells; the tonofibrils never reach the quantity noted in the preneoplastic squamous cells; cell membranes are generally closely opposed, essentially smooth, and rarely bordered by desmosomes (Akagi et al. 1980).

*Etiology*. Squamous metaplasia has been observed after pulmonary administration of various carcinogenic or irritant agents, including metals such as beryllium compounds (Groth et al. 1980) or chromium (VI) compounds (Levy and Venitt 1986), complex mixtures of organic compounds such as cigarette smoke condensate (Dagle et al. 1978) or coal tar pitch (Chang et al. 1992), polycyclic aromatic hydrocarbons (Dungworth et al. 1994b), halogenated hydrocarbons (1,2-dibromoethane; Reznik et al. 1980), and dusts (titanium dioxide; Lee et al. 1986; Dungworth 1994). With respect to its potentially preneoplastic character the development of bronchioloalveolar squamous metaplasia can as a rule be expected after treatment with substances which induce squamous cell tumors in the rat lung. Squamous metaplasia is also a consistent finding in rats fed a vitamin A deficient diet (Alexander and Bancewicz 1988). During the course of virus-induced pneumonia alveolar squamous metaplasia occurs in the reparative phase (Brownstein 1985). Nonkeratinized squamous metaplasia of the bronchi and bronchioles may be observed in rats affected by murine respiratory mycoplasmosis. This mycoplasmosis-associated squamous metaplasia is accompanied by bronchiectasis (Schoeb and Lindsay 1985).

*Frequency*. The incidence of animals affected after treatment with the substances mentioned above ranges from less than 1% to approximately 100%. A sexual predisposition for the induction of squamous metaplasia was observed for females treated with titanium dioxide dust by inhalation (Muhle et al. 1991). Squamous metaplasia is an extremely rare finding in healthy untreated rats. The RITA database of preneoplastic and neoplastic lesions of control rats (Hannover, Germany) does not contain any cases of pulmonary squamous metaplasia in 3300 male or female rats. Of these animals 2100 male and 2150 female rats were of the Wistar strain, and the remaining 1200 male and 1150 female rats were of the Sprague Dawley strain. The animals were aged 24–31 months.

## Comparison with Other Species

Compared with other rodent and nonrodent species the rat is especially sensitive to the induction of bronchioloalveolar squamous metaplasia. Of the three species rat, rabbit, and hamster, the rat developed the highest incidence of squamous metaplasia after inhalation of acrolein vapor (Feron et al. 1978). Nevertheless, many agents which have been shown to cause bronchial and bronchioloalveolar squamous metaplasia in the rat lung act in the same way on the bronchial epithelium of the hamster. Examples are mechanical injury (McDowell et al. 1979), vitamin A deficiency (McDowell and Trump 1983), and carcinogens such as benzo(a)pyrene (Becci et al. 1978). The main difference between bronchial squamous metaplasia of rat and hamster seems to be the histogenesis. In contrast to the rat, where hyperplasia of basal cells is the presumed progenitor of bronchial squamous metaplasia (Reznik-Schüller and Gregg 1981), it obviously develops from secretory hyperplasia in the hamster bronchus (McDowell et al. 1984).

Bronchioloalveolar squamous metaplasia has been induced in hamsters after systemic injection of diethylnitrosamine and dibutylnitrosamine. Histogenetically this lesion developed from hyperplasia of dense-core granulated endocrine cells (Reznik-Schüller 1976, 1977).

The preferred localization of pulmonary squamous metaplasia in mice seems to be the bronchioloalveolar region. Bronchioloalveolar squamous metaplasia has been observed in mice after treatment with carcinogens. Examples are intratracheal administration of 3-methylcholanthrene (Rehm and Kelloff 1991) and cutaneous administration of *N*-nitrosobis-(2-chloroethyl) urea (Rehm et al. 1991). It also occurred in mice repeatedly infected with influenza virus (Semkow et al. 1979). An important role is ascribed to Clara cells during histogenesis of bronchioloalveolar squamous metaplasia in mice. It has been demonstrated immunohistochemically that Clara cell antigen but not surfactant apoprotein in hyperplasia is associated with bronchioloalveolar metaplasia (Rehm et al. 1991).

In man squamous metaplasia is a common reaction to injury, toxins, and vitamin A deprivation (Basbaum and Jany 1990). The most common agent causing squamous metaplasia is cigarette smoke (Mathé et al. 1986), with a preferred localization in the larger bronchi. The histogenesis is comparable to that of squamous metaplasia in the hamster trachea. Secretory cells, specifically Goblet cells, are the main progenitors for trachobronchial squamous metaplasia (Wang et al. 1972).

## References


Adamson IYR, Bowden DH (1979) Bleomycin-induced injury and metaplasia of alveolar type 2 cells. Relationship of cellular responses to drug presence in the lung. Am J Pathol 96:531–544

Akagi G, Stanton M, Miller E, May M, Poore C (1980) Ultrastructural observations on preneoplastic epidermoid metaplasia in the lungs of rats. J Environ Pathol Toxicol 4:771–785

Alexander A, Bancewicz J (1988) Vitamin A deficiency and resistance to infection in experimental animals. Surg Res Commun 4/3:257–267

Basbaum C, Jany B (1990) Plasticity in the airway epithelium. Am J Physiol 259:L38–L46

Becci PJ, McDowell EM, Trump BF (1978) The respiratory epithelium. IV. Histogenesis of epidermoid metaplasia and carcinoma in situ in the hamster. J Natl Cancer Inst 61:577–586

Brownstein DG (1985) Sendai virus infection, lung, mouse and rat. In: Jones TC, Mohr U, Hunt RD (eds) Monographs on pathology of laboratory animals, vol I: respiratory system. Springer, Berlin Heidelberg New York, pp 195–202

Buckley LA, Jiang XZ, James RA, Morgan KT, Barrow CS (1984) Respiratory tract lesions induced by sensory irritants at the RD50 concentration. Toxicol Appl Pharmacol 74:417–429

Chang F, Wang L, Zhao Q, Zhu Q, Wu Y, Chen C, Syrjanen S, Syrjanen K (1992) Investigation on the carcinogenic effects of coal tar pitch in rat respiratory tract by intratracheal instillations. Carcinogenesis 13:233–239

Dagle GE, McDonald KE, Smith LG, Stevens DL Jr (1978) Pulmonary carcinogenesis in rats given implants of cigarette smoke condensate in beeswax pellets. J Natl Cancer Inst 61:905–910

Dungworth DL (1989) Non-carcinogenic responses of the respiratory tract to inhaled toxicants. In: Mc Clennan RO, Henderson RF (eds) Concepts in inhalation toxicology. Hemisphere, New York, pp 273–298

Dungworth DL (1994) Histopathological endpoints in the respiratory tract. In: Mohr U (ed) Monographs on the IPCS international symposium on respiratory toxicology and risk assessment 6–9 Oct 1992, Hannover, FRG (in press)

Dungworth DL, Mohr U, Heinrich U, Ernst H, Kittel B (1994) Pathologic effects of inhaled particles in rat lungs: associations between inflammatory and neoplastic processes. In: Mohr U, Dungworth DL, Mauderly JL, Oberdörster G (eds) Toxic and carcinogenic effects of solid particles in the respiratory tract. ILSI Press, Washington DC, pp 75–98

Espinosa CG, Balis JU, Saba SR, Paciga JE, Shelley SA (1984) Ultrastructural and immunohistochemical studies of bronchioalveolar carcinoma. Cancer 54:2182–2189

Feron VJ, Kruysse A, Til HP, Immel HR (1978) Repeated exposure to acrolein vapour: subacute studies in hamsters, rats and rabbits. Toxicology 9:47–57

Groth DH, Kommineni C, Mackay GR (1980) Carcinogenicity of beryllium hydroxide and alloys. Environ Res 21:63–84

Innes J, Garner F, Stookey J (1967) Respiratory diseases in rats. In: Cotchin E, Roe F (eds) Pathology of laboratory rats and mice. Davis, Philadelphia, pp 229–257

Keenan KP (1987) Cell injury and repair of tracheobronchial epithelium. In: McDowell EM (ed) Current problems in tumor pathology, vol 3: lung carcinomas. Churchill Livingstone, Edinburgh, pp 74–93

Klein-Szanto AJP, Topping DC, Heckman CA, Nettesheim P (1980a) Ultrastructural characteristics of carcinogen-induced nondysplastic changes in tracheal epithelium. Am J Pathol 98:61–82

Klein-Szanto AJP, Topping DC, Heckman CA, Nettesheim P (1980b) Ultrastructural characteristics of carcinogen-induced non-dysplastic changes in tracheal epithelium. Am J Pathol 98:83–100

Kuschner M, Laskin S (1970) Pulmonary epithelial tumors and tumor-like proliferations in the rat. Morphology of experimental carcinogenesis. Proceedings of biology division conference, Oak Ridge, National Laboratory, Gatlingburg, 13–16 May, pp 203–222

Lee KP, Henry NW III, Trochimowicz HJ, Reinhardt CF (1986) Pulmonary responses to impaired lung clearance in rats following excessive $TiO_2$ dust deposition. Environ Res 41:144–167

Levy LS, Venitt S (1986) Carcinogenicity and mutagenicity of chromium compounds: the association between bronchial metaplasia and neoplasia. Carcinogenesis 7:831–835

Mathé G, Santelli G, Gouveia J, Lemaigre G, Misset LJ, Homasson JP, Sudre MC, Gros F, Kim B, Gaget H (1986) Correlation of bronchial epidermoid metaplasia with level of tobacco consumption in heavy smokers. Cancer Detect Prev 9:79–81

McDowell EM, Trump BF (1983) Histogenesis of preneoplastic and neoplastic lesions in tracheobronchial epithelium. Surv Synth Pathol Res 2:235–279

McDowell EM, Becci PJ, Schurch W, Trump BF (1979) The respiratory epithelium. VII Epidermoid metaplasia of hamster tracheal epithelium during regeneration following mechanical injury. J Natl Cancer Inst 62:995–1008

McDowell EM, Keenan KP, Huang M (1984) Effects of vitamin A-deprivation on hamster tracheal epithelium. A quantitative morphologic study. Virchows Arch [B] Cell Pathol Incl Mol Pathol 45:197–219

Mohr U (1992) IARC international classification of rodent tumors, part I: the rat. Respiratory system. Oxford University Press, Oxford

Mohr U, Dungworth DL (1988) Relevance to humans of experimentally induced pulmonary tumors in rats and hamsters. In: Mohr U (ed) Inhalation toxicology. Springer, Berlin Heidelberg New York, pp 209–232

Muhle H, Bellmann B, Creutzenberg O, Dasenbrock C, Ernst H, Kipper R, MacKenzie JC, Morrow P, Mohr U, Takenaka S, Mermelstein R (1991) Pulmonary response to toner upon chronic inhalation exposure in rats. Fundam Appl Toxicol 17:280–299

Nettesheim P, Marchok A (1983) Neoplastic development in airway epithelium. Adv Cancer Res 39:1–70

Nolte T, Thiedemann KU, Dungworth DL, Ernst H, Paulini I, Heinrich U, Dasenbrock C, Peters L, Ueberschär S, Mohr U (1993) Morphology and histogenesis of squamous cell metaplasia of the rat lung after chronic exposure to a pyrolized pitch condensate and/or carbon black, or to combinations of pyrolized pitch condensate, carbon black and irritant gases. Exp Toxicol Pathol 45:135–144

Raick AN (1973) Ultrastructural, histological and biochemical alterations produced by 12-O-tetradecanoyl-pharbol-13-acetate on mouse epidermis and their relevance to skin tumor promotion. Cancer Res 33:269–286

Rehm S, Kelloff GJ (1991) Histologic characterization of mouse bronchiolar cell hyperplasia, metaplasia, and neoplasia induced intratracheally by 3-methylcholanthrene. Exp Lung Res 17/2:229–244

Rehm S, Lijinsky W, Singh G, Katayal SL (1991) Mouse bronchiolar cell carcinogenesis. Histologic characterization and expression of Clara cell antigen in lesions induced by N-nitrosobis-(2-choroethyl) ureas. Am J Pathol 139:413–422

Reznik G, Stinson SF, Ward JM (1980) Respiratory pathology in rats and mice after inhalation of 1,2 dibromo-3-chloropropane or 1,2-dibromoethane for 13 weeks. Arch Toxicol 46:233–240

Reznik-Schüller HM (1976) Proliferation of endocrine (APUD-type) cells during early N-diethylnitrosamine-induced lung carcinogenesis in hamsters. Cancer Lett 1:255–258

Reznik-Schüller HM (1977) Sequential morphologic alterations in the bronchial epithelium of Syrian golden hamsters during N-nitrosomorpholine-induced pulmonary tumorigenesis. Am J Pathol 89:59–66

Reznik-Schüller HM, Gregg M (1981) Pathogenesis of lung tumors induced by N-nitrosoheptamethyleneimine in F344 rats. Virch Arch [A] 393:333–343

Schoeb TR, Lindsay JR (1985) Murine respiratory mycoplasmosis, lung, rat. In: Jones TC, Mohr U, Hunt RD (eds) Monographs on pathology of laboratory animals, vol I: respiratory system. Springer, Berlin Heidelberg New York, pp 213–217

Schreiber H, Nettesheim P, Martin DH (1972) Rapid development of bronchiolo-alveolar squamous cell tumors in rats after intratracheal injection of 3-methylcholanthrene. J Natl Cancer Inst 49:541–554

Semkow R, Wilczynski J, Krus S, Bogacka-Zatorska E (1979) Squamous metaplasia of the lung alveolar epithelium in mice after influenza virus infection. Acta Virol 23:479–499

Wang NS, Huang SN, Turlbeck WM (1972) Squamous metaplasia of the opening of bronchial glands. Am J Pathol 67:571–582

Yamamoto K, Yokose Y, Nakajima A, Eimoto H, Shiraiwa K, Tamura K, Tsutsumi M, Konishi Y (1988) Comparative histochemical investigation of the glutathione S-transferase placental form and gamma-glutamyltranspeptidase during N-nitrosobis(2-hydroxypropyl)amine-induced lung carcinogenesis in rats. Carcinogenesis 9:399–404

# Pulmonary Hair Embolism, Rat

Alexander Kast

*Synonyms.* Hair fragment emboli in the pulmonary vascular system, trichoembolism, pulmonary embolism caused by hairs, microembolic pulmonary lesions, skin emboli in lungs

## Gross Appearance

Pulmonary hair emboli are not visible grossly. Yamamoto et al. (1982), using a stereomicroscope, observed the foreign bodies from the cut surface of rat lungs.

## Microscopic Features

In histological sections of lungs, foreign body granulomas are seen in medium-sized pulmonary arteries, interalveolar capillaries, and alveoli. In the center of these lesions fragments of skin, hairs, and broken-off shafts of hair follicles cut transversely, obliquely, or longitudinally may be found.

Identification of the foreign bodies is facilitated by the use of azan-Mallory stain and periodic acid–Schiff reagent (Yamamoto et al. 1982). Under polarized light this material has the same birefringent character as epidermal keratin (Innes et al. 1958; Tekeli 1974). The hair shafts have bright yellow dichroism in polarized light, and with azan they appear as a red and blue double-ring structure (Schneider and Pappritz 1976). Since the structure of the hair is often unmistakably visible in hematoxylin and eosin stained sections, no special methods are necessary to identify these structures (Figs. 326–328).

In our experience, giant cell formation begins on the 3rd day after injection. At this time the embolic hair particles are surrounded by multinucleated giant cells, fibrin, and leukocytes. At the end of subacute toxicological experiments (usually 28 days) in which material is injected intravenously, most granulomas are found in alveoli or alveolar capillaries.

Less commonly the hair particles are lodged in parietal thrombi in pulmonary vessels, where they cause partial or complete obturation of the lumen. Endovascular and perivascular inflammatory cell infiltration of vessels containing thrombi has been observed (Tekeli 1974; Yamamoto et al. 1982).

In most cases long-standing intravascular obturations become rechanneled in varying degrees. The granulation tissue often extends into the arterial wall, leading to its destruction and consequent periarterial granuloma (Schneider and Pappritz 1976). It is also striking that hair particles are often found embedded in the wall or in alveoli near to pulmonary arteries (Tsunenari and Kast 1977). This phenomenon has been explained by Johnston et al. (1981) on the basis of the ability of the macrophages to carry the foreign body through the vessel wall to reach the alveolar spaces.

Infrequently some arteries become surrounded by an abscess (Yamamoto et al. 1982). Although the injected parts of the epidermis are naturally populated with bacteria, the thromboemboli very seldom result in bacterial infection. In only six caudal thrombi or pulmonary emboli found among 1422 rats studied (Table 30) was purulent inflammation present in adjacent tissue. No pulmonary infarction has been observed. Only one exception is present in the literature; areas of hemorrhagic infarction were described in a rabbit experimentally injected with a suspension of hair (Innes et al. 1958).

## Differential Diagnosis

Problems in differential diagnosis may arise if no hair particles are detected within a granuloma, or if the granulomatous processes are extensive. In such cases drug-specific effects may be simulated. Parasitic nodules are to be differentiated in dogs (Schneider and Pappritz 1976). The virogenic giant cell pneumonia, so-called Hecht's pneumonia (Sedlmeier and Schiefer 1971; Giese 1974), may be considered. Nests of foam cells in alveoli of rat lungs are common but seem to be involved in lipid metabolism (Flodh et al. 1974; see p. 270). In none of these lesions are the granulomas found in blood vessels.

Inhaled foreign bodies, such as particles of hairs or plants, may lead to similar pulmonary granulomas,

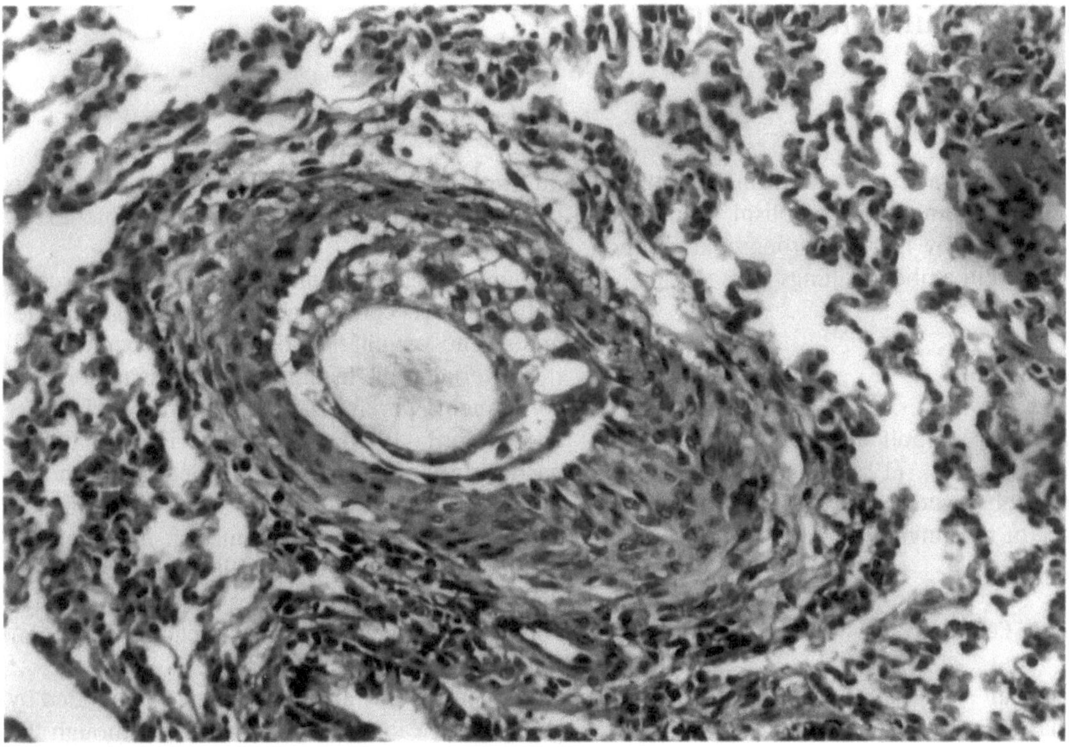

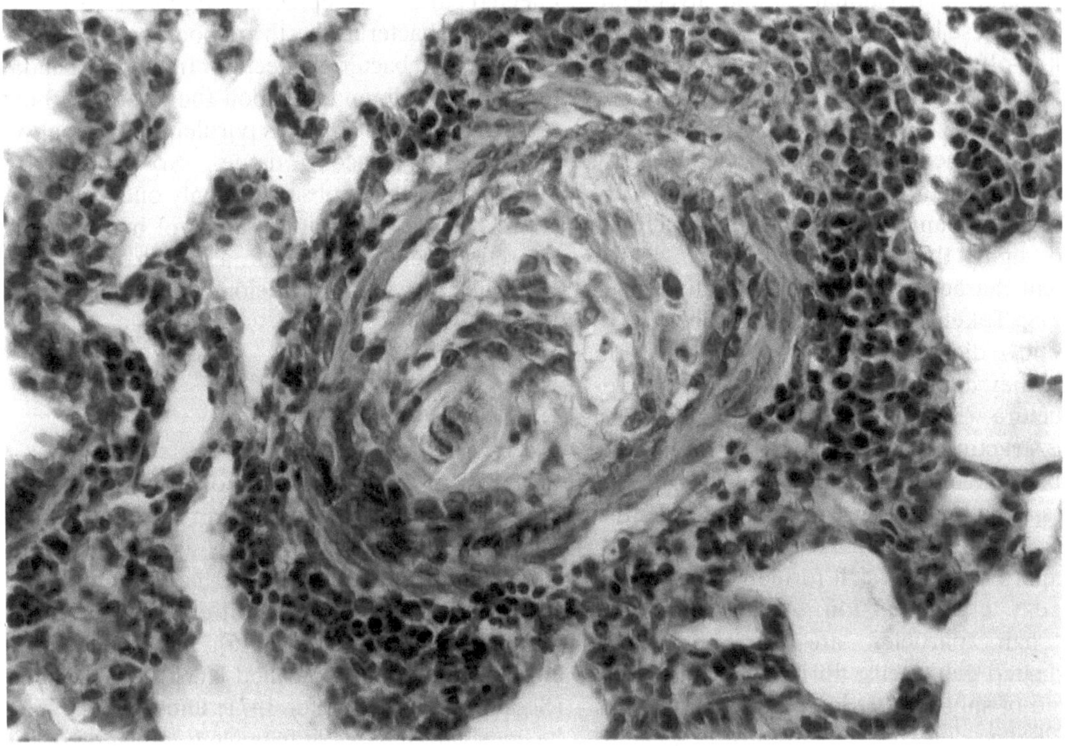

**Fig. 326.** (*above*) Transverse section of an embolic piece of hair embedded in thrombotic material in a pulmonary artery of a male rat killed after 4 weeks of daily injections into caudal veins. H&E, ×200

**Fig. 327.** (*below*) Pigmented hair segment with distinctly visible medulla cells in a thrombotic pulmonary artery of a female rabbit given 28 intravenous injections into ear veins. H&E, ×200

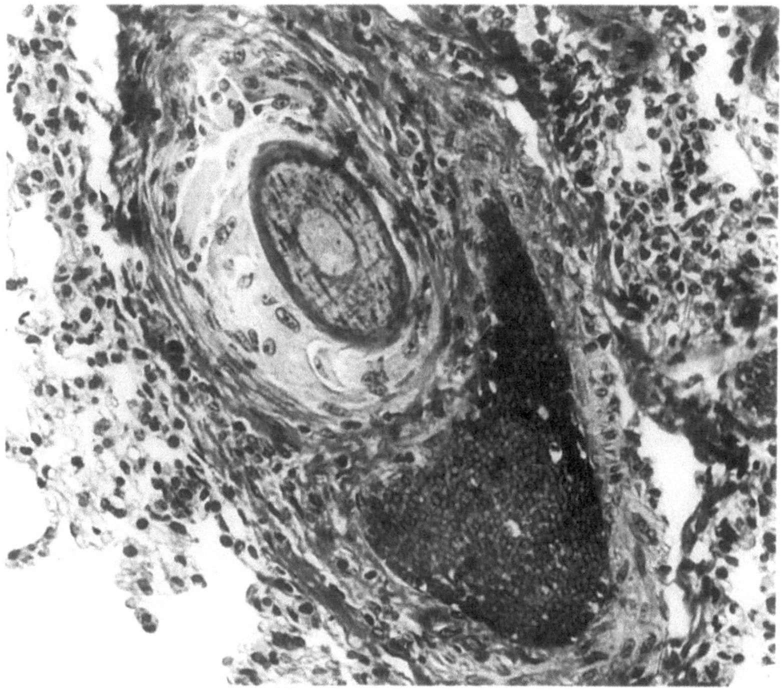

**Fig. 328.** Pulmonary artery of a beagle with embolic hair trapped in a thrombus. Note the concentric layers of the hair. Azan, ×200 (from Schneider and Pappritz 1976)

**Table 30.** Lesions in tail veins and lungs in 1422 Sprague-Dawley rats following daily intravenous injections for 28 days (from Kast and Tsunenari 1983)

| Organ | Finding | Males ($n$ = 703) | | Females ($n$ = 779) | |
|---|---|---|---|---|---|
| | | Mean ± SD[a] | Total(%) | Mean ± SC[a] | Total (%) |
| Tail veins | Total | 7.19 ± 2.69 | 374 (53.2) | 7.79 ± 2.48 | 405 (56.3) |
| | Bleeding | 2.12 ± 1.91 | 110 (15.6) | 1.81 ± 1.58 | 94 (13.1) |
| | Periphlebitis | 2.56 ± 1.88 | 133 (18.9) | 4.27 ± 2.13 | 222 (30.9) |
| | Phlebitis | 1.58 ± 1.47 | 82 (11.7) | 2.60 ± 1.91 | 135 (18.8) |
| | Swelling of intima | 1.38 ± 1.29 | 72 (10.2) | 1.27 ± 1.09 | 66 (9.2) |
| | Hair in vessel Wall | 2.10 ± 1.26 | 109 (15.5) | 2.12 ± 1.40 | 110 (15.3) |
| | Thrombophlebitis | 3.13 ± 2.32 | 163 (23.2) | 3.69 ± 2.22 | 192 (26.7) |
| | With hair particle | 1.37 ± 1.34 | 71 (10.1) | 1.40 ± 1.30 | 73 (10.2) |
| Lungs | Total | 3.75 ± 2.46 | 195 (27.7) | 3.58 ± 2.49 | 186 (25.9) |
| | Thromboarteritis | 0.56 ± 0.87 | 29 (4.1) | 0.42 ± 0.61 | 22 (3.1) |
| | With hair particle | 0.42 ± 0.70 | 22 (3.1) | 0.27 ± 0.49 | 14 (1.9) |
| | With skin particle | 0.08 ± 0.27 | 4 (0.6) | 0.06 ± 0.24 | 3 (0.4) |
| | Giant cell granuloma[b] | 3.35 ± 2.35 | 174 (24.8) | 3.29 ± 2.43 | 171 (23.8) |
| | With hair particle | 1.96 ± 1.80 | 102 (14.5) | 1.96 ± 2.10 | 102 (14.2) |
| | With skin particle | 0.12 ± 0.38 | 6 (0.9) | 0.06 ± 0.24 | 3 (0.4) |

[a] Mean number of lesions in each group of 15 rats, excluding animals which did not receive all 28 injections.
[b] In alveolar capillaries or alveoli.

including giant cell formation (Fig. 329). For example, Sahu et al. (1975) have reported giant cells in lungs of mice 30 days after the inhalation of asbestos.

Many reports have accumulated in the literature about pulmonary embolism and foreign body granulomatosis in man and experimental animals caused by the intravenous injection of particles such as cotton wool fibers, microcrystalline cellulose, cornstarch, talc, rubber, metal or glass, and other materials (Simpson 1922; Easton 1952; Garvan and Gunner 1964; Zientara and Moore

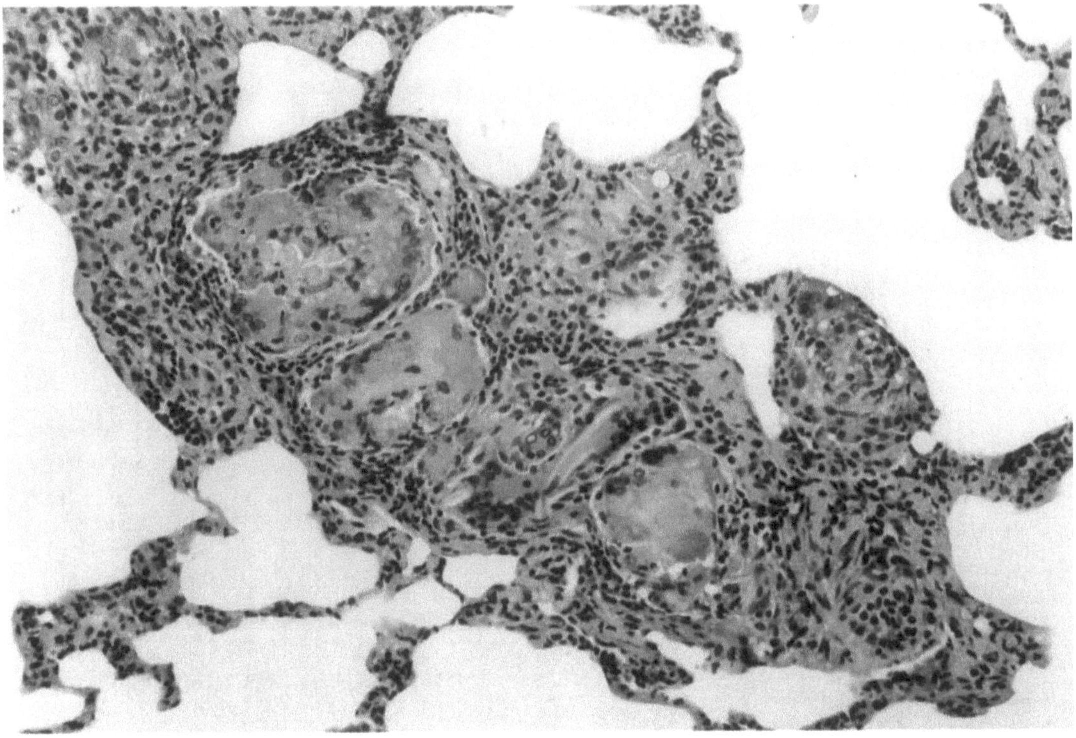

**Fig. 329.** Granuloma with foreign body giant cells phagocytosing inhaled particles of plants in pulmonary alveolus of a 2-year-old female rat. H&E, ×100

1970; Bowden 1971; Johnston and Waisman 1971; Johnston et al. 1981; Tomashefski et al. 1981).

## Biological Features

*Pathogenesis.* Intravenous injection into caudal veins of rats and mice, veins of ear of rabbits, and into veins of bigger mammals, such as dog and man, is often followed by embolism of skin particles and hair fragments. These may become part of a thrombus at the site of injection or be caught by the pulmonary filter, phagocytosed, and removed by foreign body giant cells within a few weeks. Eventually the integrity of the affected pulmonary arteries and alveoli is restored. The entire process belongs to the so-called "pathology of therapy."

In one study we examined histological sections of lung and caudal vein from each of 1422 rats that had received 28 daily intravenous injections of various test substances. Lesions in caudal veins were found at the site of injection in more than 50% of the rats (Table 30). These lesions included bleeding into the surrounding tissue, periphlebitis and phlebitis, cushionlike swellings of the intima, and thrombosis.

The frequency of hair-containing thrombi does not significantly differ between rats injected intravenously with various test substances at different dosages and their saline-treated controls. Therefore, controls and treated animals are shown together in Table 30.

The current view is that particles of hair, hair follicles, or other bits of skin are punched out by the injecting needle and tranferred through the needle into the wall or lumen of the caudal veins. At this site they may become embedded in thrombotic material (Fig. 330). If not caught in a thrombus in a vein near the site of injection, hair and skin particles are floated to the lungs, where they are stopped in the pulmonary filter. Innes et al. (1958), who were the first to describe this condition, also found a fragment of hair attached to the wall of the right ventricle in one mouse and in the right atrium of another one.

According to Purkiss (1975), the pulmonary capillaries have a diameter of 7–12 μm, and therefore particles greater than 12 μm in diameter (such as cellulose fibers with average diameter of 20.5 μm) would be trapped in the vascular bed of the lung.

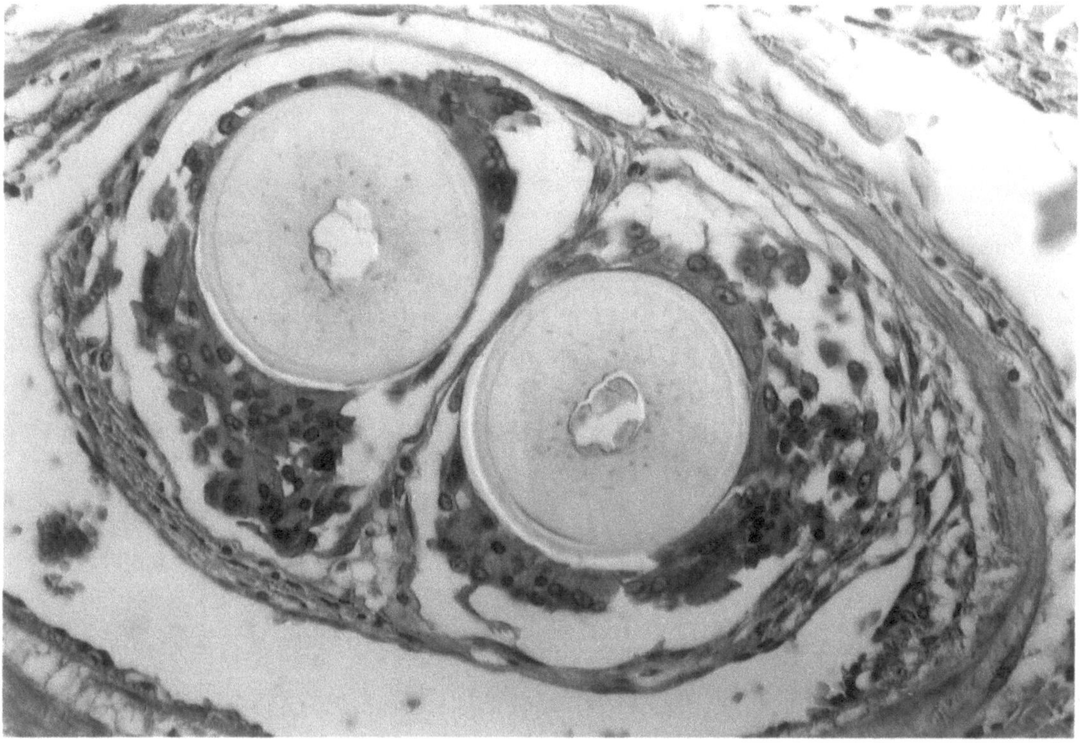

**Fig. 330.** Sections of hair embedded in parietal thrombus in the caudal vein of a male rat. H&E, ×200

However, due to the existence of arteriovenous shunts in the lungs, not all of them are so entrapped. Such shunts should enable the emboli to escape into veins and then into the systemic circulation. In our trials (Tsunenari and Kast 1977) only intravenously injected nylon 12 globules less than 10 μm in diameter have floated with the blood through the lungs into spleen, liver, and kidneys.

In an experimental study of these lesions we prepared a suspension in physiological saline solution containing about 3000 hair particles per milliliter. The hairs were taken from the backs of rats and cut into about 10-μm lengths using a cryostat (Tsunenari and Kast 1977). We injected into caudal veins of each of 50 male Sprague-Dawley rats a single dose of 0.25 ml of this rat's hair suspension for each 100 g body weight (low dose). A second group of 50 males were each given 0.75 ml/100 g body weight (high dose). Ten rats of each group were killed on days 3, 7, 14, 21, and 28 after treatment and examined histologically.

The development during the first 3 days of pulmonary granulomas that result from hair emboli after intravenous injection has not been described. Therefore, a quotation from Johnston et al. (1981) in studies of pulmonary embolism in the rat produced by cotton fibers is of interest: "Within an hour the fibres become covered by platelets and plasma proteins and neutrophil polymorphs are attracted around them. By 2 hours macrophages congregate around the emboli and, with accumulation of epitheloid cells, granulomas are formed. By 16 hours these have increased in size with the appearance of foreign body giant cells, and reach their maximum size in 3 days."

In our experiments the frequency of embolic hair fragments in lungs was dose-dependent, and most of the fragments were observed in the groups killed 3 days after the injection. The fragments at this time were located in arteries or alveolar capillaries with little adjacent leukocytic reaction, including eosinophils, but in several cases the hair fragments were already surrounded by multinucleated giant cells (Fig. 331). Giant cells sometimes appeared to originate from the endothelium of the involved capillaries.

After 7 days phagocytosis of the bits of hair is complete (Fig. 332). During the following weeks the granulomas decline in size, the hair particles and giant cells disappear gradually, and finally after 28 days the lungs are essentially free of lesions

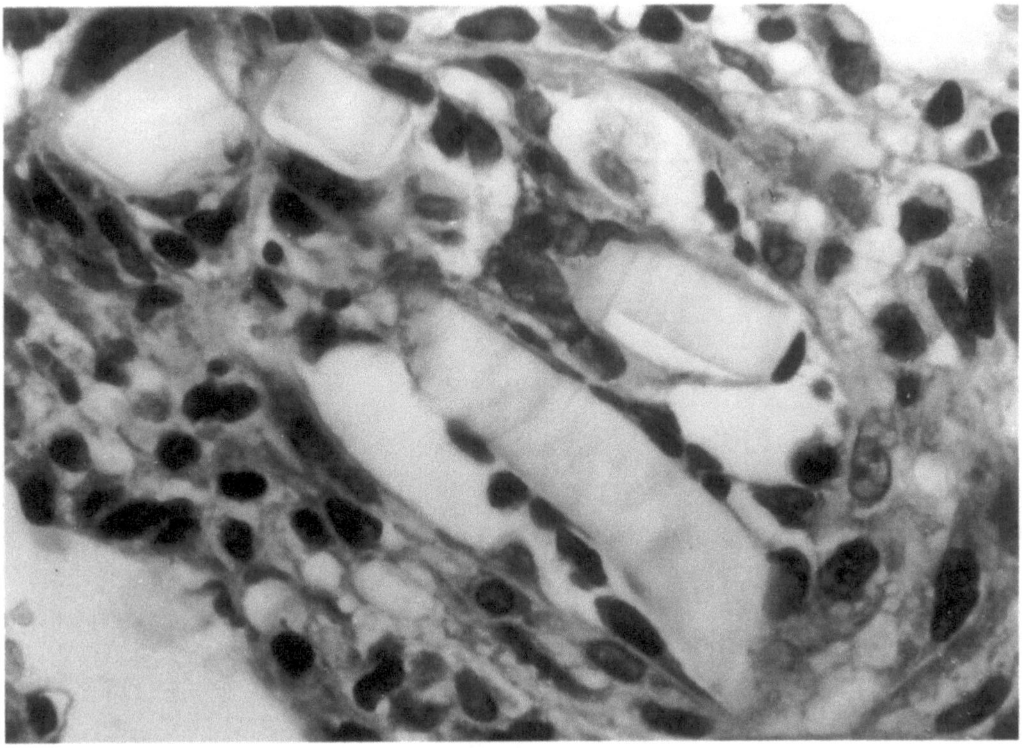

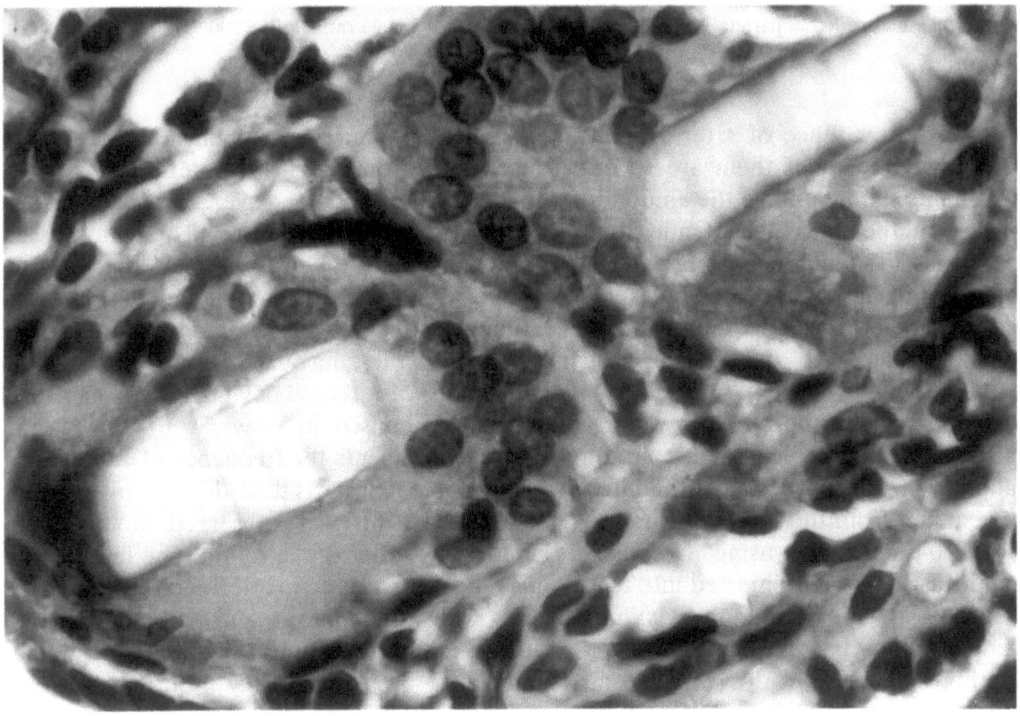

**Fig. 331.** (*above*) Hair particles in pulmonary alveolus of a male rat 3 days after the intravenous injection of a suspension of ha (for methods see Fig. 333). H&E, ×400

**Fig. 332.** (*below*) Giant cells phagocytosing hair particles in an alveolus 7 days after the intravenous injection. H&E, ×400

(Fig. 333). No hair particles are found in other organs. This confirms the statement of Tekeli (1974), who searched for but did not find keratin, fragments of hair, or hair follicles in the vessels of other organs.

*Frequency.* In our study of 1422 rats that had been injected intravenously with various materials in toxicology tests (Table 30), lesions in the lungs were observed in 381 (27%). These lesions consisted of giant cell granulomas with phagocytosed hair in alveoli and hair-containing thrombi in pulmonary blood vessels (Fig. 326). No differences were attributable to the sex of the animals. The frequency is surprisingly high when one considers that only one cross-section of about 3 μm thickness from one lobe of the lungs was studied in each animal. Schneider and Pappritz (1976) have pointed out that this frequency in such a small random sample of lung indicates the large number of hair particles that must have been injected in the course of the experiments.

Innes et al. (1958) found 22 pulmonary granulomas (28%; six containing foreign bodies) in 80 mice dosed intravenously at different periods of 5–20 days. Yamamoto et al. (1982) treated their 165 rats intravenously for 6 months and observed lesions in 28%, including such histopathological changes such as granuloma (23%), thrombus (18%), giant cells (10%), and arterial abscess

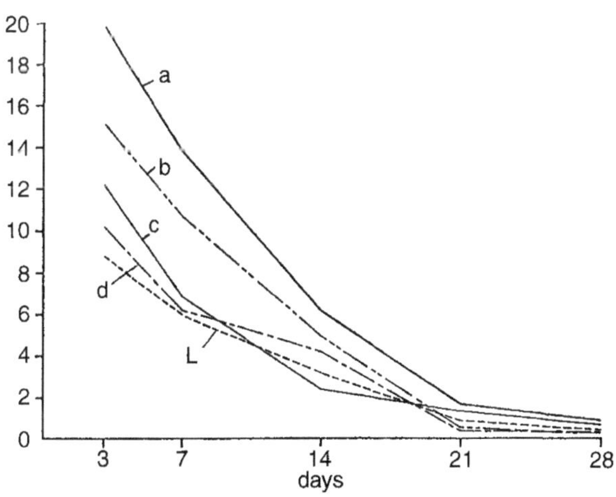


**Fig. 333.** Average number of hair-phagocytosing giant cells in lungs of rats 3, 7, 14, 21, and 28 days after a single intravenous injection (0.75 ml/100 g body weight) of a suspension containing about 3000 hair particles per milliliter cut at about 10 μm length. Right lung: *a*, apical lobe; *b*, cardiac lobe; *c*, diaphragmatic lobe; and *d*, azygos lobe. *L*, Left lung. (From Tsunenari and Kast 1977)

(4%). Tekeli (1974) has seen pulmonary embolism after 7–30 days of treatment in 26 of his 120 rats (22%).

No difference has been demonstrated in the frequency of pulmonary embolism between carrier-treated controls and test animals given various doses of injectable solutions (Innes et al. 1958; Liehn and Dahme 1975; Yamamoto et al. 1982; Kast and Tsunenari 1983). The more often the animals have been injected, the more numerous are the lesions (Innes et al. 1958); however, reparability of the lesions must be taken into consideration.

*Reparability.* In our experiments with the injection of hair suspensions (Tsunenari and Kast 1977) phagocytosis was observed rapidly progressing to nearly complete removal of the embolic hair particles within 4 weeks (Fig. 333). However, in our subacute toxicity studies, phagocytosis and removal of hairs inoculated through a needle into caudal veins was not complete after 6 weeks of recovery. The number of hair particles remaining in the lungs was significant (Table 31, Fig. 334). This suggests differences in the condition of immunity in individual rats. However, the effects are similar when different suspensions are used, one containing the rat's own hair and another made up of foreign hairs (Kast and Tsunenari 1983). It is possible that the hair of the back of the rat, used in our experiments, is more easily phagocytosed than the caudal (tail) bristles with their thicker cortex. According to Liehn and Dahme (1975), pulmonary hair emboli disappear within 8–10 weeks after the final intravenous injection.

Contrary to the views of Hottendorf and Hirth (1974) and Schneider and Pappritz (1976), who believe that the risk is minor if the hairs at the injection site are carefully clipped and the injection is carried out with care, we agree with other authors that no matter how carefully the intravenous injection is performed, pulmonary pathological changes are inevitable results of intravenous injection.

## Comparison with Other Species

Three single observations of skin embolism in humans have been published by Hirst and Toyama, (1968), Andrew (1976), and Gilbert and Borchard (1980). The skin particles in these cases were believed to have been punched out by puncture of

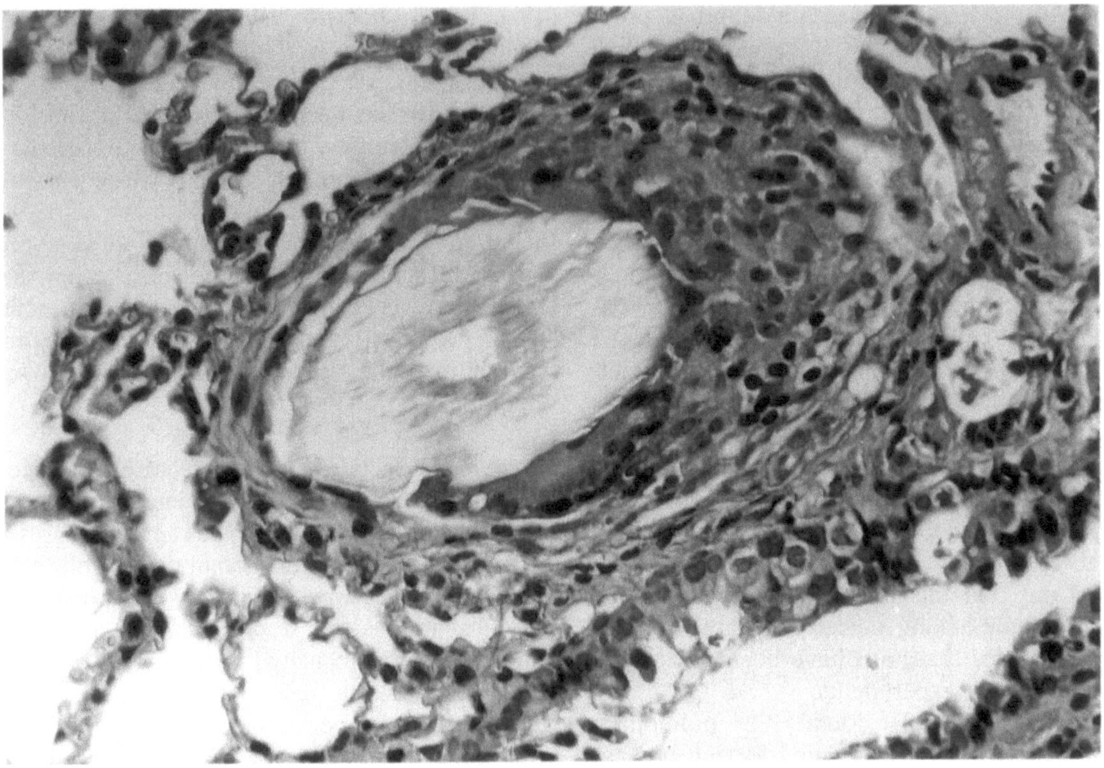

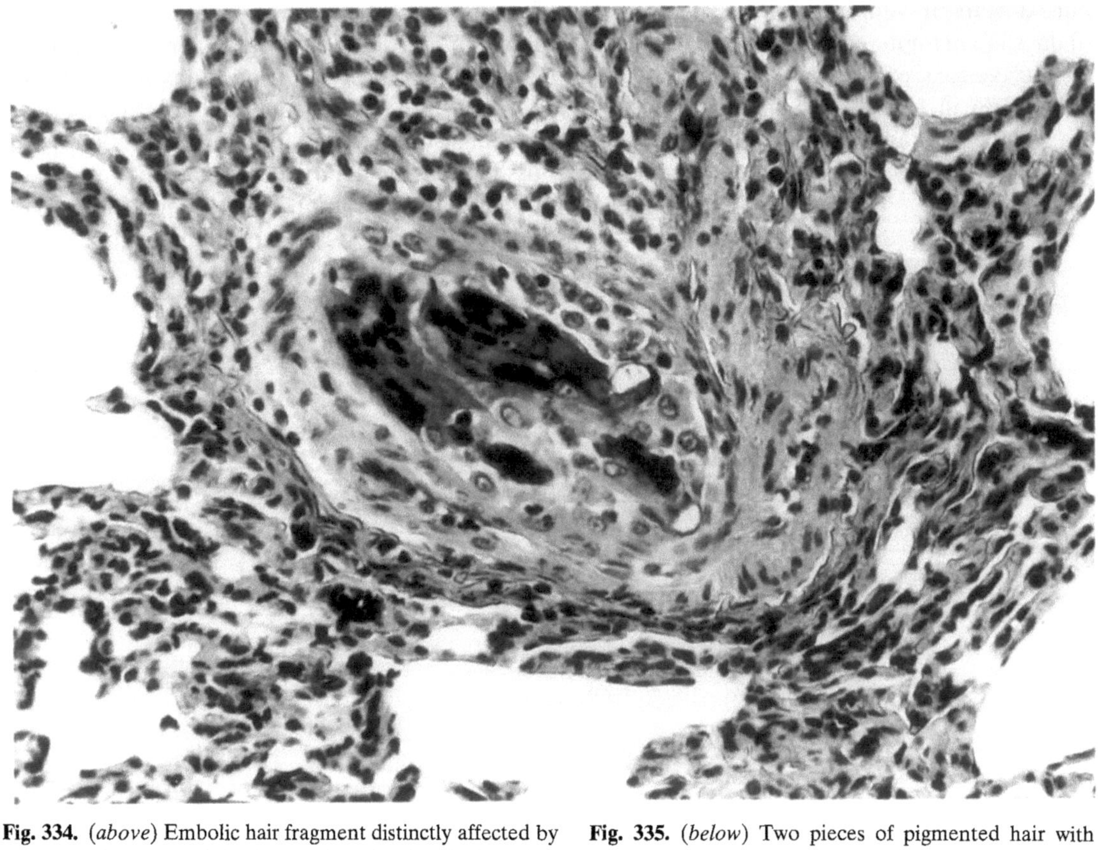

**Fig. 334.** (*above*) Embolic hair fragment distinctly affected by phagocytosis but remaining in lung 6 weeks after the last of 28 daily intravenous injections, male rat. H&E, ×200

**Fig. 335.** (*below*) Two pieces of pigmented hair with small medulla cells in a thrombotic pulmonary artery of a female rhesus monkey given 28 daily injections into cephalic or saphenous veins. Masson's trichrome, ×200

**Table 31.** Lesions in tail veins and lungs of 90 Sprague-Dawley rats injected intravenously daily for 28 days and allowed to recover for 6 weeks (from Kast and Tsunenari 1983)

| Organ | Finding | Males ($n$ = 47) | | Females ($n$ = 43) | |
|---|---|---|---|---|---|
| | | Mean ± SD[a] | Total (%) | Mean ± SD[a] | Total (%) |
| Tail veins | Total | 3.60 ± 1.52 | 18 (38.3) | 3.20 ± 1.92 | 16 (37.2) |
| | Bleeding | 0 | 0 (0) | 0 | 0 (0) |
| | Periphlebitis | 0.40 ± 0.55 | 2 (4.3) | 0 | 0 (0) |
| | Phlebitis | 1.00 ± 1.22 | 5 (10.6) | 0.80 ± 1.30 | 4 (9.3) |
| | Swelling of intima | 0.40 ± 0.55 | 2 (4.3) | 0.40 ± 0.55 | 2 (4.7) |
| | Hair in vessel wall | 1.40 ± 1.34 | 7 (14.9) | 1.40 ± 1.14 | 7 (16.3) |
| | Thrombophlebitis | 1.80 ± 1.79 | 9 (19.1) | 1.60 ± 1.52 | 8 (18.6) |
| | With hair | 0.60 ± 0.55 | 3 (6.4) | 0.80 ± 1.10 | 4 (9.3) |
| Lungs | Total | 0.80 ± 0.84 | 4 (8.5) | 0.20 ± 0.45 | 1 (2.3) |
| | Thromboarteritis | | | | |
| | With hair particle | None | | | |
| | With skin particle | | | | |
| | Giant cell granuloma[b] | 0.80 ± 0.84 | 4 (8.5) | 0.20 ± 0.45 | 1 (2.3) |
| | With hair particle | 0.40 ± 0.55 | 2 (4.3) | 0.20 ± 0.45 | 1 (2.3) |
| | With skin particle | None | | | |

[a] Mean mumber of lesions in each group of 10 rats excluding animals which did not receive all 28 injections.
[b] In alveolar capillaries or alveoli.

the cephalic vein or heart and carried by the blood to the lungs. Favara and Moores (1991) reported 14 cases of pulmonary embolism among 64 autopsies after cardiac surgery or catheterization in a pediatric hospital. After pathogenetic intervals of 2 days–8 weeks hair was found to be the embolic material in six cases. A similar but very rare finding is known in human pathology: after amniotic fluid embolism, small lanugo hairs of the human fetus are occasionally found in capillaries of maternal lungs (Scotti 1966; Adamsons et al. 1971; Morgan 1979; Rossi et al. 1989). The meconium aspiration syndrome with multinucleated giant cells phagozytosing squamous cells or keratin in the lung is also common in calves (Lopez and Bildfell 1992).

According to Schneider and Pappritz (1976), the dermal fibrosis at the point of repeated injections in beagle dogs (cephalic vein) forces many hair roots into deeper skin layers, making them more vulnerable for an excision by the needle and transfer into the puncture channel or the vein wall.

**Table 32.** Lesions in cephalic or saphenous veins and lungs of monkeys following daily intravenous injections for 28 days

| Organ | Finding | Males ($n$ = 92) | | Females ($n$ = 92) | |
|---|---|---|---|---|---|
| | | Mean ± SD[a] | Total (%) | Mean ± SD[a] | Total (%) |
| Veins | Total | 10.8 ± 1.5 | 84 (91.3) | 10.7 ± 1.7 | 83 (90.2) |
| | Bleeding | 9.0 ± 1.9 | 70 (75.0) | 9.2 ± 2.7 | 72 (78.3) |
| | Periphlebitis | 7.6 ± 1.8 | 60 (64.1) | 7.3 ± 2.9 | 57 (62.0) |
| | Phlebitis | 1.2 ± 1.6 | 9 (9.8) | 0.4 ± 0.7 | 3 (3.3) |
| | Swelling of intima | 1.0 ± 1.3 | 8 (8.7) | 0.7 ± 0.9 | 5 (5.4) |
| | Thrombophlebitis[b] | 0.7 ± 0.6 | 5 (5.4) | 0.8 ± 1.0 | 6 (6.5) |
| Lungs | Total | 0.9 ± 1.0 | 7 (7.6) | 0.9 ± 1.1 | 7 (7.6) |
| | Thromboarteritis | 0.4 ± 0.7 | 3 (3.3) | 0.1 ± 0.4 | 1 (1.1) |
| | Giant cell grannloma | 0.5 ± 0.8 | 4 (4.3) | 0.8 ± 0.9 | 6 (6.5) |

[a] Mean of 12 monkeys per study, excluding animals which did not receive 28 injections.
[b] Excluding five substance-related cases of each gender in study 7.

These authors identified hair particles within the arteries in 10 of their 30 dogs (33%) treated over 4 weeks.

In the studies of Hottendorf and Hirth (1974) eight of 67 beagles (12%) had granulomas in small pulmonary arteries. Among 64 Himalayan rabbits treated intravenously over 4 weeks, Kast and Tsunenari (1983) discovered five giant cell granulomas, two arterial thrombi (Fig. 327), and one fat cell embolus of the lungs (13%).

Of 184 rhesus and cynomolgus monkeys treated daily for 28 consecutive days by injection into cephalic or saphenous veins, 14 (7.6%) had pulmonary emboli with fragments of skin or hair in arterial thrombi (Fig. 335) or in giant cell granulomas. In 167 monkeys (91%) there were lesions at the site of injection, predominantly bleeding and chronic periphlebitis, whereas particles of skin or hair were rare around the veins (2.2%; Table 32). At 2 or 8 weeks after cessation of treatment no pulmonary lesions were observed, and healing at the sites of injection was nearly completed in 11 of 12 monkeys allowed to recover (Kast 1994). Recently, the author compared the findings at the site of injection and the skin emboli in lungs of rat, rabbit and monkey. Differences between rat and monkey may be essentially related to the anatomy of skin (Kast, 1995).

## References


Adamsons K, Mueller-Heubach E, Myers RE (1971) The innocuousness of amniotic fluid infusion in the pregnant rhesus monkey. Am J Obstet Gynecol 109:977–984

Andrew JH (1976) Pulmonary skin embolism: a case report. Pathology 8:185–187

Bowden DH (1971) The alveolar macrophage. Curr Top Pathol 55:1–36

Easton TW (1952) The role of macrophage movements in the transport and elimination of intravenous thorium dioxide in mice. Am J Anat 90:1–33

Favara B, Moores H (1991) Foreign-body pulmonary embolism. Pediatric Path 11:371–379

Flodh H, Magnusson G, Magnusson O (1974) Pulmonary foam cells in rats of different age. Z Versuchstierkd 16:299–312

Garvan JM, Gunner BW (1964) The harmful effects of particles in intravenous fluids. Med J Aust 51:1–6

Giese W (1974) Akute interstitielle Pneumonien. In: Doerr W (ed) Organpathologie, vol 1. Thieme, Stuttgart, chap 3

Gilbert P, Borchard F (1980) Hautembolie der Lunge. Pathologe 1:161–163

Hirst AE, Toyama M (1968) Skin embolism to the lung. JAMA 205:54

Hottendorf GH, Hirth RS (1974) Lesions of spontaneous subclinical disease in beagle dogs. Vet Pathol 11:240–258

Innes JRM, Donati EJ, Yevich PP (1958) Pulmonary lesions in mice due to fragments of hair, epidermis and extraneous matter accidentally injected in toxicity experiments. Am J Pathol 34:161–167

Johnston WH, Waisman J (1971) Pulmonary corn starch granulomas in a drug user. Arch Pathol 92:196–202

Johnston B, Smith P, Heath D (1981) Experimental cottonfibre pulmonary embolism in the rat. Thorax 36:910–916

Kast A (1994) Pulmonary hair embolism in monkeys. Exp Tox Path 46:183–188

Kast A (1995) Pulmonary embolism of skin and hair particles following intravenous injection. Berl Münch Tierärztl Wschr 108:61–65

Kast A, Tsunenari Y (1983) Hair embolism in lungs of rat and rabbit caused by intravenous injection. Lab Anim 17:203–207

Liehn HD, Dahme E (1975) Mikroembolische Lungenveränderungen bei Versuchstieren nach intravenöser Applikation. Med Int Congr. Proceedings of the European Society of Toxicology, Series no 345:319–323

Lopez A, Bildfell R (1992) Pulmonary inflammation associated with aspirated meconium and epithelial cells in calves. Vet Path 29:104–111

Morgan M (1979) Amniotic fluid embolism. Anaesthesia 34:20–32

Purkiss R (1975) Effects and distribution of intravenously administered cellulose particles in mice. J Pharm Pharmacol 27:290–292

Rossi E, Philipson E, Williams T, Kalhan S (1989) Meconium aspiration syndrom: intrapartum and neonatal attributes. Am J Obstet Gynecol 161:1106–1110

Sahu AP, Dogra RK, Shanker R, Zaidi S (1975) Fibrogenic response in murine lungs to asbestos. Exp Pathol 11:21–24

Schneider P, Pappritz G (1976) Hairs causing pulmonary emboli. A rare complication in long-term intravenous studies in dogs. Vet Pathol 13:394–400

Scotti TM (1966) Disturbance of body water and electrolytes, and of circulation of blood. In: Anderson W (ed) Pathology (Asian edition). Mosby, St. Louis, chap 4

Sedlmeier H, Schiefer B (1971) Entzündungen der Lunge. In: Dobberstein J, Pallaske G, Stuenzi H (eds) Handbuch der speziellen pathologischen Anatomie der Haustiere, vol 7. Parey, Berlin

Simpson M (1922) The experimental production of macrophages in the circulating blood. J Med Res 43:77–144

Tekeli S (1974) Occurrence of hair-fragment emboli in the pulmonary vascular system of rats. Vet Pathol 11:482–485

Tomashefski JF Jr, Hirsch CS, Jolly PN (1981) Microcrystalline cellulose pulmonary embolism and granulomatosis. Arch Pathol Lab Med 105:89–93

Tsunenari Y, Kast A (1977) Hair embolism in lungs of rat after intravenous injection into caudal veins. Arzneim Forsch 27:1979–1982

Yamamoto H, Imai S, Okuyama T, Tsubura Y (1982) Pulmonary lesions in rats caused by intravenous injection. Acta Pathol Jpn 32:741–747

Zientara M, Moore S (1970) Fatal talc embolism in a drug addict. Hum Pathol 1:324–327

# Goblet Cell Metaplasia, Lung, Rat

Birgit Kittel

## Gross Appearance

Goblet cell metaplasia arise in peripheral or central regions of the lung parenchyma, and only larger lesions reaching sizes of several millimeters in diameter are detected grossly if they expand subpleurally. They appear as opaque areas with a sometimes slightly raised surface due to the accumulation of mucus. Because of this inconspicuous appearance they usually escape macroscopic detection and are found only during histological examination.

## Microscopic Features

In chronically altered, particle-exposed lungs initial minimal goblet cell metaplasia is easily overlooked due to multifocal bronchioloalveolar hyperplasia and inflammation present in these lungs. These small lesions are limited to single alveoli, which are covered by one layer of distended, sometimes hypertrophic goblet cells (Fig. 336). The alveolar lumina are filled with clear, sometimes pale eosinophilic mucus originating from these cells. Mucus in goblet cells and free in alveoli is positive in the periodic acid–Schiff (PAS) reaction and in the Alcian blue stain. Application of these methods also enhances the detection of minimal goblet cell metaplasia in chronically altered lungs.

Larger foci of goblet cell metaplasia can reach sizes of up to 20mm. They are easily detected by histological examination but can be mistaken for a neoplastic lesion (Fig. 337). These focally prominent goblet cell metaplasias are often located in central areas of the lung close to or in continuity with airways, but have also been observed in the peripheral lung tissue without obvious connection to bronchi or bronchioles.

The lesion is typically composed of a small peripheral rim with epithelial lining and an inner mucus filled area.

The periphery appears as a collection of alveoli which are distended and sometimes have an opening through which the content flows into adjacent alveoli (Fig. 338). The epithelium predominantly consists of a single layer of well-differentiated columnar or cuboidal goblet cells (Fig. 339) with a basally situated nucleus and basophilic cytoplasm; apically it appears light in H&E stains due to the accumulation of numerous secretory granules. The mitotic rate is very low, and atypia is absent. In particle-exposed lungs fibrosis and chronic inflammation are prominent features that frequently occur in this localization (Fig. 338). Other epithelial elements of bronchioloalveolar hyperplasia, such as ciliated or nonciliated epithelium, can also be found in the peripheral lining of goblet cell lesions. An accumulation of mucus in dilated air spaces may cause minimal compression of adjacent alveoli.

In the central area the most prominent element is mucus, which fills the preexisting airspaces and seems to be entrapped by the peripheral rim of epithelium (Fig. 340). The central alveolar epithelium appears to be reduced to a thin fibrotic stroma, where hemorrhage and interstitial inflammation are observed. Hyperplastic or metaplastic epithelium is normally not found in these central regions, but islets of metaplastic goblet cells can be found in transitional areas close to the periphery.

## Differential Diagnosis

Small goblet cell metaplasia must be differentiated from bronchioloalveolar hyperplasia, where only insignificant amounts of goblet cells may be present, and intraluminal mucus is absent. Focally prominent goblet cell metaplasia must also be differentiated from mucinous adenomas and mucinous adenocarcinomas (Figs. 341–344). Both lesions are characterized by an increased cellularity of neoplastic cells, the accumulation of mucus, and usually the absence of a clear differentiation between outer (epithelium-lined) and inner (mucus-rich) area. The underlying alveolar architecture is distorted by neoplastic cells. Mucinous adenomas are made up of columnar epithelial cells which may form nests, tubules, or acini occasionally filled with mucus (Figs. 341, 342). Goblet cells are present but less well-differentiated and hypertrophic than in goblet cell metaplasia. Adenomas tend to compress sur-

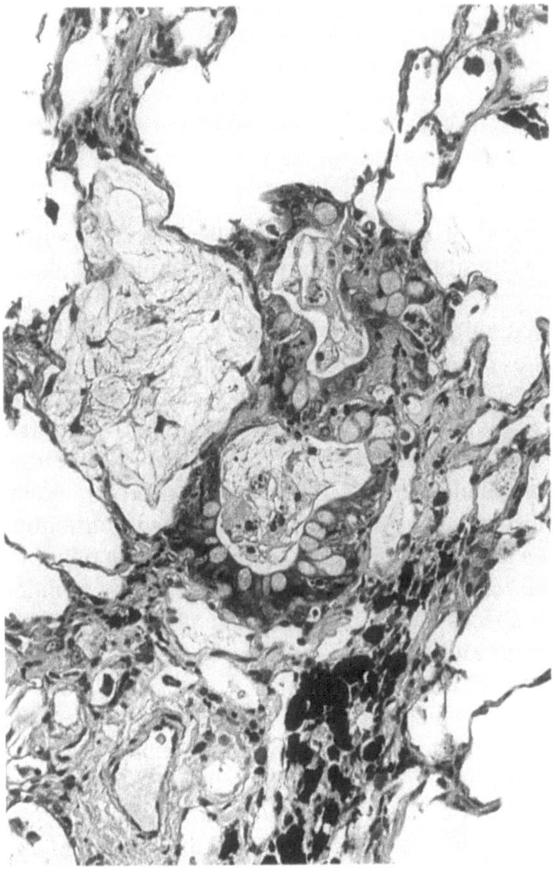
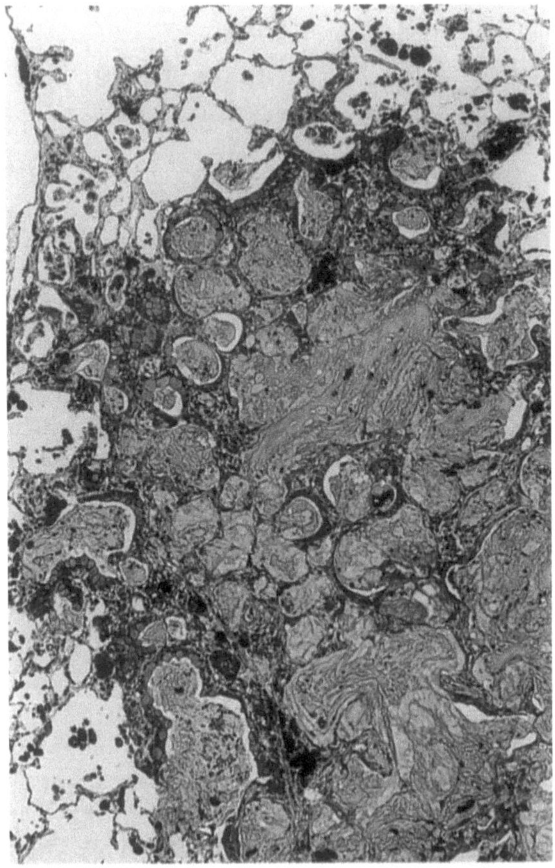
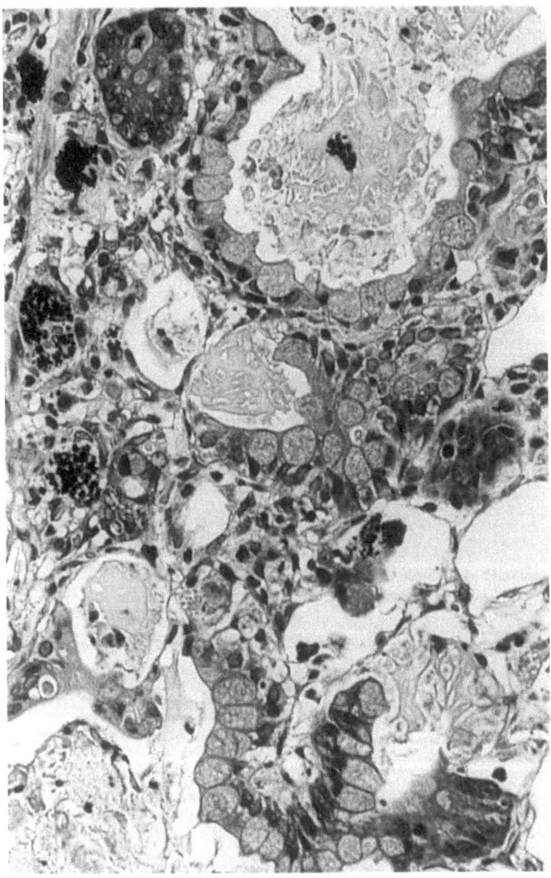
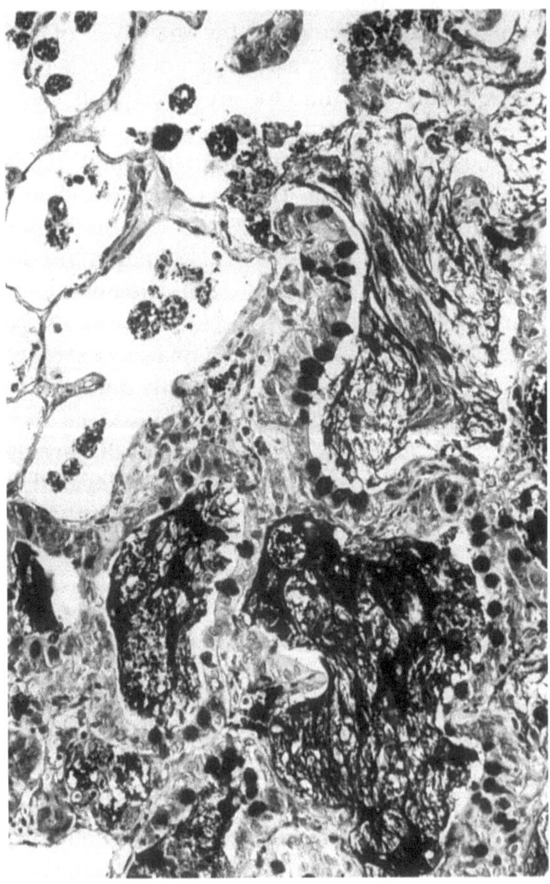

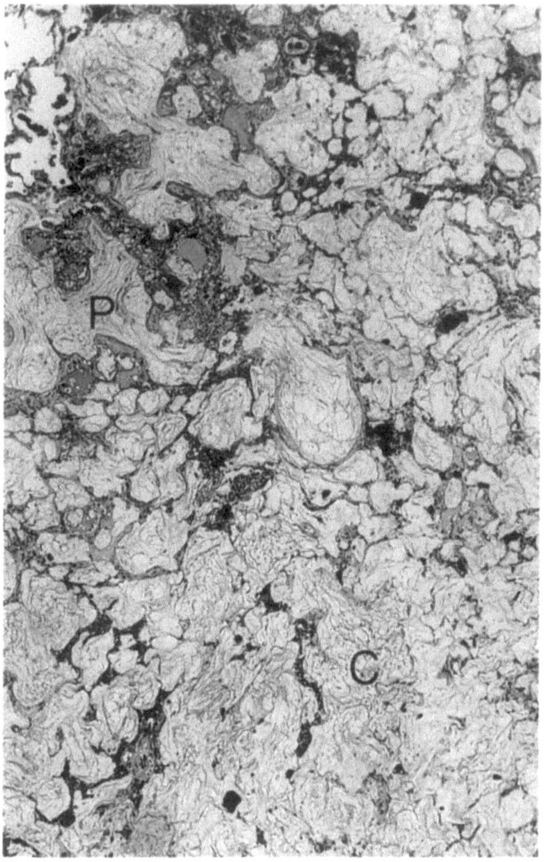


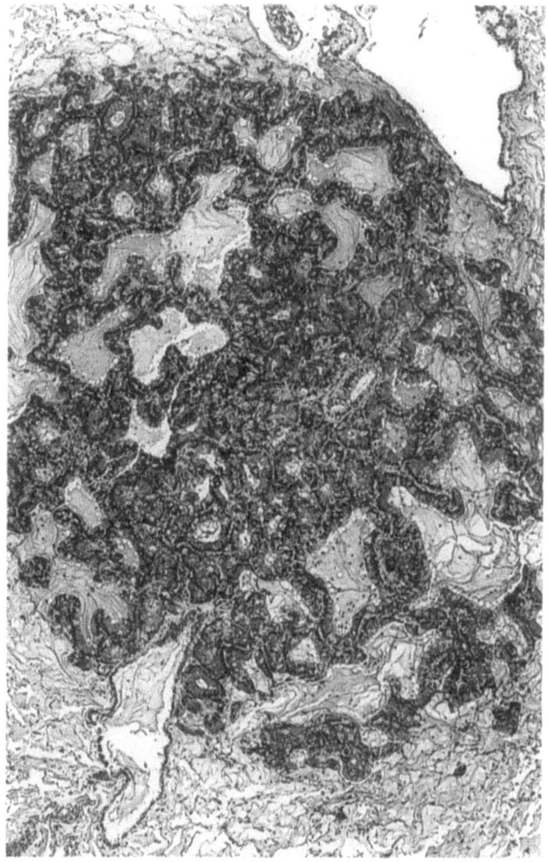

**Fig. 340.** (*upper left*) Center (*C*) of goblet cell metaplasia, characterized predominantly by mucus and sparse alveolar septa. Inflammation and epithelium in the periphery (*P*). H&E, ×100

**Fig. 341.** (*upper right*) Centrally located mucinous adenoma in a Wistar rat. H&E, ×40

**Fig. 342.** (*below*) Mucinous adenoma, lung, Wistar rat. Air spaces lined by one or two layered dense goblet epithelium. Compared to goblet cell metaplasia, the tumor goblet cells are more numerous, smaller and the typical "goblet" shape of secretory granules is absent. Air spaces are filled with mucus. H&E, ×200

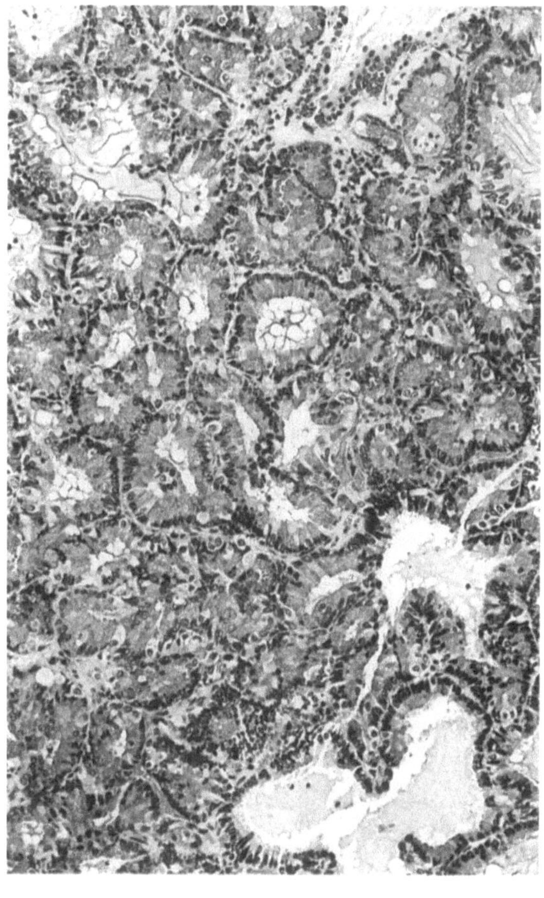

◄

**Fig. 336.** (*upper left*) Minimal focal goblet cell metaplasia comprising a few alveoli in a rat chronically exposed to carbon black particles. Several alveolar lumina are filled with mucus and debris. H&E, ×400

**Fig. 337.** (*upper right*) Focally prominent goblet cell metaplasia in lung of a rat chronically exposed to carbon black particles. Goblet cell metaplasia in continuity with a larger airway. H&E, ×100

**Fig. 338.** (*lower left*) Periphery of goblet cell metaplasia. Dilated air spaces filled with mucus and lined by a single layer of well differentiated goblet cells with prominent secretory granules. Marked inflammatory cell infiltration and particle-laden macrophages. H&E, ×400

**Fig. 339.** (*lower right*) Periphery of goblet cell metaplasia. Single epithelial layer with black appearing PAS-positive granules. Carbon-black laden macrophages are visible in the alveoli. PAS, ×200

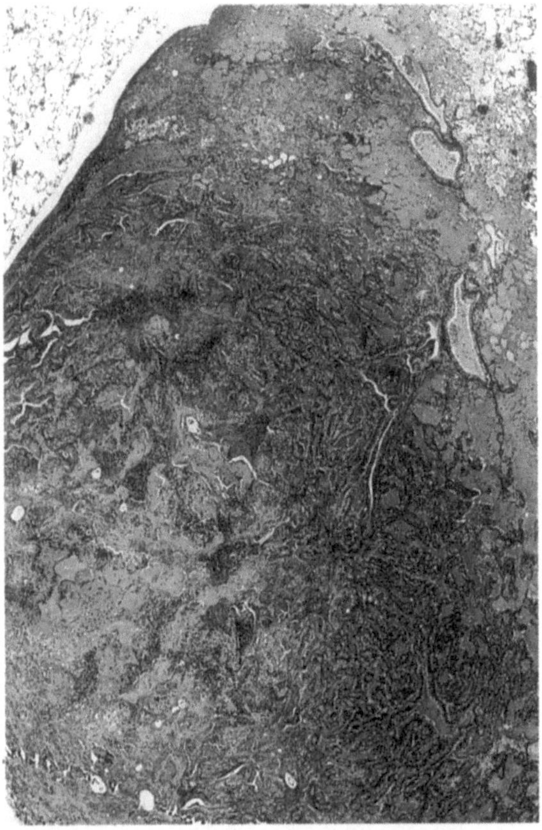

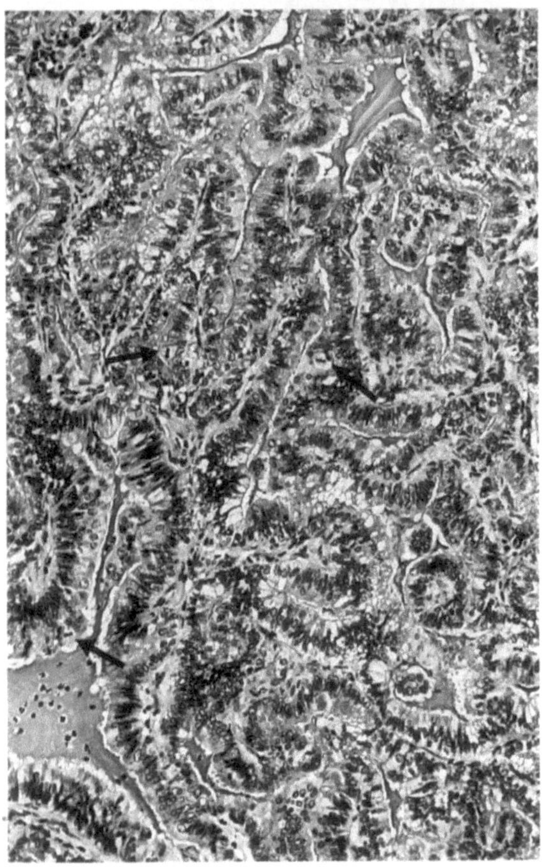

rounding alveoli and may have a thin capsule. In mucinous adenocarcinomas, obvious signs of malignancy are present, such as local invasion into the pleura, mediastinum or bronchiolar walls, numerous mitotic figures, and cellular atypia. Central portions of the tumor may undergo necrosis and fibrosis (Figs. 343, 344).

## Biological Features

*Etiology.* It is presumed that at first a few goblet cells are present which arise from metaplastic alveolar type II or Clara cells (Fig. 336), as goblet cells are normally rare or absent in distal airways of the rat. The mucous product of these goblet cells seems to lead to direct or indirect destruction of the preexisting (central) alveolar epithelium. Eventually even the alveolar septa break down, and only a thin stroma embedded in mucous substance remains. Peripheral parts of the metaplastic epithelium survive, so that the process of mucus production, central epithelial necrosis, and peripheral epithelial metaplasia is self-perpetuating (Fig. 345).

*Frequency.* Goblet cell metaplasia is a rare lesion that in most cases has been observed after chronic exposure to particles (Dungworth et al. 1992; Kittel et al. 1994), chemicals, or after infectious diseases (Boorman and Eustis 1990). The rarity of spontaneous goblet cell metaplasia is evident in the fact that at present in the Hanover Registry of Industrial Toxicology Animal Data database only two cases have been recorded among 5612 male and female control rats.

## Comparison with Other Species

Goblet cell metaplasias have been described in the pulmonary airways of humans and hamsters (Christensen et al. 1977; Karpick et al. 1970; Wang and Ying 1977). To our knowledge, goblet cell metaplasia of the lung tissue has not been described in other rodents. Mucinous

◄

**Fig. 343.** (*above*) Mucinous adenocarcinoma, lung, rat. Large lesion with peripheral compression and central scar. H&E, ×25

**Fig. 344.** (*below*) Mucinous adenocarcinoma, lung, rat. Multilayering, mitoses (arrows) and atypia. H&E, ×400

**Fig. 345.** Possible pathogenesis of goblet cell metaplasia

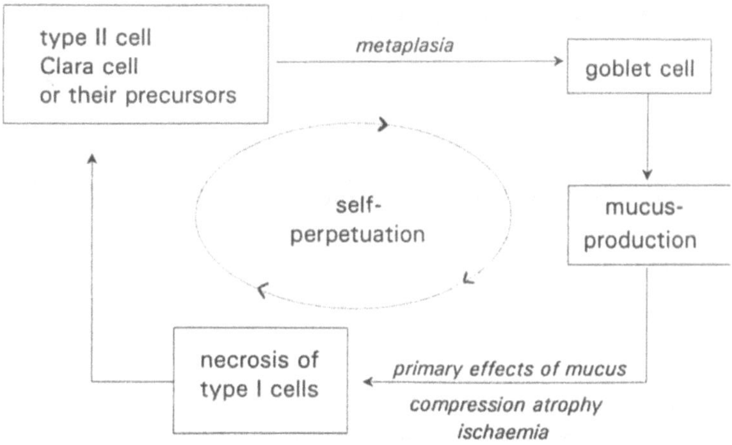


adenocarcinomas, however, have been reported in humans and horses (Higashiyama et al. 1992; Kish et al. 1989; Schultze et al. 1988).

## References

Boorman GA, Eustis SL (1990) Lung. In: Boorman GA, Eustis SL, Elwell MR, Montgomery CA Jr, MacKenzie WF (eds) Pathology of the Fischer rat. Academic, San Diego, pp 339–365

Christensen T, Korthy AL, Snider GL, Hayes JA (1977) Irreversible bronchial goblet cell metaplasia in hamsters with elastase-induced panacinar emphysema. J Clin Invest 59:377–404

Dungworth DL, Hahn FF, Hayashi Y, Keenan K, Mohr U, Rittinghausen S, Schwartz L (1992) Respiratory system. In: Mohr U, Capen CC, Dungworth DL, Griesemer RA, Ito N, Turusov VS (eds) International classification of rodent tumours, part I: the rat. IARC, Lyon (IARC scientific publications no 122)

Higashiyama M, Doi O, Kodama K, Yokouchi H, Tateishi R (1992) Cystic mucinous adenocarcinoma of the lung. Chest 101:763–766

Karpick RJ, Pratt PC, Asmundsson T, Kilburn KH (1970) Pathological findings in respiratory failure. Goblet cell metaplasia, alveolar damage and myocardial infarction. Ann Intern Med 72:189–197

Kish JK, Ro JY, Ayala AG, McMurtrey MJ (1989) Primary mucinous adenocarcinoma of the lung with signet-ring cells. Hum Pathol 20:1097–1102

Kittel B, Dungworth DL, Mohr U (1994) Goblet cell metaplasia in the peripheral lung tissue of rats after chronic exposure to particles. In: Mohr U, Dungworth DL, Mauderly JL, Oberdörster G (eds) Toxic and carcinogenic effects of solid particles in the respiratory tract. ILSI Press, Washington DC, pp 545–548

Schultze AE, Sonea I, Bell TG (1988) Primary malignant pulmonary neoplasia in two horses. J Am Vet Med Assoc 193:477–480

Wang NS, Ying WL (1977) The pattern of goblet cell hyperplasia in human airways. Hum Pathol 8:301–311

# Sendai Virus Infection, Lung, Mouse, and Rat

David G. Brownstein

*Synonyms.* Hemagglutinating virus infection of Japan, Japanese hemagglutinating virus infection, hemagglutinating virus infection of the mouse, parainfluenza virus infection.

### Gross Appearance

*Mice.* Asymptomatic or mildly affected mice usually have no gross pulmonary changes other than increased lung weight, although a few mildly affected mice have prominent bronchioles, and discrete foci of consolidation. Average increases of 50% have been reported by the 5th day and 100% by the 14th day after experimental infection of Swiss mice (Robinson et al. 1968). Overtly ill and genetically susceptible mice have more dramatic increases in lung weights (200%–300%; Parker et al. 1978). In these cases one or more lung lobes are plum-colored or contain sharply demarcated plum-colored foci which exude frothy sanguinous fluid when cut. If these mice survive into the 3rd week, consolidated foci are gray.

Extrapulmonary changes reflect local and systemic activation of the immune system. Regional lymph nodes enlarge during the 2nd week, a change most obvious in the submaxillary lymph nodes. These nodes may triple or quadruple in weight. Splenic enlargement (20%–50% in weight) also occurs during the 2nd week.

*Rats.* Asymptomatic infections are the rule and follow a pattern similar to that described for asymptomatic or mildly affected mice.

### Microscopic Features

*Mice.* Histopathological changes in experimental and natural disease can be divided into: acute phase, characterized by degeneration and necrosis of target epithelium and exudative inflammation; reparative phase, characterized by regeneration of damaged target cells and interstitial inflammation; and resolution phase, characterized by a rapid subsidence of inflammation and repair.

During the *acute phase*, which lasts from 8 to 12 days, there is a descending infection of conducting airway epithelium. This frequently extends to proximal type II and to a lesser degree to type I alveolar epithelium (Brownstein et al. 1981; Parker and Richter 1982; Richter 1970, 1973; Zurcher et al. 1977). The result is acute endobronchitis-bronchiolitis and bronchogenic alveolitis. The earliest airway changes are segmental. Infected bronchiolar epithelial cells are hypertrophied with eosinophilic foamy, granular, or homogeneous cytoplasm. The nuclei of infected cells are poorly polarized and may be enlarged and vesicular. Inflammatory infiltrates appear shortly after these initial cytological changes (Fig. 346). The lamina propria and adventitia are expanded by edema, dilated lymphatics, and cellular infiltrates. Initially these infiltrates are a mixture of polymorphonuclear leukocytes, lymphoid cells with homogeneous amphophilic or eosinophilic cytoplasm, and large round or fusiform lymphoreticular cells. The relative number of each type depends on the age and genetic composition of the host and the dose and route (intranasal versus aerosol) of viral exposure. In genetically susceptible or immature mice neutrophils often predominate as they do after exposure to large doses of virus. Peribronchiolar arterioles and venules have increased intimal cellularity. The endothelium is hypertrophied and elevated by asymmetric accumulations of leukocytes in the subendothelial layer of the intima. There is striking leukocyte pavementing. The adventitia of these vessels is also hypercellular due to leukocytic infiltrates. The adventitia is also expanded by edema.

Cytopathic changes in bronchiolar epithelium are afforded some specificity if syncytia, cytoplasmic inclusions, or intranuclear inclusions are present. The lesions may depend in part on virus and mouse strain.

These changes are usually not seen or are equivocal since infected cells tend to slough prior to their development. Syncytia usually appear as central clusters of condensed or pyknotic epithelial nuclei surrounded by foamy eosinophilic cytoplasm that crowds adjacent cells (Fig. 347). Cytoplasmic inclusions represent aggregates of redundant nucleocapsids within the cytoplasmic matrix (see "Ultrastructure"). They are most obvious as homogeneous spherical or irregular eosinophilic cytoplasmic bodies surrounded by a narrow halo. This halo is a fixation shrinkage artifact. Intranuclear inclusions are rare in Sendai virus infections but intranuclear viral particles have been described in DBA/2 mice (Richter 1970), and intranuclear inclusions have been reported in athymic nude mice (Ward et al. 1976).

Near the end of the acute phase infected epithelium has sloughed in sheets or as individual cells which lie within the lumen along with an inflammatory exudate. Because of the segmental nature of the infection some airways may be devoid of lining cells while others are lined by intact, hypertrophied epithelium. Airways with desquamating epithelium frequently have focally dense lymphoid aggregates within the lamina propria, which cause overlying epithelium to bulge into the lumen.

The alveolar component of the acute phase is characterized by accumulations of polymorphonuclear leukocytes, macrophages, lymphoid cells, and desquamated pneumocytes within alveolar spaces. Alveolar septa are thickened by edema, congested capillaries, and hypertrophied alveolar corner cells. These changes are multifocal, being oriented around infected terminal bronchioles. In severe cases foci of parenchymal inflammation may become confluent, resulting in lobar pneumonia. Alveolar spaces may fill with fibrin or extravasated blood. Foci of emphysema may occur where septal integrity has been destroyed. Near the end of the acute phase fibrin deposits have condensed along denuded alveolar surfaces or as discrete deposits in alveolar spaces. Increased cellularity of thickened alveolar septa is due to accumulating mononuclear cells (Fig. 348). Inflamed alveoli may be partially atelectatic.

The *reparative phase* is heralded by the appearance of regenerating epithelium. This may be seen as early as the 3rd day but does not predominate over degenerative airway changes until days 8–12. Initially, partially denuded airways contain continuous or interrupted patches of low cuboidal, polygonal, or squamous cells with basophilic cytoplasm and large pleomorphic vesicular nuclei which are poorly polarized and contain prominent nucleoli (Fig. 349). Mitotic figures are common in these cells. Once denuded airways are reepithelialized, lining cells become columnar and rapidly assume a normal mucociliary appearance. Sessile or pedunculated airway excrescences are extremely common during the reparative phase. These may be composed solely of epithelium or have cores of lymphoreticular cells or fibroblasts. These are ephemeral structures and are rarely seen after the 3rd week. It is common during this phase for terminal bronchioles to be lined by nonkeratinizing stratified squamous epithelium. The metaplastic epithelial cells most closely resemble spinous cells, although intercellular bridges are usually difficult to identify. The adventitia and lamina propria of segments undergoing repair are less edematous than in the acute phase, and are densely infiltrated with lymphocytes and plasma cells. The intimal cellularity of pulmonary arterioles and venules seen during the acute phase is usually absent in the reparative phase, but adventitial infiltrates of lymphocytes and plasma cells are prominent.

During the reparative phase alveolar inflammation shifts from the airspaces to the interstitium. Two forms of alveolar repair are recognized. In the first form septa are lined by cuboidal epithelium (adenomatous hyperplasia, alveolar bronchiolization, alveolar epithelialization; Fig. 350). These epithelial cells are initially undifferentiated but soon differentiate into pneumocytes or ciliated, mucous, or Clara cells. In the second form of repair sheets and nests of metaplastic squamous epithelium fill alveolar spaces (Fig. 351). There is partial or total atelectasis of affected alveoli during this phase. If fibrin has been deposited it undergoes lysis or organization. Macrophages surround and infiltrate large fibrin deposits. Plump fibroblasts may also traverse these deposits. During the 3rd week collagen bundles can be identified in organizing fibrin depositis. The reparative phase is usually complete by the end of the 3rd week.

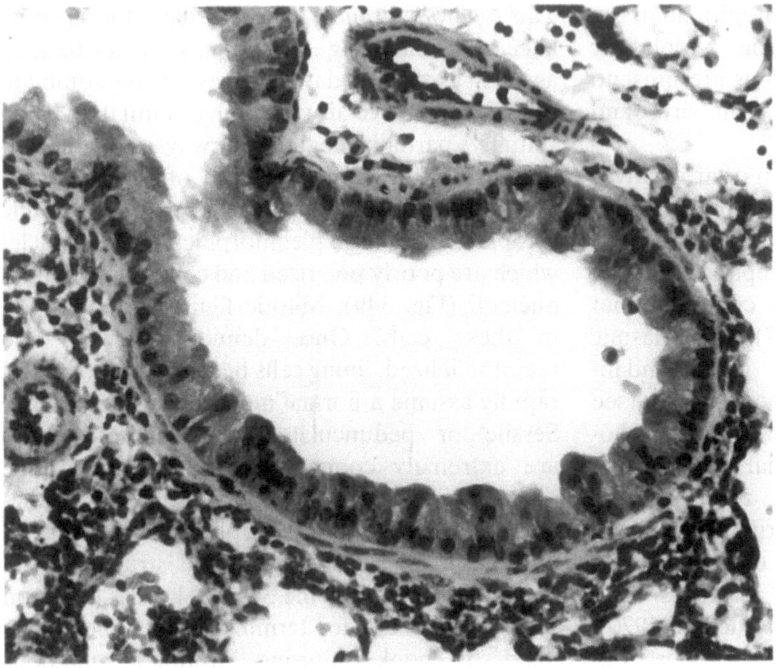

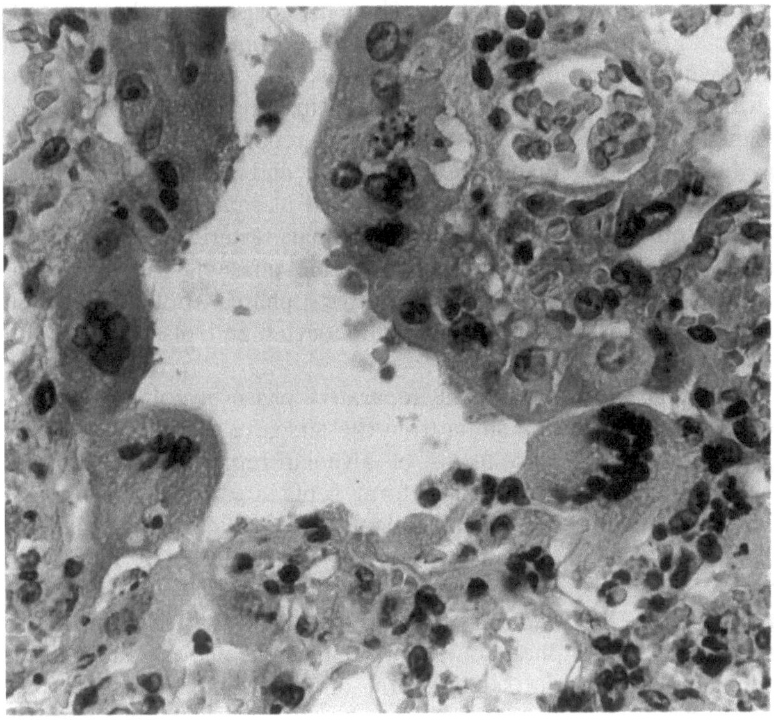

**Fig. 346.** (*above*) Sendai virus infection, acute phase. Bronchiolar epithelium is hypertrophied with some loss of nuclear polarity. The adventitia is edematous and infiltrated with lymphoid cell. H&E, ×354

**Fig. 347.** (*below*) Sendai virus infection, acute phase. Bronchiole with multiple epithelial syncytia. H&E, ×791

The *resolution phase* may be as short as 1 week, so that by the end of the 4th week residual lesions are difficult to identify. There are, however, several changes which may persist for long periods. The most severe sequela, and one that may persist for the life of the animal, is organizing alveolitis with or without bronchiolitis fibrosa obliterans (Fig. 352). This change is the end result of the organiza-

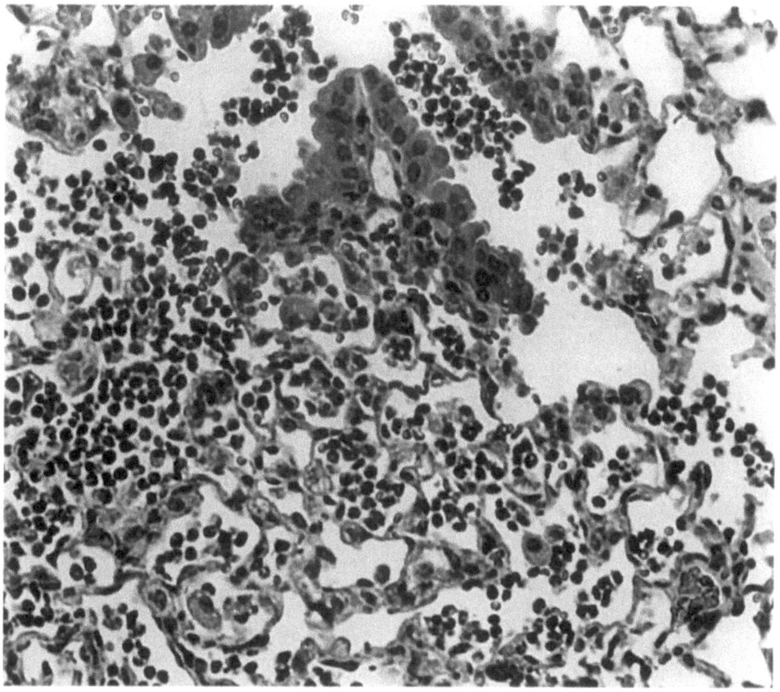

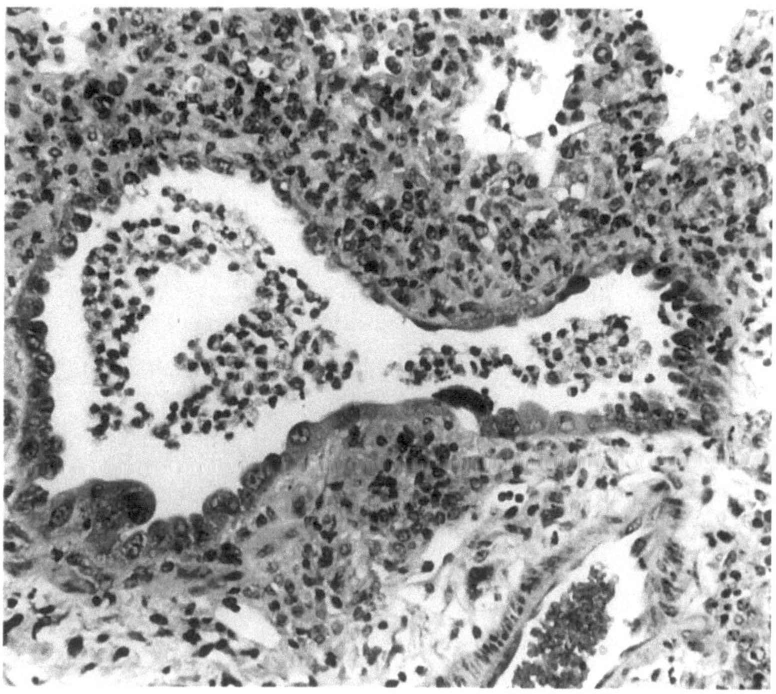

**Fig. 348.** (*above*) Sendai virus infection, acute phase. Alveoli radiating from an infected terminal bronchiole contain a mixed inflammatory exudate. Alveolar septa are edematous and infiltrated with mononuclear cells. H&E, ×345

**Fig. 349.** (*below*) Sendai virus infection, reparative phase. Bronchiole with disorganized regenerating epithelium. Nuclei are pleomorphic and vesicular with prominent nucleoli. H&E, ×245

tion of extensive fibrin deposits in denuded alveoli and terminal airways. Sheets of haphazardly arranged collagen bundles and fibroblasts in natural infections may obliterate parenchymal architecture or may fill alveolar spaces, leaving parenchymal architecture intact. Other residual lesions include foci of emphysema containing inspissated secretions, cholesterol crystals, and

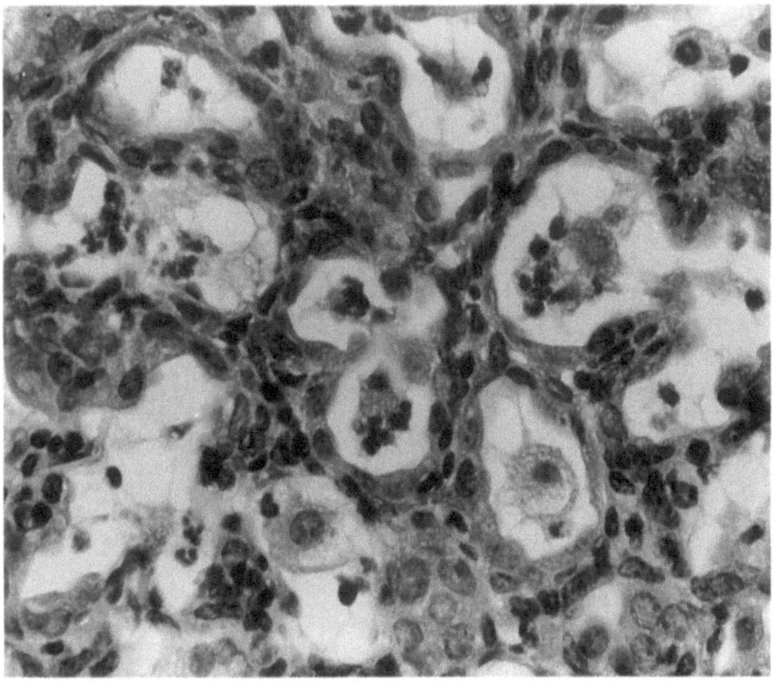

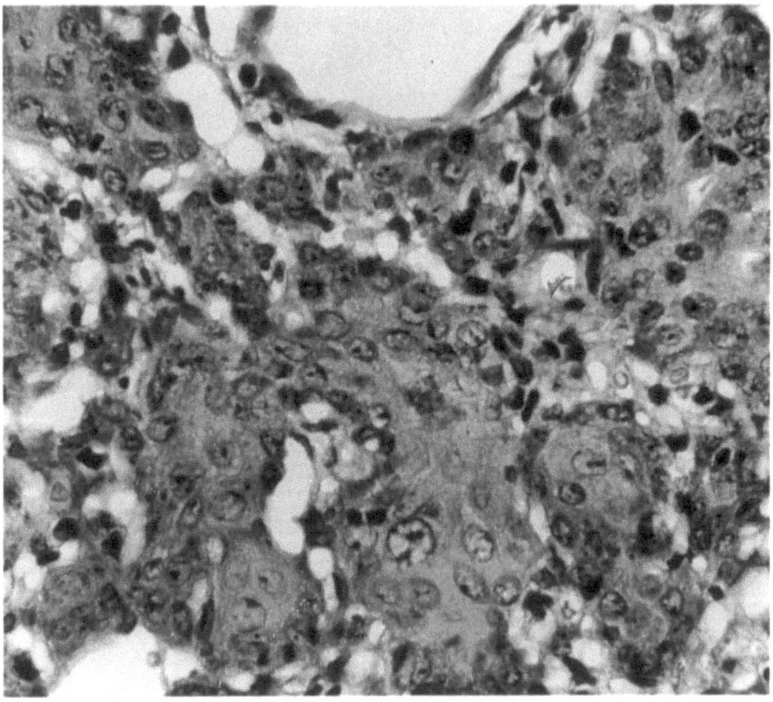

**Fig. 350.** (*above*) Sendai virus infection, reparative phase. Alveoli are lined by cuboidal epithelium and septa are infiltrated with lymphoid cells. H&E, ×600

**Fig. 351.** (*below*). Sendai virus infection, reparative phase. Alveolar squamous metaplasia. H&E, ×600

macrophages; focal aggregates of foamy, alveolar macrophages; focal thickening of alveolar septa; focal adenomatous hyperplasia of alveoli; and perivascular and peribronchiolar lymphoplasmacytic infiltrates. These changes have been identified in mice up to 1 year after infection with Sendai virus (Appel et al. 1971; Parker and Richter 1982; Robinson et al. 1968).

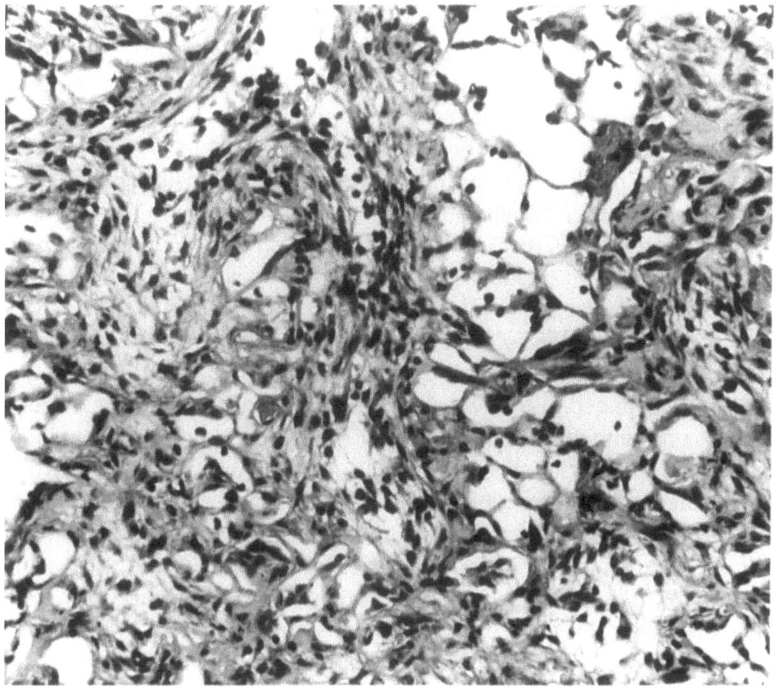

**Fig. 352.** Sendai virus infection, resolution phase. Organizing alveolitis. H&E, ×244

Athymic nude mice, unlike euthymic mice, develop progressive lung changes due to persistent infection with Sendai virus (Iwai et al. 1979; Ward et al. 1976). Pulmonary changes are most often diffuse due to extensive parenchymal involvement. Alveolar septa are thickened by edema, neutrophils, and macrophages. Alveolar epithelialization is striking and squamous metaplasia is prominent in some cases. Bronchiolar epithelium is hyperplastic with numerous mitotic figures. Airways may be filled with neutrophils. Lymphoid infiltrates are usually sparse.

*Rats.* Information on the microscopic appearance of Sendai virus induced lung lesions in rats is limited. Lesions in a colony of mixed rat strains that develop antibodies to Sendai virus have been reported but virus isolation was not attempted (Burek et al. 1977). These rats had mild to severe peribronchial and perivascular cuffing by lymphocytes and plasma cells, and interstitial pneumonia. Bronchiolar epithelium was hyperplastic and focally ulcerated. Unfortunately, the rats also developed antibodies to pneumonia virus of mice. In the author's experience this virus is capable of producing inflammatory lung disease in the rat. Necrotizing bronchitis has been reported in germ-free rats inoculated intranasally with Sendai virus (Jacoby et al. 1979).

## Ultrastructure

Limited ultrastructural pathology has been reported of experimental and spontaneous Sendai virus infections in euthymic mice (Brownstein et al. 1981; Parker and Richter 1982; Richter 1970, 1973; Zurcher et al. 1977). The ultrastructure of naturally infected athymic nude mice has also been reported (Ward et al. 1976). The primary site of replication is the epithelium of bronchi and bronchioles, and it is within ciliated and Clara cells that ultrastructural evidence of replication is most easily seen. Nucleocapsid assembly occurs in the cytosol at a rate far in excess of the rate of virus assembly. The result is massive accumulations of nucleocapsids, which appear as poorly delineated aggregates or crystalline arrays of rigid hollow fibrils 16–18 nm in diameter. Intranuclear aggregates of similar-appearing fibrils have been reported, and these apparently correspond to the intranuclear inclusions seen by light microscopy. The significance of these aggregates is not known; they are rare and appear late in infection, suggesting that they are transported from sites of synthesis in the cytosol (Choppin and Compans 1975). Nucleocapsids align beneath modified segments of plasma membrane to initiate exotrophy. These modified segments are thickened by glycoprotein surface spikes and an electron-dense layer on the inside of the plasma membrane. Budding forms may be spherical, filamentous, or pleomorphic (Darlington et al. 1970).

This appearance of productively infected cells is also seen in infected type II alveolar epithelium (Brownstein et al. 1981). An additional cytoplasmic inclusion consisting of membrane-bound, randomly arranged hollow fibrils, 15–20 nm in diameter, surrounded by 40-nm electron-dense cuffs has been reported in these cells (Zurcher et al. 1977). Incomplete reports indicate viral components in type I alveolar epithelium and septal capillary endothelium (Parker and Richter 1982; Ward et al. 1976). Only intranuclear nucleocapsids have been described in the former (nude mice). Viral assembly has not been observed in either cell type. Both of these may be examples of abortive infections.

Alveolar macrophages are susceptible to abortive infections in vitro (Eustatia et al. 1972; Mims and Murphy 1973), but ultrastructural evidence of viral replication is lacking. The author has seen numerous virions and nucleocapsids within heterophagosomes of alveolar macrophages in experimentally infected mice. This perhaps represents phagocytosis of debris containing viral particles.

## Differential Diagnosis

*Mice.* Sendai virus pneumonia must be distinguished from pneumonias caused by mouse coronaviruses, K virus, pneumonia virus, *Mycoplasma pulmonis*, and *Corynebacterium kutscheri*. The chronic wasting disease produced in athymic nude mice must be distinguished from similar syndromes caused by mouse coronarviruses, mouse adenovirus, *Pneumocystis*, *Giardia*, *Spironucleus*, and *Toxoplasma*.

*Rats.* Sendai virus pneumonia must be distinguished from pneumonias caused by rat coronavirus, pneumonia virus, *M. pulmonis*, *Streptococcus pneumoniae*, and *C. kutscheri*.

Some pulmonary changes caused by Sendai virus infection mimic those changes caused by exposure of rodents to halogenated aromatic hydrocarbons (Reid et al. 1973), oxidant gases (Stephens et al. 1974), and other toxicants which have the terminal conducting airways as target structures.

## Biological Features

*Natural History.* Sendai virus causes acute, limited infections in immunocompetent rodents. There is no evidence for latency or chronic infections (Fujiwara et al. 1976; van der Veen et al. 1974). Enzootic and epizootic forms exist. Enzootic infections occur in partially immune rodent colonies where susceptible individuals are regularly introduced to perpetuate the infection. This can occur in breeding or open colonies. In breeding colonies the susceptible population is the weaning age animals (3–6 weeks), due to their declining passive immunity (Parker and Reynolds 1968). Enzootic infections are usually subclinical. Epizootic infections occur in naive rodent colonies and either die out after 2–7 months or become enzootic if the proper conditions exist (Parker and Reynolds 1968; Parker et al. 1978). Clinical signs may be associated with epizootic infections in mice but have not been reported in rats. Such factors as strain susceptibility, age, husbandry, shipping, and copathogens are important in precipitating overt disease in mice (Jakab 1974; Jakab and Dick 1973; Parker et al. 1978; Ward 1974; Zurcher et al. 1977). Breeding colonies may exhibit neonatal or weanling mortality, prolonged gestation, fetal resorption, or runting in young mice (Bhatt and Jonas 1974; Iwai et al. 1979). Adult mice may exhibit anorexia, depression, ruffled fur, hunched posture, chattering, conjunctivitis, and photophobia.

Sendai virus is transmitted by aerosol and contact routes. Naso- and oropharyngeal secretions develop high infectivity titers during the 1st week. Some 50%–70% of mice become infected after 24 h of contact with a transmitter mouse (van der Veen et al. 1970, 1972). Attack rates are lower for aerosol transmission unless multiple transmitters are present (van der Veen et al. 1974).

Athymic nude mice infected with Sendai virus are persistently infected. Most exhibit dramatic weight loss, depression, wrinkled skin, dyspnea, and cyanosis and usually die between 2 and 10 weeks later (Iwai et al. 1979; Ward et al. 1976).

*Pathogenesis.* Viral replication is restricted to the respiratory tract in natural infections, although a low-level transient viremia may occur. Experimental evidence indicates that the strict pneumotropism of Sendai virus is partially a consequence of its dependence upon one or more respiratory serine endoproteases for activation of the viral fusion glycoprotein. Tryptase clara is one such protease, which specifically cleaves the inactive nascent fusion glycoprotein at residue arginine-116 to the active form (Tachiro et al. 1992). Pneumotropism is also a consequence of apical budding of wild-type Sendai virus (Tashiro et al. 1990). Systemic Sendai virus infections have been produced experimentally using protease-activation mutants that have additional mutations in the matrix protein which allows basolateral budding (Tashiro et al. 1990). Peak titers are reached in 3–6 days, and virus is usually not recoverable after 8–12 days (Appel et al. 1971; Parker et al. 1978; Robinson et al. 1968; Sawicki 1962; Stewart and Tucker 1978; van Nunen and van der Veen 1967). Adult mice eliminate virus earlier than suckling mice and develop lower peak titers (Sawicki 1961). Outbred mice eliminate virus earlier than inbred mice (Stewart and Tucker 1978).

Clearance of a primary Sendai virus infection is mediated by $CD8^+$ cytotoxic T cells ($T_c$) and by one or more effectors controlled by $CD4^+$ helper T cells. The latter mechanisms are delayed 24–48 h relative to the $T_c$ response (Kast et al. 1986; Hou et al. 1992). Seroconversion (hemagglutination inhibition, complement fixation) is usually detectable on days 7–9 (Appel et al. 1971; Robinson et al. 1968; Stewart and Tucker 1978; van Nunen and van der Veen 1967). Mice are usually leukopenic by the 7th day of infection; leukocytosis follows on days 8–11 (Robinson et al 1968). Offspring of naturally infected dams rapidly acquire neutralizing and complement-fixing antibodies of the $IgG_1$ and $IgG_2$ subclasses with the onset of nursing. These titers plateau on days 7–14 and then rapidly decline (Iida et al. 1973).

*Etiology.* Sendai virus is a parainfluenza 1 virus of the genus *Paramyxovirus*, family Paramyxoviridae. It is a pleomorphic, enveloped virus measuring approximately 100–300 nm in length. The helical nucleocapsid contains a continuous single strand of RNA. The envelope is studded with two types of surface-projecting glycosylated polypeptides. The larger projection has hemagglutination and neuraminidase activity; the smaller projection has hemolysin and cell fusion activity. The virus rapidly inactivates at temperatures between 20° and 37°C (Chanock et al. 1963).

*Frequency.* Sendai virus is ubiquitous in colonies of mice and rats. A survey of various institutional and commercial colonies published in 1978 indicated that 66% of mouse colonies and 63% of rat colonies had experienced infections (Parker et al. 1978). Attack rates usually exceed 50% (Parker et al. 1964, 1978).

## Comparison with Other Species

Parainfluenza viruses naturally infect humans, other primates, dogs, cattle, sheep, and birds in addition to rodents. All mammalian parainfluenza viruses replicate and cause disease primarily in the respiratory tract. They have a tropism for the epithelium of the conducting airways. Besides Sendai virus, histopathology is well described for parainfluenza 3 virus infection in calves (Dawson et al. 1965; Omar et al. 1966; Tsai and Thomson 1975). These lesions are similar to those caused by Sendai virus in rodents. Intranuclear inclusions are more prevalent and intracytoplasmic inclusions are more distinct in parainfluenza 3 virus infections.

## References


Appel LH, Kovatch RM, Reddecliff JM, Gerone PJ (1971) Pathogenesis of Sendai virus infection in mice. Am J Vet Res 32:1835–1841

Bhatt PN, Jonas AM (1974) An epizootic of Sendai infection with mortality in a barrier-maintained mouse colony. Am J Epidemiol 100:222–229

Brownstein DG, Smith AL, Johnson EA (1981) Sendai virus infection in genetically resistant and susceptible mice. Am J Pathol 105:156–163

Burek JD, Zurcher C, van Nunen MCJ, Hollander CF (1977) A naturally occurring epizootic caused by Sendai virus in breeding and aging rodent colonies. II. Infection in the rat. Lab Anim Sci 27:963–971

Chanock RN, Parrott RH, Johnson KM, Kopikian AZ, Bell JA (1963) Myxoviruses: parainfluenza. Am J Respir Dis 88 [Suppl]:152–166

Choppin PW, Compans RW (1975) Reproduction of paramyxoviruses. Compr Virol 4:95–178

Darlington RW, Portner A, Kingsbury DW (1970) Sendai virus replication: an ultrastructural comparison of productive and abortive infections in avian cells. J Gen Virol 9:169–177

Dawson PS, Darbyshire JH, Lamont PH (1965) The inoculation of calves with parainfluenza 3 virus. Res Vet Sci 6:108–113

Eustatia JM, Maase E, van Helden P, van der Veen J (1972) Viral replication in mouse macrophages. Arch Gesamte Virusforsch 39:376–380

Fujiwara K, Takenaka S, Shumiya S (1976) Carrier state of antibody and viruses in a mouse breeding colony persistently infected with Sendai and mouse hepatitis viruses. Lab Anim Sci 26:153–159

Hou S, Doherty PC, Zijlstra M, Jaenisch R, Katz JM (1992) Delayed clearance of Sendai virus in mice lacking class I MHC-restricted $CD8^+$ T cells. J Immunol 149:1319–1325

Iida T, Tajima M, Murata Y (1973) Transmission of maternal antibodies to Sendai virus in mice and its significance in enzootic infection. J Gen Virol 18:247–254

Iwai H, Goto Y, Ueda K (1979) Response of athymic nude mice to Sendai virus. Jpn J Exp Med 49:123–130

Jacoby RO, Bhatt PN, Jonas AM (1979) Viral disease. In: Baker HJ, Lindsey JR, Weisbroth SH (eds) The laboratory rat, vol 1, biology and diseases. Academic, New York, chap 11

Jakab GJ (1974) Effect of sequential inoculations of Sendai virus and *Pasteurella pneumotropica* in mice. J Am Vet Med Assoc 164:723–728

Jakab GJ, Dick EC (1973) Synergistic effect in viral-bacterial infection: combined infection of the murine respiratory tract with Sendai virus and *Pasteurella pneumotropica*. Infect Immun 8:762–768

Kast WM, Bronkhorst AM, deWaal LP, Melief CJM (1986) Cooperation between cytotoxic and helper T lymphocytes in protection against lethal Sendai virus infection. J Exp Med 164:723–738

Mims CA, Murphy FA (1973) Parainfluenza virus Sendai infection in macrophages, ependyma, choroid plexus, vascular endothelium and respiratory tract of mice. Am J Pathol 70:315–328

Omar AR, Jennings AR, Betts AO (1966) The experimental disease produced in calves by the J-121 strain of parainfluenza virus type 3. Res Vet Sci 7:379–388

Parker JC, Reynolds RK (1968) Natural history of Sendai virus infection in mice. Am J Epidemiol 88:112–125

Parker JC, Richter CB (1982) Viral diseases of the respiratory system. In: Foster HL, Small JD, Fox JG (eds) The mouse in biomedical research, vol 2, diseases. Academic, New York, chap 8

Parker JC, Tennant RW, Ward TG, Rowe WP (1964) Enzootic Sendai virus infections in mouse breeder colonies within the United States. Science 146:936–938

Parker JC, Whiteman MD, Richter CB (1978) Susceptibility of inbred and outbred mouse strains to Sendai virus and prevalence of infection in laboratory rodents. Infect Immun 19:123–130

Reid WD, Ilett KF, Glick JM, Krishna G (1973) Metabolism and binding of aromatic hydrocarbons in the lung. Relationship to experimental bronchiolar necrosis. Am Rev Respir Dis 107:539–551

Richter CB (1970) Application of infectious agents to the study of lung cancer: studies on the etiology and morphogenesis of metaplastic lung lesions in mice. USAEC Symposium Series 21:365–382

Richter CB (1973) Experimental pathology of Sendai virus infection in mice. J Am Vet Med Assoc 163:1204

Robinson TWE, Cureton RJR, Heath RB (1968) The pathogenesis of Sendai virus infection in the mouse lung. J Med Microbiol 1:89–95

Sawicki L (1961) Influence of age of mice on the recovery from experimental Sendai virus infection. Nature 192:1258–1259

Sawicki L (1962) Studies on experimental Sendai virus infection in laboratory mice. Acta Virol (Praha) 6:347–351

Stephens RJ, Sloan MF, Evans MJ, Freeman G (1974) Early response of lung to low levels of ozone. Am J Pathol 74:31–58

Stewart RB, Tucker MJ (1978) Infection of inbred strains of mice with Sendai virus. Can J Microbiol 24:9–13

Tashiro M, Yamakawa M, Tobita K, Klenk H-D, Rott R, Seto JT (1990) Organ tropism of Sendai virus in mice; proteolytic activation of the fusion glycoprotein in mouse organs and budding site at the bronchial epithelium. J Virol 64:3627–3634

Tashiro M, Yokogoshi Y, Tobita K, Seto JT, Rott R, Kido H (1992) Tryptase clara, an activating protease for Sendai virus in rat lungs, is involved in pneumopathogenicity. J Virol 66:7211–7216

Tsai KS, Thomson RG (1975) Bovine parainfluenza type 3 virus infection: ultrastructural aspects of viral pathogenesis in the bovine respiratory tract. Infect Immun 11:783–803

van Nunen MCJ, van der Veen J (1967) Experimental infection with Sendai virus in mice. Arch Gesamte Virusforsch 22:388–397

van der Veen J, Poort Y, Birchfield DJ (1970) Experimental transmission of Sendai virus infection in mice. Arch Gesamte Virusforsch 31:237–246

van der Veen J, Poort Y, Birchfield DJ (1972) Effect of relative humidity on experimental transmission of Sendai virus in mice. Proc Soc Exp Biol Med 140:1437–1440

van der Veen J, Poort Y, Birchfield DJ (1974) Study of the possible persistence of Sendai virus in mice. Lab Anim Sci 24:48–50

Ward JM (1974) Naturally occurring Sendai virus disease of mice. Lab Anim Sci 24:938–942

Ward JM, Houchens DP, Collins MJ, Young DM, Reagan RL (1976) Naturally-occurring Sendai virus infection of athymic nude mice. Vet Pathol 13:36–46

Zurcher C, Burek JD, van Nunen MCJ, Meihuizen SP (1977) A naturally occurring epizootic caused by Sendai virus in breeding and aging rodent colonies. I. Infection in the mouse. Lab Anim Sci 27:955–962

# Pneumonia Virus of Mice Infection, Lung, Mouse, and Rat

David G. Brownstein

*Synonyms.* Mouse pneumonia virus, pneumonia virus

## Gross Appearance

*Mice.* Gross lung changes are not seen in mice naturally infected with pneumonia virus of mice (PVM). Pulmonary consolidation has been produced experimentally using tissue culture adapted virus (Harter and Choppin 1967; Tennant et al. 1965) or serially blind-passed PVM-infected lung tissue (Horsfall and Hahn 1940; Curnen and Horsfall 1947). Initially, consolidation is hilar in distribution with subsequent radiation along bronchioles. Consolidated foci are dark red and exude sanguinous fluid when cut. Later these foci become gray. Athymic mice, which are susceptible to persistent PVM infection, develop lobar consolidation or diffuse pulmonary edema (Weir et al. 1988).

*Rats.* Naturally infected adult rats usually have no gross lung changes but may have focal or multifocal plum-colored to gray foci less than 2 mm in diameter. These may occur in any lobe.

## Microscopic Features

*Mice.* Histopathological lung changes are rare in naturally infected mice. Lesions produced experimentally with tissue culture adapted (Carthew and Sparrow 1980a; Vogtsberger et al. 1982) or serially blind-passed infected lung tissue (Horsfall and Hahn 1940) include both airway and parenchymal changes. PVM adapted to BHK-21 cells and inoculated at high doses ($10^4$–$10^5$ $TCID_{50}$) intranasally causes a mild erosive bronchiolitis and interstitial pneumonia. Bronchiolar epithelium first develops granular eosinophilic cytoplasm followed by lifting from the basal lamina. Desquamated epithelium and neutrophils may plug affected airways. Alveolar changes generally lag behind those in the airways. Alveolar septa are edematous, congested, and infiltrated with neutrophils and macrophages. There is some necrosis within alveolar walls. By the time bronchiolar epithelium has regenerated and returned to a normal appearance, alveolar septa are thickened by dense infiltrates of lymphocytes, macrophages, and scattered neutrophils. Alveolar spaces may contain an exudate with a similar inflammatory cell composition. Inflammatory changes in the parenchyma peak near the end of the 2nd week of experimental infection and are usually resolved by the end of the 3rd week.

Lower doses ($<10^3$ $TCID_{50}$) of tissue culture adapted PVM cause vascular-oriented inflammation and interstitial pneumonia (Vogtsberget et al. 1982). The vascular component has been described as an acute vasculitis with infiltrates of neutrophils and lymphocytes followed by a mild nonsuppurative vasculitis, which persists to the end of the 3rd week of infection. The interstitial pneumonia is acute, but its duration and histological features have not been reported.

Mild rhinitis is a constant feature in mice infected intranasally with tissue culture adapted PVM, even at doses that fail to produce pulmonary histological lesions. The nasal mucosa is edematous with multifocal erosions. Neutrophils and lymphoid cells infiltrate the lamina propria. A sparse exudate rich in neutrophils and desquamated epithelium is occasionally present.

Changes in the lung of athymic mice infected with PVM consist of thickening and hypercellularity of alveolar walls, intra-alveolar hemorrhage and fibrin deposition, and accumulations of macrophages and desquamated alveolar type II cells in alveolar spaces (Weir et al. 1988).

*Rats.* Histopathological changes in lung have been observed in naturally and experimentally infected rats. Naturally infected weanling Lewis rats develop hyperplasia of bronchus-associated lymphoid tissue (BALT), perivascular mononuclear cell infiltrates, and multifocal interstitial pneumonia (Fig. 353). Prominent germinal centers form within the expanded BALT. The overlying airway epithelium is intact but bulges into the lumen. Transepithelial lymphocytes are increased near these reactive lymphoid nodules. Pulmonary venules, small veins, and aterioles contain dense, usually symmetrical, adventitial infiltrates of plasma cells, lymphoid cells, and macrophages (Fig. 354). The endothelium of these vessels may be hypertrophied, and leukocyte pavementing may be prominent. Perivascular infiltrates often occur in areas of interstitial inflammation. Alveolar septa are congested, edematous, and infiltrated with lymphocytes, plasma cells, and macrophages. Alveolar lining cells are swollen or hypertrophied. Alveolar spaces contain variable numbers of foamy macrophages, desquamated pneumocytes, lymphocytes, and neutrophils (Fig. 355).

Multifocal nonsuppurative vasculitis and acute interstitial pneumonia have been described in experimentally infected Fischer 344 rats (Vogtsberger et al. 1982).

## Ultrastructure

The fine structure of PVM infection has been described in cell cultures (Compans et al. 1967; Berthiaum et al. 1974) and in naturally infected athymic mice (Weir et al. 1988). Nucleocapsid assembly occurs in the cytosol. Pleomorphic inclusions, which may be seen by light microscopy in the vicinity of the nucleus, are composed of electron-dense dots or threads approximately 12 nm in diameter. Virus maturation occurs at the plasma membrane, where budding particles have round or filamentous profiles about 80–120 nm in diameter, with filamentous forms predominating. The viral envelope contains surface projections approximately 12 nm in length. Within the envelope are four to eight electron-dense dots or strands identical to those seen in the cytosol. Strands are usually coiled in filamentous forms. Terminal swellings 150–300 nm in diameter are usually present on filamentous forms.

In negatively stained preparations filamentous forms predominate with lengths up to 3 μm and diameters of approximately 100 nm. Alveolar type II cells, the principal targets of PVM infection, degenerate and detach. Most budding virions can be seen in detached and degenerate alveolar type II cells.

## Differential Diagnosis

*Mice.* Naturally occurring PVM apparently rarely causes pneumonia. Until there is evidence to the contrary, PVM should be considered an unlikely cause of inflammatory lung disease in mice under natural conditions, but should be regarded as a cause of mild erosive rhinitis. PVM is one of the causes of "wasting disease" in athymic mice and must be distinguished from other causes which include infections with Sendai virus or mouse hepatitis virus (Hou et al. 1992).

*Rats.* The pulmonary changes in PVM infection must be distinguished from those caused by Sendai virus, rat coronaviruses, *Mycoplasma pumonis*, and pathogenic bacteria. The lesions caused by PVM most closely resemble those caused by pneumotropic strains of rat coronaviruses (Parker's rat coronavirus). Generally the latter causes milder lesions than PVM.

## Biological Features

*Natural History.* PVM causes acute, limited infections in immunocompetent rodents. Virus peristence (over 20 days) has been reported in germ-free athymic (nu/nu) mice (Carthew and Sparrow 1980b). Enzootic and epizootic forms exist, and both are asymptomatic in mouse and rat colonies.

Transmissibility in mouse colonies is low; infections may therefore be focal (Tennant et al. 1966). Attack rates in 59% of infected mouse colonies are reported to be 25% or less. This is the lowest attack rate for any indigenous murine virus (Tennant et al. 1966). Various age groups may harbor the infection, depending on management practices. In one colony antibody was first detected in 8-week-old mice, while in a second colony mice did not seroconvert until the age of 7 months (Parker et al. 1966).

Attack rates are apparently higher in rat colonies. We frequently find a 100% prevalence of serum antibodies (hemagglutination inhibition test) in weanling rats from enzootically infected colonies.

Clinical signs have not been reported for naturally infected mice or rats. Depression, anorexia, weight loss, ruffled fur, hunched posture, and labored respiration have been reported in experimentally infected mice (Horsfall and Hahn 1940).

*Pathogenesis.* Viral replication is restricted to the epithelium of the respiratory tract (Carthew and

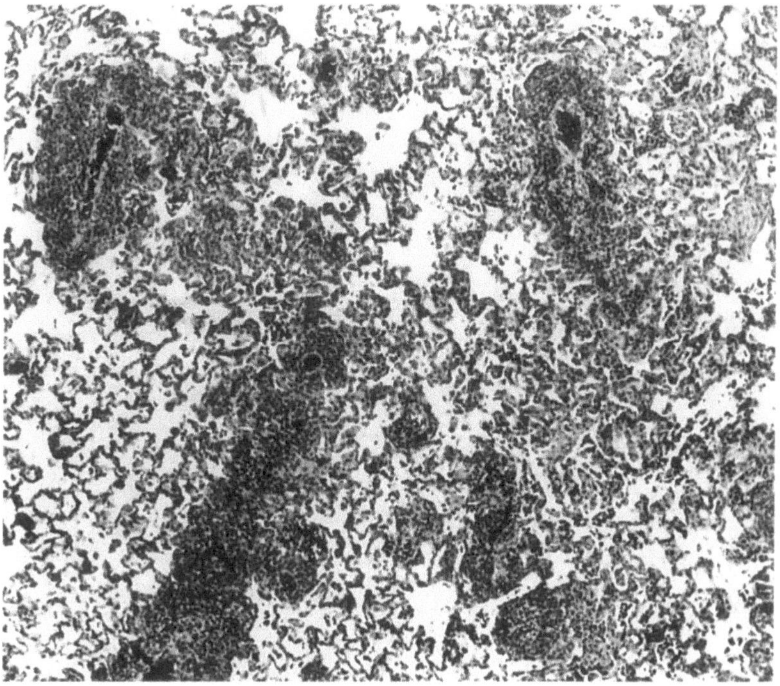

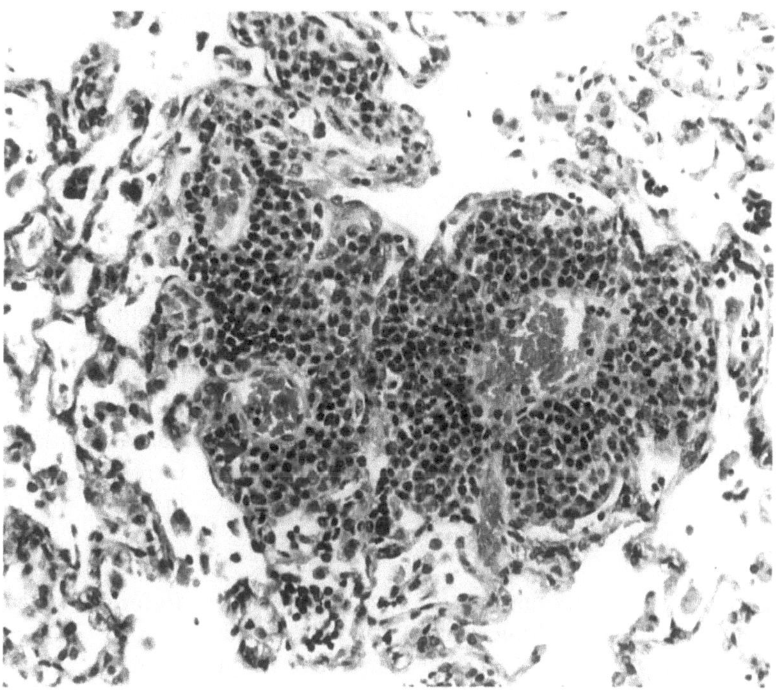

**Fig. 353.** (*above*) Perivascular infiltrates and interstitial pneumonia in a rat naturally infected with PVM. H&E, ×64

**Fig. 354.** (*below*). Perivascular plasma cell infiltrates in a naturally PVM-infected rat. H&E, ×217

Sparrow 1980a,b). Infectious virus can be detected up to 10 days after exposure (A.L. Smith and V.A. Carrano, personal communication). Viral antigens have not been detected in lung sections beyond day 7 in mice (Carthew and Sparrow 1980a). Virus is isolated most consistently from nasal washes in experimentally or naturally infected rodents (A.L. Smith and V.A. Carrano, personal communication).

Seroconversion [hemagglutination inhibition (HAI) complement fixation (CF)] usually occurs 9 or 10 days after exposure. CF antibody titers begin

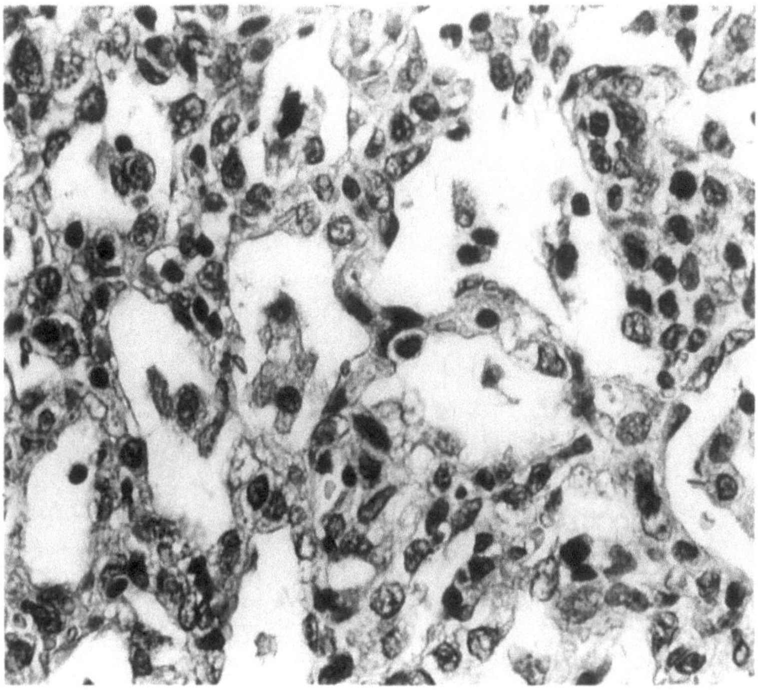

**Fig. 355.** Intersitial pneumonia in a naturally PVM-infected rat. Alveolar septa are congested, edematous, and infiltrated with mixed mononuclear cells. Alveolar lining cells are hypertrophied. Alveolar spaces contain large foamy mononuclear cells – probably desquamated pneumocytes and macrophages. H&E, ×536

to decline during the 3rd week of infection, while HAI antibody titers remain elevated for at least 4 months (Tennant et al. 1966).

*Etiology*. Pneumonia virus of mice is a *Pneumovirus* of the family Paramyxoviridae. It shares this genus with respiratory syncytial virus, which has structural and biological but not antigenic similarities (Joncas et al. 1969; Berthiaume et al. 1974). PVM is a predominantly filamentous enveloped virus containing a single-stranded RNA genome. The hemagglutinins probably occur within the fringe of envelope projections. The virus is labile in the environment and rapidly inactivates at room temperature.

*Frequency*. Pneumonia virus of mice is prevalent in mouse and rat colonies throughout the world. In a recent survey 63% of mouse and 68% of rat colonies from institutional and commercial sources were infected (Parker and Richter 1982).

## Comparison with Other Species

Pneumonia virus of mice and respiratory syncytial virus (RSV) are the sole representatives of the genus *Pneumovirus*. PVM infects rodents naturally; RSV infects children, cattle, and sheep, and experimentally infects ferrets and cotton rats. Both of these viruses have potentially broad respiratory epitheliotropism that is expressed differently depending on the host, host age, and infecting dose of virus. Experimentally, PVM causes rhinitis, bronchiolitis, or interstital pneumonia in mice. Naturally occuring PVM infection in rats causes interstital pneumonia. RSV in humans and cattle causes rhinitis, bronchiolitis, or interstital pneumonia (Aherne et al. 1970; Mohanty et al. 1975). Experimental RSV produces rhinitis and interstitial pneumonia in infant ferrets (Prince and Porter 1976) and bronchiolitis in cotton rats (Prince et al. 1978).

## References


Aherne W, Brid T, Court SD, Gardner PS, McQuillin J (1970) Pathological changes in virus infections of the lower respiratory tract in children. J Clin Pathol 23:7–18

Berthiaume L, Joncas J, Pavilanis V (1974) Comparative structure, morphogenesis and biological characteristics of the respiratory syncytial (RS) virus and the pneumonia virus of mice (PVM). Arch Virusforsch 45:39–51

Carthew P, Sparrow S (1980a) A comparison in germ-free mice of the pathogenesis of Sendai virus and mouse pneumonia virus infections. J Pathol 130:153–158

Carthew P, Sparrow S (1980b) Persistence of pneumonia virus of mice and Sendai virus in germ-free (nu/nu) mice. Br J Pathol 61:172–175

Compans RW, Harter DH, Choppin PW (1967) Studies on pneumonia virus of mice (PVM) in cell culture. II. Structure and morphogenesis of the virus particle. J Exp Med 126:267–276

Curnen EC, Horsfall FL Jr (1947) Properties of pneumonia virus of mice (PVM) in relation to its state. J Exp Med 85:39–53

Harter DH, Chopping PW (1967) Studies on pneumonia virus of mice (PVM) in cell culture. I. Replication in baby hamster kidney cells and properties of the virus. J Exp Med 126:251–266

Horsfall FL, Hahn RG (1940) A latent virus in normal mice capable of producing pneumonia in its natural host. J Exp Med 71:391–408

Hou S, Doherty PC, Zijlstra M, Jaenisch R, Katz JM (1992) Delayed clearance of Sendai virus in mice lacking class I MHC-restricted $CD8^+$ T cells. J Immunol 149:1319–1325

Joncas J, Berthiaume L, Pavilanis V (1969) The structure of the respiratory syncytial virus. Virology 38:493–496

Mohanty SB, Ingling AL, Lillie MG (1975) Experimentally induced respiratory syncytial viral infection in calves. Am J Vet Res 36:417–419

Parker JC, Richter CB (1982) Viral diseases of the respiratory system. In: Foster HL, Small JD, Fox JG (eds) The mouse in biomedical research, vol 2, diseases. Academic, New York, chap 8

Parker JC, Tennant RW, Ward TG (1966) Prevalence of viruses in mouse colonies. Natl Cancer Inst Monogr 20:25–36

Prince GA, Porter DD (1976) The pathogenesis of respiratory syncytial virus infection in infant ferrets. Am J Pathol 82:339–352

Prince GA, Jenson AB, Horswood RL, Camargo E, Chanock RM (1978) The pathogenesis of respiratory syncytial virus infection in cotton rats. Am J Pathol 93:771–791

Tennant RW, Parker JC, Ward TG (1965) Virus studies with germ-free mice. II. Comparative responses of germ-free mice to virus infection. JNCI 34:381–387

Tennant RW, Parker JC, Ward TG (1966) Respiratory virus infections of mice. Natl Cancer Inst Monogr 20:93–104

Vogtsberger LM, Stromberg PC, Rice JM (1982) Histological and serological response of $B_6C_3F_1$ mice and F344 rats to experimental pneumonia virus of mice infection. Lab Anim Sci 32:419 (abstract)

Weir EC, Brownstein DG, Smith AL, Johnson EA (1988) Respiratory disease and wasting in athymic mice infected with pneumonia virus of mice. Lab Anim Sci 38:133–137

# Rat Coronavirus Infection, Lung, Rat

David G. Brownstein

*Synonym.* Parker's rat coronavirus, rat submaxillary gland virus, sialodacryoadenitis virus intranasal inoculation (Wojcinski and Percy 1986).

## Gross Appearance

Naturally infected adult rats rarely have grossly observable lung changes. Elsewhere macroscopic lesions are absent or confined to salivary glands and periglandular tissue. Ocular changes may also occur as a consequence of keratitis sicca. Axenic rats experimentally infected with Parker's rat coronavirus (PRC) develop gross lesions in the lung on postinnoculation days 6 and 7, which consist of randomly dispersed red-brown to gray foci less than 1mm in diameter (Bhatt and Jacoby 1977). Although PRC may cause fatal pneumonia in a high percentage of newborn and day-old rats, gross pulmonary lesions have not been described (Parker et al. 1970). Outbred young adult SPF Wistar rats experimentally infected with sialodacryoadenitis virus (SDAV) develop mild randomly dispersed red foci 5–7 days after

## Microscopic Features

Lung changes in young adult rats are mild and short-lived irrespective of the infecting strain. Nonsialotropic strains such as PRC produce hyperplasia of bronchusassociated lymphoid tissue (Fig. 356), perivenular lymphoid infiltrates (Fig. 357), and patchy interstitial pneumonia (Fig. 358; Bhatt and Jacoby 1977). Sialotropic strains such as SDAV produce more severe acute inflammatory changes in bronchioles and lung parenchyma (Wojcinski and Percy 1986). Random patches of bronchiolar epithelium undergo necrosis in conjunction with infiltration and exudation by neutrophils. Acute inflammation may extend from terminal bronchioles into adjacent alveoli. Affected alveolar septa are edematous, infiltrated by leukocytes, and alveolar spaces contain desquamated pneumocytes, macrophages,

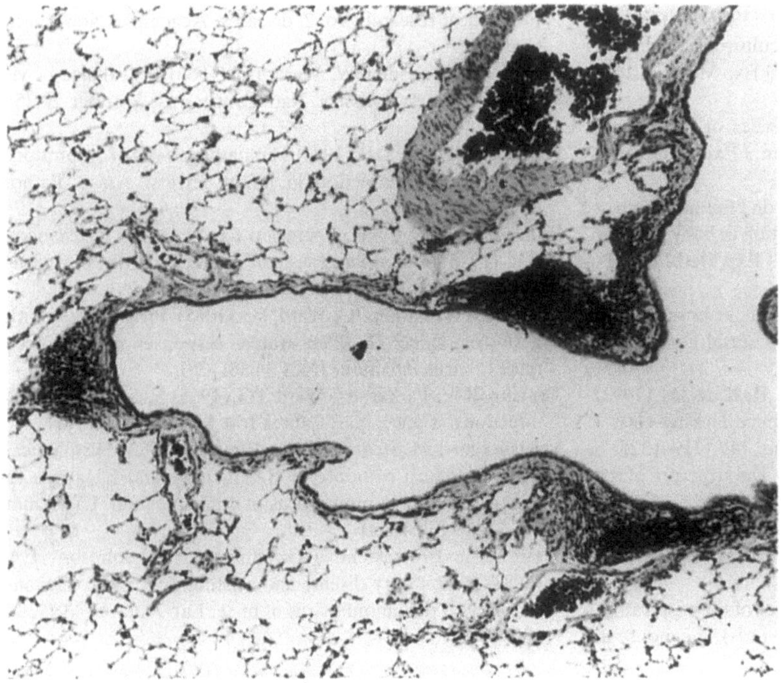

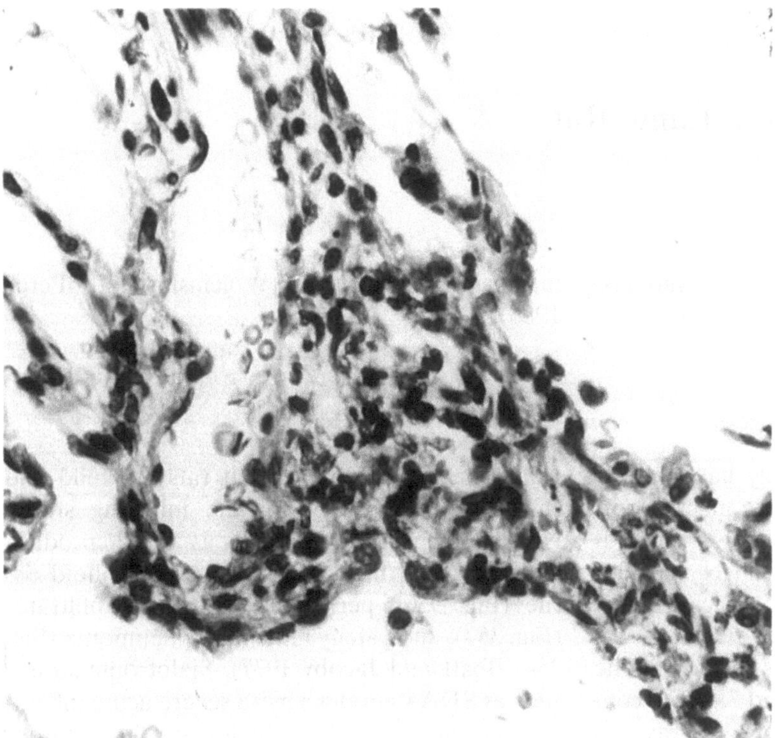

**Fig. 356.** (*above*) Rat coronavirus infection, lung. Bronchiole with mildly hyperplastic lymphoid nodules following experimental infection. H&E, ×58

**Fig. 357.** (*below*) Rat coronavirus infection, lung. Perivenular lymphoid cells in an experimentally infected rat. H&E, ×536

**Fig. 358.** Interstital pneumonia following experimental infection with rat coronavirus. Alveoli contain foamy macrophages and lymphoid cells. Septa are infiltrated with mononuclear cells. H&E, ×536

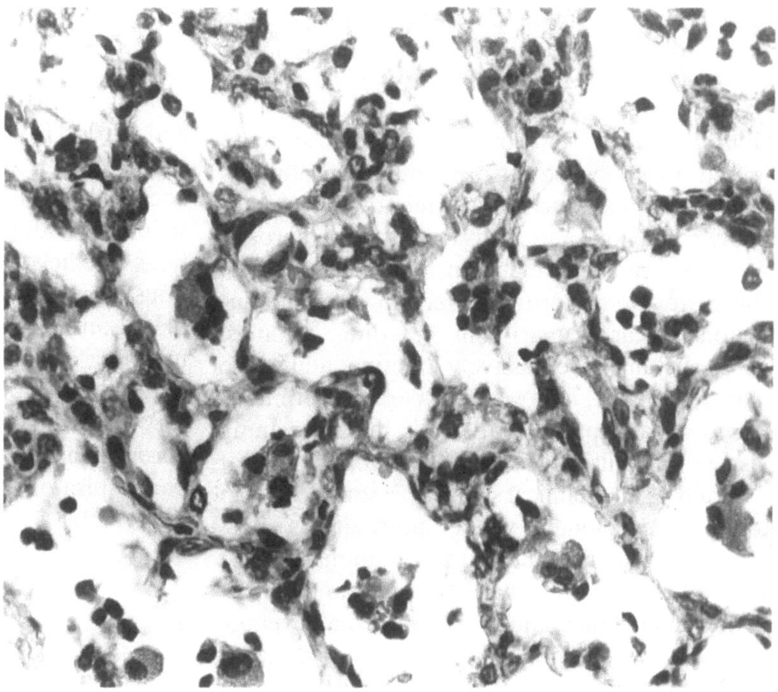

and neutrophils. The reparative phase is characterized by hyperplasia of bronchiolar epithelium and pneumocytes, infiltration by lymphoid cells, hyperplasia of bronchus-associated lymphoid tissue, and perivenular lymphoid infiltrates (Wojcinski and Percy 1986).

Transient rhinotracheitis also occurs which is more severe with SDAV than with PRC. In the former there is epithelial erosion and necrosis of perilaryngeal glands and ducts (Wojcinski and Percy 1986). In the latter there may be segmental erosion of epithelium covering nasal turbinates. In both cases lamina propria of the nasal cavity is edematous and infiltrated by lymphocytes and neutrophils. Some nasal respiratory surfaces are covered with exudate consisting of mucus, neutrophils, desquamated epithelium, and detritus.

Lesions of salivary glands are common with SDAV and uncommon or mild with PRC. With SDAV severe inflammatory changes occur in mixed or serous salivary glands, exorbital glands, and harderian glands. Mild parotitis and submaxillary sialoadenitis may occur with PRC. Description of these changes is beyond the scope of this chapter. The reader is referred to several excellent studies of sequential changes in these tissues (Innes and Stanton 1961; Jacoby et al. 1975, 1979; Bhatt and Jacoby 1977).

### Ultrastructure

Infected epithelial cells have focally dilated cisternae of endoplasmic reticulum and cytoplasmic vacuoles which contain spherical dense cores 60–70nm in diameter (Parker et al. 1970; Jonas et al. 1969). The characteristic corona, seen in negatively stained preparations, is not seen by transmission ultramicroscopy.

### Differential Diagnosis

Respiratory tract lesions must be differentiated from those caused by Sendai virus, pneumonia virus, *Mycoplasma pulmonis*, and pathogenic bacteria. Identification of the infecting agent is necessary for definitive diagnosis.

### Biological Features

*Etiology*. Rat coronaviruses are typical members of the Coronaviridae; pleomorphic, enveloped RNA viruses with plump, pedunculated surface projections (corona) measure 76–98nm in diameter in negatively stained preparations 12–25nm surface projections (Parker et al. 1970). Viruses are formed in cytoplasmic vesicles and cisternae of endoplasmic reticulum. The viruses are closely related to mouse hepatitis virus (Bhatt and Jacoby 1977).

*Natural History*. Rat coronaviruses cause acute limited infections except in immunologically disabled individuals such as athymic rats. They are highly contagious and are transmitted by aerosol, by direct contact, and transiently by fomites. There are two patterns of infection. Enzootic infections occur primarily in breeding colonies, where sucklings are passively immune, adults are actively immune, and weanlings are a continuous source of susceptible individuals due to waning passive immunity. It is therefore weanlings that generally exhibit clinical signs. Epizootics occur in nonimmune colonies, where morbidity is most likely to occur in young or aged animals. With SDAV the signs are usually transient and consist of intermandibular and cervical edema, swelling of submaxillary glands, sneezing, nasal and ocular discharges which are often red-tinged due to a high content of porphyrin, photophobia, and keratoconjunctivitis and its sequelae. Some complications of keratoconjunctivitis, such as glaucoma and phthisis, cause permanent disfigurement (Jacoby et al. 1979). Subclinical infections are the rule for PRC and are common for SDAV. Extensive host range studies have not been carried out but SDAV can be used to infect mice by the respiratory route (Bhatt et al. 1977).

*Pathogenesis*. Rat coronaviruses are epitheliotropic and replicate at all levels of the respiratory tract during the 1st week of infection. The highest respiratory titers are reached in the nasal cavity and trachea. SDAV but not PRC replicates extensively in certain exocrine tissues of the head. Neutralizing antibodies are detectable on day 6 or 7. Complement-fixing antibodies appear later and cross react with mouse hepatitis viral antigens (Bhatt and Jacoby 1977; Parker et al. 1970; Jacoby et al. 1979).

*Frequency*. Coronavirus infections are common in institutional rat colonies and in some commercial colonies. Different strains of rat coronavirus cannot be distinguished serologically.

## Comparison with Other Species

Coronaviruses are ubiquitous in humans, animals, and birds (Bohl 1981). They cause enteritis in swine, cattle, dogs, mice, turkeys, and humans; encephalomyelitis in swine and mice; sialodacryoadenitis in rats; and respiratory infections in chickens, rats, and humans. Avian infectious bronchitis virus infects the trachea and lungs of chickens, causing respiratory distress, especially in young chicks. The virus also replicates in kidneys, bursae, and oviducts, producing inflammatory disease at these sites. Human respiratory coronaviruses are apparently restricted to the upper respiratory tract, causing rhinotracheitis and pharyngitis.

## References


Bhatt PN, Jacoby RO (1977) Experimental infection of adult axenic rats with Parker's rat coronavirus. Arch Virol 54:345–352

Bhatt PN, Percy DH, Jonas AM (1972) Characterization of the virus of sialodacryoadenitis of rats: a member of the coronavirus group. J Infect Dis 126:123–130

Bhatt PN, Jacoby RO, Jonas AM (1977) Respiratory infection in mice with sialodacryoadenitis virus, a coronavirus of rats. Infect Immun 18:823–130

Bohl EH (1981) Coronavirus: diagnosis of infections. In: Kurstak E, Kurstak C (eds) Comparative diagnosis of viral diseases, vol 4. Academic, New York, chap 7

Innes JRM, Stanton MF (1961) Acute diseases of the submaxillary and harderian glands (sialodacryoadenitis) of rats with cytomegaly and no inclusion bodies. Am J Pathol 38:455–468

Jacoby RO, Bhatt PN, Jonas AM (1975) Pathogenesis of sialodacryoadenitis in gnotobiotic rats. Vet Pathol 12:196–209

Jacoby RO, Bhatt PN, Jonas AM (1979) Viral diseases. In: Baker HJ, Lindsey JR, Weisbroth SH (eds) The laboratory rat, vol 1. Academic, New York, chap 13

Jonas AM, Craft J, Black L, Bhatt PN, Hilding D (1969) Sialodacryoadenitis in the rat. A light and electron microscopic study. Arch Pathol 88:613–622

Parker JC, Cross SS, Rowe WP (1970) Rat coronavirus (RCV): a prevalent, naturally occurring pneumotropic virus of rats. Arch Gesamte Virusforsch 31:293–302

Wojcinski ZW, Percy DH (1986) Sialodacryoadenitis virus-associated lesions in the lower respiratory tract of rats. Vet Pathol 23:278–286

# Cilia-Associated Respiratory Bacillus Infection, Rat, Mouse, and Rabbit

Trenton R. Schoeb and J. Russell Lindsey

*Synonyms.* Murine chronic respiratory disease (?), enzootic bronchiectasis (?)

## Gross Appearance

Gross lesions in rats with cilia-associated respiratory (CAR) bacillus infection are not always present. Most commonly observed are purple, depressed patches of atelectasis, which usually contain yellow-tan, slightly elevated foci representing exudate-filled bronchi and bronchioles. In many cases these lesions affect entire lung lobes, with severe dilation of bronchi and bronchioles. Pulmonary abscesses up to several millimeters in diameter, especially in the periphery of the lung lobes, are a somewhat distinctive feature (Fig. 359). These lesions can occur in rats as young as 1 month of age (Lindsey et al. 1991).

Only one report describes gross lesions in mice; these were well demarcated, tan, firm areas in the cranial-ventral parts of the lungs (Griffith et al. 1988). Rabbits (*Oryctolagus cuniculus*) with natural CAR bacillus infection usually have no gross lesions, although single or multiple, 1–5mm, raised, tan nodules are present in some cases (Kurisu et al. 1990; Waggie et al. 1987).

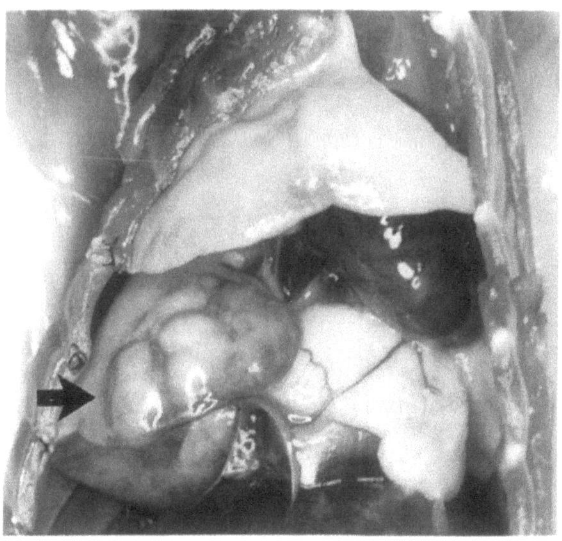

**Fig. 359.** Lungs of rat with natural CAR bacillus infection. Pneumonia in the right middle and right caudal lobes, with severe bronchiolectasis and peripheral abscesses in the right middle lobe (*arrow*). ×2

## Microscopic Features

Microscopic lesions of CAR bacillus infection in rats include suppurative inflammation of the respiratory mucosa with accumulation of lymphoid cells in the submucosa and hyperplasia of the bronchus-associated lymphoid tissue (Ganaway et al. 1985; MacKenzie et al. 1981; Matsushita 1986; Shoji et al. 1988b; van Zwieten et al. 1980; Figs. 360–362). These changes vary greatly in extent and severity from case to case and within the lungs of individual rats. In severe lesions epithelial changes include hypertrophy, hyperplasia, increased numbers of goblet cells, and accumulation of neutrophils and lymphocytes within the epithelium (Fig. 362). In some cases there also is bronchial and bronchiolar epithelial ulceration (Fig. 363). This is especially common in bronchioles that are severely dilated and appears to lead to formation of pulmonary abscesses. A granulomatous and fibrosing response often accompanies these ulcerations, and scarring or bronchiolitis obliterans sometimes occur. Alveolitis is not common but can occur in severely affected lobes, usually in patches around affected bronchioles. In such lesions bronchiolar and alveolar lumina can be filled with accumulations of mucin with admixed macrophages and neutrophils (Fig. 364). CAR bacilli also occur on ciliated surfaces throughout the upper respiratory tract, including the nasal passages, middle ears, larynx, and trachea. Lesions in these organs are similar to those in the intrapulmonary airways.

Microscopic lesions in naturally and experimentally infected mice include suppurative bronchopneumonia with epithelial hyperplasia and extensive peribronchiolar accumulation of lymphocytes and plasma cells (Ganaway et al. 1985; Griffith et al. 1988; Matsushita et al. 1989; Shoji et al. 1988b, 1992; Shoji-Darkye et al. 1991).

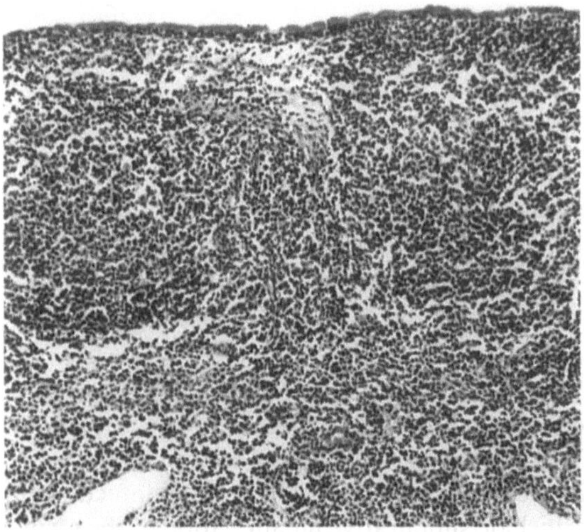

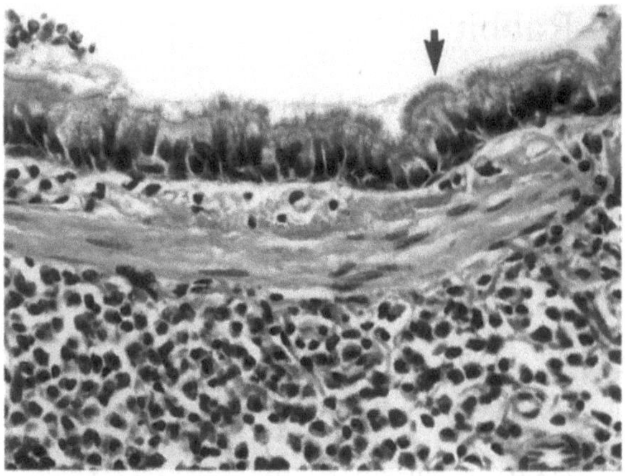

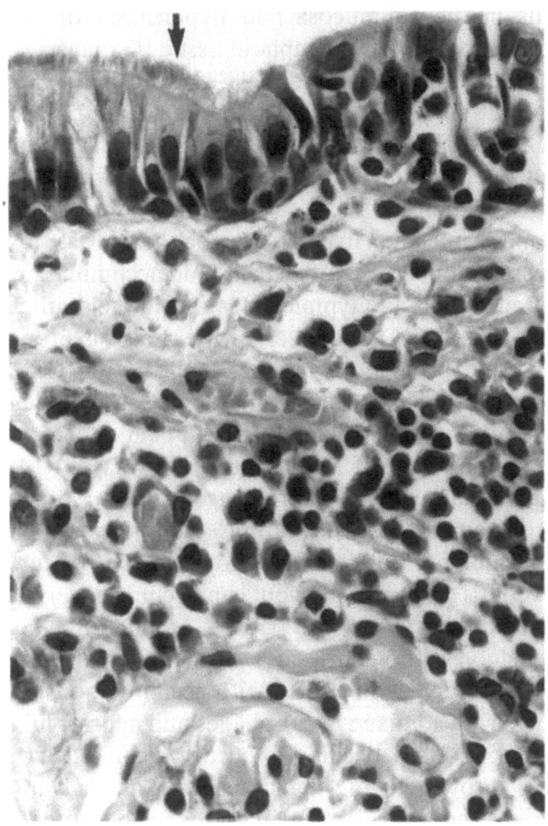

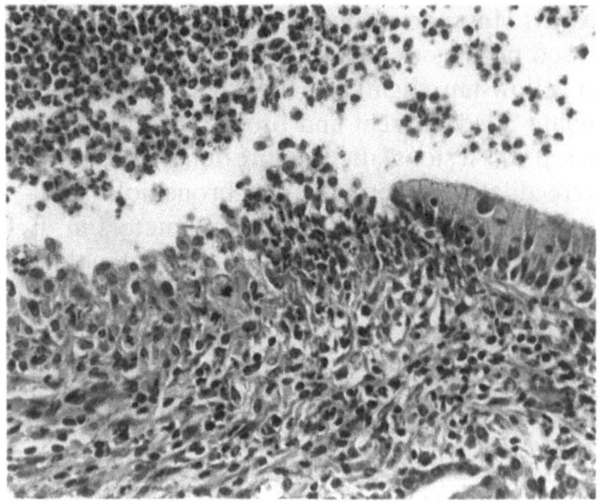

**Fig. 360.** (*upper left*) Mainstem bronchus of rat with CAR bacillus infection. Severe accumulation of lymphocytes and plasma cells, with profound hyperplasia of bronchus-associated lymphoid tissue. H&E, ×70

**Fig. 361.** (*upper right*) Mainstem bronchus of rat with CAR bacillus infection. CAR bacilli on epithelial surface (*arrow*), moderate epithelial hypertrophy, and accumulation of lymphocytes and plasma cells. H&E, ×220

**Fig. 362.** (*lower left*) Bronchial mucosa of rat with CAR bacillus infection. Severe epithelial hypertrophy, with increased numbers of goblet cells; lymphoid cells and neutrophils within epithelium; CAR bacilli on epithelial surface (*arrow*). H&E, ×500

**Fig. 363.** (*lower right*) Bronchiole of rat with CAR bacillus infection. Luminal neutrophilic exudate, epithelial hypertrophy, ulceration with neutrophil, macrophage, and fibroblastic response. H&E, ×170

Rabbits typically have milder lesions than those in rats and mice, but the general characteristics are similar, including epithelial hyperplasia and accumulation of heterophils, lymphocytes, and plasma cells affecting the mucosa of the larynx, trachea, bronchi, and bronchioles (Kurisu et al. 1990; Cundiff et al. 1995). Usually only a few scattered airways are affected. Bronchiolectasis has been observed in a few cases (Waggie et al. 1987). Nasal mucosal lesions in mice and rabbits have not been described, but in our experience the bacilli are present in the caudal ventral nasal passages of many rabbits, in most cases in association with mild suppurative and lymphocytic rhinitis. We also have observed that CAR bacilli, or morphologically similar organisms, can be found in the larynx of some rabbits that do not have laryngitis or other lesions associated with CAR bacillus infection.

In all three host species CAR bacilli are found among and parallel to the cilia in areas of inflamed respiratory mucosa. In some cases they also can be found free in luminal exudates. They are most effectively demonstrated in sections by silver impregnation stains (Fig. 365), but in H&E stained sections, they can be seen where they are numerous as basophilic areas of the ciliated surface (Fig. 361).

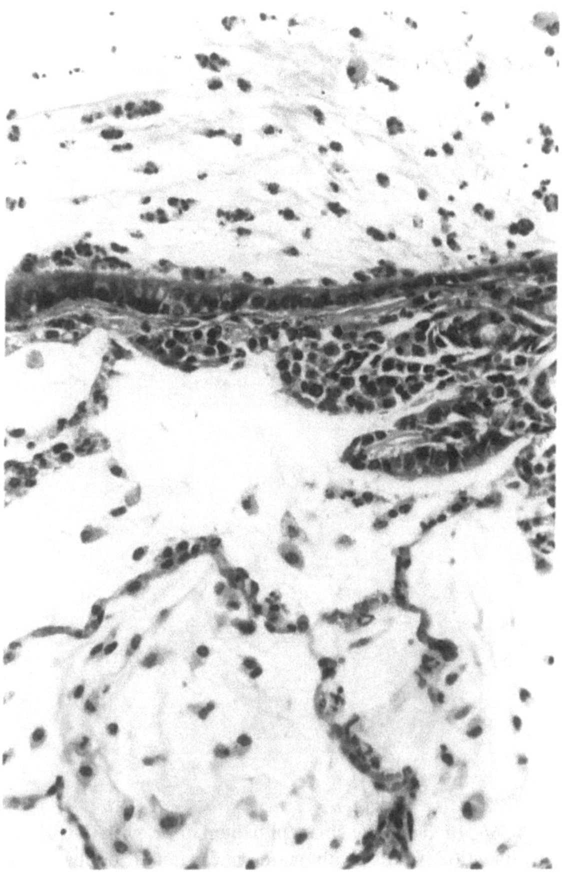

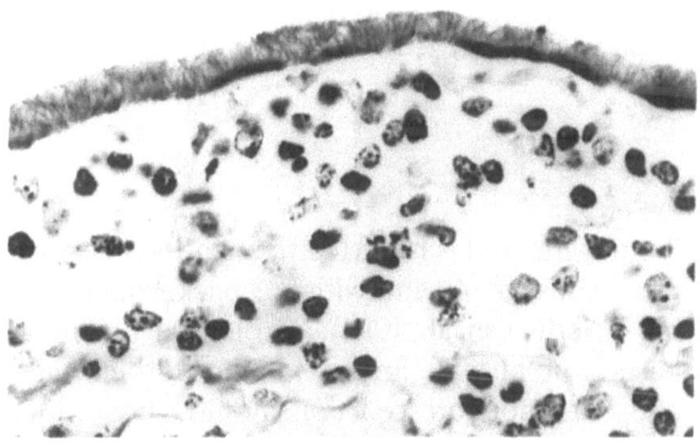

**Fig. 364.** (*above*) Terminal bronchiole and alveoli of rat with CAR bacillus infection. Mucinous exudate with macrophages, neutrophils, and cell debris. H&E, ×200

**Fig. 365.** (*below*) Bronchial epithelium of rat with CAR bacillus infection. Numerous CAR bacilli on epithelial surface. Warthin-Starry, ×500

## Ultrastructure

Ultrastructural findings in CAR bacillus infection are as would be expected from light microscopy. Epithelial cells are increased in height, with fewer Clara cells and more goblet cells than normal (Matsushita 1991). CAR bacilli are found on both ciliated and nonciliated cells. Ciliated cells may have reduced numbers of cilia, with basal bodies scattered in the apical cytoplasm. The bacilli are located among and parallel to the cilia, with one end of the bacterial cell on or near the cell membrane (Ganaway et al. 1985; Matsushita 1991; Matsushita and Joshima 1989; van Zwieten et al. 1980; Fig. 366). CAR bacilli of rats are 0.15–0.35 μm in diameter, 3.5–9 μm long, and somewhat fusiform, with a slight taper toward each end, and rounded, slightly knobbed ends. Their cell walls have the trilaminar structure characteristic of gram bacteria (Fig. 367), and they have no specialized structures such as filaments, flagella, or pili. In some cases fine fibrils of unknown composition can be observed between the bacilli and the host cell membrane (Matsushita 1991).

## Differential Diagnosis

Definitive diagnosis of CAR bacillus infection is most easily made by histological examination of sections stained by a silver impregnation method such as that of Warthin-Starry. A microwave

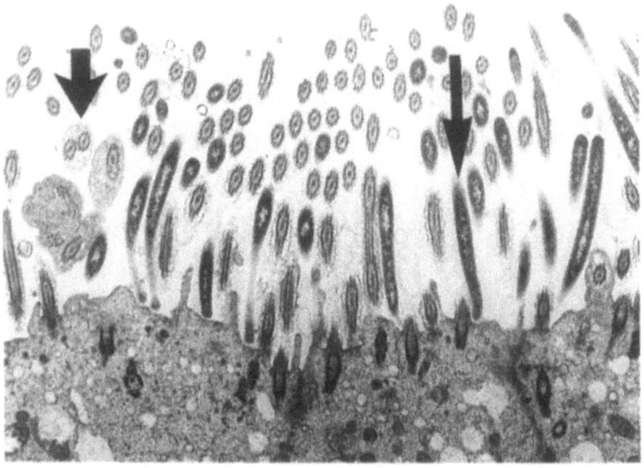

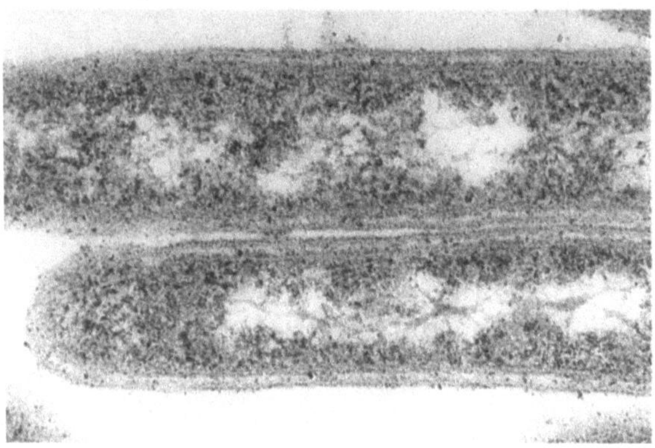

**Fig. 366.** (*above*) Bronchial epithelium of rat with CAR bacillus infection. CAR bacilli among and parallel to cilia on cell surfaces (*long arrows*). Cell at left has lost cilia, with fusion of remaining cilia (*short arrow*). TEM, ×7600

**Fig. 367.** (*below*) CAR bacilli cultured in cell culture medium. Trilaminar wall characteristic of gram-negative bacteria. TEM, ×79 000

Steiner method is reported to stain the organisms more consistently and with less background staining (Medina et al. 1994). Serological techniques based on enzyme-linked immunosorbent assay and immunofluorescence assay have been developed (Ganaway et al. 1985; Matsushita et al. 1987; Shoji et al. 1988a), and tests based on such methods are commercially available. However, the significance of negative results, or positive results in the absence of histologically evident infection, is unclear, inasmuch as studies verifying the sensitivity and specificity of these tests have not been reported. CAR bacillus can be isolated from rats, mice, and rabbits by culture in embryonated eggs, cell cultures, and various cell culture media (Cundiff et al. 1994a; Ganaway et al. 1985; Schoeb et al. 1993; Shoji et al. 1992). The sensitivity of these methods is unknown, and they are not practical for routine diagnostic use. A method for detecting CAR bacillus of rats by amplification of 16S ribosomal RNA (rRNA) gene sequences by polymerase chain reaction has been developed (Cundiff et al. 1994b), offering greatly improved sensitivity and specificity over other methods.

The most important differential diagnosis for CAR bacillus infection in rats and mice is respiratory disease caused by *Mycoplasma pulmonis* (p. 117, this volume). Lesions of CAR bacillus infection so closely resemble those of mycoplasmosis that distinction cannot be made on morphological grounds, although severe bronchiectasis and bronchiolectasis, pulmonary abscesses, bronchiolar epithelial ulceration, and mucinous bronchoalveolar exudate are more commonly found in rats with CAR bacillus infection. Although natural CAR bacillus disease in rats and mice without cultural or serological evidence of *M. pulmonis* infection has been reported (Brogden et al. 1993; Cundiff and Besch-Williford 1992; Griffith et al. 1988; Medina et al. 1994), in our experience it is much less common than concurrent infection with both agents. To date, we have examined 199 rats from 12 different colonies with CAR bacillus infection; rats from each source had positive results on *M. pulmonis* enzyme-linked immunosorbent assay, and in most cases *M. pulmonis* infection was confirmed by culture. Thus both agents should be sought when characteristic lesions are found.

CAR bacillus infection in rats has been reported to occur only in conventionally housed colonies. In naturally occurring disease in such settings various other bacteria, such as *Streptococcus pneumoniae*, *Corynebacterium kutscheri*, *Bordetella bronchiseptica*, *Pasteurella pneumotropica*, *Streptobacillus moniliformis*, *Pseudomonas aeruginosa*, and *Klebsiella pneumoniae* often can be cultured from the respiratory tract. Other than *S. pneumoniae* and *C. kutscheri*, these organisms are regarded as opportunistic, rather than primary, pathogens (Weisbroth 1979). Disease caused by either *S. pneumoniae* or *C. kutscheri* is distinctly different from that associated with CAR bacillus. Multifocal suppurative pneumonia is characteristic of *C. kutscheri* infection, whereas fibrinopurulent bronchopneumonia, pleuritis, and pericarditis are typical of *S. pneumoniae*. Both organisms are gram positive and are readily demonstrated in sections stained with tissue gram stains.

Rats and mice with natural CAR bacillus infection usually also have either serological or histological evidence of infection with respiratory viruses such as Sendai virus or sialodacryoadenitis virus, although cases in rats with no evidence of concurrent infections have been observed (Medina et al. 1994). These viruses cause mild acute necrosis of bronchial and bronchiolar epithelium, and in some cases mild multifocal interstitial pneumonia (Jacoby et al. 1979), which are easily differentiated from the lesions associated with CAR bacillus infection.

In our experience, the only reliable method of diagnosis of CAR bacillus infection in rabbits is detailed examination of silver impregnation stained sections of respiratory tract tissues; results of serological tests utilizing rat CAR bacilli as the antigen source are poorly correlated with results of histological examination. Analysis of rabbit CAR bacilli 16S rRNA sequences indicate that rat and rabbit CAR bacilli are distinctly different organisms (Cundiff et al. 1995). This information will lead to techniques based on polymerase chain reaction and other methods appropriate for diagnosis of CAR bacillus infection in rabbits.

The only significant differential diagnosis for CAR bacillus infection in rabbits is *Pasteurella multocida* infection. It commonly causes purulent or mucopurulent rhinitis and otitis media and occasionally spreads to the lungs, with resultant purulent or fibrinopurulent bronchopneumonia. Lesions caused by *P. multocida* are more exudative than those of CAR bacillus infection and lack the peribronchiolar lymphoid cell accumulations characteristic of CAR bacillus infection. *P. multocida* is readily identified by routine bacteriological methods. *Bordetella bronchiseptica* is sometimes isolated from the nasal passages of rabbits. It is not considered an important pathogen of rabbits, although it has been found in a few cases of fulminating pneumonia. *Pasteurella pneumotropica* also is occasionally found in the nasal passages but is considered at most an opportunistic organism.

## Biological Features

CAR bacilli from rats are gram-negative, filamentous, flexing, and gliding bacteria (Cundiff et al. 1994a; Ganaway et al. 1985; Schoeb et al. 1993). CAR bacilli from rabbits are morphologically similar but shorter, about 3–5 μm in length (Cundiff et al. 1994a; Schoeb et al. 1993). Neither can be grown with any bacteriological medium tested to date, and most reported isolates have been obtained in embryonated eggs or cell cultures. However, both rat and rabbit CAR bacilli can be grown in certain cell culture media (Schoeb et al. 1993; Shoji et al. 1992), and CAR bacilli are cultured equally well from rats and mice by culture of tracheal lavage samples in 3T3 cell cultures and in cell culture medium supplemented with fetal calf serum (Schoeb et al. 1993). We have since found that a 50:50 mixture of Dulbecco's minimal essential medium and Coon's modified F12 medium provides more rapid growth than Dulbecco's medium alone. The major practical difficulty in culturing CAR bacillus from naturally infected animals is that antibiotics have not been identified that prevent overgrowth by other bacteria without inhibiting growth of CAR bacilli.

Despite similarities in other respects 16S rRNA sequences of CAR bacilli from rats and rabbits are very dissimilar. Reported sequences of rat CAR bacilli, one determined from a stock of the original isolate (Ganaway et al. 1985; Schoeb et al. 1993) and the other a consensus sequence derived from three different rat isolates (Cundiff et al. 1994b), have affinities with members of the flavobacteria subdivision of the flavobacteria-bacteroid eubacterial phylum, particularly *Flavobacterium ferrugineum*. However, the organisms clearly are distinct from previously known members of this group, and the two sequences are different enough to suggest that there may be considerable genetic variation among CAR bacilli from rats. The consensus sequence derived from the highly homologous sequences of six rabbit CAR bacillus isolates is most closely related to *Helicobacter* species (Cundiff et al. 1995). The organisms also differ in host preferences. CAR bacilli from rats or mice readily infect the other host. Rabbit CAR bacilli cause typical lesions in young rabbits but are not infective for mice, and cause only seroconversion without lesions in rats (Cundiff et al. 1994a, 1995).

CAR bacillus infection has been identified in conventional laboratory rats, mice, or both in Europe, North America, and Japan and has been found in wild rats in the United States. It appears to be rather common among conventional rats, mice, and rabbits in some institutional colonies (Cundiff and Besch-Williford 1992), and in our experience is common among rabbits from commercial vendors. CAR bacillus has not been reported to occur in rats or mice from modern barrier-maintained vendor colonies, but its true prevalence in rats and mice is unknown. No surveys for CAR bacillus infection have been reported, and it is not known how efficiently existing serological tests detect infection. We have observed that CAR bacilli could be isolated up to 8 weeks after inoculation from mice that did not develop lesions, seroconvert, or have histologically detectable CAR bacilli in their tissues. If such inapparent infections occur naturally, they would be very difficult to detect.

## Comparison with Other Species

Naturally occurring CAR bacillus infection has been found in African white-tailed hamsters (*Mystromys albicaudatus*) with "chronic respiratory disease" (MacKenzie et al. 1981), but the lesions were not described. CAR bacillus infection in cattle was identified by finding the organisms in samples of trachea collected at slaughter for studies of cilia (Hastie et al. 1993). It is not known whether bovine infection is associated with any lesions, but reduced yields of ciliary axonemes from preparations of infected tracheas suggest that the organisms can cause epithelial injury. Syrian hamsters (*Mesocricetus auratus*) are susceptible to experimental CAR bacillus infection (Shoji-Darkye et al. 1991), but spontaneous infection in that species has not been reported. Inoculated hamsters had mild rhinitis, tracheitis, and bronchitis characterized by lymphoid cellular accumulation and epithelial hypertrophy. Guinea pigs inoculated with CAR bacilli from mice appeared to be only transiently infected and did not develop any lesions (Shoji-Darkye et al. 1991).

## References


Brogden KA, Cutlip RC, Lehmkuhl HD (1993) Cilia-associated respiratory bacillus in wild rats in central Iowa. J Wildl Dis 29:123–126

Cundiff DD, Besch-Williford C (1992) Respiratory disease in a colony of rats. Lab Anim 21:16–19

Cundiff DD, Besch-Williford CL, Hook RR Jr, Franklin CL, Riley LK (1994a) Characterization of cilia-associated respiratory bacillus isolates from rats and rabbits. Lab Anim Sci 44:305–312

Cundiff DD, Besch-Williford CL, Hook RR Jr, Franklin CL, Riley LK (1994b) Detection of cilia-associated respiratory bacillus by PCR. J Clin Microbiol 32:1930–1934

Cundiff DD, Besch-Williford CL, Hook RR Jr, Franklin CL, Riley LK (1995) Characterization of cilia-associated respiratory bacillus in rabbits and analysis of the 16S rRNA gene sequence. Lab Anim Sci 45:22–26

Ganaway JR, Spencer TH, Moore TD, Allen AM (1985) Isolation, propagation, and characterization of a newly recognized pathogen, cilia-associated respiratory bacillus of rats, an etiological agent of chronic respiratory disease. Infect Immun 47:472–479

Griffith JW, White WJ, Danneman PJ, Lang CM (1988) Cilia-associated respiratory (CAR) bacillus infection of obese mice. Vet Pathol 25:72–76

Hastie AT, Evans LP, Allen AM (1993) Two types of bacteria adherent to bovine respiratory tract ciliated epithelium. Vet Pathol 30:12–19

Jacoby RO, Bhatt PN, Jonas AM (1979) Viral diseases. In: Baker HJ, Lindsey JR, Weisbroth SH (eds) The laboratory rat, vol I. Biology and diseases. Academic, New York, pp 284–296

Kurisu K, Kyo S, Shiomoto Y, Matsushita S (1990) Cilia-associated respiratory bacillus infection in rabbits. Lab Anim Sci 40:413–415

Lindsey JR, Boorman GA, Collins MJ Jr, Hsu CK, Van Hoosier GL Jr, Wagner JE (1991) Infectious diseases of mice and rats. National Academy Press, Washingtion DC

MacKenzie WF, Magill LS, Hulse M (1981) A filamentous bacterium associated with respiratory disease in wild rats. Vet Pathol 18:836–839

Matsushita S (1986) Spontaneous respiratory disease associated with cilia-associated respiratory (CAR) bacillus in a rat. Nippon Juigaku Zasshi 48:437–440

Matsushita S (1991) Ultrastructure of respiratory tract epithelium of rats experimentally infected with the CAR bacillus. J Vet Med Sci 53:361–363

Matsushita S, Joshima H (1989) Pathology of rats intranasally inoculated with the cilia-associated respiratory bacillus. Lab Anim 23:89–95

Matsushita S, Kashima M, Joshima H (1987) Serodiagnosis of cilia-associated respiratory bacillus infection by the indirect immunofluorescence assay technique. Lab Anim 21:356–359

Matsushita S, Joshima H, Matsumoto T, Fukutsu K (1989) Transmission experiments of cilia-associated respiratory bacillus in mice, rabbits and guinea pigs. Lab Anim 23:96–102

Medina LV, Fortman JD, Bunte RM, Bennett BT (1994) Respiratory disease in a rat colony: identification of CAR bacillus without other respiratory pathogens by standard diagnostic screening methods. Lab Anim Sci 44:521–525

Schoeb TR, Dybvig K, Davidson MK, Davis JK (1993) Cultivation of cilia-associated respiratory bacillus in artificial medium and determination of the 16S rRNA gene sequence. J Clin Microbiol 31:2751–2757

Shoji Y, Itoh T, Kagiyama N (1988a) Enzyme-linked immunosorbent assay for detection of serum antibody to CAR bacillus. Jikken Dobutsu 37:67–72

Shoji Y, Itoh T, Kagiyama N (1988b) Pathogenicities of two CAR bacillus strains in mice and rats. Jikken Dobutsu 37:447–453

Shoji-Darkye Y, Itoh T, Kagiyama N (1991) Pathogenesis of CAR bacillus in rabbits, guinea pigs, Syrian hamsters, and mice. Lab Anim Sci 41:567–571

Shoji Y, Itoh T, Kagiyama N (1992) Propagation of CAR bacillus in artificial media. Jikken Dobutsu 41:231–234

van Zwieten MJ, Solleveld HA, Lindsey JR, de Groot FG, Zurcher C, Hollander CF (1980) Respiratory disease in rats associated with a filamentous bacterium: a preliminary report. Lab Anim Sci 30:215–221
Waggie KS, Spencer TH, Allen AM (1987) Cilia associated respiratory (CAR) bacillus infection in New Zealand white rabbits. Abstract 89, annual meeting of the American Association for Laboratory Animal Science. Lab Anim Sci 37: 533
Weisbroth SH (1979) Bacterial and mycotic diseases. In: Baker HJ, Lindsey JR, Weisbroth SH (eds) The laboratory rat, vol I. Academic, New York, pp 193–241

# Pneumocystosis, Lung, Rat

J.K. Frenkel

*Synonym.* Interstitial plasma cell pneumonia

## Gross Appearance

Heavily infected lungs are focally to diffusely consolidated, but the infiltrate never involves an entire lobe. The alveoli are filled with grayish material. The intervening pinkish alveolar walls can be seen with a hand lens (Fig. 368). If tissue necrosis or abscesses are present, another organism should also be considered. The lungs are not hyperemic and are less voluminous than seen in other consolidated lungs. No fibrinous

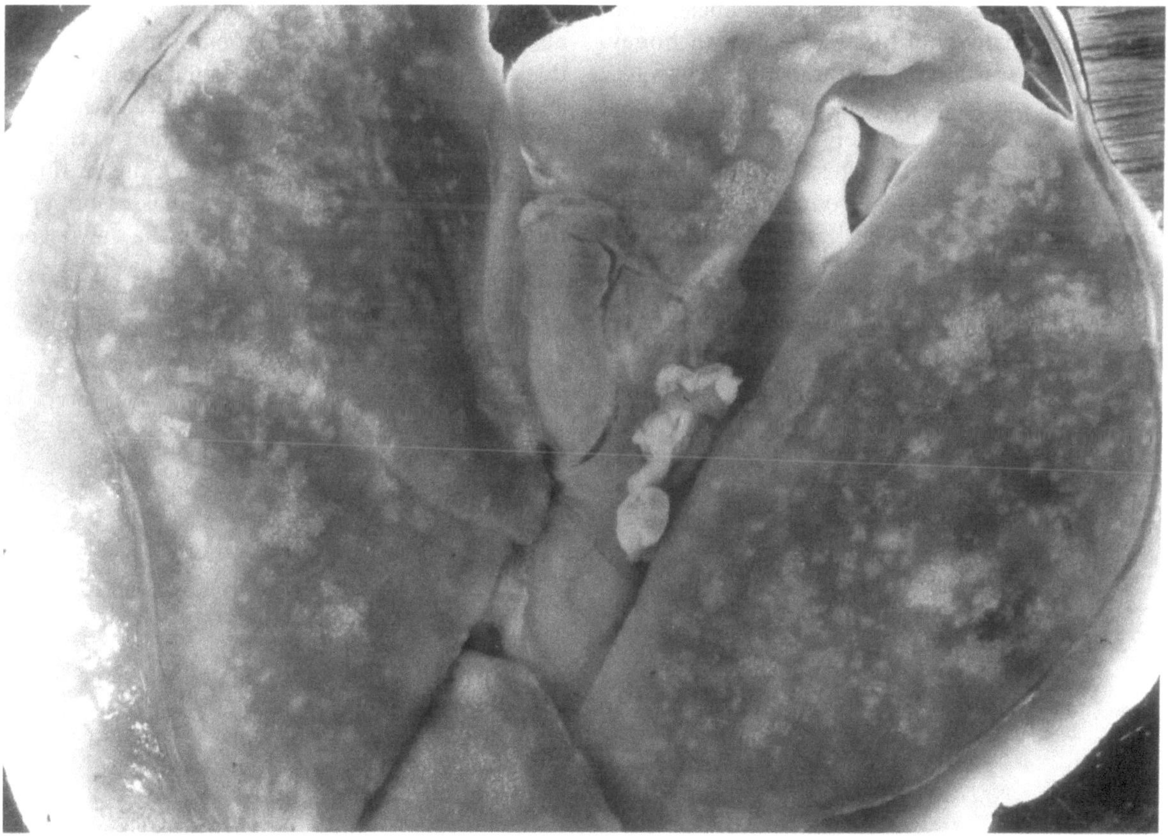

**Fig. 368.** Pneumocystosis, lung of rat. The dorsal aspect of both lungs is diffusely pale pink opaque with only few alveoli containing trapped air (light, refractile areas). Rat was treated with 25 mg cortisone acetate twice weekly and with 1 mg amphotericin subcutaneously three times weekly for 75 days

pleuritis occurs unless bacterial or fungal pneumonia is present.

## Microscopic Features

*Pneumocystis* organisms have a nucleus, and a covering membrane and can occur individually or within cysts. All or parts of these structures may be stained in different ways depending on the staining technique used. The alveoli are filled with masses of *Pneumocystis* organisms, usually with a few accompanying macrophages (Figs. 369, 370). In hematoxylin and eosin (H&E) stained sections the intraalveolar masses appear regularly vacuolated, comparable to a honeycomb (Fig. 370). With the periodic acid–Schiff (PAS) technique the honeycombed material is more intensely stained; H&E-stained nuclei are less distinct (Fig. 371). Using the Grocott modification of Gomori's methenamine silver technique, black yeastlike cysts measuring 3–5 µm in diameter are found individually or in groups in some of the alveolar masses (Fig. 372). The number of these cysts is variable; it is less than the number of nuclei staining with hematoxylin. Many alveoli with honeycombed masses contain few or no cysts. The silver technique generally demonstrates only the cyst wall, not the enclosed nuclei (Fig. 373). The cysts are best identified in Giemsa-stained imprints, where they appear as clear, round spaces against a dark-staining protein background with eight dark-staining nuclei. Methyl violet, toluidine blue, and related dyes also stain the cyst walls. Several rapid staining techniques have been described using Diff-Quick, monoclonal antibody and calcofluor white stains. The sensitive polymerase chain reaction has been used for diagnosis and for differentiation of candidate species (Keely et al. 1994).

## Ultrastructure

Trophozoites are ameboid in shape and measure 1–5 µm with a 20–30 nm pellicle, apparently composed of a double layer. Filopodia extend from the surfaces. The nucleus is bordered by a single- or double-layered poorly defined membrane. The cytoplasm contains mitochondria, ribosomes, endoplasmic reticulum, some vacuoles, lipid globules, and granules, some of which stain for glycogen (Campbell 1972). A precyst, limited by a semirigid trilayered membrane, contains one to several masses of nucleoplasm.

Cysts measure 3.5–5 µm in diameter and are also limited by a trilayered wall, 50–300 nm in thickness. An inner unit type membrane is 5–7 nm thick. A middle granular electrolucent layer usually measure 30–40 nm in diameter, with occasional thicker portions. The outer layer is granular, electron dense, and 20–75 nm in thickness. It contains several nuclear masses or separate intracystic bodies, mitochondria, glycogen,

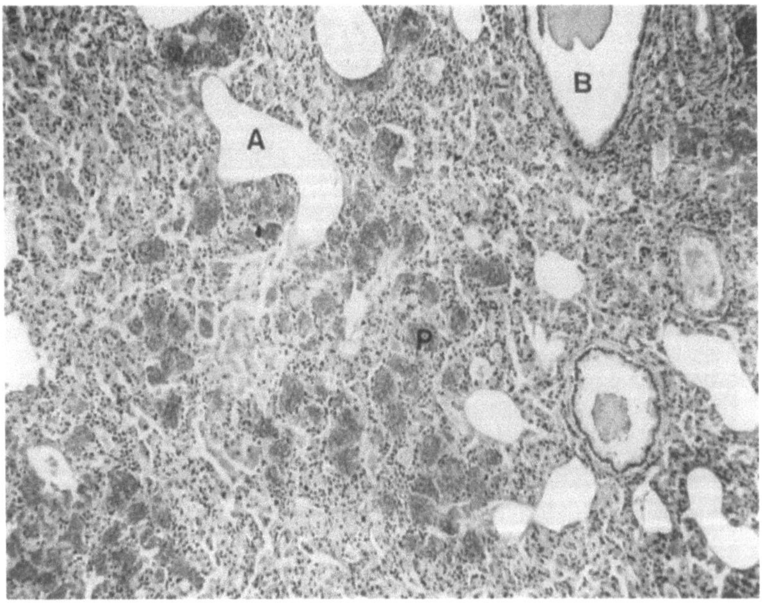


**Fig. 369.** Rat lung. Most alveoli filled with masses of *Pneumocystisis carinii* (*P*); trapped air in some alveoli (*A*). The bronchi (*B*) contain a small amount of fluid, devoid of *Pneumocystis*. PAS and H, ×80

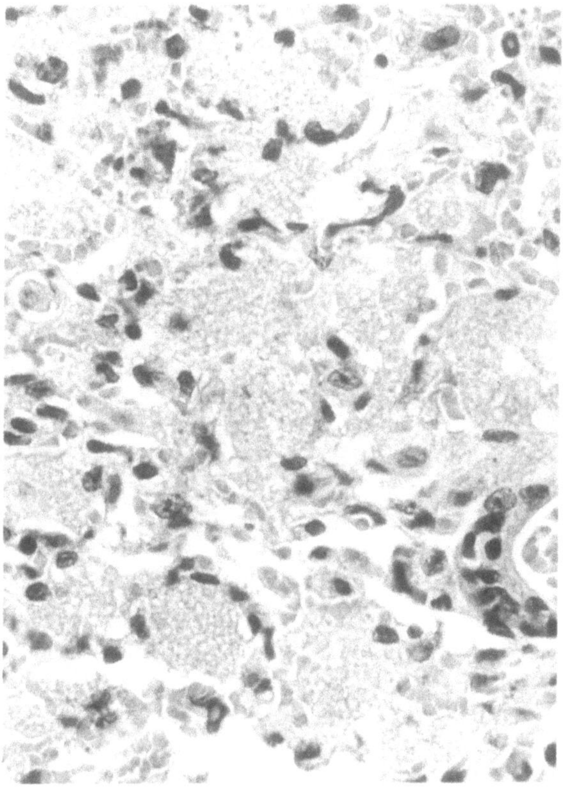

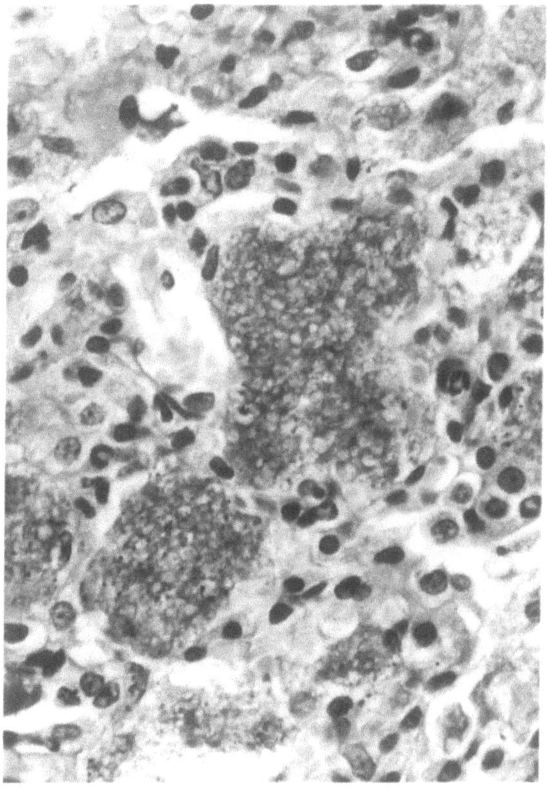

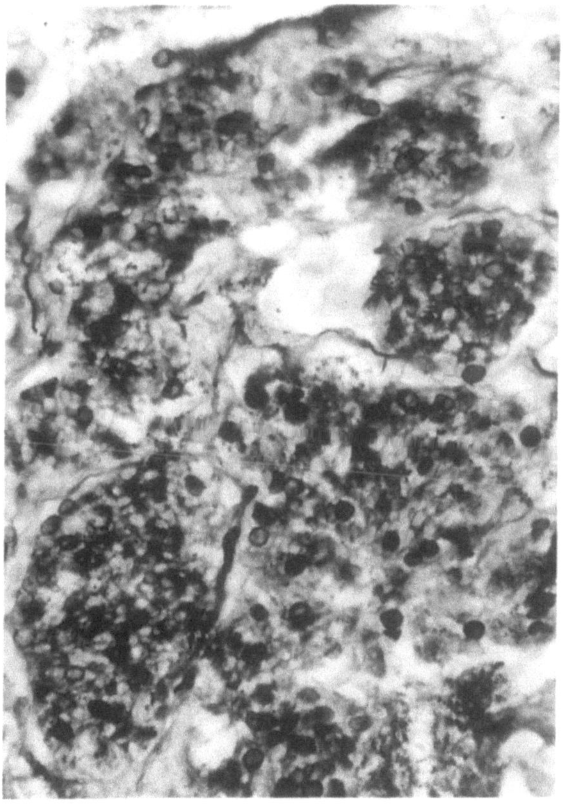

**Fig. 370.** (*upper left*) Alveolar filling with *Pneumocystis*. Rat was treated with 25 mg cortisone acetate twice weekly, subcutaneously, for 64 days. With H&E the organisms appear as faintly hematoxylin-staining nuclei in a foamy eosinophilic material. A few inflammatory macrophages are present. H&E, ×630

**Fig. 371.** (*upper right*) Same lung as in Fig. 370. With the PAS-hematoxylin technique the foamy matrix is emphasized, but the hematoxylin-staining nuclei can also be seen. PAS and H, ×630

**Fig. 372.** (*below*) Same lung as in Fig. 370. With the Grocott methenamine silver technique the cysts resemble spherical or collapsed yeasts, such as *Histoplasma* or *Torulopsis*; this technique is useful mainly to identify candidate forms which much be confirmed by Giemsa staining in smears; some collagen and reticulum fibers are also present. Grocott methenamine silver, ×630

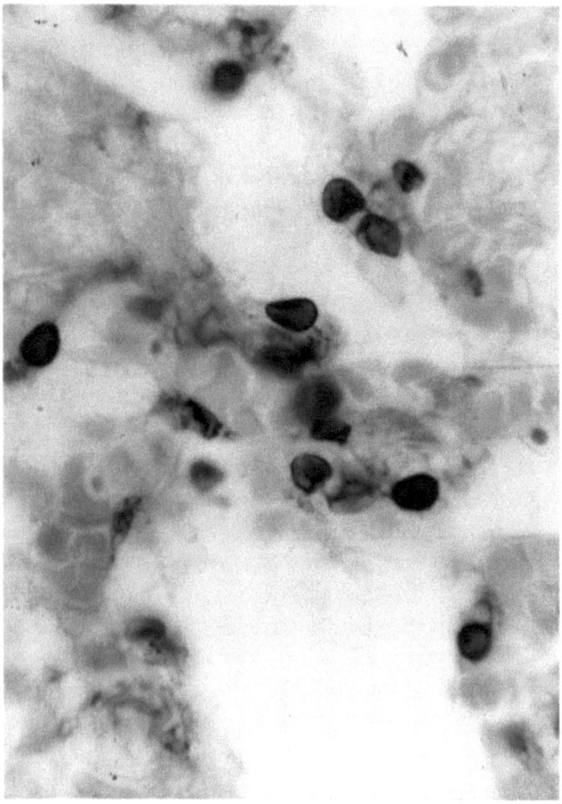

**Fig. 373.** *Pneumocystis carinii* cysts in section of lung impregnated with silver appear as flattened, wrinkled, or folded yeastlike bodies. Grocott methenamine silver, ×1500

and vacuoles. Filopodia arising from the surface of trophzoites and cysts anchor the organisms to the alveolar wall lining cells and to each other (Campbell 1972).

Intracystic bodies measure 1–2 μm in diameter and are enclosed by a double-layered membrane 20–30 nm thick. Their nuclei measure less than 1 μm. The nuclear envelope is sometimes continuous with the endoplasmic reticulum and ribosomes are often attached to the external surface. Intracystic bodies develop into extracystic trophoblasts.

Empty cysts are irregular in shape and often appear crescentic because of collapse of the wall.

## Differential Diagnosis

Since the intraalveolar accumulations of *Pneumocystis* appear honeycombed and contain trophozoite nuclei, this lesion can be easily differentiated from pulmonary edema, which often accompanies it and may be the primary finding after inhalation of toxic substances. Depending on the immune defect present, a small number of inflammatory cells, usually macrophages, may be found. Alveolar wall infiltration is usually slight; however, in the presence of associated bacterial or fungal infection it may be severe.

*Pneumocystis* must be differentiated from other organisms. Their nuclei stain with hematoxylin, but are less densely stained than most gram-positive bacteria, which also stain with hematoxylin. Cyst walls stained with silver, methyl violet, or toluidine blue must be differentiated from fungi, especially *Candida (Torulopsis) glabrata* (Fig. 374). The finding of crescentic or cup-shaped cysts is characteristic of *Pneumocystis*, as is the irregular wrinkling of the intact cyst. Budding is characteristic for yeast; *Candida glabrata*, which is the most common source of confusion, can be cultured. When present, the eight-nucleated cyst in Giemsa-stained imprints confirms the diagnosis.

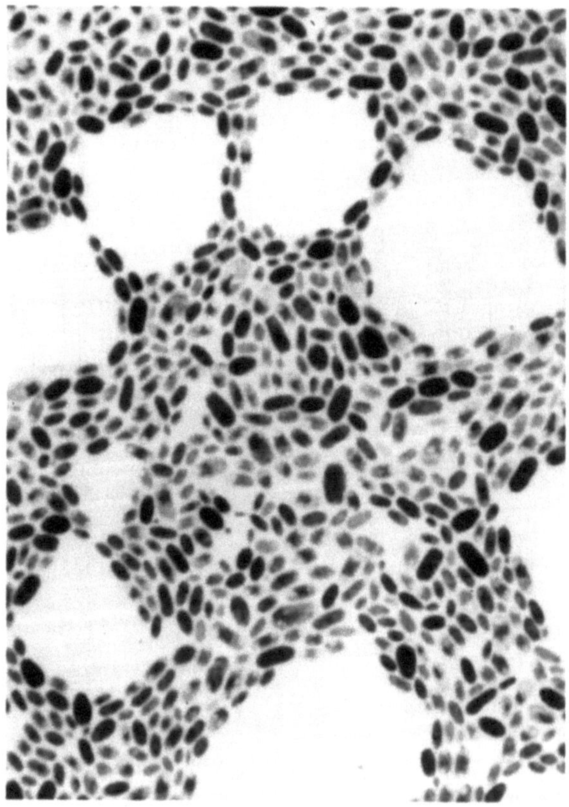

**Fig. 374.** Fungal yeasts. This strain [of *Candida* (*Torulopsis*) *glabrata*] has ovoid singular nuclei and would not easily be confused with *Pneumocystis*, but round yeasts could be easily confused. Smear from culture. Giemsa, ×1500

**Biological Features**

*Natural History*. Most colonies of rats are naturally infected with *Pneumocystis*, as are some colonies of mice and rabbits. Normally infections are subclinical and iatrogenic immunosuppression, usually with corticosteroids or cyclophosphamide, or profound malnutrition is necessary to give rise to clinically significant pulmonary involvement (Frenkel et al. 1966; Frenkel 1976; Robbins et al. 1976). Athymic nude mice are also susceptible (Walzer and Rutledge 1980). Spontaneous instances of pneumocystosis have been described in cats, horses, goats, pigs, dogs, hares, owl monkeys, chimpanzees, ferrets, shrews (*Sorex*), and others (Chandler et al. 1976).
The presence of significant pulmonary involvement with *Pneumocystis* is an indication of immunosuppression. Hughes (1982) showed that naturally infected lung tissue is not infectious unless given intratracheally (Bartlett et al. 1988), and that rats become infected from contaminated air. Presence of an aerosolized stage has been shown by polymerase chain reaction (Bartlett et al. 1994; Wakefield 1994), but its morphological or other biological properties have not been clarified.

*Pathogenesis*. In normal rats *Pneumocystis* organisms are quite scarce, and the and Delanoë (1912), who described and named *Pneumocystis*, reported searching three or four impression smears before finding a single cyst in normal rats. In athymic rats, athymic mice, and SCID mice small focal infiltrates may be found. Only after cortisone became available was massive pulmonary involvement produced in rats (Frenkel et al. 1966; Chandler et al. 1979). Earlier workers encountered *Pneumocystis* accompanied by pneumonia and abscesses from *Corynebacterium kutscheri*, staphylococci, *Pseudomonas*, *Proteus*, *Streptobacillus moniliformis*, *Pasteurella pneumotropica*, coliforms, and fungi. The use of chlortetracycline in drinking water (50mg/dl) and of amphotericin B, 1mg three times weekly subcutaneously, prevented most bacterial and fungal infections and permitted the study of relatively pure *Pneumocystis* infection. The following other regimes have led to clinical pneumocystosis in 200g, 6- to 8-week old rats: 25mg cortisone acetate given subcutaneously twice weekly alternating with cortisol; dexamethasone sodium phosphate, 1mg/l in drinking water; placing 250g rats on 8% protein diet; cyclophosphamide, 240mg/kg body weight orally three times weekly; aminopterin and chlorambucil together with subeffective doses of cortisone acetate; and cyclosporin A 10mg/kg per day orally.
Masses of *Pneumocystis* tachyzoites fill the alveoli, leading to anoxia in immunosuppressed hosts (Fig. 370). Ordinarily, little inflammatory reaction is present, in part because the organism is not highly chemotactic, and in part because the immunosuppressive state is accompanied by an impaired inflammatory response. Inflammation appears when immunocompetence returns, for example when corticosteroid administration is stopped. Inflammation also appears when the organisms are killed by the administration of pentamidine or by sulfonamide and a dihydrofolate reductase inhibitor (Frenkel et al. 1966; Hughes et al. 1974), even though corticosteroids are still administered. All of these causes of resurgent inflammatory reaction may initially result in further impaired alveolocapillary diffusions and increased anoxia, until some of the *Pneumocystis* are eliminated.
The organisms are essentially confined to the alveoli, where they are closely attached to type I pneumocytes, which later degenerate (Walzer et al. 1980; Yoneda and Walzer 1981). They are sometimes phagocytized and may be carried to hilar lymph nodes but have not been reported to multiply there in laboratory animals. Because of their tight attachment to type I pneumocytes the organisms are not expectorated and are not found in the bronchi, except after the administration of chemotherapy with sulfadiazine-pyrimethamine, sulfamethoxazole-trimethoprim, or pentamidine.

*Etiology*. Carlos Chagas first recognized the eight-nucleated cysts in lungs of guinea pigs infected with *Trypanosoma cruzi* and, believing it to indicate schizogony and to be part of the trypanosomal cycle, named the genus *Schizotrypanum* (Chagas 1909). *Pneumocystis carinii* was described as a separate organism by Delanoë and Delanoë (1912) in the lungs of rats and later in guinea pigs from Paris. The organism had generally been regarded as a protozoan, although in the absence of characteristic organelles, its affinity to protozoan orders, remains obscure. On the basis of the study of its ultrastructure Vavra and Kucera (1970) stressed the similarity of this organism to fungi. The most salient nonfungal features of

*Pneumocystis* are the lack of ergosterol in the plasma membrane, unusually fastidious growth requirement, a very low copy number nuclear genes encoding ribosomal RNA (Guintoli et al. 1994) and resistance to amphotericin B, ketoconazole, 5-fluorocytosine, and miconazole (Frenkel et al. 1990). One should consider that assignment to either protozoa or fungi should be based not only on DNA relatedness and sequences, but should be accompanied by some predictive value. Because either assignment does not tell us much about *Pneumocystis*, it makes more sense to regard it as a phylogenetically old parasite without close relative (Frenkel et al. 1990).

*Frequency*. All conventional rats examined in 1964 and 1965 and even five or six lines advertised as "specific-pathogen-free" (SPF) developed pneumocystosis when treated with cortisone acetate, 25 mg twice weekly. Sources of rats free of *Pneumocystis* infection in 1987 have been published (Bartlett et al. 1987).

## Comparison with Other Species

Pneumocystosis in man was recognized in institutionalized premature babies and in infants at the end of World War II in Europe. The histological picture was of an interstitial plasma cell pneumonia with masses of *Pneumocystis* filling the alveoli.

Plasma cell pneumonia has not been observed in experimental animals. In an immunosuppressed baby with congenital rubella both plasma cells and large mononuclear cells were present. However, no significant interstitial inflammation, as in the experimental models, is found in children with agammaglobulinemia due to deficiency of B cells (Bruton's disease), in patients with leukemia or lymphoma treated with appropriate chemotherapy, or in organ-transplant recipients immunosuppressed with corticosteroids and azathioprine and in patients with the acquired immunodeficiency syndrome. Because there are serological differences to *P. carinii* of rats, the human organism is designated *P. jiroveci* (Frenkel 1976).

The genetic diversity of *Pneumocystis* spp. from various hosts is sometimes greater than is seen in fungi that have been placed in different genera. Nonetheless, it is not clear whether genetic diversity was the result of clonal diversity from uniparental reproduction or from true speciation (Stringer 1994). A trinomial nomenclature appeared to be a suitably conservative approach for the designation of *Pneumocystis* from rat, 1 prototype and 1 variant (Cushion et al. 1993), man, ferret, mouse, horse, pig, and rabbit, all of which are considered special forms of *P. carinii* (Stringer 1994). Until the degree of mating between different forms has been studied, a free-living stage has been better characterized, and until the expediency of a binomial over a trinomial system has been recognized, this system will likely persist.

Athymic nude mice are sometimes observed with focal *Pneumocystis* accumulations; cortisone-treated rabbits and mice are also found to be infected (Sheldon 1959; Walzer et al. 1980).

Since *Pneumocystis* has been recognized as an important, and often first, manifestation of the acquired immunodeficiency syndrome, research in all aspects of this field has received a major stimulus. Because cell culture is of limited use, the rat model remains in general use, especially for chemotherapeutic evaluation.

## References


Bartlett MS, Durkin MM, Jay MA, Queener SF, Smith JW (1987) Sources of rats free of latent Pneumocystis carinii. J Clin Microbiol 25:1794–1795

Bartlett MS, Fishman JA, Queener SF, Durkin MM, Jay MA, Smith JW (1988) New rat model of Pneumocystis carinii infection. J Clin Microbiol 26:1100–1102

Bartlett MS, Lee CH, Luj J, Bauer NL, Betts JF, McLaughlin GL, Smith JW (1994) Pneumocystis carinii detected in air. J Eukaryot Microbiol 41:75S

Campbell WG Jr (1972) Ultrastructure of Pneumocystis in human lung. Life cycle in human pneumocystis. Arch Pathol 93:312–324

Chagas C (1909) Nova tripanozomiaza human. Estudos sobre a morfolojia e o ciclo evolutivo de Schizotrypanum cruzi n.gen., n. sp. ajenta etiologio de nova entidade morbida de homan. Mem Inst Oswaldo Cruz 1:159–164

Chandler FW, McClure HM, Campbell WG Jr, Watts JC (1976) Pulmonary pneumocystosis in nonhuman primates. Arch Pathol Lab Med 100:163–167

Chandler FW Jr, Frenkel JK, Campbell WG Jr (1979) Pneumocystis pneumonia. Animal model: pneumocystis carinii pneumonia in the immunosuppressed rat. Am J Pathol 95:571–574

Cushion MT, Kaselis M, Stringer SL, Stringer JR (1993) Genetic stability and diversity of Pneumocystis carinii infecting rat colonies. Infect Immun 61:4801–4813

Delanoë P, Delanoë M (1912) Sur les rapports des kystes de Carini du poumon des rats avec le Trypanosoma lewisii. CR Seq Acad Sci 155:658–664

Frenkel JK (1976) Pneumocystis jiroveci n.sp. from man: morphology, physiology, and immunology in relation to pathology. Natl Cancer Inst Monogr 43:13–30
Frenkel JK, Good JT, Shultz JA (1966) Latent Pneumocystis infection of rats, relapse and chemotherapy. Lab Invest 15:1559–1577
Frenkel JK, Bartlett MS, Smith JW (1990) RNA homology and the reclassification of Pneumocystis. Diagn Microbiol Infect Dis 13:1–2
Giuntoli D, Stringer SL, Stringer JR (1994) Extraordinarily low number of ribosomal RNA genes in P. carinii. J Eukaryot Microbiol 41:88S
Hughes WT (1982) Natural mode of acquisition for de novo infection with Pneumocystis carinii. J Infect Dis 145:842–848
Hughes WT, McNabb PC, Makres TD, Feldman S (1974) Efficacy of trimethoprim and sulfamethoxazole in the prevention and treatment of Pneumocystis carinii pneumonitis. Antimicrob Agents Chemother 5:289–293
Keely S, Pai H, Baughman R, Sidman C, Sunkin SM, Stringer JR, Stringer SL (1994) Pneumocystis species inferred from analysis of multiple genes. J Eukaryot Microbiol 41:94S
Robbins JB, DeVita VT Jr, Dutz W (eds) (1976) Symposium on pneumocystis carinii infection. National Cancer Institute, Bethesda (National Cancer Institute monography, vol 43)
Sheldon WH (1959) Experimental pulmonary Pneumocystis carinii infection in rabbits. J Exp Med 110:147–160
Stringer JR (1994) Pneumocystis workshop. Revised nomenclature for Pneumocystis carinii. J Eukaryot Microbiol 41:121S-122S
Vavra J, Kucera K (1970) Pneumocystis carinii delanoe, its ultrastructure and ultrastructural affinities. J Protozool 17:463–483
Wakefield AE (1994) Detection of DNA sequences identical to Pneumocystis carinii in samples of ambient air. J Eukaryot Microbiol 41, 116S
Walzer PD, Rutledge ME (1980) Comparison of rat, mouse, and human Pneumocystis carinii by immunofluorescence. J Infect Dis 142:449
Walzer PD, Powell RD Jr, Yoneda K, Rutledge ME, Milder JE (1980) Growth characteristics and pathogenesis of experimental Pneumocystis carinii pneumonia. Infect Immun 27:928–937
Yoneda K, Walzer PD (1981) Mechanism of pulmonary alveolar injury in experimental Pneumocystis carinii pneumonia in the rat. Br J Exp Pathol 62:339–346

# Toxoplasmosis, Lung, Mouse, and Hamster

J.K. Frenkel

*Synonyms.* None

### Gross Appearance

Focal to confluent pneumonias, often with serous pleural exudate, are seen at necropsy of animals which succumb to acute infection. In immunosuppressed animals in which a chronic infection relapses white to yellowish necrotic foci surrounded by hemorrhage are seen in the lungs in addition to diffuse pneumonia and encephalitis.

### Microscopic Features

*Toxoplasma* tachyzoites, the rapidly multiplying forms, are found in the alveolar walls, in cells of alveolar exudate, and in many other cells of the body (Fig. 375). Diffuse interstitial pneumonia is the usual picture. More rarely, focal necrosis involves segments of the alveolar wall. Intracellular and free tachyzoites, a mixed mononuclear cell infiltration, and serofibrinous exudate accompany both (Fig. 376). In immunosuppressed animals larger focal lesions involving several alveoli may be found, with diffuse cellular infiltration and necrosis or early organization by fibroblasts (Fig. 377). Focal fibrinous pleuritis is present with parenchymal lesions reaching the pleura. Rarely *Toxoplasma* cysts comtaining bradyzoites or slowly multiplying forms are found in the lungs without inflammatory reaction.

### Ultrastructure

The ultrastructure of *Toxoplasma* is useful to distinguish it from some other small organisms that may be encountered in the lungs. *Toxoplasma* tachyzoites are banana shaped to ovoid and carry an apical complex at the anterior end composed of a conoid, a polar ring, and rhoptries, which contain enzymes that apparently aid their active penetration of host cells. Also, a vesicular nucleus,

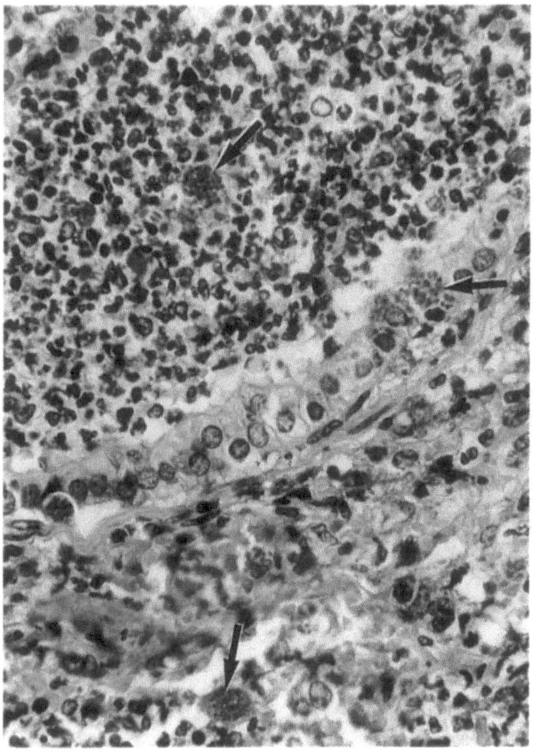

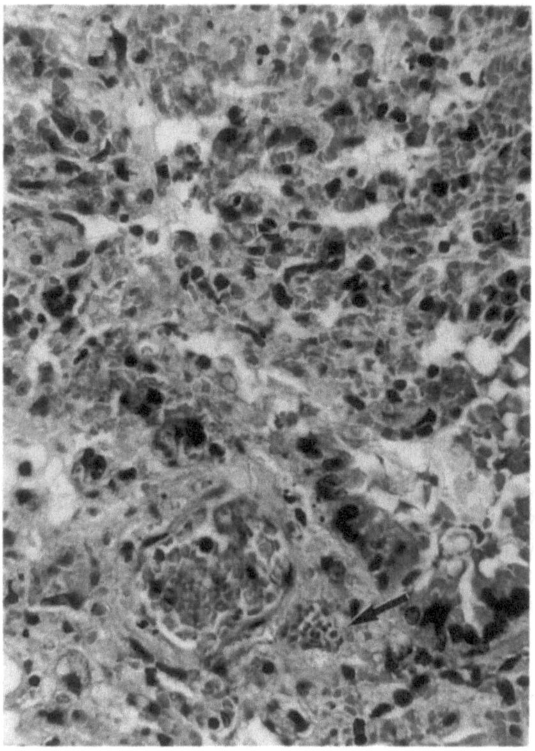

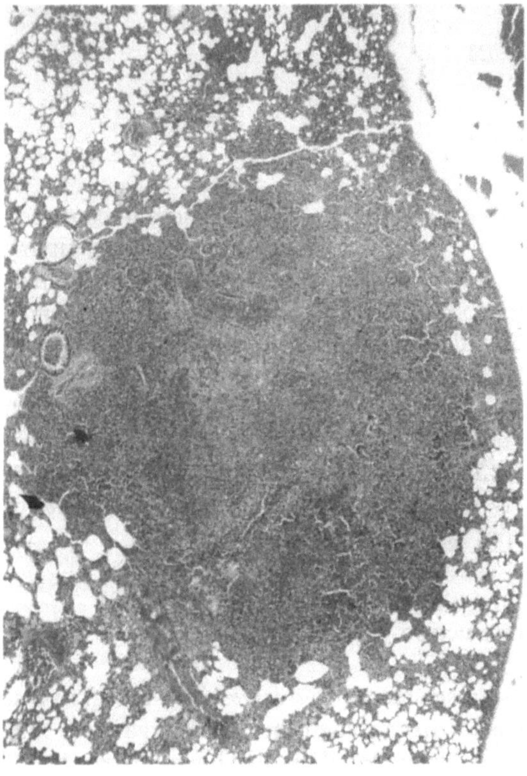

**Fig. 375.** (*upper left*) Focal toxoplasmic pneumonia, hamster (Fig. 377) with tachyzoites in parenchyma, bronchial epithelium, and exudate. Groups of tachyzoites (*arrows*). H&E, ×450

**Fig. 376.** (*upper right*) Toxoplasmic pneumonia. Nude mouse with partially functioning thymic transplant, died 22 days after subcutaneous inoculation with *Toxoplasma* tachyzoites. Group of tachyzoites (*arrow*). H&E, ×400

**Fig. 377.** (*below*) Focal toxoplasmic pneumonia. Syrian golden hamster latently infected with *Toxoplasma* for several months. Immunosuppression with subcutaneously administered cortisol, 2.5 mg twice weekly, was then begun. Forty-five days later this animal died with focal pneumonia and focal encephalitis. H&E, ×25

mitochondria, endoplasmic reticulum, microtubules, and micronemes are enclosed in a pellicle (Chobotar and Scholtyseck 1982).

## Differential Diagnosis

The apical complex is present in other Sporozoa, such as intestinal and cyst-forming coccidia, which has led to a redefinition of the phylum as the Apicomplexa. Members of this group need to be differentiated by their cycle and cyst structure. However, because of their small size they must also be distinguished from *Leishmania* spp. and *Trypanosoma cruzi*, which have a kinetoplast; from *Encephalitozoon*, which contains a spiral polar filament; from *Pneumocystis*, which lacks of a special organelle; and from *Histoplasma* and other fungal yeasts with their PAS-positive cell wall.

## Biological Features

*Natural History*. *Toxoplasma gondii* is an intestinal coccidian of cats with an enteroepithelial cycle that leads to the development of oocysts that are shed in the feces. Oocysts sporulate outside the host. Ground-feeding animals and herbivores become infected by ingesting vegetation mixed with soil contaminated with cat feces. These animals constitute the intermediate host; all mammals and birds investigated have been found to be susceptible. During acute infection tachyzoites multiply actively, giving rise to necrosis of infected cells. Coincident with the development of immunity, bradyzoites slowly develop within tissue cysts, with cells of the brain, muscle, and other organs supporting large numbers of organisms. The cysts appear in the chronic, persisting stage of infection, and when eaten by a carnivore, produce tachyzoites. Only in felines do they initiate an intraepithelial and a sexual cycle in the gut. Laboratory animals are likely to become infected by the ingestion of oocysts from either contaminated food or bedding. Cats are known to cover their feces and sometimes defecate in open sacks or bins containing feed and cage bedding (Fig. 378). Brooms contaminated with feces of exhibited or ferel cats may bring the infectious oocyst to susceptible zoo animals.

*Pathogenesis*. The tachyzoites of acute infection multiply by successive division (endodiogeny),

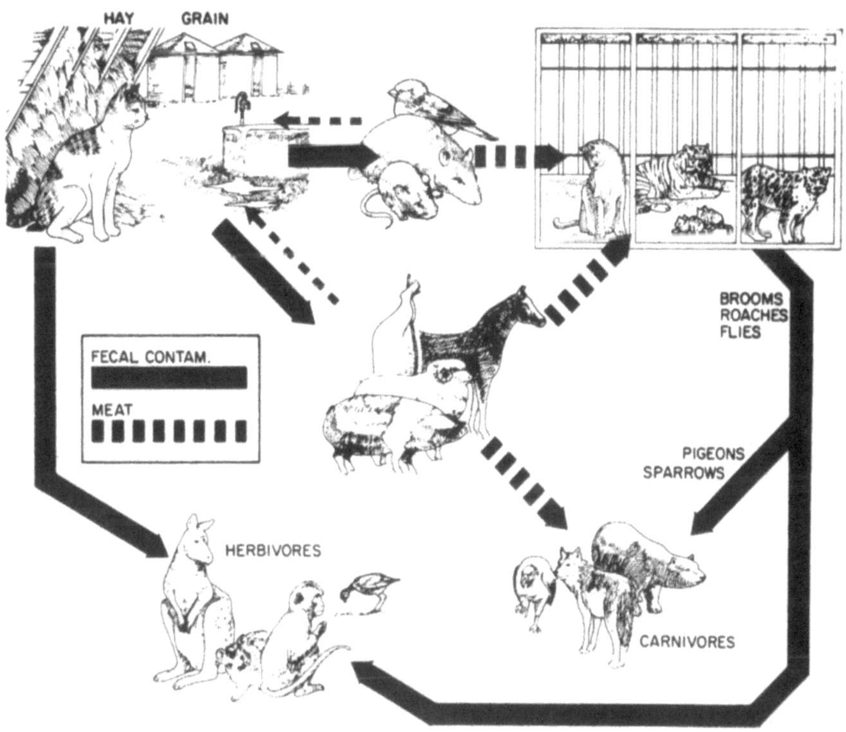


**Fig. 378.** Transmission of toxoplasmosis in zoos and animal colonies

reaching 8–32 organisms per cell, at which time the cell usually disintegrates, and the tachyzoites infect other cells. Bradyzoites develop in mice 4–5 days after infection with tachyzoites, 7–9 days after infection with bradyzoites, and 9–10 days after infection with sporozoites from oocysts.

The slow multiplication of bradyzoites leads to accumulations of tens to hundreds of organisms within intracellular cysts. These cysts contain organisms in resting stages, awaiting ingestion by a carnivore, and have little pathogenicity to the host cell, which maintains the cyst for months to years. However, disintegration of a cyst may lead to tissue necrosis in the presence of delayed hypersensitivity (type IV). This is of clinical importance when cyst rupture occurs in the retina, because function is concentrated in a few cells which do not regenerate. The liberated organisms are usually destroyed by immune mechanisms. Minimal pathogenicity is also associated with the proliferation of stages A, B, C, D, and E and the development of gametocytes in the intestinal epithelial cells of cats, because they coincide more or less with the natural turnover of epithelial cells which mature while migrating from the crypts to the tips of the villi where they are shed.

*Etiology*. *Toxoplasma gondii* was originally described as a *Leishmania* or related organism in 1908, both in North Africa and South America. Nicolle and Manceaux found it in gondis, wild rodents used in studies of *Lesihmania* and typhus at the Pasteur Institute in Tunis. These animals presumably became infected in the laboratory. Splendore found *Toxoplasma* in laboratory rabbits in San Paulo, Brazil. The absence of a kinetoplast separated it from *Leishmania*. In 1909 it was named *Toxoplasma gondii* by Nicolle and Manceaux (reviewed by Frenkel 1973). The organism was suspected to give rise to human disease sporadically, but it was not definitely linked with human disease until Wolf, Cowan, and Paige, starting in 1937, identified *Toxoplasma* in newborn babies in New York, isolated it by 1940, and linked it to intrauterine infection from an asymptomatic mother. At first the organism was called *Encephalitozzon*, as in a case described by Janku in 1923 (Frenkel 1973). But by 1940, when the organism had been isolated from an infected baby, it was recognized by Sabin as identical with *Toxoplasma* isolated from animals (Frenkel 1973). This was followed by characterization of the neonatal infection by Sabin, the development of serological tests, especially the dye test by Sabin and Feldman, and the recognition of ocular, encephalitic, and lymph node syndromes, apart from generalized infection in children and adults. *Toxoplasma* was found to give rise to disease in many domestic, wild, zoo, and laboratory animals, without—because of its size and number—causing serious errors in the interpretation of laboratory experiments (Frenkel 1973).

Although it was realized that carnivorism could be responsible for transmitting toxoplasmosis, it did not become clear how herbivores became infected till 1965, when Hutchison discovered the infectivity of the feces of a cat that had eaten *Toxoplasma*-infected mice. In 1967 he described the supposed transmission in nematode eggs. Between 1969 and 1970 transmission without the nematode was established, and a small *Toxoplasma* oocyst was recognized in cat feces (reviewed by Frenkel 1973). *Toxoplasma* is now classified in the protozoan phylum Apicomplexa, as a cyst-forming, heteroxenous coccidian in the family Sarcocystidae, subfamily Toxoplasmatina (Frenkel 1977). *Toxoplasma* differs from the genera *Besnoitia*, *Hammondia*, *Cystoisospora*, *Sarcocystis*, *Neospora*, and *Frenkelia* by the characteristics of the cysts and the transmission cycle (Frenkel 1973, 1977; Frenkel et al. 1979).

*Frequency*. Naturally occurring toxoplasmosis with illness and sometimes death has been observed in gondis, rabbits, guinea pigs, neotropical primates, chincilles, hyraxes, Australian marsupials, Madegascan lemurs, and pigeons. Asymptomatic infection has been observed in guinea pigs, rats, chickens, and goats. Cats were formally given free run in some animal colonies to catch wild and accidentally escaped mice. Disposition of the feces of these cats was not considered important, and it is likely that some of the feces were deposited in grain bins and bedding. With improved practices in handling animal feed and bedding and exclusion of pet and stray cats, the opportunity for infection has been diminished. Experimental toxoplasmosis has been widely studied in mice, rabbits, and hamsters. These animals are more susceptible than rats and guinea pigs, which develop an age-dependent resistance. In these laboratory studies direct transmission does not occur from animal to animal except by oocasional cannibalism and congenital infection. However, experimental infection with oocysts from cat feces must be conducted with care, because a portion of the fed oocysts may be passed intact in the feces, where they withstand drying and are thus capable of infecting other animals. Bedding should be changed and autoclaved 1 day and 2 days after the administration of oocysts. Food and bedding are the fomites; there is no evidence of airborne infection.

### Comparison with Other Species

Generalized toxoplasmosis is similar in animals and man, keeping in mind their different degrees of resistance and strains of *Toxoplasma* which differ in pathogenicity. Well-adapted laboratory strains may convey a distorted impression, killing mice 3–4 days after intraperitoneal inoculation of a large number of organisms. However, of 31 recent natural isolates 90% gave rise to inapparent infections in mice (Ruiz and Frenkel 1980) and fatal infections could be transformed to chronic infections when mice were treated prophylactically with 15–60 mg% sulfadiazine or sulfamerazine in the drinking water. Adult rats are resistant even to strains pathogenic to mice, as are adult guinea pigs, adult humans, and most children. Ocular toxoplasmosis in humans has been reproduced in hamsters; after subcutaneous inoculation, followed by sulfadiazine treatment, the retinas of many of these animals became infected (Frenkel 1961). Relapsing chronic toxoplasmosis seen in humans has also been reproduced in hamsters treated with pharmacological doses of cortico-steroids or cyclophosphamide (Frenkel et al. 1978). Most experimental infections are produced by injection, the intraperitoneal route being much more effective than the subcutaneous. Oral infection is the usual route in animals and man, either with oocysts from cat faces or with tissue cysts from infected meat (Dubey and Frenkel 1973). The course of the disease and the development of immunity may differ according to the route of infection and, of course, the animal host.

### References

Chobotar B, Scholtyseck E (1982) Ultrastructure. In: Long PL (ed) The biology of the coccidia. University Park, Baltimore, chap 4

Dubey JP, Frenkel JK (1973) Experimental toxoplasma infection in mice with strains producing oocysts. J Parasitol 59:505–512

Frenkel JK (1961) Pathogenesis of toxoplasmosis with a consideration of cyst rupture in *Besnoitia* infection. Surv Ophthalmol 6:799–825

Frenkel JK (1973) Toxoplasma in and around us. Bioscience 23:343–352

Frenkel JK (1977) *Bensoitia wallacei* of cats and rodents: with a reclassification of other cyst-forming isosporoid coccidia. J Parasitol 63:611–628

Frenkel JK, Amare M, Larsen W (1978) Immune competence in a patient with Hodgkin's disease and relapsing toxoplasmosis. Infection 6(2):84–91

Frenkel JK, Heydorn AO, Mehlhorn H, Rommel M (1979) Sarcocystinae: *Nomina dubia* and available names. Z Parasitenkd 58:115–139

Ruiz A, Frenkel JK (1980) Intermediate and transport hosts of *Toxoplasma gondii* in Costa Rica. Am J Trop Med Hyg 29:1161–1166

# Aspergillosis and Mucormycosis, Lung, Rat

J.K. Frenkel

*Synonyms.* Aspergillosis: none; mucormycosis: phycomycosis, zygomycosis, hyphomycosis

### Gross Appearance

Members of fungal species give rise to focal and diffuse pneumonia, which often progresses to necrosis, vascular invasion, and infarction in immunosuppressed rats and occasionally in mice and hamsters. The affected areas are raised, with white, necrotic centers surrounded by gray, consolidated tissue and hyperemic borders (Fig. 379). Fibrinous pleuritis usually accompanies the lesions.

### Microscopic Features

Diffuse pneumonia is accompanied by fungal hyphae, generally with tissue necrosis and infarction.

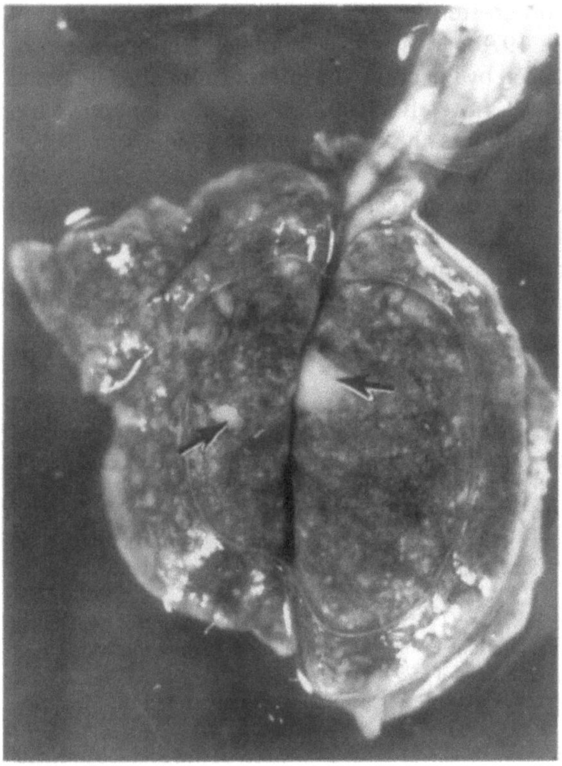

**Fig. 379.** Rat lung with two white plaques (*arrows*) covering the pleural surface. The rat was treated with 25 mg cortisone acetate subcutaneously twice weekly for 64 days

The fungi may exhibit nonseptate hyphae, characteristic of *Mucor*, or septate hyphae, compatible with *Aspergillus*. Fungal bronchitis is common with *Candida*, a fungal yeast, but *Aspergillus* and *Mucor* also give rise to bronchitis. *Aspergillus* infection next to a bronchus may erode into it, forming an ulcer, a cavity, and sometimes a fungal ball. Growth of the fungus may occur through the pleura into the pleural sac (Figs. 380, 381).

The cellular exudate contains mononuclear cells and granulocytes, which occasionally leads to granuloma formation. *Aspergillus* hyphae are of approximately constant width, are septate, and often undergo dichotomous branching. In the presence of a bronchus or a cavity conidia (fruiting bodies) may be formed. The agent of *Mucor* has hyphae of greatly varied width which are sparsely septate with haphazard branching; the hyphae sometimes appear twisted or folded, misleadingly suggesting septation (Fig. 382). Vascular invasion is common, and blood vessels often serve as conduits for the spread of the fungi.

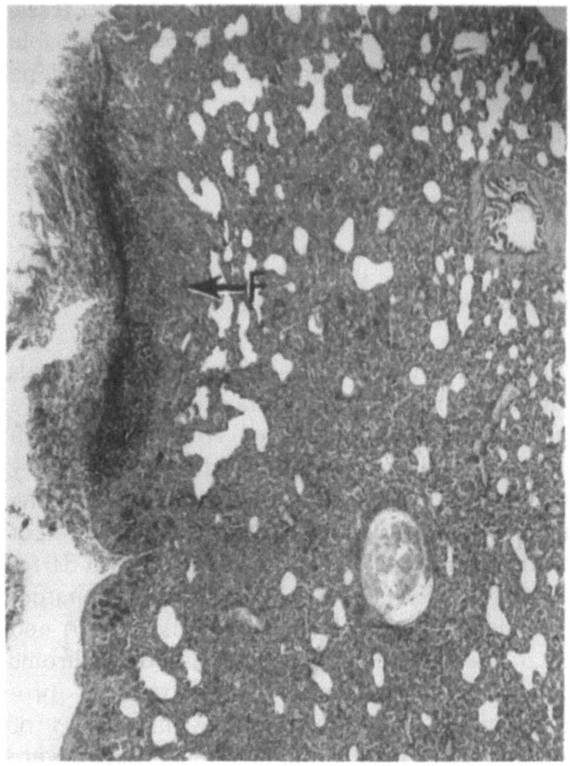


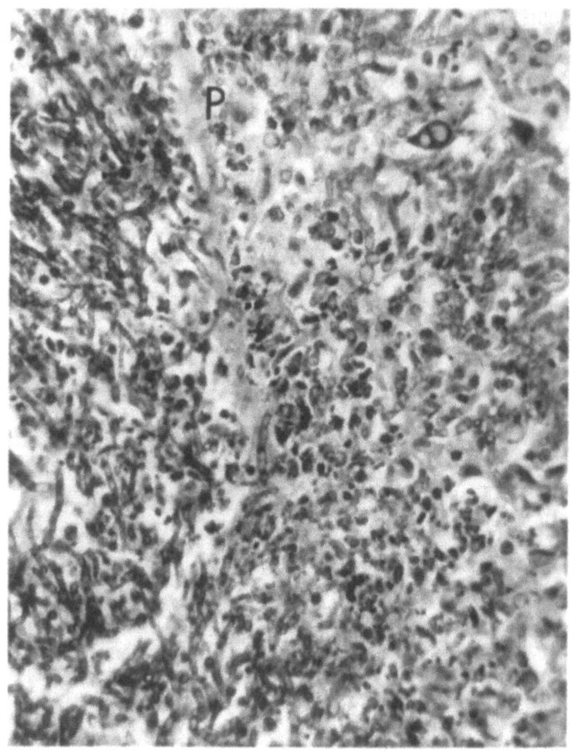


**Fig. 380.** (*above*) Lung with fungal hyphae growing from parenchyma into pleura (*F*). Some of the nearby blood vessels contain similar fungi, but the bronchi are free. PAS and H, ×25

**Fig. 381.** (*below*) *Aspergillus terreus* (identified by culture) in pleura of rat. Septate fungal hyphae of constant bore and with occasional spores in pleura (*P*) and subpleural area. PAS and H, ×400

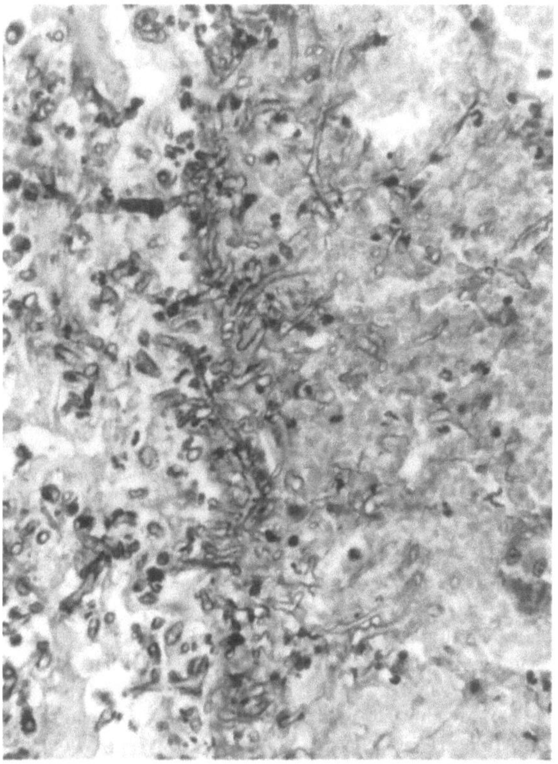

**Fig. 382.** Mucormycosis, lung, rat. Nonseptate fungal hyphae of irregular diameter. Blood vessels were also involved, turning this area of lung into a hemorrhagic infarct. This fungus was not cultured. PAS and H, ×400

## Ultrastructure

The ultrastructure is rarely examined because the organisms are readily visible by light microscopy and their identification depends on culture. The fungal hyphae appear as tubules with prominent cell walls.

## Differential Diagnosis

Fungal granulomas, abscesses, and pneumonias must be differentiated from bacterial abscesses and pneumonias using impression smears, histological sections, and cultures. Fungal and bacterial infections may both be present, sometimes even with viral infections and *Pneumocystis* in immunosuppressed animals. Because fungal contaminants are so common, one cannot rely on culture alone, and the isolated organisms must be shown by evidence in histological sections to be related to the lesion.

## Biological Features

*Natural History.* The fungi are widely distributed in the environment, especially in moist feed and bedding (Emmons 1962), and the spores are readily inhaled by animals. Immunocompetent animals control the infection by means of their macrophages (deRepentigny et al. 1993). Occasionally a single aspergilloma is found, sometimes with cavitation. This is not the case in the immunosuppressed animal, where focal fungal bronchitis leads to necrotizing bronchopneumonia, vascular invasion, dissemination in the lung and occasionally to the other organs, and extension to the pleura. Thrombi form in the infected vessels and may give rise to infarcts without fungi, which are mainly aerobic.

*Pathogenesis.* In both aspergillosis and mucormycosis tissue invasion from the bronchi and vascular invasion are predominant. It is likely that proteolytic enzymes favor fungi penetration through the connective tissue; collagenases and elastases have been isolated from some of the Mucorales. Acidosis markedly lowers natural resistance of hosts to mucormycosis, as has been observed clinically in humans, usually those with diabetes. This has been studied in rabbits that received injections of alloxan (Sheldon and Bauer 1962). Acidosis temporarily decreased the levels of an inhibitory serum factor. Athymic mice appear to be resistant (Corbel and Eades 1977), but corticosteroids markedly depress the capacity to react to these fungi (Frenkel 1962). Endotoxin, hemolysins, and other factors from these fungi have been described but do not appear to play an obvious role in the pathogenesis of clinical illness.
Aflatoxin is produced by *Aspergillosis flavus* in culture, but in the course of infection by the organism it is unknown whether sufficient toxin is produced to give rise to lesions. In a sufficient dose aflatoxin does cause acute liver necrosis and scarring in many animals, the effective dose varying according to species. It is also a potent carcinogen, again with wide variations in sensitivity according to species and hormonal states (Goodall and Butler 1969).

*Etiology.* Several species of *Aspergillus (A. flavus, A. niger, A. fumigatus)* and species of *Mucor, Absidia, Rhizopus*, and *Mortierella* may be found in laboratory animals. The diagnosis is often difficult because some of the Mucorales do not grow easily in culture. Experimental infections with *A. fumigatus*, *A. flavus*, *A. niger*, and *Rhizopus oryzae* are commonly fatal.

*Frequency*. Infections are rare in normal animals unless they are exposed to very large doses of fungi, as from moist and moldy feed. The frequency of illness is directly related to the degree of immunosuppression. The infection can be suppressed by the administration of amphotericin B, 6mg/kg body weight (rat) administered intramuscularly three times weekly (Frenkel et al. 1966). A model of recurrent pulmonary aspergillosis has been described in rats (Niki et al. 1991).

## Comparison with Other Species

The tissue lesions described are quite similar in rats and humans. Mice and hamsters appear more resistant than rats. *Aspergillus* bronchitis is common in certain birds, often leading to disseminated infection. Spontaneous allergic bronchitis due to fungi is rare in experimental animals but does occur in man. A murine model has recently been described (Kurup et al. 1992). Mucorales have been reported to give rise to illness in animals fed moist and moldy food, with generalized infection common at the time of death (Jones and Hunt 1983). The rhinofacial mucormycosis of humans has also been seen in a rhesus monkey (Martin et al. 1969) but appears to be rare in small laboratory animals.

## References

Corbel MJ, Eades SM (1977) Experimental mucormyosis in congenitally athymic (nude) mice. Mycopathologia 62:117–120

deRepentigny L, Petitbois S, Boushira M, Michaliszyn E, et al. (1993) Acquired immunity in experimental murine aspergillosis is mediated by macrophages. Infect Immun 61:3791–3802

Emmons CW (1962) Natural occurrence of opportunistic fungi. Lab Invest 11:1026–1032

Frenkel JK (1962) Role of corticosteroids as predisposing factors in fungal diseases. Lab Invest 11:1192–1208

Frenkel JK, Good JT, Shultz JA (1966) Latent *Pneumocystis* infection of rats, relapse and chemotherapy. Lab Invest 15:1559–1577

Goodall CM, Butler WH (1969) Aflatoxin carcinogenesis: inhibition of liver cancer induction in hypophysectomized rats. Int J Cancer 4:422–429

Jones TC, Hunt RD (1983) Veterinary pathology, 5th edn. Lea and Febiger, Philadelphia

Kurup VP, Mauze S, Choi H, Seymour BW, Coffman RL (1992) A murine model of allergic bronchopulmonary aspergillosis with elevated eosinophils and IgE. J Immunol 148:3783–3788

Martin JE, Kroe DJ, Bostrom RE, Johnson DJ, Whitney RA Jr (1969) Rhino-orbital phycomycosis in a rhesus monkey (*Macaca mulatta*). J Am Vet Med Assoc 155:1253–1257

Niki Y, Bernard EM, Edwards FF, Schmitt HJ, et al. (1991) Model of recurrent pulmonary aspergillosis in rats. J Clin Microbiol 29:1317–1322

Sheldon WH, Bauer H (1962) The role of predisposing factors in experimental fungus infections. Lab Inves 11:1184–1191

# Subject Index*



* Page numbers in **boldface** indicate the principal discussion; figures are designated by the letter "f" following the page number; Tables are found on page numbers followed by the letter "t".

# Springer-Verlag and the Environment

We at Springer-Verlag firmly believe that an international science publisher has a special obligation to the environment, and our corporate policies consistently reflect this conviction.

We also expect our business partners – paper mills, printers, packaging manufacturers, etc. – to commit themselves to using environmentally friendly materials and production processes.

The paper in this book is made from low- or no-chlorine pulp and is acid free, in conformance with international standards for paper permanency.

MIX
Papier aus verantwortungsvollen Quellen
Paper from responsible sources
FSC® C105338

If you have any concerns about our products,
you can contact us on
**ProductSafety@springernature.com**

In case Publisher is established outside the EU,
the EU authorized representative is:
**Springer Nature Customer Service Center GmbH**
**Europaplatz 3, 69115 Heidelberg, Germany**

Printed by Libri Plureos GmbH
in Hamburg, Germany